Handbook of Parasitology

Handbook of Parasitology

Edited by Madelyn Goodman

hayle medical
New York

Hayle Medical,
750 Third Avenue, 9th Floor,
New York, NY 10017, USA

Visit us on the World Wide Web at:
www.haylemedical.com

ISBN: 978-1-63241-649-0

The publisher's policy is to use permanent paper from mills that operate a sustainable forestry policy. Furthermore, the publisher ensures that the text paper and cover boards used have met acceptable environmental accreditation standards.

Printed in China.

Cataloging-in-Publication Data

Handbook of parasitology / edited by Madelyn Goodman.
p. cm.
Includes bibliographical references and index.
ISBN 978-1-63241-649-0
1. Medical parasitology. 2. Parasitology. 3. Parasitic diseases. I. Goodman, Madelyn.
RC119 .H36 2019
616.9--dc23

Table of Contents

Preface

This book has been an outcome of determined endeavour from a group of educationists in the field. The primary objective was to involve a broad spectrum of professionals from diverse cultural background involved in the field for developing new researches. The book not only targets students but also scholars pursuing higher research for further enhancement of the theoretical and practical applications of the subject.

The in-depth study of parasites along with their hosts is known as parasitology. The study of the relationship between the parasite and the host is also within the scope of this field. As a sub-field of biology, parasitology forms a synthesis of various other disciplines and integrates their techniques. Some of these disciplines include bioinformatics, immunology, genetics, molecular biology, etc. Medical parasitology is a subset of parasitology, which is concerned with the parasites that affect humans. It studies the diseases caused by parasites in humans and the clinical response of humans against them. The diagnosis, control, prevention and treatment of such parasitic diseases are also under the scope of this field. This book attempts to understand the multiple branches that fall under the discipline of parasitology and how such concepts have practical applications. While understanding the long-term perspectives of the topics, this book makes an effort in highlighting their impact as a modern tool for growth of the medical science. Researchers and students in this field will be assisted by this book.

It was an honour to edit such a profound book and also a challenging task to compile and examine all the relevant data for accuracy and originality. I wish to acknowledge the efforts of the contributors for submitting such brilliant and diverse chapters in the field and for endlessly working for the completion of the book. Last, but not the least; I thank my family for being a constant source of support in all my research endeavours.

Editor

1

A bite so sweet: the glycobiology interface of tick-host-pathogen interactions

Pavlina Vechtova[1,2*†], Jarmila Sterbova[1,2†], Jan Sterba[1,2], Marie Vancova[1,2], Ryan O. M. Rego[1,2], Martin Selinger[1,2], Martin Strnad[1,2], Maryna Golovchenko[1], Nataliia Rudenko[1] and Libor Grubhoffer[1,2]

Abstract

Vector-borne diseases constitute 17% of all infectious diseases in the world; among the blood-feeding arthropods, ticks transmit the highest number of pathogens. Understanding the interactions between the tick vector, the mammalian host and the pathogens circulating between them is the basis for the successful development of vaccines against ticks or the tick-transmitted pathogens as well as for the development of specific treatments against tick-borne infections. A lot of effort has been put into transcriptomic and proteomic analyses; however, the protein-carbohydrate interactions and the overall glycobiology of ticks and tick-borne pathogens has not been given the importance or priority deserved. Novel (bio)analytical techniques and their availability have immensely increased the possibilities in glycobiology research and thus novel information in the glycobiology of ticks and tick-borne pathogens is being generated at a faster pace each year. This review brings a comprehensive summary of the knowledge on both the glycosylated proteins and the glycan-binding proteins of the ticks as well as the tick-transmitted pathogens, with emphasis on the interactions allowing the infection of both the ticks and the hosts by various bacteria and tick-borne encephalitis virus.

Keywords: Tick, Pathogen, Host, Glycan, Lectin, Glycobiology, *Borrelia*, *Anaplasma*, TBEV, Carbohydrate-binding

Background

Vector-borne diseases constitute 17% of all infectious diseases in the world [1]. Pathogenic viruses, bacteria, and protozoa are carried by blood-feeding arthropods on just about all the continents and both livestock and people tend to be affected by these. This becomes a large economic burden on the animal health sector and on the public health system of various countries. Ticks are the first among blood-feeding vectors in terms of the number of pathogens that they can transmit. Unfortunately, there are next to no vaccines against the tick-transmitted bacterial and protozoan diseases and very few against tick-borne viruses [2]. The only successful anti-tick vaccine, based on the glycoprotein Bm86 from the cattle tick *Rhiphicephalus microplus*, has been shown to be efficient against ticks of the genus *Rhiphicephalus* and Bm86 homologue vaccines have had some efficiency against at least two species of the genus *Hyalomma*, but this is not the case for other ticks and the pathogens they transmit [3]. The European Centre for Disease Prevention and Control suggests that there will be a rise in tick-borne diseases based on changes in various factors including the environment and socio-economics [4]. Research efforts to combat tick-borne diseases have usually centred, as with most other infectious diseases, on determining the Achilles' heel of the pathogen. Most endeavours have focussed on understanding host-pathogen interactions, primarily at the vertebrate level. Protein-carbohydrate interactions between the pathogen and the host cell are of primary importance, in terms of attachment and/or invasion of the cell, whether in an invertebrate or vertebrate host. The observation that there is conservation in the protein-carbohydrate recognition strategies can be used as part of novel approaches for intervention [5]. It has been shown that many regulatory mechanisms are mediated by post-translational modifications (PTM). One example of a PTM that regulates protein degradation and signaling in eukaryotes is ubiquitination. Pathogens are known to exploit ubiquitination to infect mammalian cells and it

* Correspondence: vechtp00@jcu.cz
†Pavlina Vechtova and Jarmila Sterbova contributed equally to this work.
[1]Institute of Parasitology, Biology Centre, Czech Academy of Sciences, Branišovská 31, CZ-37005 České Budějovice, Czech Republic
[2]Faculty of Science, University of South Bohemia, Branišovská 1760, CZ-37005 České Budějovice, Czech Republic

has been shown that the ubiquitination machinery is present in the tick *Ixodes scapularis*. It was identified that the E3 ubiquitin ligase XIAP restricted bacterial colonization of the vector and *xiap* silencing significantly increased tick colonization by the bacterium *Anaplasma phagocytophilum*, the causative agent of human granulocytic anaplasmosis [6].

Over the last decade, there has been a slow increase in the knowledge of vector-host-pathogen interactions which start from the time a pathogen invades the vector within a blood meal and attaches to the tick midgut lumen. Later it traverses to the tick salivary glands and completes its life-cycle by transmission to a new mammalian host during the subsequent tick feeding [2].

Four possible routes that may facilitate pathogen survival and transmission by most arthropod vectors including ticks have been pointed out. These include: (i) pathogen carbohydrate-binding adhesins that attach to receptors in the tick midgut; (ii) the attachment of carbohydrate-binding proteins of the arthropod to the pathogen as part of its innate immunity; (iii) carbohydrate-binding proteins that are soluble and form a link between the pathogen and midgut surfaces; and (iv) the use of co-receptors to enhance the interactions within the vector [5].

In this review, we would like to highlight the glycobiological aspects of all four of these specific mechanisms that come into play when looking at the vector-pathogen interactions as well as glycobiology-associated processes between the mammalian host and the pathogen (see Fig. 1). Glycobiology of ticks and tick-borne pathogens is developing together with the increased availability and sensitivity of analytical methods; a short overview is listed below, together with some relevant references for readers seeking deeper knowledge.

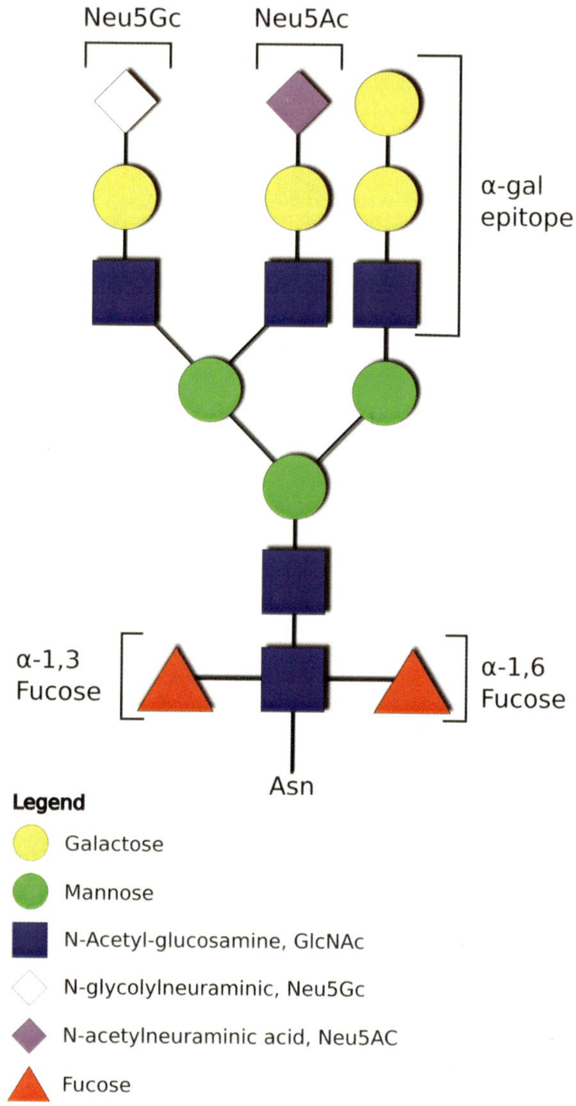

Fig. 1 Pathogen-tick and pathogen-host interactions. The scheme represents carbohydrate mediated interactions depicting in particular the most well-known interacting partners of *Borrelia*, tick vector and host (**a**) and *Anaplasma*, tick vector and host (**b**). Both *Borrelia* and *Anaplasma* produce adhesion molecules recognizing either a specific glycoprotein (such as TROSPA, decorin) or a specific glycan (core α1,3-fucose, sialylated glycans) in the tick and the host. Furthermore, *Borrelia* produce proteins interacting with host glycoproteins regulating its immune system. Two examples of the recognized glycans are shown in (**b**): an *O*-glycan bearing both α1,3-bound fucose and also a sialic acid, and an *N*-glycan with its core modified by the α1,3-bound fucose. The used symbol nomenclature is based on the Consortium for Functional Glycomics (http://www.functionalglycomics.org/)

Importance of glycosylation for protein functions

Post-translational modifications can be found in both prokaryotic and eukaryotic organisms; among them, glycosylation is one of the most abundant and most important. Protein glycosylation affects all the functions of proteins - their structure, activity, interactions with other molecules, half-life in the cell or organism; immune recognition is also dependent on the interaction of immune cells and receptors with glycosylated molecules. A wide variety of possible glycan structures and linkages increases the functionality of proteins [7].

The importance of carbohydrates for the function of proteins can be simply shown on complement proteins. The complement system comprises of more than 30 plasma- or membrane-bound components. Most of them are glycosylated to the various extent and the type of glycosylation generates tissue- or cell-specific population of glycoforms of each complement molecule. The specific glycoform population then secures functions that are required for a particular cell type or tissue. The repertoire of functions secured by glycans ranges from the control of protein folding, proper assembly within the endoplasmic reticulum, mechanistic shielding of the protein backbone against protease degradation, preventing inappropriate protein-protein interactions or formation of proper spatial protein conformation or participation in recognition epitope formation [8]. Specific examples show interesting ways in which glycans influence or modulate the complement cascade.

C1q is a recognition molecule of classical complement pathway and mediates initiation of the pathway by binding to the antibody-antigen complexes. The proper function of the C1q is conditioned by the appropriate triple helix formation within C1q monomer and the formation of C1q hexamer whose spatial conformation may be secured by the presence of N-linked glycan of each monomer [9].

Glycosylation was also proven important in complement regulatory factors where factor H (fH) glycosylation mediates its proper folding within the endoplasmic reticulum (ER). The absence of glycosylation or its malfunctioning leads to in fH misfolding and retention in ER causing clinical symptoms in children in form of hypocomplementemic renal disease [10].

C1-inhibitor is a plasma glycoprotein and, along with other members of the serpin proteases, its inhibitory activities are enhanced by binding of negatively charged polysaccharides. Most of the polysaccharides binding to the C1-inhibitor induce allosteric changes of the inhibitor molecule causing potentiation of the attachment to the C1 proteases or, as in case of dermatan sulphate, the potentiation is caused by the formation of a negatively charged polysaccharide-mediated linkage between positively charged portions of the C1-inhibitor and C1 protease molecules [11]. Structural characterization of the C1-inhibitor reveals extensive O-glycosylation with a high number of sialylated glycans. The trials for functional characterization of C1-inhibitor glycosylation showed an increased resistance of highly O-glycosylated region against proteolytic degradation [12] and highlighted the importance of sialylation for prolonged serum half-life [13].

Advances in bioanalytical methods for glycobiology

The most frequently used methods in glycobiology are mass spectrometry in combination with chromatography or capillary electrophoresis, glycan/lectin microarrays, or lectin staining. All of these developed greatly recently; for example, the increasing number of mass spectrometers available throughout the world and the development of more sensitive instruments and specifically the introduction of the Orbitrap mass spectrometers, greatly advanced the possibilities for glycan and glycoprotein analysis [14, 15]. The number of commercially available microarrays is also increasing and nowadays allows more or less specific detection of almost any kind of glycan. The availability of lectins together with the possibility to synthesize specific glycan molecules allows also the preparation of in-house glycan- or lectin-arrays; another possibility is the service provided by the Consortium for Functional Glycomics (http://www.functionalglycomics.org/).

Here, we review the current knowledge on how pathogens have evolved "sweet" strategies to overcome the immune responses within the vector and the mammalian host and the use of carbohydrate-binding properties to perpetuate their transmission and dissemination into a vertebrate host (Tables 1 and 2). We also provide a near comprehensive catalogue of all carbohydrate molecules that play a part in the disease cycle that have been characterized to date, be it within the tick or the mammalian host. We would like this to be the start of a renewed interest in the glycobiology of ticks and tick-borne diseases.

Glycosylation in the *Borrelia* infection cycle

Compared to eukaryotes, glycosylation in bacteria produces a much more diverse repertoire of glycoconjugate structures which are often species- or strain-specific. Most of the bacterial glycoconjugates are an integral part of the bacterial cell wall and provide the bacterial cell structural integrity. Additionally, the bacterial glycosylated cell surface structures mediate adhesion and interaction with its environment or host. Although the structural features of bacterial surface glycans have been well described, the function of many of them, including those in pathogenic bacteria, remain unexplored. In principle, pathogenic bacteria use glycosylation for two reasons; they synthesize host-like glycan structures to hide from the host immune system and, conversely, they produce glycosylated proteins that are able to bind more effectively the host immune molecules and thus influence their activity [16].

Since all *Borrelia* species are host-propagated bacteria that shuttle between a vertebrate host and an arthropod vector, these spirochetes have developed strategies to adjust to these diverse environments [17]. This is achieved by regulating the level of gene expression in response to changes in temperature, pH, salts, nutrient content, and other host- and vector-dependent factors. A significant number of *Borrelia* proteins mediate the interactions with host/vector molecules and thus enable *Borrelia* to complete its infectious cycle. Recent findings highlight the importance of carbohydrate moieties in these interactions and in the overall pathogenesis of this infectious spirochete.

Borrelia/tick glycosylated interactions

When entering the vertebrate host during tick-feeding, *Borrelia* must overcome several barriers to successfully invade and disseminate in the host body. The invasion of the host is difficult as it requires the interaction of the existing *Borrelia* surface structures with host tissues without being noticed by the host immune system. *Borrelia* have developed many elaborate strategies to recognize diverse host molecules and cell types to promote

Table 1 Summary of carbohydrate-binding proteins of *Borrelia* spp. recognizing tick or host receptors. The carbohydrate-binding proteins from *Borrelia* spp. are listed together with the recognized molecule from the vector or the host. Glycoproteins or glycans are listed as the recognized molecules depending on the available information. Majority of proteins from Lyme borreliosis spirochetes are listed; in the case of relapsing fever *Borrelia*, the bacterial species is defined

Borrelia spp. protein	Tick binding partner	Reference
Borrelia vs tick		
OspA	TROSPA	[236]
OspC	SALP15	[27]
TSLPI/P8	Mannose binding lectin (MBL)	[42]
Vsp33 (*B. hermsii*)	Unknown receptor in tick SG	[62]
Borrelia vs host		
Bgp (p26)	GAG	[294]
DbpA (p20)	Decorin/dermatansulfate	[48, 295]
DbpB (p19)	Decorin/dermatansulfate/chondroitinsulfate	[48, 295]
Bbk32	Fibronectin /heparansulfate/dermatansulfate	[63]
P66	Integrins	[87]
OspA	Plasminogen	[296]
OspC	Plasminogen	[297, 298]
Enolase	Plasminogen	[299]
Erps (OspE/F related proteins)	Factor H or FHL protein	[105]
CRASPs	Factor H	[105]
PAMPs	Mannose receptor on dendritic cells	[300]
Unknown	Neolacto-(Gal4GlcNAc3Gal4Glc1)-carrying glycoconjugates in human erythrocytes	[301]
VspB (*B.turicatae*)	GAG	[61]

Table 2 Summary of carbohydrate-binding proteins of *Anaplasma* recognizing tick or host receptors. The carbohydrate-binding proteins from *Anaplasma* are listed together with the recognized molecule from the vector or the host. Glycoproteins or glycans are listed as the recognized molecules depending on the available information

Anaplasma protein	Binding partner	Reference
MSP1a (MSP1 complex)	Vector binding partner: Unknown receptor in IDE8 tick cells	[189, 190]
Unknown molecule	Vector binding partner: Core α 1,3-fucose glycoprotein	[203]
Unknown adhesin-like molecule	Host binding partner: 1,3-Fuc and Sia in sialyl Lewis X, PSGL-1 in human neutrophils	[199, 200]
Unknown adhesin-like molecule	Host binding partner: 1,3-Fuc and Sia in sialyl Lewis X, PSGL-1 in murine neutrophils	[199]
Unknown adhesin-like molecule	Host binding partner: 1,3-Fuc and Sia in sialyl Lewis X, PSGL-1 in human myeloid HL-60 cells	[197, 201]
Unknown molecule of *A. phagocytophilum* NCH-1 strain	Host binding partner: 1,3-fucose in murine bone marrow-derived mast cells (BMMCs), murine peritoneal mast cells	[198]
Unknown molecule of *A. phagocytophilum* NCH-1 strain	Host binding partner: α 1,3-Fuc in human skin-derived mast cells	[198]
AmOmpA	Host binding partner: α2,3-sialylated and α1,3-fucosylated glycan of the sialyl Lewis x in myeloid cells	[182]
AmOmpA	Host binding partner: α2,3-sialylated and α1,3-fucosylated glycan of the 6- sulfo-sialyl Lewis x in endothelial cells	[180, 182]
AmOmpA	Host binding partner: α2,3-sialylated, α2,6-sialylated, α1,3-fucosylated glycan receptors in human and murine myeloid HL-60 cells, 6- sulpho-sialyl Lewis x in endothelial cells	[180–182]
Unknown	Host binding partner: α1,3-fucose	[203]

dissemination and chronic infection [18], and to overcome host immune system surveillance [19]. The concerted action of these structurally and functionally diverse *Borrelia* surface molecules helps the spirochete to successfully adapt and multiply in the host body.

The interacting molecules of *Borrelia* and the tick are often modified by glycosylation producing a diverse pool of structures. Moreover, glycosylation is a dynamic modification and can be readily altered upon environmental cues [20].

The presence of glycoconjugates on the surface of cultured *B. burgdorferi* has been demonstrated by the ability of *Borrelia* to bind a number of lectins [21]. In search of *B. burgdorferi* glycosylation patterns, increased attention has been paid to outer surface proteins that are produced at different stages of the *Borrelia* transmission cycle and represent points of interaction between the spirochetes and their hosts/vectors.

Borrelia outer surface proteins

Borrelia outer surface proteins A and B (*osp*A and *osp*B) are encoded on a bicistronic operon and extensively expressed on the surface of spirochetes in unfed ticks. OspA is one of the major and most comprehensively studied *Borrelia* proteins. While OspA mediates *Borrelia* attachment to the tick midgut when spirochetes are acquired by ticks during blood-feeding, OspB plays a key role in successful colonization of the tick midgut. OspA downregulation is important for *Borrelia* detachment, multiplication, and migration from the tick midgut to salivary glands [22–25]. When ticks are fed to engorgement, *Borrelia* clears OspA and OspB from the surface expressing instead another outer surface protein C (OspC) [22, 26].

OspC, encoded by *bbb19* mapped to the cp26 plasmid, is one of the most divergent genes in *Borrelia* genome, and is crucial for the early stages of mammalian host infection by the spirochete, but not required for acquisition of spirochetes by tick, tick colonization or migration from salivary glands to the gut [27–32].

Erps (OspE/F-related proteins) are a family of surface integrins with high affinity to factor H and encoded by *erp*-loci localised on each of the cp32 plasmids. Lyme disease spirochetes control Erp synthesis throughout the bacterial infectious tabacycle, producing the proteins during the infection of the host but downregulating their synthesis during tick infection stage. The best-characterized members are OspE and OspF proteins [33], their paralogues OspE/F-related proteins [34] and a group of OspE/F-like leader peptides (Elps) [35].

OspA, OspB and TROSPA

Earlier work had indicated that OspA and OspB are the major *Borrelia* glycosylated proteins [36], yet a later study showed that the suggested *N*-linked glycosylation does not occur [37]. Colonization of ticks by spirochetes requires the involvement of tick receptor(s). Although a tick receptor for OspB has not yet been identified, the tick receptor for OspA (TROSPA) is located in the tick gut and is heavily glycosylated. The blockade of TROSPA by TROSPA antisera or by downregulation of TROSPA *via* RNAi reduced *B. burgdorferi* adherence to the tick gut, hampering the spirochete transmission to the mammalian host. The number of potential posttranslational modification sites in TROSPA is unusually high (> 30), with a predominance of *O*-glycosylation sites [25].

OspC and Salp15

When transmitted from the tick vector to the host, *Borrelia* are delivered within the tick saliva. Tick saliva contains a plethora of bioactive molecules, which have been shown to be important for immunosuppression of the host responses [28]. One of the secreted salivary proteins is *Salp15* [29]. This protein specifically interacts with *B. burgdorferi* OspC which results in the protection of *Borrelia* from antibody-mediated killing and plays a critical role in establishing *B. burgdorferi* infection [27]. Whereas no data exists about the potential glycosylation of OspC, the glycosylation of Salp15 was demonstrated experimentally [30]. Salp15 from *I. ricinus* did not deliver the same protection to *B. garinii* and *B. afzelii* against antibody-mediated killing [31], presumably suggesting that the Salp15 binding for some species is an advantage for surviving in nature [31]. An explanation may lie in a different structural or spatial organization of the OspC or Salp15 molecule causing better access to the binding sites of each of the molecules in *B. burgdorferi.* Another hypothesis claims that *B. burgdorferi* OspC holds differently charged areas which interact in a way that favour formation of OspC multimers or even a lattice [38]. This structure, along with bound Salp15, might form a protective coating on the bacteria preventing an access of anti-OspC antibodies or *B. burgdorferi* antiserum [27]. In addition to the direct interplay between Salp15 and *B. burgdorferi*, Salp15 indirectly facilitates the host invasion by inhibiting dendritic cell activation by binding to the receptor/lectin DC-SIGN, localized on the surface of macrophages and dendritic cells [32].

Ixofin3D and Ixodes scapularis dystroglycan-like protein

Ixofin3D and *I. scapularis* dystroglycan-like protein (ISDLP) are glycoproteins expressed on the surface of midgut cells which were identified as candidate tick midgut binding partners of *B. burgdorferi* using a yeast surface display assay [39]. The expression of both Ixofin3D and ISDLP was elevated in *Borrelia*-infected tick midgut during feeding. Ixofin3D and ISDLP interact with spirochete cells as was confirmed *in vitro* by immunofluorescence assay and RNA interference. The RNAi-mediated reduction in expression of Ixofin3D and ISDLP resulted in decreased spirochete burdens in the tick salivary glands and in the murine host as well [39, 40]. The full-length Ixofin3D contains four putative fibronectin type III domains. Ixofin3D is glycosylated as shown experimentally by periodic-acid Schiff's staining of a recombinant protein produced in *Drosophila* cells. Even though the importance of Ixofin3D for *Borrelia* infection was shown, the borrelial binding partner for Ixofin3D has not yet been identified [39].

The binding partner for ISDLP is also yet to be discovered. Like Ixofin3D, ISDLP silencing did not reduce the spirochete numbers in the gut but the transmigration process from gut to salivary glands was impaired. The mechanism remains unknown although the collected evidence implies that ISDLP may facilitate gut tissue remodelling or reduced barrier for spirochete transfer to salivary glands [40].

TSLPI

Tick salivary lectin pathway inhibitor (TSLPI) is a secreted salivary protein that protects *Borrelia* from complement-mediated killing. TSLPI facilitates spirochete transmission and acquisition through interference with the host mannose-binding lectin (MBL) and inhibition of the host lectin complement pathway [41]. *N*-linked glycosylation of recombinant *Drosophila*-expressed TSLPI appeared to be vital for its function as a lectin pathway inhibitor, suggesting that TSLPI *N*-glycans are involved in its binding to MBL carbohydrate recognition domains [42, 43].

Borrelia adhesins and extracellular matrix

Adhesion is the first and basic event in establishing an infection. The *Borrelia* cell surface is, at the time of host invasion, covered by adhesion proteins that can recognize and bind to various host cell types and/or extracellular matrix (ECM) components and thus promote *Borrelia* dissemination and settlement in various corners of the host body. Although *Borrelia* adhesins are not glycosylated, the presence of glycosylation has been confirmed in their tick receptors, suggesting a significant role of glycosylation in adhesin-receptor interaction.

Borrelia burgdorferi encodes a variety of adhesins and their characterization and role in the *Borrelia* infection cycle using different approaches was thoroughly described in a review by Coburn et al. [44]. With regard to their overlapping roles in *Borrelia* adhesion to the host tissue, it is important to note that only the concerted action of various adhesins guarantees an effective adhesion and transmigration of spirochetes to different hosts and their tissues [44].

A short overview of host ECM proteins

Glycosaminoglycans

Several ECM-associated molecules are specifically targeted by *Borrelia* adhesins. Exceptionally important seem to be the glycosaminoglycans (GAGs), large linear polysaccharides constructed of repeating disaccharide units (e.g. hyaluronan, chondroitin, dermatan, heparan, keratan) that decorate the ECM proteins. GAG chains are abundantly modified by sulphurylation, which imparts them a strong negative charge [45]. Numerous studies have shown that binding of GAGs by *B. burgdorferi* enables colonization of the host [46].

Fibronectin

A relevant ECM-associated molecule for *B. burgdorferi* attachment is fibronectin (Fn), a high-molecular weight, dimeric glycoprotein found in body fluids and in the ECM. *Borrelia burgdorferi* fails to bind to the ECM *in vitro* upon exposure to an anti-Fn antibody, implicating the Fn involvement in *Borrelia* attachment [47].

Decorins

Decorins are ubiquitous ECM proteoglycans, which are associated with collagen fibrils in the mammalian connective tissues [48]. Decorins are complex glycoproteins; apart from serine linked GAG chain, they are also modified by up to 3 N-glycans [49, 50]. Numerous studies associate decorins with *Borrelia* adhesin attachment and interestingly, the binding is promoted by intact decorin proteoglycan molecule rather than its protein core or GAG chain itself [48].

Laminin

Laminin is a large extracellular matrix multidomain glycoprotein. It is a critical molecule in the basement membrane assembly and, by extension, in tissue formation in the developing organism [51]. Besides its role in basement membrane architecture, it also mediates cellular interactions and provides a dense network for various cellular signalling and attachment events. The existence of different laminin isoforms gives space to developmental regulations mediated by differential responses to cells and newly forming tissues. Laminin, as well as other ECM forming molecules, possesses numerous glycosylation sites and its molecule is modified up to 32 % by N-linked glycans [52].

The carbohydrate portion of Laminin was proven to be a mediator of attachment in several bacterial species [53]. Laminin is also a potent target of several borrelial adhesins [54–56] although the direct involvement of the laminin carbohydrate moiety has not been reported yet.

Integrins

Integrins are glycosylated cell surface receptors mediating cell adhesions to the extracellular matrix and some important cell-cell interactions [57]. The presence of *N*-linked glycans in integrin molecule proves integral for the stability of the domain conformation and consequently affects integrin adhesive properties [58]. Integrins possess a typical heterodimeric structure combining different α and β polypeptide chains and their combination determines the specificity of integrins [59]. Integrins are expressed on all mammalian cells except erythrocytes. The expression of different integrin subtypes produces unique cell surface signature of each cell type [60].

Borrelia adhesins

Vsps

Relapsing fever *Borrelia*, unlike Lyme disease-causing *Borrelia*, are vectored by soft ticks of the genus *Ornithodoros*. They are present in the blood of the mammalian host in high numbers which lead to high fevers followed by bouts of relapses. They recognize glycosaminoglycans (GAG), which mediates the attachment of *Borrelia* to mammalian cells. GAG recognition is partly dependent on the presence of some of the variable small proteins (Vsps). *Borrelia turicatae*, a relapsing fever borrelia that is vectored by *O. turicata*, recognizes GAGs *via* VspB which allows binding of *B. turicatae* to cultured mammalian cells as well as increased spread and replication in the mammalian host. *Borrelia hermsii* also attaches to cultured mammalian cells *via* GAGs; however, Vsps are not essential for this binding [61].

After the feeding of *O. hermsi* with *B. hermsii*-infected blood, the bacteria switched from expression of many bloodstream outer surface variable major proteins (Vmps) to a unique protein, variable tick protein (Vtp, Vsp33) [62].

BBK32, RevA and C1-inhibitor

Borrelia burgdorferi expresses at least two fibrinogen-binding proteins, BBK32 [63] and RevA [64]. BBK32 is a protein, whose attenuation does not block the spirochete transmission from the tick to the host [65], but lowers the bacterial loads in different tissues at different time points of infection [66]. *Borrelia burgdorferi* also attaches to endothelium in the vascular system through fibrinogen (Fn) and this interaction becomes stronger with increasing blood flow, allowing the spirochete to overcome fluid shear stress [67]. These stabilizing interactions are sustained by catch bond properties of BBK32 [68]. Following the binding to Fn, BBK32 binds to various kinds of GAGs, including heparin sulphates and dermatan sulphates of the host ECM [69–71]. It also seems to be involved in the modulation of the innate immunity. In particular, BBK32 binds the C1 complex of the classical innate immunity pathway, preventing its activation and thus obstructing classical pathway-mediated *Borrelia* lysis [72].

As *B. burgdorferi* BBK32 mutants are still able to bind fibronectin, an additional Fn-binding protein, RevA, was identified [58]. RevA expression on the *Borrelia* cell surface was upregulated in mammalian host compared to the tick vector. Furthermore, *Borrelia*-infected patients produced anti-RevA antibodies throughout various stages of Lyme disease suggesting its involvement in Lyme disease establishment and persistence in the host. RevA appears to have multiple binding sites which *Borrelia* uses to bind host cells *via* Fn [46, 73].

DbpA/DbpB

Decorin-binding proteins A and B (DbpA and DbpB) are adhesins found on the surface of *B. burgdorferi* [20, 45]. These proteins are critical for the virulence of *B. burgdorferi* [74, 75]. New data suggests that the decorin-binding proteins actually do not bind directly to the decorin protein core but interact with decorin *via* GAGs that are attached to the protein [76–78]. The binding studies of DbpA and DbpB from different *Borrelia* genospecies showed that there are clear differences in the decorin binding activity and that these differences may ultimately lead to the differences in tissue tropism and clinical manifestations associated with particular *Borrelia* genospecies [76, 79]. *In vivo* functional studies demonstrated the importance of DbpA/B adhesins for *Borrelia* invasion of the mammalian host especially in the early stages of infection [80].

Bgp

Borrelia burgdorferi glycosaminoglycan binding protein (Bgp) is a surface-exposed protein on intact spirochetes [70]. Recombinant Bgp bound the same GAG as the whole spirochete, agglutinated erythrocytes and inhibited binding of *B. burgdorferi* to the mammalian cells. A transposon mutant of the *Bgp* gene had less ability to adhere to host endothelial and epithelial cells *in vitro* and to colonize host target tissues leading to the reduced inflammatory manifestation of Lyme disease in the mouse model. The adherence was not fully disrupted due to the existence of other GAG-binding adhesins which facilitate host colonization and also highlights the importance of *Borrelia* GAG-binding ability for the completion of the infection cycle [81]. Although the Bgp attachment to GAG is not essential for disease establishment, the protein appears to be involved in the formation of an initial infectious niche in the host. Different spirochetes strains possess different GAG-binding preferences and their binding ability to multiple cells depends on the GAGs that they express [76].

BmpA

BmpA (*Borrelia* membrane protein A) and its three paralogues B, C, and D are all laminin-binding borrelial outer surface proteins [82]. Like other *Borrelia* surface proteins, BmpA is also antigenic. All bmp genes are located on the *Borrelia* chromosome, arranged in clusters that are differentially regulated [83]. The involvement in the development of arthritis in the mouse model was described for two Bmp proteins, BmpA and BmpB [84].

Borrelia adhesins and integrin-mediated interactions

Borrelia binds to host endothelial cells *via* the interaction of integrins $\alpha_{IIb}\beta_3$, $\alpha_V\beta_3$, and $\alpha_V\beta_1$ with *Borrelia* surface adhesins [59, 85]. It was also described that the causative agent of relapsing fever, *B. hermsii*, binds to human platelets promoted by the platelet glycoprotein integrin $\alpha_{IIb}\beta_3$ and is diminished by $\alpha_{IIb}\beta_3$ antagonists or by a genetic defect in this integrin [86].

P66

P66 is one of the candidate ligands for β_3-chain integrins (e.g. $\alpha_{IIb}\beta_3$, $\alpha_V\beta_3$) [87]. P66 also functions as a porin [88, 89], and structural predictions, as well as some experimental data, present the molecule as porin assuming the structure of β-barrel [90].

P66 mutants showed a dramatically reduced ability to attach to integrin $\alpha_V\beta_3$ [91]. Endothelial cells responded to wild-type *Borrelia* infection by upregulation of endothelial growth factor compared to a control infection with a P66 deletion mutant. The ability of P66 mutants to transmigrate through the cell monolayer was impaired, which suggests the role of P66 in *Borrelia* transendothelial migration, although its porin function does not play a role in the migration process [92].

Mammalian integrins typically contain an RGD (Arg--Gly-Asp tripeptide) consensus sequence in their binding domain, where aspartic acid is a key binding amino acid. P66 lacks this sequence; however, residues 205 and 207 of its 203–209 binding region are both aspartic acid [93]. P66 deletion mutants applied subcutaneously are readily cleared out of the site of infection, which refers to the possible involvement of the innate immune system and confirms the importance of this protein for host colonization together with other studies [94]. However, tick colonization is shown to be P66-independent [94].

BB0172

BB0172 is an outer membrane protein containing von Willebrand factor A domain which mediates intercellular and protein-protein interactions in ECM. It is, for example, involved in the attachment of platelets to the ECM in the site of damaged endothelial epithelium *via* platelet surface glycoprotein [95]. BB0172 showed a weak interaction with ECM-associated fibronectin. Importantly, a strong affinity was observed in the attachment of BB0172 to $\alpha_{III}\beta_1$ integrin. Moreover, the affinity was much stronger than the one observed in the interaction of borrelial P66 adhesins with β_3 chain integrins [95].

Borrelia adhesins interacting with mammalian complement

Mammalian innate immunity is alerted by a variety of surface-exposed molecules of invading pathogens. The first encounter of host antibodies with potentially harmful intruder activates the complement system which assists in tagging of the pathogen for destruction and also acts on pathogen clearance itself by the formation of membrane attack complex. Different pathways of the complement system progress in a cascade-like manner and its brisk response to pathogen invasion must be under the control of regulating mechanisms preventing complement from attacking host cells.

Invading a host organism, the pathogens have evolved different strategies to circumvent the immune response. Many of these strategies are in fact directed against components of the complement system. The most widespread strategy employs molecules recruiting or mimicking the complement regulators, including the direct interaction of pathogens with complement proteins leading to the modulation or inhibition of their function or indirectly to the activation of complement proteins enzymatic degradation [96].

The complement regulators are represented by several serum proteins that are able to dampen the activity of complement and prevent host self-destruction. Two of them, complement factor H (FH) and its splice homologue Factor H-like (FHL) inhibit the alternative complement pathway response using host-|specific surface patterns like sialic acid or GAGs and thus promoting self-recognition processes [97, 98].

FH is a plasma glycoprotein containing 9 glycosylation sites [99] bearing complex, predominantly diantennary disialylated, fucosylated, and nonfucosylated glycans at eight of the nine glycosylation sites [100]. Similarly, FHL is also a plasma glycoprotein [101]. Both proteins possess a RGD motif which is assigned cell adhesive properties and thus can modulate cell adhesion. Additionally, FHL promotes anchorage-dependent cell attachment and spreading [102].

CRASPs and ERPs

The two complement regulators, FH and FHL are bound by *Borrelia* surface proteins hence preventing the activation at the central step of the complement cascade. Serum resistant *Borrelia* express adhesins on their surface, which are capable of interfering with different components of the host complement system leading to the modulation of host immune response and hampering the complement-mediated spirochete lysis [103, 104].

The two well-characterized types of complement interfering adhesins, complement regulator-acquiring surface proteins (CRASP) 1 and 2 [105], control the complement activity by binding complement regulating molecules such as FH and FHL-1 [104, 106]. Up to now, five different CRASPs (CRASP-1 to CRASP-5) have been described and each of them presents a different binding ability to FH, FHL-1, or plasminogen [98, 104, 106].

CRASP-1 (CspA, BBA68) has been studied the most extensively. It shows a strong affinity to the complement regulators which inactivate the complement response very efficiently [106, 107].

The expression of CRASP-1 is repressed in the tick vector and increases in the mammalian host, which suggests its role in spirochete transmission and evasion of the host immune response [108, 109]. CRASP-1 also confers serum resistance to *B. burgdorferi*. The role of CRASP-1 in complement inactivation is evident in the CRASP-1 knockout-mutants which inefficiently bound human FHL and attracted complement constituents more readily [110, 111].

Apart from *B. bavariensis*, all studied *Borrelia* species possess CRASP-1 orthologues conferring complement inactivation [112, 113]. The orthologues belong to the same protein family although the encoding genes do not share the same locus with the *B. burgdorferi* CspA [98].

CRASP-2 (CspZ) is another *Borrelia* adhesin binding both FH and FHL-1 independently of CRASP-1 and reinforcing *Borrelia* complement resistance [114, 115]. The CRASP-2 expression fluctuates in a somewhat similar manner to CRASP-1 during the *Borrelia* infectious cycle. Like CRASP-1, CRASP-2 is also upregulated during an established mammalian infection and is able to activate antibody-mediated immune response [116], which makes this adhesin important for the diagnosis of Lyme disease infection. The triggered immune response does not, however, provide the host with protective immunity and has no effect on spirochete dissemination [117].

Three members of the polymorphic Erp (OspE/F-related protein) protein family, ErpA (BBP38, CRASP-5), ErpC (CRASP-4) and ErpP (BBN38, CRASP-3), are plasminogen binding proteins that can simultaneously bind to FH and FH-related proteins [103, 107, 118–122].

The Erp proteins are most probably involved in different reservoir hosts infection due to differential binding abilities of particular Erp paralogues [123, 124]. Despite their complement regulator binding properties, none of the Erp proteins are necessary for the protection of *Borrelia* spirochetes against complement-mediated killing; CRASP-1/CRASP-2 deletion mutants expressing all Erp proteins were susceptible to serum mediated lysis [119, 120, 125].

Erps are not upregulated during *Borrelia* transmission but their expression gradually increases during Lyme disease progression, suggesting their role during mammalian infection [125]. Interestingly, *Borrelia* can regulate the expression of both Erps and CRASPs very dynamically as different isolates of *B. burgdorferi* (*s.l.*) reacted differently to complement-mediated killing [56, 126]. Moreover, some of the Erp members present multiple functions during *Borrelia* infection. For example, ErpX ability to bind complement regulators is complemented by its laminin binding properties [56]. The overlapping activities of *Borrelia* surface molecules enhance the overall infectious potential of the spirochete.

Borrelia-specific host pattern-recognition receptors and lectins

Toll-like receptors

Recognition of pathogens is mediated by a set of pattern-recognition receptors (PRRs). The group of glycosylated proteins that comprise the Toll or Toll-like receptors family (TLRs) are transmembrane receptors that function as PRRs in mammals [127]. So far, eleven members that potentially participate in the recognition of invading pathogens have been identified in mammalian genomes [128] and glycosylation was shown to have a critical role in TLR presentation on the cell surface [129, 130].

There are several TLR members, whose role in spirochete recognition has been identified. The well-characterized TLR2 is presented on antigen-presenting cells, epithelial and endothelial cells [131]. It was able to recognize a variety of ligands and was important for macrophage activation and further triggering of the immune response in *Borrelia*-infected mammalian hosts when stimulated by OspA [132]. The signal transduction through TLR1/2 in response to *B. burgdorferi* invasion can elicit opposite immunoregulatory effects in the blood and CNS immune cells, affecting the different susceptibility of these compartments to infection [127].

TLR4 is expressed in macrophages and dendritic cells [130] and is upregulated upon *Borrelia* infection or stimulation by OspC [133, 134] and its main ligands are lipopolysaccharides (LPS) from gram-negative bacteria [135]. The role of TLR4 in *Borrelia* recognition remains unclear as *B. burgdorferi* does not express LPS on its surface.

TLR9 is responsible for recognition and further endosomal/lysosomal internalization of CpG motifs in bacterial DNA [136]. This process has been observed in sonicated *Borrelia*, which promoted the activation of murine cells *via* TLR9 [137].

Nucleotide-oligomerization domain-like receptors

Nucleotide-oligomerization domain-like receptors (NOD-like receptors or NLR) are a group of intracellular PRRs, capable of binding bacterial muropeptides, the molecules derived from bacterial peptidoglycans [138]. Together with TLRs, NOD-like receptors are crucial for recognition of *Borrelia* species. Contrary to other PRR families, NLRs bind bacterial ligands intracellularly, i.e. they are able to recognize the pathogen-associated molecular patterns (PAMPs) that enter the cell *via* phagocytosis or through the membrane pores induced during cellular stress [139].

There are several NLR protein members that can bind carbohydrate-associated PAMPs, although only a few of them were directly observed to be involved in Lyme disease. NOD1 and NOD2 receptors are the most extensively investigated major PRRs [138, 140].

Borrelia-infected primary murine astrocytes upregulated NOD-proteins upon exposure to some TLR-ligands [138], while murine primary microglia infected by *Borrelia* only upregulated NOD2 and not the NOD1 [141]. NOD2 activation by *Borrelia* stimulated inflammatory cytokines release. Their activities are assigned to a host proinflammatory response, although their particular role in Lyme disease establishment remains unknown [142]. NOD2 stimulation by *Borrelia* induces inflammation during the early stages of Lyme disease but induces tolerance and suppresses *B. burgdorferi*-mediated Lyme arthritis and carditis in mice during later phases of infection [143]. *Borrelia* recognition in the host is conferred by the combined action of TLR and NOD2. The activation of both receptors at a time by *Borrelia* species is essential for an effective cytokine release. It has been concluded that TLR2 and NOD2 co-recognition of *Borrelia* surface receptors leads to both induction of a proper immune response and to inflammatory-induced pathology [144].

C-type lectin receptors

A family of calcium-dependent receptors that bind carbohydrate ligands include both soluble and cell-associated (transmembrane) lectins in vertebrates. C-type lectin receptors (CLRs) expressed by dendritic cells are crucial for tailoring immune response to pathogens. The transmembrane type is predominantly expressed by antigen-presenting cells functioning as PRRs recognizing PAMPs in bacteria [128]. Currently, 17 CLR subfamilies are described in vertebrates.

Mannose receptor represents a subgroup of CLRs binding mannose-containing bacterial transmembrane PAMPs. CLRs are involved in the recognition and phagocytosis of several microorganisms including *B. burgdorferi*. In particular, CLRs were upregulated in dendritic cells after *B. burgdorferi* activation and facilitated phagocytosis of *B. burgdorferi* by monocytes and macrophages [128]. However, the recognized borrelial protein is yet to be identified.

Surface glycolipids of *Borrelia burgdorferi*

Borrelia have an unusual composition of glycolipids in their outer membrane; they synthesize mono-α-galactosyl-diacylglycerol (MGalD) and cholesterol derived glycolipids cholesteryl-β-D-galacto-pyranoside, cholesteryl 6-O-acyl-β-D-galactopyranoside (ACG), or cholesteryl 6-O-palmitoyl-β-D-galactopyranoside (ACGal/BbGL-1) [145–147].

The *Borrelia* glycolipids induce inflammatory reactions; in particular, two glycolipids ACGal/BbGL-I and MGalD/BbGL-II, are probably immunogenic [145, 148]. The immunogenic epitope is recognized in the lipid part of the glycolipids [149]. An important constituent of the immunogenic epitope is the α-linked terminally bound galactose which is recognized by the T-cell receptor of invariant natural killer T cells (NKT) [150]. This then promotes their activation as well as the proliferation of Lyme disease-directed antibodies [151–153] which recognize glycolipids in the cell membrane of *Borrelia* but also *Ehrlichia* [154]. Importantly, the induced antibodies against the glycolipid fraction cross-react with gangliosides, which explains the phenomenon of neuroborreliosis [155].

The glycolipid recognition by invariant NKT cells seems to be an alternative system for innate immune system activation by bacteria lacking LPS, an otherwise typical antigenic determinant of most gram-negative bacteria [156].

Borrelia bind to GalCer (galactosylceramide) on Schwan cells [157], LacCer (lactosylceramide), ceramide trihexoside and gangliosides GD1a and GT1b. Moreover, *Borrelia* displays a specific affinity to disialoganglioside GD1a and trisialoganglioside GT1b carrying sialic acid. The ability to bind such a wide range of glycosphingolipids might provide an explanation for its ability to adhere to a wide spectrum of different cell types [158]. *Borrelia* did not bind gangliosides GM1, GD1b, GM2, GM3 and asialo-GM1 implying the requirement for terminally bound sialic acid in ganglioside recognized epitope and demonstrates the specific character of *Borrelia* and acidic gangliosides interaction. Interestingly, adhesion to GD1a and GT1b, as well as GalCer or LacCer was not compromised by free sialic acid, galactose or lactose, respectively [158, 159]. Conversely, GalCer-binding sites were saturable using free GalCer in CHO-K1 cells preventing spirochetes from attachment [148].

Vector-host glycosylated interactions

Similarly to *Borrelia*, the tick's successful evasion of the host response depends on its ability to conceal its activities from the host immune system. The pursuit of successful feeding drove ticks to equip their saliva with multiple pharmacologically active molecules which feature immunomodulatory activities. The myriad of diverse functions include cytolysis, vasodilatation, anticoagulation, anti-inflammation and immunosuppression. The comprehensive list of tick pharmacologically active salivary gland molecules is presented in a recent review [28].

P672 and CCL8

P672 is a chemokine binding protein (evasin). Evasins bind to multiple chemokines of different origin and their effects are thus pleiotropic. To date, several evasins originating in tick saliva have been identified [160, 161] and they inhibit responses of many chemokine sensitive molecules including neutrophiles or macrophages, which have been demonstrated in several tick species [28]. P672 was originally identified in *Rhipicephalus pulchellus* and its promiscuous binding abilities assign it 13 different chemokine partners showing different dissociation constants.

Mass spectrometric characterisation revealed the presence of several *N*-linked glycans and their deprival negatively influences the affinity of P672 to CCL8, although the underlying mechanism of this observation is yet to be uncovered [162].

Protease inhibitors

Many of the tick salivary proteins are glycosylated [163]. While the exact structure of the glycans attached to these proteins has not been studied, research has concentrated on the role of glycosylation with regard to the recognition of glycans by host immune systems. The importance of the glycan part for antibody recognition was shown for several proteins, such as AamS6 serpin [164], *R. microplus* serpins [165] or evasins 1 and 3 [166] confirming the need to use of glycosylated recombinant proteins in anti-tick vaccine preparations.

For proteins, where the role of glycosylation for the protein function was not confirmed, masking of the tick proteins antigenic epitopes and thus minimization of the immune response was speculated as the role of glycosylation [166].

Serpin 19

Serpin 19 is a serine protease inhibitor identified in the saliva of *Amblyomma americanum*. Serpin 19 displays a broad range of inhibitory activities: it interferes with the host homeostasis, coagulation and the development of inflammatory response. Importantly, the activity of many serine proteases is both positively and negatively regulated when bound to GAGs [167–169] and serpin 19 also contains several predicted GAG binding motives [170]. The functional validation further confirmed its GAG-binding properties and also extended the list of binding partners with heparin sulphate and heparin [170].

Variegin

The inhibition of blood coagulation cascade represents an important property of tick saliva that facilitates successful engorgement on the host. Variegin is a small thrombin-binding oligopeptide isolated from *A. variegatum* salivary glands. During tick feeding, variegin binds thrombin and disables its fibrinolytic activity and thus blocks the blood coagulation cascade. Despite its small size, variegin possesses a single *O*-linked glycan [171]. The synthetic *O*-glycosylated variegin analogues show significantly higher affinity to thrombin and consequently lower reaction kinetics of thrombin-mediated fibrinogenolysis compared to the non-glycosylated form, confirming the importance of its glycosylation. The functional analysis of the inhibition mechanism using macromolecular docking revealed the formation of some favourable hydrogen bonds between hydroxyl groups of the glycan and the allosterically important sites of thrombin [172].

Glycosylation in the *Anaplasma* infection cycle

Anaplasma is a genus of gram-negative rickettsial bacteria. They are obligate intracellular parasites infecting mammals including many domestic animals. The infection causes a reduction of the animal's body weight, abortions, reduces milk production and frequently leads to death [173–175]. In humans, *A. phagocytophilum* is the only confirmed pathogenic species causing human granulocytic anaplasmosis. Patients suffer from fever, headache, myalgias, chills, leukopenia, thrombocytopenia and liver damage manifested by elevated liver enzymes in serum [176]. The symptoms are usually mild but for some individuals, e.g. patients with a weakened immune system, it can be fatal. The infected vertebrate host serves as a reservoir where the bacterium can proliferate for many years and infect naïve ticks [177].

The main vectors of the genus *Anaplasma* are ticks, especially species of the genera *Ixodes, Dermacentor, Rhipicephalus* and *Amblyomma* [178, 179]. The initial phase of the infection during colonization of the host is the recognition of a suitable cell, attachment onto this cell, and entry into it. This process is facilitated by several specialized bacterial proteins (adhesins/invasins) that can recognize host surface molecules including glycans and glycoproteins and initiate signalling cascades to promote pathogen internalization. *Anaplasma* spp. express several surface proteins which are involved in binding to glycosylated host cells receptors and thus in the infection of the host and tick cells. These differ in glycan specificity and importance for the infection of various hosts and host cell types.

Anaplasma glycoprotein-binding surface proteins

As an intracellular pathogen, *Anaplasma* depends on a host cell to survive. *Anaplasma* infects two different types (groups) of organisms: the tick vector and the mammalian hosts, with various cell types being infected by the pathogen. Recognition of the cell type and of the infected organism is provided through binding of surface glycan epitopes or even several epitopes on a glycoprotein molecules.

Two groups of *Anaplasma* surface proteins were shown to recognize tick or host glycoproteins: outer membrane proteins (Omps) and major surface proteins (MSPs).

OmpA belongs to highly conserved genes among *A. phagocytophilum* isolates and is transcriptionally induced during feeding of *A. phagocytophilum*-infected ticks on mice and also during the invasion of mammalian but not tick cells [180, 181]. Pre-treatment of *A. phagocytophilum* or *A. marginale* bacteria with the respective OmpA antiserum reduces their ability to infect mammalian cells [181, 182]. Also, preincubation of mammalian cells with a recombinant ApOmpA effectively inhibits *A. phagocytophilum* infection of host cells.

Glycoproteins containing α1,3-fucose and either sLex or 6-sulfo sLex on host cells are recognized by the outer membrane protein A (ApOmpA) of *A. phagocytophilum* [180, 181]. On the other hand, OmpA of *A. marginale* (AmOmpA), a species non-pathogenic for humans, binds only α1,3-fucose and sLex but not 6-sulfo-sLex glycans. *Anaplasma marginale* also produces AmOmpA in both the infected mammalian and tick cells. Pre-treatment of host cells with sialidase or trypsin reduces or nearly eliminates OmpA adhesion. Therefore, AmOmpA interacts with sialylated glycoproteins *via* an adhesin-receptor pair. Thus, both AmOmpA and ApOmpA recognize different receptor molecules even though these receptors share some structural similarity and thus provide a similar function to these two bacterial species [182].

Structures of *A. marginale* and *A. phagocytophilum* OmpA proteins are very similar and their binding domains are structurally conserved. The OmpA binding domain was identified within amino acids 59 to 74 and it is responsible for the recognition of α2,3-bound sialic acid and α1,3-fucose [180]. A recent study by Hebert et al. [182] describes the OmpA receptor-binding domain between the amino acids 19 to 74.

Another group of surface proteins interacting with host (glycosylated) molecules are the major surface proteins (MSPs) that are involved in the adhesion of host cells and the immunological reaction of the host [183–187]. MSP1 protein with its variants α, β1, and β2 and the MSP3 protein are present in *A. marginale*, while MSP2 and MSP4 in both *A. marginale* and *A. phagocytophilum* [188]. The MSP1 complex consists of two polypeptides MSP1a and MSP1b and both polypeptides participate in adhesion processes to both tick cells and bovine erythrocytes [183–186].

Similarly to OmpA, these proteins show glycan-binding activity. *Anaplasma marginale* MSP1 and MSP2 can hemagglutinate bovine erythrocytes [184] suggesting recognition of some erythrocyte surface saccharide molecules. Recombinant forms of the MSP1 isoforms are glycosylated; MSP1a recombinant glycoprotein contains glucose, galactose, mannose and xylose, while MSP1b contains glucose, galactose and mannose. The functional domain of MSP1a contains tandemly repeated peptides that are important for adhesion to tick cells and bovine erythrocytes. The MSP1a polypeptide backbone alone shows binding to tick cell extract proteins and the glycan in its N-terminus enhances this binding [189, 190]. The MSP2 protein binds to the mammalian PSGL-1 [191] and thus can be responsible for the above mentioned *Anaplasma* recognition of sialic acid on this protein. A hypervariable region is present in the middle of the MSP2 gene which allows the bacterium to express various paralogs of the protein on its surface, possibly enhancing immune system evasion [192, 193]. However, the glycan binding abilities of the various MSP2 paralogs were not studied.

In addition to the above-described receptor molecules, two other proteins, Asp14 and AipA, were found to be acting together with OmpA during the infection of host cells. However, neither of these two proteins were shown to bind glycans nor to be glycosylated [180]. Finally, during the past ten years, other novel *A. phagocytophilum* surface proteins Asp55, Asp62 and APH_1235, with possible function as adhesins and invasins have been identified [194–196]; however, their receptor molecules remain unknown.

Anaplasma-host interactions

A confirmation of *Anaplasma* recognition of host-surface glycans came by Goodman et al. [197] showing binding of *A. phagocytophilum* to the cell surface of the promyelocytic leukaemia cell line HL-60. Bacterial binding to the cell surface correlates with the expression of the sialyl Lewis x (sLex) or a closely related 6-sulpho sLex glycan-containing molecules glycan and α1,3-fucosylated molecules. On the other hand, α1,3-fucosylated glycans but not sialylated glycans, are essential for the infection of murine and human mast cells by *A. phagocytophilum* [180, 198]. These glycan epitopes are important for *Anaplasma in vivo* as has been shown by Carlyon et al. [199].

The protein part bearing the recognized glycans can be also important; thus, not any glycan molecule is recognized, only the one found on a specific protein. In humans and animal hosts, *A. phagocytophilum* exhibits, amongst others, a tropism for myeloid cells. As an adhesion molecule involved in the binding to the surface of human neutrophils, the P-selectin glycoprotein ligand-1, PSGL-1, has been identified [197, 199–202]. In the case of human PSGL-1, *A. phagocytophilum* cooperatively binds to a short amino acid sequence in its *N*-terminal region and an *O*-glycan containing a sialyl Lewis x (sLex) on PSGL-1 (NeuAcα2,3Galβ1,4[Fucα1,3]GlcNac) [202] or on another molecule. On the other hand, PSGL-1 is not the major ligand in mice [199, 200]. Thus, the terminal or core α1,3-fucosylated glycans seem to be a generally recognized receptor, while sialylated glycans and PSGL-1 enhance the infection of diverse types of mammalian host cells.

Anaplasma-vector interactions

In the pathogen-tick relationship, several tick glycosylated molecules can be induced in the presence of a pathogen in the tick tissues and help the pathogen to colonize the tick or enhance its infection. For example, α1,3-core-fucosylated glycans are required for tick colonization by *A. phagocytophilum* and silencing of the responsible fucosyltransferases results in the absence of *Anaplasma* in the infected ticks. To increase the number of its receptors in the tick, *A. phagocytophilum* induces the expression of α1,3-fucosyltransferases to enhance the colonization of *I. scapularis* ticks. Therefore, α 1,3-fucose is a unifying determinant that *A. phagocytophilum* targets to infect its natural murine and arthropod reservoirs and accidental human hosts as well. In addition, the presence or absence of these glycans does not affect the transmission of the pathogen from the tick vector to the vertebrate host. While the infection of the tick by *Anaplasma* depends on the presence of α1,3-core-fucosylated glycans, these epitopes do not seem to be important for the infection by another tick-borne pathogen, *B. burgdorferi* [203].

Furthermore, tandem repeat peptides of the MSP1a functional domain are important for the adhesion of bacteria to tick cells and the glycosylation of MSP1a probably plays a role during the adhesion of *A. marginale* to tick cells [189, 190].

Colonization of the tick by pathogens depends on the tick life-cycle; one of the crucial steps is the colonization of the midgut or survival in the midgut in the process of the blood meal digestion. For successful colonization, the tick midgut peritrophic matrix (PM) and bacterial biofilms formed in the midgut are critical. The PM forms a barrier between the midgut lumen and the epithelial cells lining the luminal side of the midgut and is formed by a thick matrix of mostly chitin with various proteins, such as chitin deacetylase, and glycoproteins [204]. One of the bacteria depending on the biofilm formation in the *I. scapularis* tick midgut is *A. phagocytophilum*. The presence of this bacterium affects the midgut microbial community and biofilm composition and it also decreases the expression of several genes for the glycoprotein peritrophin, one of the major PM components. This results also in decreased PM thickness. Furthermore, RNAi silencing of these genes significantly enhanced *Anaplasma* colonization of the tick [205]. *Anaplasma* further enhances its chances for a successful colonization of *I. scapularis* ticks by induction of an antifreeze protein (IAFGP) during the infection of ticks [205]. This secreted antifreeze glycoprotein inhibits bacterial biofilm formation through binding to the D-alanine residue of some bacteria peptidoglycan and was induced in response to *Anaplasma* infection [206, 207]. IAFGP expression resulted in thinning of the tick midgut PM and RNAi silencing of *iafgp* gene resulted in the absence of *Anaplasma* in the tick midgut [205].

Tick lectins

Ticks, like other arthropods, lack specific adaptive immunity. To defend themselves against invading microorganisms, ticks use the evolutionarily older nonspecific innate immune system, including both cellular and humoral immune responses. Cellular immune reactions involve haemocytes capable of phagocytosis, encapsulation or nodulation of foreign microorganisms and particles. The humoral immune response involves a range of non-specific pathogen-recognizing defence systems: PRRs, lectins, complement-like molecules, pro-phenoloxidase activation, haemolymph coagulation factors, antimicrobial peptides, reactive oxygen species, etc. Some of these molecules which function as mediators in the innate immune response are glycosylated and/or may recognize glycan-containing epitopes, e.g. recognition receptors for pathogens, complement-related molecules, or lectins (Table 3). In mammals, lectins play an important role in the recognition of specific glycosylated surface molecules of a variety of pathogens (PAMPs) and subsequent activation of the lectin pathway [208, 209]. MBL or ficolins known to recognize *N*-acetyl groups [210] serve as the recognition molecules, which are further integrated with the MBL-associated serine proteases to trigger the complement activation.

Fibrinogen-related proteins

Invertebrates contain a variety of fibrinogen-related proteins (FRePs), all of them sharing structural similarity with fibrinogen. A common feature of FRePs is their glycan-binding activity as they recognize the invading pathogen through its specific glycan epitopes. Their expression increases upon infection of the invertebrate by parasites or by pathogens [211, 212] with possibly a specific role in complement activation [213]. However, some of the tick FRePs family proteins (such as ixoderins described below) may have various other functions (Table 3).

Dorin M from the soft tick *Ornithodoros moubata*, the first lectin purified and characterized from any tick species, shows a strong similarity to ficolins but lacks the N-terminal collagen domain [214, 215]. Dorin M and its closest homologue OMFREP, also from *O. moubata*, share sequence similarity with the innate immune FRePs Tachylectin 5A and B from the horseshoe crab, *Tachypleus tridentatus* [215, 216]. It has a binding activity for sialic acid [214], its conjugates and *N*-acetyl-hexosamines. The protein has three *N*-glycosylation sites modified by high-mannose type glycans and core-fucosylated paucimannose glycans [217]. Other FRePs were later identified in the haemolymph of *D. marginatus*, *R. appendiculatus*, *R. pulchellus* and *R. sanguineus* based on the cross-reactivity with sera directed against Dorin M [218].

The hard tick *I. ricinus* contains several FReP encoding sequences in its genome (ixoderins A, B and C) and their analogues are present in *I. scapularis* as well. While proteins similar to ixoderins A and C are present also in other tick species, ixoderin B-like proteins are found only in the genus *Ixodes*. All these proteins contain predicted glycosylation sites and they contain the fibrinogen-like domain with carbohydrate-binding properties [213, 215]. In *I. ricinus*, the expression of ixoderin A is restricted to haemocytes, salivary glands, and midgut while ixoderin B is only expressed in salivary glands [215]. As expected based on published information on other invertebrate

Table 3 Overview of identified tick lectins. Lectins identified in different tick species are listed including the tissue where the lectin was identified. Lectin binding specificity, its function and molecular weight are also listed if known

Lectin	Species	Tick tissue	Specificity	MW (kDa)	Function	Reference
Galectins (OmGalec)	*O. moubata*	Haemocytes, midgut, SG, ovaries	Lactosamine-like disaccharides	37.4	Putative functions in tick development, immunity, and vector-pathogen interaction	[221]
Dorin M	*O. moubata*	Haemocytes	*N*-acetyl-D-hexosamines and Sialic acid specific	na	Pattern recognition molecules	[214]
OMFREP	*O. moubata*	Hemolymph, salivary glands	Probably similar to Dorin M	na	Probably similar to Dorin M	[215]
Ixoderin A	*I. ricinus*	Hemolymph, salivary glands, midgut	Peptidoglycan recognition protein?	na	Putative defence protein, identification of self-/non-self tissues	[215, 219]
Ixoderin B	*I. ricinus*	Salivary glands	Unknown	na	Unknown putative immunomodulatory function	[215, 219]
Hemelipoglycoprotein	*D. marginatus*	Haemocytes, salivary glands, gut	Galactose- and mannose-binding specificity	290, 2 subunits	Putative innate immunity	[220]
Unknown lectin	*I. ricinus*	Gut, hemolymph	Sialic acid, *N*-acetyl-glucosamine	85	Putative recognition molecule	[233]
Unknown lectin	*I. ricinus*	SGs	Sialic acid	70	Unknown	[233]
TSLPI	*I. scapularis*	Unknown	Mannan	na	Unknown	[42]
HlCLec	*H. longicornis*	Midgut, ovary	Unknown	60.2	Unknown	[223]
Serpin 19	*A. americanum*	Saliva	GAGs	43.0	Serine protease inhibitor	[170]

Abbreviations: *MW* molecular weight, *na* not available

FRePs, ixoderins are also involved in defence against pathogens. Namely, ixoderins A and B are involved in phagocytosis of some pathogens as shown for *Candida albicans* [219]. On the other hand, knockdown of these two ixoderins did not affect the phagocytosis of the tick-transmitted *B. afzelii* and knockdown of all three ixoderins does not affect its transmission [219]. The reason can be the missing protein glycosylation and thus the binding site for these lectins on the *Borrelia* surface [37]. Ixoderins and FRePs can be involved in other processes as well; ixoderin B may be involved in the matrix attachment processes and angiogenesis inhibition. Alternatively, it may antagonize the effect of host ficolin [215].

Finally, one of the tick storage proteins, hemelipoglycoprotein, from several hard tick species seems to share a structural similarity to FRePs with its primary sequence showing a high similarity to the fibrinogen domain [218, 220].

Other tick lectins

OmGalec from the soft tick *O. moubata* is the first member of galectin family identified in ticks with the specificity towards β1-3 and β1-4 bound galactose to GlcNAc, and Glc and α1-3 bound galactose to GalNAc [221]. Similar proteins are also present in *R. appendiculatus* and *I. scapularis* [188]. OmGalec contains two carbohydrate-binding domains which share low sequence similarity and thus possibly possesses a different saccharide-specificity. The protein is expressed in various life-stages and tissues, with the highest expression in haemocytes, midguts and ovaries [221]. It has been shown that galectins play a vital role in immune homeostasis by being pathogen recognition receptors [222].

C-type lectins are also present in the available tick genomes and transcriptomes [223, 224]. The only characterized C-type lectin from *Haemaphysalis longicornis* (HlCLec) contains three various carbohydrate-binding domains. Each of them has been shown to recognize the bacteria *E. coli* and *S. aureus* and participate in the tick defence against gram-negative bacteria, but they do not have a direct effect on bacterial growth. HlCLec also affects the blood-feeding process and affects larvae hatching and mortality. Expression of this lectin is increased during blood-feeding and is the highest in the midgut and ovary [223]. In mosquitoes, C-type lectins influence the midgut colonization by bacteria midgut microbiome [225] and facilitate infection with West Nile and dengue viruses [226, 227].

Calreticulin (CRT), a lectin chaperone responsible mainly for the control and proper folding of glycoproteins, is conserved in all tick species and is even used as the biomarker for human tick bites in *I. scapularis* [228]. In blood-feeding parasites, CRTs participate in evasion of the host defence mechanisms, namely the complement by binding the initiator of this pathway, the C1q protein, or factor Xa participating in the blood coagulation [229]. In mammals, CRT on the surface of neutrophils also binds C1q as well as other immune-related lectins [230]. Similarly, the salivary secreted CRT from *A. americanum* binds host C1q. On the other hand, it does not bind the factor Xa and does not inhibit the activation of the classical complement cascade and host haemostasis. The *A. americanum* CRT shares a very high sequence similarity with other tick CRTs and thus similar functions of tick CRT can be expected [231].

Several other lectins are characterized in *I. ricinus*, but have not been identified to date: the 37, 60, 65, and 73 kDa lectins from midgut showing haemagglutination activity [163, 232]. The 37 kDa lectin has a binding specificity towards β1-3 glucan, while the 65 kDa protein binds bovine submaxillary mucin, containing a complicated mixture of various glycan structures and more specifically binds free sialic acid. Another lectin is present in haemolymph/haemocytes with a molecular weight of 85 kDa. It is a C-type lectin with specificity towards sialic acid and GlcNAc [233]. Several other lectins with haemagglutination activity have also been described in other ticks including *R. appendiculatus* [234, 235], *O. tartakovskyi, O. tholozani* and *A. polonicus* [233].

Tick glycans

Regarding the glycans and glycoproteins of blood-feeding arthropods, several studies describe these molecules using lectin staining and other indirect methods. Lectin studies show the presence of both *N*- and *O*-glycosylated proteins in tick tissues and some glycoproteins have been shown to be antigenic determinants for the immune response of the host [236–239]. In recent years, the direct determination of glycan structures and composition, mostly using mass spectrometry, has also been published, either from tick tissues and cells [203, 240] or purified proteins [220]. The three most interesting glycan structures related to host-parasite interaction and host immune system reaction are described below; representation of these structures in a glycan molecule is shown in Fig. 2. An overview of tick glycans with known structures is listed in Table 4.

Alpha-galactose epitope

Alpha-galactose epitopes (Galα1-3Gal; αGal) are abundant on glycolipids and glycoproteins of plants, arthropods and non-primate mammals [241]. αGal is a novel allergen identified first during clinical trials in 2004 in patients treated with cetuximab, a medical preparation for metastatic colorectal cancer treatment. Several cases of hypersensitivity reaction were registered soon after cetuximab administration into the blood due to the presence of αGal in its structure. The majority of sensitive individuals come from a population in south-eastern USA [242]. Furthermore, the geographical distribution of cases with cetuximab hypersensitivity corresponded to the distribution of red meat allergy cases and tick prevalence. Additionally, patients with red meat allergy experienced a tick bite in the months preceding the allergy symptoms. The causative agent of the αGal sensitization in the south-eastern region of the USA is the lone star tick *A. americanum* [243]. Red meat allergy is also linked with *I. holocyclus* tick bite in the Australian population [244] . Conversely, a bite by the *I. scapularis* tick from the same genus in the USA does not seem to result in red meat allergy [243]. Lastly, Chinuki et al. [245] described the allergy development upon *H. longicornis* bite in Japan. Direct evidence on αGal epitopes presence in *I. ricinus* is provided by Hamsten et al. [246], specifically in the tick midgut. However, the presence of αGal just in the tick saliva is what is important for patient sensitization. In this regard, the presence of undigested complete host proteins and glycoproteins was described in the tick body and, importantly, in the tick saliva [240, 246, 247] and thus the presence of αGal originating in the blood of non-mammalian hosts from the previous blood-feeding can be expected in the saliva. The αGal epitope is only known to be present in the saliva of *A. sculptum*, a tick that until now has not been connected with red meat allergy cases [248].

Core α1,3-fucosylation

The allergenic core α1,3-fucose (α1,3-Fuc) attached on the proximal GlcNAc residue is widely present in plants and arthropods and is one of the well-known possible human allergens as it is usually absent in mammals. It can induce production of specific IgE antibodies associated with IgE-mediated allergic immune responses, which is mostly described for schistosomes or venoms of some species of the order Hymenoptera. However, such a response is not described after a tick bite [249–251]. It is rather surprising, as α1,3-fucosylated structures are present in the tick salivary glands as well as in saliva of both *I. ricinus* and *I. scapularis* [203, 252]. This can be explained by the structural features of the allergenic epitopes; for example, in the case of core α1,3-Fuc, terminal GlcNAc weakens the immune response [253]. Additionally, more than one epitope has to be present to trigger the allergic reaction and the presence of blocking IgG4 antibodies against this epitope can lower the immune reaction [249].

The α1,3-Fuc modification of the *N*-linked glycan core mediates an entrance of one of the tick-transmitted pathogens, *A. phagocytophilum*, into *I. scapularis* midgut cells, but it is not required for the transmission of the pathogen to a vertebrate host. Furthermore, *Anaplasma* increases the expression of α1,3-fucosyltransferases in the tick, further increasing its ability to infect the tick. On the other hand, the infection of the tick by *B. burgdorferi* was not affected by the presence or absence of core α1,3-Fuc [203].

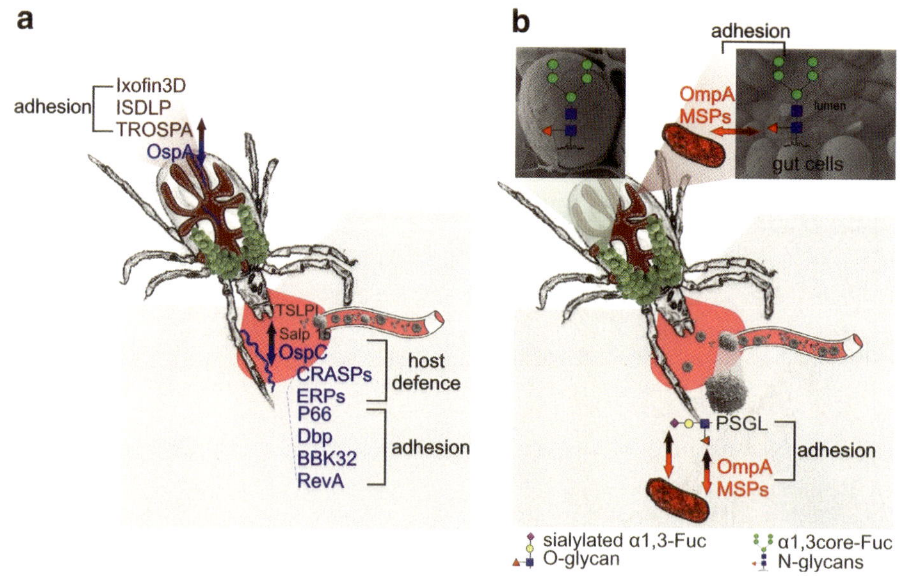

Fig. 2 Scheme of a model complex-type glycan showing presented oligosaccharide structures. An example of an *N*-glycan bearing the three glycoepitopes immunogenic in the mammalian hosts are shown. The αGal epitope is formed by a terminal galactose bound to another galactose *via* an α1-3 bond. In the case of the core α1,3-fucose, both the specific α1,3 bond and the core (not terminal localization of fucose are important for the immunogenicity in mammals. Two types of sialic acid are present in Eukaryotes: the *N*-acetylneuraminic acid (Neu5Ac) and the *N*-glycolylneuraminic acid (Neu5Gc). As humans do not possess the enzymatic apparatus for the production of Neu5Gc into glycans, glycans terminated with this type of sialic acid are immunogenic in humans. The used symbol nomenclature is based on the Consortium for Functional Glycomics (http://www.functionalglycomics.org/)

Sialic acids

Sialic acids (Sia) are found typically in the terminal position of vertebrate complex *N*- or *O*-linked glycans. In insects, some studies have shown the ability of sialylation [254, 255] and the importance of sialylation for insect-development, even though the abundance of sialylated glycans is very low [256].

N-glycans terminated with Sia are present also in the organs of the tick *I. ricinus*, namely in the gut, salivary glands, ovary and Malpighian tubules [240, 257]. However, the sialylated proteins in the adult ticks originate most probably from the host blood [258]. Hypothetically, sialoglycans present in the tick organs and in the secreted tick saliva can be engaged in molecular mimicry. We suppose that sialic acid is produced also by the tick itself in the ovary and eggs and later in larvae; the exact role of the tick sialylated proteins for the physiology and development of ticks is not yet known (unpublished results). Both eukaryotic types of sialic acids, *N*-acetyl-neuraminic acid and *N*-glycolyl-neuraminic acid (Fig. 2), were detected in the ticks [240].

N-linked glycans of flaviviruses

Tick-borne encephalitis virus (TBEV), a member of the genus *Flavivirus*, can cause serious infections in humans, which may result in encephalitis/meningoencephalitis. The viral single-stranded genomic RNA of positive polarity contains one open reading frame, which encodes a single polyprotein that is co-translationally and post-translationally cleaved by viral and cellular proteases into three structural and seven non-structural proteins (Table 4) [259].

Flaviviral non-structural proteins

Non-structural proteins of the flavivirus family (NS1, NS2A, NS2B, NS3, NS4A, NS4B and NS5) do not have their precise role elucidated, but they are generally considered as the effectors of viral replication, which occurs in close association with cellular membranes. Dramatic changes in the intracellular membrane structures including convoluted membranes, vesicle packets or paracrystalline arrays were observed as a result of dengue virus (DENV), TBEV or West Nile virus (WNV) replication [260–262]. Recently, NS1, NS4A and possibly also NS2A, were described to be involved in the formation of vesicle packets [263, 264]. Moreover, novel functions in terms of virus-host interactions were recently described for particular NS proteins; for example, TBEV NS5 protein acts as an inhibitor of interferon-activated Jak-STAT signalling [265].

Flaviviral structural proteins

Apart from seven non-structural proteins, the flaviviral genome encodes three structural proteins (C, M, E). The flaviviral nucleocapsid is composed of (+) ssRNA genome and the capsid protein (C), whereas the host-derived

Table 4 Overview of identified tick glycan structures composition. Monosaccharide compositions of the identified N-glycans are shown. Note that in some cases, the same composition can define various structures. For each glycan, the protein or the tick samples is listed, in which it was identified by mass spectrometry

Glycan composition				Protein/sample	Reference
Paucimannose glycans					
HexNAc	Hex	dHex	Sia		
2	3	0	0	Dorin M (position ^{41}NHS, ^{171}NGS, ^{129}NHS) from *O. moubata*	[217]
				I. ricinus fed female salivary glands	[240]
				I. ricinus fed female midgut	[240]
				I. scapularis salivary gland	[203]
2	4	0	0	Dorin M (position ^{41}NHS, ^{171}NGS, ^{129}NHS) from *O. moubata*	[217]
				I. ricinus fed female salivary glands	[240]
				I. ricinus fed female midgut	[240]
				I. scapularis salivary gland	[203]
High-mannose glycans					
HexNAc	Hex	dHex	Sia		
2	5	0	0	Dorin M (position ^{41}NHS, ^{129}NHS) from *O. moubata*	[217]
				I. ricinus fed female salivary glands	[240]
				I. ricinus fed female midgut	[240]
				I. scapularis salivary gland	[203]
2	6	0	0	Dorin M (position ^{41}NHS, ^{129}NHS) from *O. moubata*	[217]
				I. ricinus fed female salivary glands	[240]
				I. ricinus fed female midgut	[240]
				I. scapularis salivary gland	[203]
2	7	0	0	Dorin M (position ^{41}NHS, ^{129}NHS) from *O. moubata*	[217]
				I. ricinus fed female midgut	[240]
				I. scapularis salivary gland	[203]
2	8	0	0	Dorin M (position ^{41}NHS, ^{129}NHS) from *O. moubata*	[217]
				I. ricinus fed female midgut	[240]
				I. scapularis salivary gland	[203]
2	9	0	0	Dorin M (position ^{41}NHS, ^{129}NHS) from *O. moubata*	[217]
				I. ricinus fed female salivary glands	[240]
				I. ricinus fed female midgut	[240]
				D. marginatus Hemelipoglycoprotein	[220]
				I. scapularis salivary gland	[203]
2	10	0	0	*D. marginatus* Hemelipoglycoprotein	[220]
				I. scapularis salivary gland	[203]
Core-fucosylated glycans					
HexNAc	Hex	dHex	Sia		
2	3	1	0	Dorin M (position ^{171}NGS) from *O. moubata*	[217]
				I. ricinus fed female salivary glands	[240]
				I. ricinus fed female midgut	[240]
				I. scapularis salivary gland	[203]
2	4	1	0	Dorin M (position ^{171}NGS) from *O. moubata*	[217]
				I. ricinus fed female salivary glands	[240]
				I. ricinus fed female midgut	[240]

Table 4 Overview of identified tick glycan structures composition. Monosaccharide compositions of the identified N-glycans are shown. Note that in some cases, the same composition can define various structures. For each glycan, the protein or the tick samples is listed, in which it was identified by mass spectrometry *(Continued)*

Glycan composition				Protein/sample	Reference
				I. scapularis salivary gland	[203]
2	5	1	0	Dorin M (position [171]NGS) from *O. moubata*	[217]
				I. ricinus fed female salivary glands	[240]
				I. ricinus fed female midgut	[240]
				I. scapularis salivary gland	[203]
3	2	1	0	*I. ricinus* fed female salivary glands	[240]
3	3	1	0	*I. ricinus* fed female salivary glands	[240]
				I. ricinus fed female midgut	[240]
				I. scapularis salivary gland	[203]
4	3	1	0	*I. ricinus* fed female midgut	[240]
				I. scapularis salivary gland	[203]
4	4	1	0	*I. scapularis* salivary gland	[203]
4	5	1	0	*I. ricinus* fed female midgut	[240]
				I. scapularis salivary gland	[203]
4	6	1	0	*I. ricinus* fed female midgut	[240]
5	3	1	0	*I. ricinus* fed female salivary glands	[240]
				I. scapularis salivary gland	[203]
5	5	1	0	*I. ricinus* fed female midgut	[240]
6	6	1	0	*I. ricinus* fed female midgut	[240]
Complex glycans					
HexNAc	Hex	dHex	Sia		
3	4	0	0	*I. ricinus* fed female salivary glands	[240]
4	5	0	0	*I. ricinus* fed female salivary glands	[240]
				I. ricinus fed female midgut	[240]
4	6	0	0	*I. ricinus* fed female midgut	[240]
4	7	0	0	*D. marginatus* Hemelipoglycoprotein	[220]
4	8	0	0	*D. marginatus* Hemelipoglycoprotein	[220]
5	6	0	0	*I. ricinus* fed female midgut	[240]
6	2	0	0	*I. ricinus* fed female midgut	[240]
Sialylated glycans (containing either Neu5Ac or Neu5Gc)					
HexNAc	Hex	dHex	Sia		
4	5	0	1	*I. ricinus* fed female salivary glands	[240]
				I. ricinus fed female midgut	[240]
4	5	0	2	*I. ricinus* fed female midgut	[240]
5	6	0	1	*I. ricinus* fed female midgut	[240]
5	6	0	2	*I. ricinus* fed female midgut	[240]

Abbreviations: *HexNAc* N-acetyl-hexosamine (*N*-acetyl-glucosamine or *N*-acetyl-galactosamine), *Hex* hexose (mannose, glucose, galactose), *dHex* deoxyhexose (fucose), *Sia* sialic acid (*N*-acetyl-neuraminic acid, *N*-glycolyl-neuraminic acid)

envelope contains two glycoproteins, the membrane (prM/M) protein and the envelope (E) protein [266].

The E glycoprotein is localized in the viral envelope and is the main antigenic determinant of TBEV inducing a humoral immune response. It mediates fusion of TBEV with host cell membrane and thus facilitates the virus entry to the host cell. It forms heterodimers with the prM protein; the prM-E protein interaction is essential for proper folding of E protein [267]. The heterodimers then migrate to the ER membrane and eventually bud off as nucleocapsid-containing immature virions [260, 268].

The M glycoprotein is an integral part of the viral envelope together with E protein. It forms heterodimers with the E protein and functions as a chaperon ensuring proper folding of E protein [267]. Non-infectious immature virions containing prM/E homodimers undergo maturation process in late trans-Golgi network by cleavage of pr part from the prM protein by host protease furin. The cleavage produces protein M and triggers re-organization of protein E to form homodimers [268, 269].

TBEV proteins glycosylation

The glycosylation of viral proteins increases their folding efficiency and promotes their intracellular transport by the interaction with host lectins [270]. In several viruses that cross the endoplasmic reticulum during their life-cycle, the protein glycosylation was proven important for virus growth, budding, secretion, and pathogenicity (reviewed in [271–273]). So far, only membrane glycoproteins prM/M and E are known to be *N*-glycosylated in TBEV (Table 5) [274–276]. α1,3-core fucosylated, high-mannose and hybrid N-glycans were shown to be present in the E protein of TBEV produced in chicken embryos by affinoblots [277]. E protein glycosylation was also confirmed recently also using cryo-electron microscopy, even though the exact glycan structure was not defined [278]. Another two sites (N130 and N207) in the NS1 protein are *N*-glycosylated in the case of dengue virus [274, 279]. One of these two *N*-glycosylation sites (N207) is present also in the TBEV NS1 protein; however, its glycosylation has not yet been shown (Table 5).

The E glycoprotein is a viral surface protein and thus contains major antigenic epitopes responsible for triggering the host immune system [280]. The *N*-glycosylation site at position N154 is present in the majority of TBEV strains and other flaviviruses. Moreover, a potential N361 glycosylation site is present in TBEV E protein as well. Depending on the strain, zero to two glycans are attached [280, 281]. The investigation of the presence and position of E protein glycans showed that an increased number of E protein glycans elevate its expression. Conversely, the E protein glycosylation deletion mutants showed reduced E protein production, suggesting the importance of glycosylation for the viral life-cycle [276].

Importantly, the absence of E-protein glycosylation affects the E protein conformation and further the TBEV infectivity only in the mammalian host, but not in the tick vector. Different temperatures in the host (37 °C) and the vector (23 °C) do not affect the stability of the deglycosylated E protein [282]. In light of this evidence, the E protein glycosylation seems to represent one of the factors conferring different vector and host competence. Interestingly, the investigation of mosquito-borne flaviviruses, DENV and WNV, shows that glycans modifying E protein are important for virus propagation in both vector and host cells. However, the role of the particular *N*-linked glycosylation site varies depending on the invertebrate/vertebrate host [283–285]. For example, the importance of *N*-linked glycan at 154 aa of WNV E protein was proved in case of the vector (*Culex pipiens* and *Cx. tarsalis* mosquitoes) as well as the bird host (*Gallus gallus*) [286, 287].

The prM protein encodes for the precursor of membrane protein M and also contains one *N*-linked glycosylation consensus sequence in N32 position (Table 5) [267, 276]. During TBEV maturation, the structural proteins prM and E form heterodimer, where prM has a chaperone-like role in the folding and maturation of E protein [267], although the biological role of TBEV prM glycosylation, has not yet been elucidated. However, Goto et al. [279] suggest the participation of carbohydrate-mediated interaction for prM-E heterodimer formation; glycosylation-deficient mutant of prM reduces the secretion of E protein to 60% in comparison to the wild-type prM. Further evidence for the crucial role of prM glycan was described in the case of WNV.

Table 5 TBEV protein glycosylation overview. List of TBEV proteins and their functions. Identified or predicted N-linked glycosylation sites are listed as well. NetNGlyc 1.0 Server was used for N-linked glycosylation site prediction

	Protein	Function	*N*-linked glycosylation	Reference
Structural	C	Capsid protein; forming of nucleocapsid	None	
	prM/M	Envelope protein; E protein chaperone	N32	[265, 302]
	E	Envelope protein; binding and fusion	N154, N361	[263–265]
Non-structural	NS1	Replication	Predicted: N85, N207	
	NS2A	Assembly, replication	None	
	NS2B	NS3 serine-protease cofactor	None	
	NS3	Serine-protease, helicase, replication RNA triphosphatase	Predicted: N160, N499, N555	
	NS4A	Assembly, replication	None	
	NS4B	Assembly, induction of membrane rearrangements	Predicted: N188	
	NS5	Methyltransferase, RNA-dependent RNA polymerase	Predicted: N18, N175, N215	

The prM glycosylation-deficient mutants decreased the formation and release of virus-like particles as well as genome copies. However, the infectivity of prM glycosylation-deficient mutants was not affected in mosquito, avian or mammalian cell lines [284].

In summary, *N*-linked glycosylation of TBEV prM and E proteins represents a multifaceted factor which is involved in many steps of the viral life-cycle, especially in virion assembly/secretion, and host/vector competence. Despite various studies, there are many aspects which need to be elucidated, especially the role of viral protein *N*-linked glycans within tick vectors. Moreover, the presence of other *N*-linked glycans in predicted sites of NS1, NS3, NS4B, and NS5 remains to be determined as well as their potential function.

Conclusions

The recent decades have provided an outstanding amount of new data about glycoconjugates and a growing line of evidence highlights the importance of carbohydrate-based interactions in the complex pathogen-host environment [288]. Glycoconjugates have an enormous structural diversity in the glycan moieties and therefore fulfil a variety of biological roles [289]. Given the fact that glycoconjugates are the major components of the outer surface of animal cells [290], it is likely that all interactions of microbial pathogens with their hosts/vectors are affected to a certain degree by the pattern of glycans and glycan-binding molecules that each produces. Despite the fact that protein glycosylation in the field of tick-borne pathogens has become a subject of increased attention in the last decade [37, 218, 291], there is still a deep knowledge gap regarding the nature and the specific roles of the glycoconjugates in the infectious cycle of these pathogens. All the findings mentioned in this review have tackled the important, yet still inadequately explored, the field of the carbohydrate-based interactions at the pathogen-tick-host interface. The basis of these interactions needs to be further addressed to gain clearer insights into the intricate strategies that the parasites employ to successfully finish their life-cycles. Ultimately, the common goal of scientists working in any field dealing with infectious diseases is to find an effective countermeasure against the particular threat. Ticks transmit a great variety of bacterial, viral and protozoan pathogens and therefore the search for a potent vaccine against each of these parasites costs an enormous amount of effort and money. One of the most promising strategies to cope with all pathogens transmitted by ticks is the development of a general anti-tick vaccine [292]. The potentially important role of sugar moieties in such a tick vaccine has already been suggested, showing, for instance, the tick midgut protein Bm86 to be more immunogenic in glycosylated form than non-glycosylated [291]. However, the progress in this matter is still insufficient and intense analysis of glycosylation needs to be addressed in future studies in order to be applied to the development of new therapeutics. Modern glycan sequencing technologies and strategies that allow site-specific mass-spectrometric identification of proteins with glycan modifications in a complex biological sample have shown that glycosylation could be much more extensive than previously thought [293].

Abbreviations

ACG: Cholesteryl 6-O-acyl-β-D-galactopyranoside; ACGal/Bb-GL-1: Cholesteryl 6-O-palmitoyl-β-D-galactopyranoside; AmOmp: *Anaplasma marginale* outer membrane protein; AP: Alternative complement pathway; ApOmp: *Anaplasma phagocytophilum* outer membrane protein; Bgp: *Borrelia* GAG-binding protein; CLR: C-type lectin receptor; CP: Classical complement pathway; CRASP: Complement regulator-acquiring surface protein; CRT: Calreticulin; DAF: Decay accelerating factor; DbpA: Decorin-binding protein; DENV: Dengue virus; ECM: Extracellular matrix; Erp: OspE/F-related proteins; FH: Complement factor H; FHL: Factor H-like; Fn: Fibrinogen; FREP: Fibrinogen-related protein; Fuc: Fucose; GAG: Glycosaminoglycan; GalCer: Galactosylceramide; IAFGP: *Ixodes scapularis* antifreeze glycoprotein; ISDLP: *Ixodes scapularis* dystroglycan-like protein; LacCer: Lactosylceramide; LP: Lectin complement pathway; LPS: Lipopolisaccharides; MAC: Membrane attack complex; MBL: Mannose-binding lectin; MGalD: Mono-α-galactosyl-diacylglycerol; MSP: Major surface proteins; MW: Molecular weight; na: Not available; NKT: Natural killer T cells; NLR/NOD-like receptors: Nucleotide-oligomerization domain-like receptors; Omp: Outer membrane protein; Osp: Outer surface protein; PAMP: Pathogen-associated molecular pattern; PM: Peritrophic matrix; PRR: Pattern recognition receptor; PSGL–1: P-selectin glycoprotein ligand-1; RGD: Arg-Gly-Asp tripeptide, a binding motif of fibronectin; Salp: Salivary protein; SG: Salivary glands; Sia: Sialic acid; TBEV: Tick-borne encephalitis virus; TLR: Toll-like receptors; TROSPA: Tick receptor for OspA; TSLPI: Tick salivary lectin pathway inhibitors; Vmp: Variable major protein; Vsp: Variable small protein; Vtp: Variable tick protein; WNV: West Nile virus

Funding

This work was supported by the Ministry of Education, Youth and Sports of the Czech Republic projects Postdok_BIOGLOBE (CZ.1.07/2.3.00/30.0032), C4SYS (LM2015055), and Czech-BioImaging (LM2015062), by the Czech Science Foundation (15-03044S), INTER-ACTION project No. LTARF18021, and by the European Union FP7 projects ANTIDotE (602272-2) and ANTIGONE (278976).

Authors' contributions

All authors contributed to the manuscript preparation. PV and JS contributed to this work equally. All authors read and approved the final manuscript.

Competing interests

The authors declare that they have no competing interests.

References

1. WHO. http://www.who.int/en/. 1948. Accessed 28 Mar 2018.
2. de la Fuente J, Antunes S, Bonnet S, Cabezas-Cruz A, Domingos AG, Estrada-Pena A, et al. Tick-pathogen interactions and vector competence:

identification of molecular drivers for tick-borne diseases. Front Cell Infect Microbiol. 2017;7:114.
3. Coumou J, Wagemakers A, Trentelman JJ, Nijhof AM, Hovius JW. Vaccination against Bm86 homologues in rabbits does not impair *Ixodes ricinus* feeding or oviposition. PLoS One. 2014;10:e0123495.
4. Semenza JC, Suk JE. Vector-borne diseases and climate change: a European perspective. FEMS Microbiol Lett. 2018;365:2.
5. Dinglasan RR, Jacobs-Lorena M. Insight into a conserved lifestyle: protein-carbohydrate adhesion strategies of vector-borne pathogens. Infect Immun. 2005;73:7797–807.
6. Severo MS, Choy A, Stephens KD, Sakhon OS, Chen G, Chung DW, et al. The E3 ubiquitin ligase XIAP restricts *Anaplasma phagocytophilum* colonization of *Ixodes scapularis* ticks. J Infect Dis. 2013;208:1830–40.
7. Varki ACR, Esko JD, et al. Essentials of Glycobiology. 3rd ed. Cold Spring Harbor: Cold Spring Harbor Laboratory Press; 2017.
8. Ritchie GE, Moffatt BE, Sim RB, Morgan BP, Dwek RA, Rudd PM. Glycosylation and the complement system. Chem Rev. 2002;102:305-20-19.
9. Bann JG, Bachinger HP. Glycosylation/hydroxylation-induced stabilization of the collagen triple helix. 4-trans-hydroxyproline in the Xaa position can stabilize the triple helix. J Biol Chem. 2000;275:24466–9.
10. Ault BH, Schmidt BZ, Fowler NL, Kashtan CE, Ahmed AE, Vogt BA, et al. Human factor H deficiency. Mutations in framework cysteine residues and block in H protein secretion and intracellular catabolism. J Biol Chem. 1997;272:25168–75.
11. Dijk M, Holkers J, Voskamp P, Giannetti BM, Waterreus WJ, van Veen HA, et al. How dextran sulfate affects C1-inhibitor activity: a model for polysaccharide potentiation. Structure. 2016;24:2182–9.
12. Stavenhagen K, Kayili HM, Holst S, Koeleman C, Engel R, Wouters D, et al. *N*- and *O*-glycosylation analysis of human C1-inhibitor reveals extensive mucin-type *O*-glycosylation. Mol Cell Proteomics. 2017;17:1225–38.
13. Minta JO. The role of sialic acid in the functional activity and the hepatic clearance of C1-INH. J Immunol. 1981;126:245–9.
14. Novotny MV, Alley WR. Recent trends in analytical and structural glycobiology. Curr Opin Chem Biol. 2013;17:832–40.
15. Oswald DM, Cobb BA. Emerging glycobiology tools: a Renaissance in accessibility. Cell Immunol. 2018; https://doi.org/10.1016/j.cellimm.2018.04.010.
16. Tytgat HL, van Teijlingen NH, Sullan RM, Douillard FP, Rasinkangas P, Messing M, et al. Probiotic gut microbiota isolate interacts with dendritic cells *via* glycosylated heterotrimeric pili. PLoS One. 2016;11:e0151824.
17. Barbour AG, Hayes SF. Biology of *Borrelia* species. Microbiol Rev. 1986; 50:381–400.
18. Coburn J, Fischer JR, Leong JM. Solving a sticky problem: new genetic approaches to host cell adhesion by the Lyme disease spirochete. Mol Microbiol. 2005;57:1182–95.
19. Berndtson K. Review of evidence for immune evasion and persistent infection in Lyme disease. Int J Gen Med. 2013;6:291–306.
20. Cohen M. Notable aspects of glycan-protein interactions. Biomolecules. 2015;5:2056–72.
21. Vancova M, Nebesarova J, Grubhoffer L. Lectin-binding characteristics of a Lyme borreliosis spirochete *Borrelia burgdorferi sensu stricto*. Folia Microbiol. 2005;50:229–38.
22. Stevenson B, Schwan TG, Rosa PA. Temperature-related differential expression of antigens in the Lyme disease spirochete, *Borrelia burgdorferi*. Infect Immun. 1995;63:4535–9.
23. Pal U, de Silva AM, Montgomery RR, Fish D, Anguita J, Anderson JF, et al. Attachment of *Borrelia burgdorferi* within *Ixodes scapularis* mediated by outer surface protein A. J Clin Invest. 2000;106:561–9.
24. Schwan TG, Piesman J. Vector interactions and molecular adaptations of Lyme disease and relapsing fever spirochetes associated with transmission by ticks. Emerg Infect Dis. 2002;8:115–21.
25. Fikrig E, Pal U, Chen M, Anderson JF, Flavell RA. OspB antibody prevents *Borrelia burgdorferi* colonization of *Ixodes scapularis*. Infect Immun. 2004;72:1755–9.
26. Schwan TG, Piesman J, Golde WT, Dolan MC, Rosa PA. Induction of an outer surface protein on *Borrelia burgdorferi* during tick feeding. Proc Natl Acad Sci USA. 1995;92:2909–13.
27. Ramamoorthi N, Narasimhan S, Pal U, Bao F, Yang XF, Fish D, et al. The Lyme disease agent exploits a tick protein to infect the mammalian host. Nature. 2005;436:573–7.
28. Simo L, Kazimirova M, Richardson J, Bonnet SI. The essential role of tick salivary glands and saliva in tick feeding and pathogen transmission. Front Cell Infect Microbiol. 2017;7:281.
29. Anguita J, Ramamoorthi N, Hovius JWR, Das S, Thomas V, Persinski R, et al. Salp15, an *Ixodes scapularis* salivary protein, inhibits CD4(+) T cell activation. Immunity. 2002;16:849–59.
30. Kolb P, Vorreiter J, Habicht J, Bentrop D, Wallich R, Nassal M. Soluble cysteine-rich tick saliva proteins Salp15 and Iric-1 from *E. coli*. FEBS Open Bio. 2015;5:42–55.
31. Hovius JW, Schuijt TJ, de Groot KA, Roelofs JJ, Oei GA, Marquart JA, et al. Preferential protection of *Borrelia burgdorferi sensu stricto* by a Salp15 homologue in *Ixodes ricinus* saliva. J Infect Dis. 2008;198:1189–97.
32. Hovius JW, de Jong MA, den Dunnen J, Litjens M, Fikrig E, van der Poll T, et al. Salp15 binding to DC-SIGN inhibits cytokine expression by impairing both nucleosome remodeling and mRNA stabilization. PLoS Pathog. 2008;4:e31.
33. Lam TT, Nguyen TP, Montgomery RR, Kantor FS, Fikrig E, Flavell RA. Outer surface proteins E and F of *Borrelia burgdorferi*, the agent of Lyme disease. Infect Immun. 1994;62:290–8.
34. Casjens S, van Vugt R, Tilly K, Rosa PA, Stevenson B. Homology throughout the multiple 32-kilobase circular plasmids present in Lyme disease spirochetes. J Bacteriol. 1997;179:217–27.
35. Akins DR, Caimano MJ, Yang X, Cerna F, Norgard MV, Radolf JD. Molecular and evolutionary analysis of *Borrelia burgdorferi* 297 circular plasmid-encoded lipoproteins with OspE- and OspF-like leader peptides. Infect Immun. 1999;67:1526–32.
36. Sambri V, Stefanelli C, Cevenini R. Detection of glycoproteins in *Borrelia burgdorferi*. Arch Microbiol. 1992;157:205–8.
37. Sterba J, Vancova M, Rudenko N, Golovchenko M, Tremblay TL, Kelly JF, et al. Flagellin and outer surface proteins from *Borrelia burgdorferi* are not glycosylated. J Bacteriol. 2008;190:2619–23.
38. Eicken C, Sharma V, Klabunde T, Lawrenz MB, Hardham JM, Norris SJ, et al. Crystal structure of Lyme disease variable surface antigen VlsE of *Borrelia burgdorferi*. J Biol Chem. 2002;277:21691–6.
39. Narasimhan S, Coumou J, Schuijt TJ, Boder E, Hovius JW, Fikrig E. A tick gut protein with fibronectin III domains aids *Borrelia burgdorferi* congregation to the gut during transmission. PLoS Pathog. 2014;10:e1004278.
40. Coumou J, Narasimhan S, Trentelman JJ, Wagemakers A, Koetsveld J, Ersoz JI, et al. *Ixodes scapularis* dystroglycan-like protein promotes *Borrelia burgdorferi* migration from the gut. J Mol Med (Berl). 2016;94:361–70.
41. Narasimhan S, Santiago F, Koski RA, Brei B, Anderson JF, Fish D, et al. Examination of the *Borrelia burgdorferi* transcriptome in *Ixodes scapularis* during feeding. J Bacteriol. 2002;184:3122–5.
42. Schuijt TJ, Coumou J, Narasimhan S, Dai J, Deponte K, Wouters D, et al. A tick mannose-binding lectin inhibitor interferes with the vertebrate complement cascade to enhance transmission of the Lyme disease agent. Cell Host Microbe. 2011;10:136–46.
43. Schuijt TJ, Narasimhan S, Daffre S, DePonte K, Hovius JW, Van't Veer C, et al. Identification and characterization of *Ixodes scapularis* antigens that elicit tick immunity using yeast surface display. PLoS One. 2011;6:e15926.
44. Coburn J, Leong J, Chaconas G. Illuminating the roles of the *Borrelia burgdorferi* adhesins. Trends Microbiol. 2013;21:372–9.
45. Leong JM, Robbins D, Rosenfeld L, Lahiri B, Parveen N. Structural requirements for glycosaminoglycan recognition by the Lyme disease spirochete, *Borrelia burgdorferi*. Infect Immun. 1998;66:6045–8.
46. Brissette CA, Gaultney RA. That's my story, and I'm sticking to it - an update on *B. burgdorferi* adhesins. Front Cell Infect Microbiol. 2014;4:41.
47. Szczepanski A, Furie MB, Benach JL, Lane BP, Fleit HB. Interaction between *Borrelia burgdorferi* and endothelium *in vitro*. J Clin Invest. 1990;85:1637–47.
48. Guo BP, Norris SJ, Rosenberg LC, Hook M. Adherence of *Borrelia burgdorferi* to the proteoglycan decorin. Infect Immun. 1995;63:3467–72.
49. Choi HU, Johnson TL, Pal S, Tang LH, Rosenberg L, Neame PJ. Characterization of the dermatan sulfate proteoglycans, DS-PGI and DS-PGII, from bovine articular cartilage and skin isolated by octyl-sepharose chromatography. J Biol Chem. 1989;264:2876–84.
50. Rosenberg LC, Choi HU, Tang LH, Johnson TL, Pal S, Webber C, et al. Isolation of dermatan sulfate proteoglycans from mature bovine articular cartilages. J Biol Chem. 1985;260:6304–13.
51. Sasaki T, Fassler R, Hohenester E. Laminin: the crux of basement membrane assembly. J Cell Biol. 2004;164:959–63.
52. Kumar AP, Nandini CD, Salimath PV. Structural characterization of N-linked oligosaccharides of laminin from rat kidney: changes during diabetes and modulation by dietary fiber and butyric acid. FEBS J. 2011;278:143–55.
53. Singh B, Fleury C, Jalalvand F, Riesbeck K. Human pathogens utilize host extracellular matrix proteins laminin and collagen for adhesion and invasion of the host. FEMS Microbiol Rev. 2012;36:1122–80.

54. Cabello FC, Hulinska D, Godfrey HP. Molecular Biology of Spirochetes. Amsterdam: IOS Press; 2006.
55. Brissette CA, Verma A, Bowman A, Cooley AE, Stevenson B. The *Borrelia burgdorferi* outer-surface protein ErpX binds mammalian laminin. Microbiology. 2009;155:863–72.
56. Brissette CA, Cooley AE, Burns LH, Riley SP, Verma A, Woodman ME, et al. Lyme borreliosis spirochete Erp proteins, their known host ligands, and potential roles in mammalian infection. Int J Med Microbiol. 2008;298(Suppl. 1):257–67.
57. Hynes RO. Integrins: a family of cell surface receptors. Cell. 1987;48:549–54.
58. Cai X, Thinn AMM, Wang Z, Shan H, Zhu J. The importance of *N*-glycosylation on β3 integrin ligand binding and conformational regulation. Sci Rep. 2017;7:4656.
59. Coburn J, Magoun L, Bodary SC, Leong JM. Integrins αvβ3 and α5β1 mediate attachment of Lyme disease spirochetes to human cells. Infect Immun. 1998;66:1946–52.
60. Hynes RO. Integrins: versatility, modulation, and signaling in cell adhesion. Cell. 1992;69:11–25.
61. Magoun L, Zuckert WR, Robbins D, Parveen N, Alugupalli KR, Schwan TG, et al. Variable small protein (Vsp)-dependent and Vsp-independent pathways for glycosaminoglycan recognition by relapsing fever spirochaetes. Mol Microbiol. 2000;36:886–97.
62. Porcella SF, Raffel SJ, Anderson DE Jr, Gilk SD, Bono JL, Schrumpf ME, et al. Variable tick protein in two genomic groups of the relapsing fever spirochete *Borrelia hermsii* in western North America. Infect Immun. 2005;73:6647–58.
63. Probert WS, Johnson BJ. Identification of a 47 kDa fibronectin-binding protein expressed by *Borrelia burgdorferi* isolate B31. Mol Microbiol. 1998;30:1003–15.
64. Brissette CA, Bykowski T, Cooley AE, Bowman A, Stevenson B. *Borrelia burgdorferi* RevA antigen binds host fibronectin. Infect Immun. 2009; 77:2802–12.
65. Li X, Liu X, Beck DS, Kantor FS, Fikrig E. *Borrelia burgdorferi* lacking BBK32, a fibronectin-binding protein, retains full pathogenicity. Infect Immun. 2006;74:3305–13.
66. Hyde JA, Weening EH, Chang M, Trzeciakowski JP, Hook M, Cirillo JD, et al. Bioluminescent imaging of *Borrelia burgdorferi in vivo* demonstrates that the fibronectin-binding protein BBK32 is required for optimal infectivity. Mol Microbiol. 2011;82:99–113.
67. Niddam AF, Ebady R, Bansal A, Koehler A, Hinz B, Moriarty TJ. Plasma fibronectin stabilizes *Borrelia burgdorferi*-endothelial interactions under vascular shear stress by a catch-bond mechanism. Proc Natl Acad Sci USA. 2017;114:E3490–E8.
68. Ebady R, Niddam AF, Boczula AE, Kim YR, Gupta N, Tang TT, et al. Biomechanics of *Borrelia burgdorferi* vascular interactions. Cell Rep. 2016;16:2593–604.
69. Lin YP, Chen Q, Ritchie JA, Dufour NP, Fischer JR, Coburn J, et al. Glycosaminoglycan binding by *Borrelia burgdorferi* adhesin BBK32 specifically and uniquely promotes joint colonization. Cell Microbiol. 2015;17:860–75.
70. Parveen N, Robbins D, Leong JM. Strain variation in glycosaminoglycan recognition influences cell-type-specific binding by Lyme disease spirochetes. Infect Immun. 1999;67:1743–9.
71. Moriarty TJ, Shi M, Lin YP, Ebady R, Zhou H, Odisho T, et al. Vascular binding of a pathogen under shear force through mechanistically distinct sequential interactions with host macromolecules. Mol Microbiol. 2012;86:1116–31.
72. Garcia BL, Zhi H, Wager B, Hook M, Skare JT. *Borrelia burgdorferi* BBK32 inhibits the classical pathway by blocking activation of the C1 complement complex. PLoS Pathog. 2016;12:e1005404.
73. Brissette CA, Rossmann E, Bowman A, Cooley AE, Riley SP, Hunfeld KP, et al. The borrelial fibronectin-binding protein RevA is an early antigen of human Lyme disease. Clin Vaccine Immunol. 2010;17:274–80.
74. Shi Y, Xu Q, McShan K, Liang FT. Both decorin-binding proteins A and B are critical for the overall virulence of *Borrelia burgdorferi*. Infect Immun. 2008;76:1239–46.
75. Salo J, Jaatinen A, Soderstrom M, Viljanen MK, Hytonen J. Decorin binding proteins of *Borrelia burgdorferi* promote arthritis development and joint specific post-treatment DNA persistence in mice. PLoS One. 2015;10:e0121512.
76. Benoit VM, Fischer JR, Lin YP, Parveen N, Leong JM. Allelic variation of the Lyme disease spirochete adhesin DbpA influences spirochetal binding to decorin, dermatan sulfate, and mammalian cells. Infect Immun. 2011;79:3501–9.
77. Morgan A, Sepuru KM, Feng W, Rajarathnam K, Wang X. Flexible linker modulates glycosaminoglycan affinity of decorin binding protein A. Biochemistry. 2015;54:5113–9.
78. Wang X. Solution structure of decorin-binding protein A from *Borrelia burgdorferi*. Biochemistry. 2012;51:8353–62.
79. Salo J, Loimaranta V, Lahdenne P, Viljanen MK, Hytonen J. Decorin binding by DbpA and B of *Borrelia garinii*, *Borrelia afzelii*, and *Borrelia burgdorferi sensu stricto*. J Infect Dis. 2011;204:65–73.
80. Imai DM, Samuels DS, Feng S, Hodzic E, Olsen K, Barthold SW. The early dissemination defect attributed to disruption of decorin-binding proteins is abolished in chronic murine Lyme borreliosis. Infect Immun. 2013;81:1663–73.
81. Schlachter S, Seshu J, Lin T, Norris S, Parveen N. The *Borrelia burgdorferi* glycosaminoglycan binding protein Bgp in the B31 strain is not essential for infectivity despite facilitating adherence and tissue colonization. Infect Immun. 2018;86:e00667–17.
82. Verma A, Brissette CA, Bowman A, Stevenson B. *Borrelia burgdorferi* BmpA is a laminin-binding protein. Infect Immun. 2009;77:4940–6.
83. Antonara S, Ristow L, Coburn J. Adhesion mechanisms of *Borrelia burgdorferi*. Adv Exp Med Biol. 2011;715:35–49.
84. Pal U, Wang P, Bao F, Yang X, Samanta S, Schoen R, et al. *Borrelia burgdorferi* basic membrane proteins A and B participate in the genesis of Lyme arthritis. J Exp Med. 2008;205:133–41.
85. Coburn J, Barthold SW, Leong JM. Diverse Lyme disease spirochetes bind integrin $\alpha_{IIb}\beta_3$ on human platelets. Infect Immun. 1994;62:5559–67.
86. Alugupalli KR, Michelson AD, Barnard MR, Robbins D, Coburn J, Baker EK, et al. Platelet activation by a relapsing fever spirochaete results in enhanced bacterium-platelet interaction *via* integrin $\alpha_{IIb}\beta_3$ activation. Mol Microbiol. 2001;39:330–40.
87. Coburn J, Chege W, Magoun L, Bodary SC, Leong JM. Characterization of a candidate *Borrelia burgdorferi* β3-chain integrin ligand identified using a phage display library. Mol Microbiol. 1999;34:926–40.
88. Skare JT, Mirzabekov TA, Shang ES, Blanco DR, Erdjument-Bromage H, Bunikis J, et al. The Oms66 (p66) protein is a *Borrelia burgdorferi* porin. Infect Immun. 1997;65:3654–61.
89. Barcena-Uribarri I, Thein M, Sacher A, Bunikis I, Bonde M, Bergstrom S, et al. P66 porins are present in both Lyme disease and relapsing fever spirochetes: a comparison of the biophysical properties of P66 porins from six *Borrelia* species. Biochim Biophys Acta. 1798;2010:1197–203.
90. Kenedy MR, Luthra A, Anand A, Dunn JP, Radolf JD, Akins DR. Structural modeling and physicochemical characterization provide evidence that P66 forms a β-barrel in the *Borrelia burgdorferi* outer membrane. J Bacteriol. 2014;196:859–72.
91. Coburn J, Cugini C. Targeted mutation of the outer membrane protein P66 disrupts attachment of the Lyme disease agent, *Borrelia burgdorferi*, to integrin αVβ3. Proc Natl Acad Sci USA. 2003;100:7301–6.
92. Ristow LC, Bonde M, Lin YP, Sato H, Curtis M, Wesley E, et al. Integrin binding by *Borrelia burgdorferi* P66 facilitates dissemination but is not required for infectivity. Cell Microbiol. 2015;17:1021–36.
93. Defoe G, Coburn J. Delineation of *Borrelia burgdorferi* p66 sequences required for integrin αIIbβ3 recognition. Infect Immun. 2001;69:3455–9.
94. Ristow LC, Miller HE, Padmore LJ, Chettri R, Salzman N, Caimano MJ, et al. The β3-integrin ligand of *Borrelia burgdorferi* is critical for infection of mice but not ticks. Mol Microbiol. 2012;85:1105–18.
95. Wood E, Tamborero S, Mingarro I, Esteve-Gassent MD. BB0172, a *Borrelia burgdorferi* outer membrane protein that binds integrin α3β1. J Bacteriol. 2013;195:3320–30.
96. Lambris JD, Ricklin D, Geisbrecht BV. Complement evasion by human pathogens. Nat Rev Microbiol. 2008;6:132–42.
97. Ricklin D, Hajishengallis G, Yang K, Lambris JD. Complement: a key system for immune surveillance and homeostasis. Nat Immunol. 2010;11:785–97.
98. Kraiczy P. Hide and seek: how Lyme disease spirochetes overcome complement attack. Front Immunol. 2016;7:385.
99. Rodriguez de Cordoba S, Esparza-Gordillo J, Goicoechea de Jorge E, Lopez-Trascasa M, Sanchez-Corral P. The human complement factor H: functional roles, genetic variations and disease associations. Mol Immunol. 2004;41:355–67.
100. Fenaille F, Le Mignon M, Groseil C, Ramon C, Riande S, Siret L, et al. Site-specific *N*-glycan characterization of human complement factor H. Glycobiology. 2007;17:932–44.
101. Kraiczy P, Wallich R. Borrelial complement-binding proteins. In: Embers ME, editor. The Pathogenic Spirochetes: Strategies for Evasion of Host Immunity and Persistence. Boston: Springer US; 2012. p. 63–88.

102. Hellwage J, Kuhn S, Zipfel PF. The human complement regulatory factor-H-like protein 1, which represents a truncated form of factor H, displays cell-attachment activity. Biochem J. 1997;326:321–7.
103. Metts MS, McDowell JV, Theisen M, Hansen PR, Marconi RT. Analysis of the OspE determinants involved in binding of factor H and OspE-targeting antibodies elicited during *Borrelia burgdorferi* infection in mice. Infect Immun. 2003;71:3587–96.
104. Wallich R, Pattathu J, Kitiratschky V, Brenner C, Zipfel PF, Brade V, et al. Identification and functional characterization of complement regulator-acquiring surface protein 1 of the Lyme disease spirochetes *Borrelia afzelii* and *Borrelia garinii*. Infect Immun. 2005;73:2351–9.
105. Kraiczy P, Skerka C, Kirschfink M, Brade V, Zipfel PF. Immune evasion of *Borrelia burgdorferi* by acquisition of human complement regulators FHL-1/reconectin and Factor H. Eur J Immunol. 2001;31:1674–84.
106. Kraiczy P, Hellwage J, Skerka C, Becker H, Kirschfink M, Simon MM, et al. Complement resistance of *Borrelia burgdorferi* correlates with the expression of BbCRASP-1, a novel linear plasmid-encoded surface protein that interacts with human factor H and FHL-1 and is unrelated to Erp proteins. J Biol Chem. 2004;279:2421–9.
107. Haupt K, Kraiczy P, Wallich R, Brade V, Skerka C, Zipfel PF. Binding of human factor H-related protein 1 to serum-resistant *Borrelia burgdorferi* is mediated by borrelial complement regulator-acquiring surface proteins. J Infect Dis. 2007;196:124–33.
108. von Lackum K, Miller JC, Bykowski T, Riley SP, Woodman ME, Brade V, et al. *Borrelia burgdorferi* regulates expression of complement regulator-acquiring surface protein 1 during the mammal-tick infection cycle. Infect Immun. 2005;73:7398–405.
109. Bykowski T, Woodman ME, Cooley AE, Brissette CA, Brade V, Wallich R, et al. Coordinated expression of *Borrelia burgdorferi* complement regulator-acquiring surface proteins during the Lyme disease spirochete's mammal-tick infection cycle. Infect Immun. 2007;75:4227–36.
110. Kenedy MR, Vuppala SR, Siegel C, Kraiczy P, Akins DR. CspA-mediated binding of human factor H inhibits complement deposition and confers serum resistance in *Borrelia burgdorferi*. Infect Immun. 2009;77:2773–82.
111. Hallstrom T, Siegel C, Morgelin M, Kraiczy P, Skerka C, Zipfel PF. CspA from *Borrelia burgdorferi* inhibits the terminal complement pathway. MBio. 2013;4: e00481-13.
112. Bhide MR, Travnicek M, Levkutova M, Curlik J, Revajova V, Levkut M. Sensitivity of *Borrelia* genospecies to serum complement from different animals and human: a host-pathogen relationship. FEMS Immunol Med Microbiol. 2005;43:165–72.
113. Herzberger P, Siegel C, Skerka C, Fingerle V, Schulte-Spechtel U, van Dam A, et al. Human pathogenic *Borrelia spielmanii* sp. nov. resists complement-mediated killing by direct binding of immune regulators factor H and factor H-like protein 1. Infect Immun. 2007;75:4817–25.
114. Hartmann K, Corvey C, Skerka C, Kirschfink M, Karas M, Brade V, et al. Functional characterization of BbCRASP-2, a distinct outer membrane protein of *Borrelia burgdorferi* that binds host complement regulators factor H and FHL-1. Mol Microbiol. 2006;61:1220–36.
115. Siegel C, Schreiber J, Haupt K, Skerka C, Brade V, Simon MM, et al. Deciphering the ligand-binding sites in the *Borrelia burgdorferi* complement regulator-acquiring surface protein 2 required for interactions with the human immune regulators factor H and factor H-like protein 1. J Biol Chem. 2008;283:34855–63.
116. Kraiczy P, Seling A, Brissette CA, Rossmann E, Hunfeld KP, Bykowski T, et al. *Borrelia burgdorferi* complement regulator-acquiring surface protein 2 (CspZ) as a serological marker of human Lyme disease. Clin Vaccine Immunol. 2008;15:484–91.
117. Coleman AS, Yang X, Kumar M, Zhang X, Promnares K, Shroder D, et al. *Borrelia burgdorferi* complement regulator-acquiring surface protein 2 does not contribute to complement resistance or host infectivity. PLoS One. 2008;3:3010e.
118. Alitalo A, Meri T, Lankinen H, Seppala L, Lahdenne P, Hefty PS, et al. Complement inhibitor factor H binding to Lyme disease spirochetes is mediated by inducible expression of multiple plasmid-encoded outer surface protein E paralogs. J Immunol. 2002;169:3847–53.
119. Hammerschmidt C, Hallstrom T, Skerka C, Wallich R, Stevenson B, Zipfel PF, et al. Contribution of the infection-associated complement regulator-acquiring surface protein 4 (ErpC) to complement resistance of *Borrelia burgdorferi*. Clin Dev Immunol. 2012;2012:349657.
120. Siegel C, Hallstrom T, Skerka C, Eberhardt H, Uzonyi B, Beckhaus T, et al. Complement factor H-related proteins CFHR2 and CFHR5 represent novel ligands for the infection-associated CRASP proteins of *Borrelia burgdorferi*. PLoS One. 2010;5:e13519.
121. Hovis KM, Tran E, Sundy CM, Buckles E, McDowell JV, Marconi RT. Selective binding of *Borrelia burgdorferi* OspE paralogs to factor H and serum proteins from diverse animals: possible expansion of the role of OspE in Lyme disease pathogenesis. Infect Immun. 2006;74:1967–72.
122. McDowell JV, Wolfgang J, Tran E, Metts MS, Hamilton D, Marconi RT. Comprehensive analysis of the factor H binding capabilities of *Borrelia* species associated with Lyme disease: delineation of two distinct classes of factor H binding proteins. Infect Immun. 2003;71:3597–602.
123. Stevenson B, Bono JL, Schwan TG, Rosa P. *Borrelia burgdorferi* erp proteins are immunogenic in mammals infected by tick bite, and their synthesis is inducible in cultured bacteria. Infect Immun. 1998;66:2648–54.
124. Fikrig E, Narasimhan S. *Borrelia burgdorferi*-traveling incognito? Microbes Infect. 2006;8:1390–9.
125. Brooks CS, Vuppala SR, Jett AM, Alitalo A, Meri S, Akins DR. Complement regulator-acquiring surface protein 1 imparts resistance to human serum in *Borrelia burgdorferi*. J Immunol. 2005;175:3299–308.
126. van Dam AP, Oei A, Jaspars R, Fijen C, Wilske B, Spanjaard L, et al. Complement-mediated serum sensitivity among spirochetes that cause Lyme disease. Infect Immun. 1997;65:1228–36.
127. Sun J, Duffy KE, Ranjith-Kumar CT, Xiong J, Lamb RJ, Santos J, et al. Structural and functional analyses of the human Toll-like receptor 3. Role of glycosylation. J Biol Chem. 2006;281:11144–51.
128. Berende A, Oosting M, Kullberg BJ, Netea MG, Joosten LA. Activation of innate host defense mechanisms by *Borrelia*. Eur Cytokine Netw. 2010;21:7–18.
129. Leifer CA, Medvedev AE. Molecular mechanisms of regulation of Toll-like receptor signaling. J Leukocyte Biol. 2016;100:927–41.
130. Medzhitov R, Preston-Hurlburt P, Janeway CA Jr. A human homologue of the *Drosophila* Toll protein signals activation of adaptive immunity. Nature. 1997;388:394–7.
131. Muzio M, Bosisio D, Polentarutti N, D'Amico G, Stoppacciaro A, Mancinelli R, et al. Differential expression and regulation of toll-like receptors (TLR) in human leukocytes: selective expression of TLR3 in dendritic cells. J Immunol. 2000;164:5998–6004.
132. Wooten RM, Ma Y, Yoder RA, Brown JP, Weis JH, Zachary JF, et al. Toll-like receptor 2 is required for innate, but not acquired, host defense to *Borrelia burgdorferi*. J Immunol. 2002;168:348–55.
133. Bernardino AL, Myers TA, Alvarez X, Hasegawa A, Philipp MT. Toll-like receptors: insights into their possible role in the pathogenesis of Lyme neuroborreliosis. Infect Immun. 2008;76:4385–95.
134. Salazar JC, Pope CD, Moore MW, Pope J, Kiely TG, Radolf JD. Lipoprotein-dependent and -independent immune responses to spirochetal infection. Clin Diagn Lab Immunol. 2005;12:949–58.
135. Hoshino K, Takeuchi O, Kawai T, Sanjo H, Ogawa T, Takeda Y, et al. Cutting edge: Toll-like receptor 4 (TLR4)-deficient mice are hyporesponsive to lipopolysaccharide: evidence for TLR4 as the Lps gene product. J Immunol. 1999;162:3749–52.
136. Hacker H, Mischak H, Miethke T, Liptay S, Schmid R, Sparwasser T, et al. CpG-DNA-specific activation of antigen-presenting cells requires stress kinase activity and is preceded by non-specific endocytosis and endosomal maturation. EMBO J. 1998;17:6230–40.
137. Hemmi H, Takeuchi O, Kawai T, Kaisho T, Sato S, Sanjo H, et al. A Toll-like receptor recognizes bacterial DNA. Nature. 2000;408:740–5.
138. Inohara N, Nunez G. NODs: intracellular proteins involved in inflammation and apoptosis. Nat Rev Immunol. 2003;3:371–82.
139. Franchi L, Warner N, Viani K, Nunez G. Function of Nod-like receptors in microbial recognition and host defense. Immunol Rev. 2009;227:106–28.
140. Kanneganti TD, Lamkanfi M, Nunez G. Intracellular NOD-like receptors in host defense and disease. Immunity. 2007;27:549–59.
141. Sterka D Jr, Marriott I. Characterization of nucleotide-binding oligomerization domain (NOD) protein expression in primary murine microglia. J Neuroimmunol. 2006;179:65–75.
142. Sterka D Jr, Marriott I. Functional expression of NOD2, a novel pattern recognition receptor for bacterial motifs, in primary murine astrocytes. Glia. 2006;53:322–30.
143. Petnicki-Ocwieja T, DeFrancesco AS, Chung E, Darcy CT, Bronson RT, Kobayashi KS, et al. Nod2 suppresses *Borrelia burgdorferi* mediated murine Lyme arthritis and carditis through the induction of tolerance. PLoS One. 2011;6:e17414.
144. Oosting M, Berende A, Sturm P, Ter Hofstede HJ, de Jong DJ, Kanneganti TD, et al. Recognition of *Borrelia burgdorferi* by NOD2 is central for the induction of an inflammatory reaction. J Infect Dis. 2010;201:1849–58.

145. Stubs G, Fingerle V, Wilske B, Gobel UB, Zahringer U, Schumann RR, et al. Acylated cholesteryl galactosides are specific antigens of *Borrelia* causing Lyme disease and frequently induce antibodies in late stages of disease. J Biol Chem. 2009;284:13326–34.
146. Ben-Menachem G, Kubler-Kielb J, Coxon B, Yergey A, Schneerson R. A newly discovered cholesteryl galactoside from *Borrelia burgdorferi*. Proc Natl Acad Sci USA. 2003;100:7913–8.
147. Radolf JD, Caimano MJ, Stevenson B, Hu LT. Of ticks, mice and men: understanding the dual-host lifestyle of Lyme disease spirochaetes. Nat Rev Microbiol. 2012;10:87–99.
148. Jones KL, Seward RJ, Ben-Menachem G, Glickstein LJ, Costello CE, Steere AC. Strong IgG antibody responses to *Borrelia burgdorferi* glycolipids in patients with Lyme arthritis, a late manifestation of the infection. Clin Immunol. 2009;132:93–102.
149. Comstock LE, Fikrig E, Shoberg RJ, Flavell RA, Thomas DD. A monoclonal antibody to OspA inhibits association of *Borrelia burgdorferi* with human endothelial cells. Infect Immun. 1993;61:423–31.
150. Wang J, Li Y, Kinjo Y, Mac TT, Gibson D, Painter GF, et al. Lipid binding orientation within CD1d affects recognition of *Borrelia burgorferi* antigens by NKT cells. Proc Natl Acad Sci USA. 2010;107:1535–40.
151. Garcia Monco JC, Wheeler CM, Benach JL, Furie RA, Lukehart SA, Stanek G, et al. Reactivity of neuroborreliosis patients (Lyme disease) to cardiolipin and gangliosides. J Neurol Sci. 1993;117:206–14.
152. Garcia-Monco JC, Seidman RJ, Benach JL. Experimental immunization with *Borrelia burgdorferi* induces development of antibodies to gangliosides. Infect Immun. 1995;63:4130–7.
153. Weller M, Stevens A, Sommer N, Dichgans J, Kappler B, Wietholter H. Ganglioside antibodies: a lack of diagnostic specificity and clinical utility? J Neurol. 1992;239:455–9.
154. Venkataswamy MM, Porcelli SA. Lipid and glycolipid antigens of CD1d-restricted natural killer T cells. Semin Immunol. 2010;22:68–78.
155. Hossain H, Wellensiek HJ, Geyer R, Lochnit G. Structural analysis of glycolipids from *Borrelia burgdorferi*. Biochimie. 2001;83:683–92.
156. Smith DG, Williams SJ. Immune sensing of microbial glycolipids and related conjugates by T cells and the pattern recognition receptors MCL and Mincle. Carbohydr Res. 2016;420:32–45.
157. Garcia Monco JC, Fernandez Villar B, Rogers RC, Szczepanski A, Wheeler CM, Benach JL. *Borrelia burgdorferi* and other related spirochetes bind to galactocerebroside. Neurology. 1992;42:1341–8.
158. Backenson PB, Coleman JL, Benach JL. *Borrelia burgdorferi* shows specificity of binding to glycosphingolipids. Infect Immun. 1995;63:2811–7.
159. Kaneda K, Masuzawa T, Yasugami K, Suzuki T, Suzuki Y, Yanagihara Y. Glycosphingolipid-binding protein of *Borrelia burgdorferi sensu lato*. Infect Immun. 1997;65:3180–5.
160. Hajnicka V, Kocakova P, Slavikova M, Slovak M, Gasperik J, Fuchsberger N, et al. Anti-interleukin-8 activity of tick salivary gland extracts. Parasite Immunol. 2001;23:483–9.
161. Frauenschuh A, Power CA, Deruaz M, Ferreira BR, Silva JS, Teixeira MM, et al. Molecular cloning and characterization of a highly selective chemokine-binding protein from the tick *Rhipicephalus sanguineus*. J Biol Chem. 2007;282:27250–8.
162. Eaton JRO, Alenazi Y, Singh K, Davies G, Geis-Asteggiante L, Kessler B, et al. The N-terminal domain of a tick evasin is critical for chemokine binding and neutralization and confers specific binding activity to other evasins. J Biol Chem. 2018; https://doi.org/10.1074/jbc.RA117.000487.
163. Uhlir J, Grubhoffer L, Borsky I, Dusbabek F. Antigens and glycoproteins of larvae, nymphs and adults of the tick *Ixodes ricinus*. Med Vet Entomol. 1994;8:141–50.
164. Mulenga A, Kim T, Ibelli AM. *Amblyomma americanum* tick saliva serine protease inhibitor 6 is a cross-class inhibitor of serine proteases and papain-like cysteine proteases that delays plasma clotting and inhibits platelet aggregation. Insect Mol Biol. 2013;22:306–19.
165. Tirloni L, Kim TK, Coutinho ML, Ali A, Seixas A, Termignoni C, et al. The putative role of *Rhipicephalus microplus* salivary serpins in the tick-host relationship. Insect Biochem Mol Biol. 2016;71:12–28.
166. Deruaz M, Frauenschuh A, Alessandri AL, Dias JM, Coelho FM, Russo RC, et al. Ticks produce highly selective chemokine binding proteins with antiinflammatory activity. J Exp Med. 2008;205:2019–31.
167. Pratt CW, Church FC. Heparin binding to protein C inhibitor. J Biol Chem. 1992;267:8789–94.
168. Rein CM, Desai UR, Church FC. Serpin-glycosaminoglycan interactions. Methods Enzymol. 2011;501:105–37.
169. Tollefsen DM. Heparin Cofactor II. In: Church FC, Cunningham DD, Ginsburg D, Hoffman M, Stone SR, Tollefsen DM, editors. Chemistry and Biology of Serpins (Advances in Experimental Medicine and Biology, Vol. 425). New York: Springer Science+Business Media; 1997.
170. Radulovic ZM, Mulenga A. Heparan sulfate/heparin glycosaminoglycan binding alters inhibitory profile and enhances anticoagulant function of conserved *Amblyomma americanum* tick saliva serpin 19. Insect Biochem Mol Biol. 2017;80:1–10.
171. Koh CY, Kazimirova M, Trimnell A, Takac P, Labuda M, Nuttall PA, et al. Variegin, a novel fast and tight binding thrombin inhibitor from the tropical bont tick. J Biol Chem. 2007;282:29101–13.
172. Shabareesh PRV, Kumar A, Salunke DM, Kaur KJ. Structural and functional studies of differentially *O*-glycosylated analogs of a thrombin inhibitory peptide - variegin. J Pept Sci. 2017;23:880–8.
173. Stuen S, Bergstrom K, Palmer E. Reduced weight gain due to subclinical *Anaplasma phagocytophilum* (formerly *Ehrlichia phagocytophila*) infection. Exp Appl Acarol. 2002;28:209–15.
174. Splitter EJ, Twiehaus MJ, Castro ER. Anaplasmosis in sheep in the United States. J Am Vet Med Assoc. 1955;127:244–5.
175. Melendez RD. Future perspectives on veterinary hemoparasite research in the tropics at the start of this century. Ann N Y Acad Sci. 2000;916:253–8.
176. Dumler JS, Bakken JS. Human ehrlichioses: newly recognized infections transmitted by ticks. Annu Rev Med. 1998;49:201–13.
177. Keesing F, Hersh MH, Tibbetts M, McHenry DJ, Duerr S, Brunner J, et al. Reservoir competence of vertebrate hosts for *Anaplasma phagocytophilum*. Emerg Infect Dis. 2012;18:2013–6.
178. Parola P, Raoult D. Ticks and tickborne bacterial diseases in humans: an emerging infectious threat. Clin Infect Dis. 2001;32:897–928.
179. Stafford KC, Station CAE. Tick management handbook: an integrated guide for homeowners, pest control operators, and public health officials for the prevention of tick-associated disease. New Haven: Connecticut Agricultural Experiment Station; 2007.
180. Seidman D, Hebert KS, Truchan HK, Miller DP, Tegels BK, Marconi RT, et al. Essential domains of *Anaplasma phagocytophilum* invasins utilized to infect mammalian host cells. PLoS Pathog. 2015;11:e1004669.
181. Ojogun N, Kahlon A, Ragland SA, Troese MJ, Mastronunzio JE, Walker NJ, et al. *Anaplasma phagocytophilum* outer membrane protein A interacts with sialylated glycoproteins to promote infection of mammalian host cells. Infect Immun. 2012;80:3748–60.
182. Hebert KS, Seidman D, Oki AT, Izac J, Emani S, Oliver LD Jr, et al. *Anaplasma marginale* outer membrane protein A is an adhesin that recognizes sialylated and fucosylated glycans and functionally depends on an essential binding domain. Infect Immun. 2017;85:e00968-16.
183. Barbet AF, Allred DR. The msp1β multigene family of *Anaplasma marginale*: nucleotide sequence analysis of an expressed copy. Infect Immun. 1991;59:971–6.
184. McGarey DJ, Allred DR. Characterization of hemagglutinating components on the *Anaplasma marginale* initial body surface and identification of possible adhesins. Infect Immun. 1994;62:4587–93.
185. de la Fuente J, Garcia-Garcia JC, Blouin EF, Kocan KM. Differential adhesion of major surface proteins 1a and 1b of the ehrlichial cattle pathogen *Anaplasma marginale* to bovine erythrocytes and tick cells. Int J Parasitol. 2001;31:145–53.
186. McGarey DJ, Barbet AF, Palmer GH, McGuire TC, Allred DR. Putative adhesins of *Anaplasma marginale:* major surface polypeptides 1a and 1b. Infect Immun. 1994;62:4594–601.
187. Contreras M, Alberdi P, Mateos-Hernandez L, Fernandez de Mera IG, Garcia-Perez AL, Vancova M, et al. *Anaplasma phagocytophilum* MSP4 and HSP70 proteins are involved in interactions with host cells during pathogen infection. Front Cell Infect Microbiol. 2017;7:307.
188. NCBI. 1988. https://www.ncbi.nlm.nih.gov/. Accessed 30 Nov 2017.
189. de la Fuente J, Garcia-Garcia JC, Blouin EF, Kocan KM. Characterization of the functional domain of major surface protein 1a involved in adhesion of the rickettsia *Anaplasma marginale* to host cells. Vet Microbiol. 2003;91:265–83.
190. Garcia-Garcia JC, de la Fuente J, Bell-Eunice G, Blouin EF, Kocan KM. Glycosylation of *Anaplasma marginale* major surface protein 1a and its putative role in adhesion to tick cells. Infect Immun. 2004;72:3022–30.
191. Park J, Choi KS, Dumler JS. Major surface protein 2 of *Anaplasma phagocytophilum* facilitates adherence to granulocytes. Infect Immun. 2003;71:4018–25.
192. Rejmanek D, Foley P, Barbet A, Foley J. Antigen variability in *Anaplasma phagocytophilum* during chronic infection of a reservoir host. Microbiology. 2012;158:2632–41.

193. Rejmanek D, Foley P, Barbet A, Foley J. Evolution of antigen variation in the tick-borne pathogen *Anaplasma phagocytophilum*. Mol Biol Evol. 2012;29:391–400.
194. Ge Y, Rikihisa Y. Identification of novel surface proteins of *Anaplasma phagocytophilum* by affinity purification and proteomics. J Bacteriol. 2007;189:7819–28.
195. Mastronunzio JE, Kurscheid S, Fikrig E. Postgenomic analyses reveal development of infectious *Anaplasma phagocytophilum* during transmission from ticks to mice. J Bacteriol. 2012;194:2238–47.
196. Troese MJ, Kahlon A, Ragland SA, Ottens AK, Ojogun N, Nelson KT, et al. Proteomic analysis of *Anaplasma phagocytophilum* during infection of human myeloid cells identifies a protein that is pronouncedly upregulated on the infectious dense-cored cell. Infect Immun. 2011;79:4696–707.
197. Goodman JL, Nelson CM, Klein MB, Hayes SF, Weston BW. Leukocyte infection by the granulocytic ehrlichiosis agent is linked to expression of a selectin ligand. J Clin Invest. 1999;103:407–12.
198. Ojogun N, Barnstein B, Huang B, Oskeritzian CA, Homeister JW, Miller D, et al. *Anaplasma phagocytophilum* infects mast cells *via* α1,3-fucosylated but not sialylated glycans and inhibits IgE-mediated cytokine production and histamine release. Infect Immun. 2011;79:2717–26.
199. Carlyon JA, Akkoyunlu M, Xia L, Yago T, Wang T, Cummings RD, et al. Murine neutrophils require α1,3-fucosylation but not PSGL-1 for productive infection with *Anaplasma phagocytophilum*. Blood. 2003;102:3387–95.
200. McEver RP, Cummings RD. Role of PSGL-1 binding to selectins in leukocyte recruitment. J Clin Invest. 1997;100(Suppl. 11):S97–103.
201. Yago T, Leppanen A, Carlyon JA, Akkoyunlu M, Karmakar S, Fikrig E, et al. Structurally distinct requirements for binding of P-selectin glycoprotein ligand-1 and sialyl Lewis x to *Anaplasma phagocytophilum* and P-selectin. J Biol Chem. 2003;278:37987–97.
202. Herron MJ, Nelson CM, Larson J, Snapp KR, Kansas GS, Goodman JL. Intracellular parasitism by the human granulocytic ehrlichiosis bacterium through the P-selectin ligand, PSGL-1. Science. 2000;288:1653–6.
203. Pedra JH, Narasimhan S, Rendic D, DePonte K, Bell-Sakyi L, Wilson IB, et al. Fucosylation enhances colonization of ticks by *Anaplasma phagocytophilum*. Cell Microbiol. 2010;12:1222–34.
204. Kariu T, Smith A, Yang X, Pal U. A chitin deacetylase-like protein is a predominant constituent of tick peritrophic membrane that influences the persistence of Lyme disease pathogens within the vector. PLoS One. 2013;8:e78376.
205. Abraham NM, Liu L, Jutras BL, Yadav AK, Narasimhan S, Gopalakrishnan V, et al. Pathogen-mediated manipulation of arthropod microbiota to promote infection. Proc Natl Acad Sci USA. 2017;114:E781–E90.
206. Heisig M, Abraham NM, Liu L, Neelakanta G, Mattessich S, Sultana H, et al. Antivirulence properties of an antifreeze protein. Cell Rep. 2014;9:417–24.
207. Neelakanta G, Sultana H, Fish D, Anderson JF, Fikrig E. *Anaplasma phagocytophilum* induces *Ixodes scapularis* ticks to express an antifreeze glycoprotein gene that enhances their survival in the cold. J Clin Invest. 2010;120:3179–90.
208. Ip WK, Takahashi K, Ezekowitz RA, Stuart LM. Mannose-binding lectin and innate immunity. Immunol Rev. 2009;230:9–21.
209. Matsushita M. Ficolins: complement-activating lectins involved in innate immunity. J Innate Immun. 2010;2:24–32.
210. Krarup A, Thiel S, Hansen A, Fujita T, Jensenius JC. L-ficolin is a pattern recognition molecule specific for acetyl groups. J Biol Chem. 2004;279:47513–9.
211. Kairies N, Beisel HG, Fuentes-Prior P, Tsuda R, Muta T, Iwanaga S, et al. The 2.0-A crystal structure of tachylectin 5A provides evidence for the common origin of the innate immunity and the blood coagulation systems. Proc Natl Acad Sci USA. 2001;98:13519–24.
212. Hanington PC, Zhang SM. The primary role of fibrinogen-related proteins in invertebrates is defense, not coagulation. J Innate Immun. 2011;3:17–27.
213. Kopacek P, Hajdusek O, Buresova V. Tick as a model for the study of a primitive complement system. Adv Exp Med Biol. 2012;710:83–93.
214. Kovar V, Kopacek P, Grubhoffer L. Isolation and characterization of Dorin M, a lectin from plasma of the soft tick *Ornithodoros moubata*. Insect Biochem Mol Biol. 2000;30:195–205.
215. Rego ROM, Hajdusek O, Kovar V, Kopacek P, Grubhoffer L, Hypsa V. Molecular cloning and comparative analysis of fibrinogen-related proteins from the soft tick *Ornithodoros moubata* and the hard tick *Ixodes ricinus*. Insect Biochem Mol Biol. 2005;35:991–1004.
216. Rego ROM, Kovar V, Kopacek P, Weise C, Man P, Sauman I, et al. The tick plasma lectin, Dorin M, is a fibrinogen-related molecule. Insect Biochem Mol Biol. 2006;36:291–9.
217. Man P, Kovar V, Sterba J, Strohalm M, Kavan D, Kopacek P, et al. Deciphering Dorin M glycosylation by mass spectrometry. Eur J Mass Spectrom. 2008;14:345–54.
218. Sterba J, Dupejova J, Fiser M, Vancova M, Grubhoffer L. Fibrinogen-related proteins in ixodid ticks. Parasit Vectors. 2011;4:127.
219. Honig Mondekova H, Sima R, Urbanova V, Kovar V, Rego ROM, Grubhoffer L, et al. Characterization of *Ixodes ricinus* fibrinogen-related proteins (Ixoderins) discloses their function in the tick innate immunity. Front Cell Infect Microbiol. 2017;7:509.
220. Dupejova J, Sterba J, Vancova M, Grubhoffer L. Hemelipoglycoprotein from the ornate sheep tick, *Dermacentor marginatus*: structural and functional characterization. Parasit Vectors. 2011;4:4.
221. Huang X, Tsuji N, Miyoshi T, Nakamura-Tsuruta S, Hirabayashi J, Fujisaki K. Molecular characterization and oligosaccharide-binding properties of a galectin from the argasid tick *Ornithodoros moubata*. Glycobiology. 2007;17:313–23.
222. Vasta GR, Ahmed H, Nita-Lazar M, Banerjee A, Pasek M, Shridhar S, et al. Galectins as self/non-self recognition receptors in innate and adaptive immunity: an unresolved paradox. Front Immunol. 2012;3:199.
223. Maeda H, Miyata T, Kusakisako K, Galay RL, Talactac MR, Umemiya-Shirafuji R, et al. A novel C-type lectin with triple carbohydrate recognition domains has critical roles for the hard tick *Haemaphysalis longicornis* against Gram-negative bacteria. Dev Comp Immunol. 2016;57:38–47.
224. Smith AA, Pal U. Immunity-related genes in *Ixodes scapularis* - perspectives from genome information. Front Cell Infect Microbiol. 2014;4:116.
225. Pang X, Xiao X, Liu Y, Zhang R, Liu J, Liu Q, et al. Mosquito C-type lectins maintain gut microbiome homeostasis. Nat Microbiol. 2016;1:16023.
226. Cheng G, Cox J, Wang P, Krishnan MN, Dai J, Qian F, et al. A C-type lectin collaborates with a CD45 phosphatase homolog to facilitate West Nile virus infection of mosquitoes. Cell. 2010;142:714–25.
227. Neelakanta G, Sultana H. Viral receptors of the gut: vector-borne viruses of medical importance. Curr Opin Insect Sci. 2016;16:44–50.
228. Alarcon-Chaidez F, Ryan R, Wikel S, Dardick K, Lawler C, Foppa IM, et al. Confirmation of tick bite by detection of antibody to *Ixodes* calreticulin salivary protein. Clin Vaccine Immunol. 2006;13:1217–22.
229. Schroeder H, Skelly PJ, Zipfel PF, Losson B, Vanderplasschen A. Subversion of complement by hematophagous parasites. Dev Comp Immunol. 2009;33:5–13.
230. Eggleton P, Lieu TS, Zappi EG, Sastry K, Coburn J, Zaner KS, et al. Calreticulin is released from activated neutrophils and binds to C1q and mannan-binding protein. Clin Immunol Immunopathol. 1994;72:405–9.
231. Kim TK, Ibelli AM, Mulenga A. *Amblyomma americanum* tick calreticulin binds C1q but does not inhibit activation of the classical complement cascade. Ticks Tick Borne Dis. 2015;6:91–101.
232. Uhlir J, Grubhoffer L, Volf P. Novel agglutinin in the midgut of the tick *Ixodes ricinus*. Folia Parasitol (Praha). 1996;43:233–9.
233. Grubhoffer L, Kovar V, Rudenko N. Tick lectins: structural and functional properties. Parasitology. 2004;129:S113–S25.
234. Kamwendo SP, Ingram GA, Musisi FL, Molyneux DH. Haemagglutinin activity in tick (*Rhipicephalus appendiculatus*) haemolymph and extracts of gut and salivary gland. Ann Trop Med Parasitol. 1993;87:303–5.
235. Kamwendo SP, Ingram GA, Musisi FL, Trees AJ, Molyneux DH. Characteristics of tick, *Rhipicephalus appendiculatus*, glands distinguished by surface lectin binding. Ann Trop Med Parasitol. 1993;87:525–35.
236. Pal U, Li X, Wang T, Montgomery RR, Ramamoorthi N, Desilva AM, et al. TROSPA, an *Ixodes scapularis* receptor for *Borrelia burgdorferi*. Cell. 2004;119:457–68.
237. Grubhoffer L, Dusbabek F. Lectin binding analysis of *Argas polonicus* tissue glycoproteins. Vet Parasitol. 1991;38:235–47.
238. Vancova M, Zacharovova K, Grubhoffer L, Nebesarova J. Ultrastructure and lectin characterization of granular salivary cells from *Ixodes ricinus* females. J Parasitol. 2006;92:431–40.
239. Grubhoffer L, Hajdusek O, Vancova M, Sterba J, Rudenko N. Glycobiochemistry of ticks, vectors of infectious diseases: carbohydrate-binding proteins and glycans. FEBS J. 2009;276:141.
240. Vancova M, Sterba J, Dupejova J, Simonova Z, Nebesarova J, Novotny MV, et al. Uptake and incorporation of sialic acid by the tick *Ixodes ricinus*. J Insect Physiol. 2012;58:1277–87.
241. Thall A, Galili U. Distribution of Galα1-3Galβ1-4GlcNAc residues on secreted mammalian glycoproteins (thyroglobulin, fibrinogen, and immunoglobulin G) as measured by a sensitive solid-phase radioimmunoassay. Biochemistry. 1990;29:3959–65.
242. Chung CH, Mirakhur B, Chan E, Le QT, Berlin J, Morse M, et al. Cetuximab-induced anaphylaxis and IgE specific for galactose-α-1,3-galactose. N Engl J Med. 2008;358:1109–17.

243. Commins SP, James HR, Kelly LA, Pochan SL, Workman LJ, Perzanowski MS, et al. The relevance of tick bites to the production of IgE antibodies to the mammalian oligosaccharide galactose-α-1,3-galactose. J Allergy Clin Immunol. 2011;127:1286–93.e6.
244. Van Nunen SA, O'Connor KS, Clarke LR, Boyle RX, Fernando SL. An association between tick bite reactions and red meat allergy in humans. Med J Aust. 2009;190:510–1.
245. Chinuki Y, Ishiwata K, Yamaji K, Takahashi H, Morita E. *Haemaphysalis longicornis* tick bites are a possible cause of red meat allergy in Japan. Allergy. 2016;71:421–5.
246. Hamsten C, Starkhammar M, Tran TA, Johansson M, Bengtsson U, Ahlen G, et al. Identification of galactose-α-1,3-galactose in the gastrointestinal tract of the tick *Ixodes ricinus*; possible relationship with red meat allergy. Allergy. 2013;68:549–52.
247. Wang H, Nuttall PA. Excretion of host immunoglobulin in tick saliva and detection of IgG-binding proteins in tick haemolymph and salivary glands. Parasitology. 1994;109:525–30.
248. Valenzuela JG, Francischetti IMB, Pham VM, Garfield MK, Mather TN, Ribeiro JMC. Exploring the sialome of the tick *Ixodes scapularis*. J Exp Biol. 2002;205:2843–64.
249. Araujo RN, Franco PF, Rodrigues H, Santos LCB, McKay CS, Sanhueza CA, et al. *Amblyomma sculptum* tick saliva: α-Gal identification, antibody response and possible association with red meat allergy in Brazil. Int J Parasitol. 2016;46:213–20.
250. Altmann F. The role of protein glycosylation in allergy. Int Arch Allergy Immunol. 2007;142:99–115.
251. van Die I, Gomord V, Kooyman FN, van den Berg TK, Cummings RD, Vervelde L. Core α1->3-fucose is a common modification of *N*-glycans in parasitic helminths and constitutes an important epitope for IgE from *Haemonchus contortus* infected sheep. FEBS Lett. 1999;463:189–93.
252. Altmann F. Coping with cross-reactive carbohydrate determinants in allergy diagnosis. Allergo J Int. 2016;25:98–105.
253. Vancova M, Nebesarova J. Correlative fluorescence and scanning electron microscopy of labelled core fucosylated glycans using cryosections mounted on carbon-patterned glass slides. PLoS One. 2015;10:e0145034.
254. Bencurova M, Hemmer W, Focke-Tejkl M, Wilson IB, Altmann F. Specificity of IgG and IgE antibodies against plant and insect glycoprotein glycans determined with artificial glycoforms of human transferrin. Glycobiology. 2004;14:457–66.
255. North SJ, Koles K, Hembd C, Morris HR, Dell A, Panin VM, et al. Glycomic studies of *Drosophila melanogaster* embryos. Glycoconjugate J. 2006;23:345–54.
256. Koles K, Irvine KD, Panin VM. Functional characterization of *Drosophila* sialyltransferase. J Biol Chem. 2004;279:4346–57.
257. Repnikova E, Koles K, Nakamura M, Pitts J, Li H, Ambavane A, et al. Sialyltransferase regulates nervous system function in *Drosophila*. J Neurosci. 2010;30:6466–76.
258. Sterba J, Vancova M, Sterbova J, Bell-Sakyi L, Grubhoffer L. The majority of sialylated glycoproteins in adult *Ixodes ricinus* ticks originate in the host, not the tick. Carbohydr Res. 2014;389:93–9.
259. Gritsun TS, Lashkevich VA, Gould EA. Tick-borne encephalitis. Antiviral Res. 2003;57:129–46.
260. Welsch S, Miller S, Romero-Brey I, Merz A, Bleck CK, Walther P, et al. Composition and three-dimensional architecture of the dengue virus replication and assembly sites. Cell Host Microbe. 2009;5:365–75.
261. Gillespie LK, Hoenen A, Morgan G, Mackenzie JM. The endoplasmic reticulum provides the membrane platform for biogenesis of the flavivirus replication complex. J Virol. 2010;84:10438–47.
262. Offerdahl DK, Dorward DW, Hansen BT, Bloom ME. A three-dimensional comparison of tick-borne flavivirus infection in mammalian and tick cell lines. PLoS One. 2012;7:e47912.
263. Miorin L, Romero-Brey I, Maiuri P, Hoppe S, Krijnse-Locker J, Bartenschlager R, et al. Three-dimensional architecture of tick-borne encephalitis virus replication sites and trafficking of the replicated RNA. J Virol. 2013;87:6469–81.
264. Yu L, Takeda K, Gao Y. Characterization of virus-specific vesicles assembled by West Nile virus non-structural proteins. Virology. 2017;506:130–40.
265. Best SM, Morris KL, Shannon JG, Robertson SJ, Mitzel DN, Park GS, et al. Inhibition of interferon-stimulated JAK-STAT signaling by a tick-borne flavivirus and identification of NS5 as an interferon antagonist. J Virol. 2005;79:12828–39.
266. Lindenbach BD, Rice CM. Molecular biology of flaviviruses. Adv Virus Res. 2003;59:23–61.
267. Lorenz IC, Allison SL, Heinz FX, Helenius A. Folding and dimerization of tick-borne encephalitis virus envelope proteins prM and E in the endoplasmic reticulum. J Virol. 2002;76:5480–91.
268. Mackenzie JM, Westaway EG. Assembly and maturation of the flavivirus Kunjin virus appear to occur in the rough endoplasmic reticulum and along the secretory pathway, respectively. J Virol. 2001;75:10787–99.
269. Stadler K, Allison SL, Schalich J, Heinz FX. Proteolytic activation of tick-borne encephalitis virus by furin. J Virol. 1997;71:8475–81.
270. Mandl CW. Steps of the tick-borne encephalitis virus replication cycle that affect neuropathogenesis. Virus Res. 2005;111:161–74.
271. Heinz FX, Allison SL. Flavivirus structure and membrane fusion. Adv Virus Res. 2003;59:63–97.
272. Hammond C, Braakman I, Helenius A. Role of *N*-linked oligosaccharide recognition, glucose trimming, and calnexin in glycoprotein folding and quality control. Proc Natl Acad Sci USA. 1994;91:913–7.
273. Yoshii K, Yanagihara N, Ishizuka M, Sakai M, Kariwa H. *N*-linked glycan in tick-borne encephalitis virus envelope protein affects viral secretion in mammalian cells, but not in tick cells. J Gen Virol. 2013;94:2249–58.
274. Winkler G, Heinz FX, Kunz C. Studies on the glycosylation of flavivirus E proteins and the role of carbohydrate in antigenic structure. Virology. 1987;159:237–43.
275. Rey FA, Heinz FX, Mandl C, Kunz C, Harrison SC. The envelope glycoprotein from tick-borne encephalitis virus at 2 A resolution. Nature. 1995;375:291–8.
276. Lorenz IC, Kartenbeck J, Mezzacasa A, Allison SL, Heinz FX, Helenius A. Intracellular assembly and secretion of recombinant subviral particles from tick-borne encephalitis virus. J Virol. 2003;77:4370–82.
277. Grubhoffer L, Guirakhoo F, Heinz F, Kunz C. Interaction of tick-borne encephalitis virus protein E with labelled lectins. In: Lectins: Biology, Biochemistry and Clinical Biochemistry, vol. 7. St Louis: Sigma Chemical Company; 1990. p. 313–9.
278. Fuzik T, Formanova P, Ruzek D, Yoshii K, Niedrig M, Plevka P. Structure of tick-borne encephalitis virus and its neutralization by a monoclonal antibody. Nat Commun. 2018;9:436.
279. Goto A, Yoshii K, Obara M, Ueki T, Mizutani T, Kariwa H, et al. Role of the *N*-linked glycans of the prM and E envelope proteins in tick-borne encephalitis virus particle secretion. Vaccine. 2005;23:3043–52.
280. Putnak JR, Charles PC, Padmanabhan R, Irie K, Hoke CH, Burke DS. Functional and antigenic domains of the dengue-2 virus nonstructural glycoprotein NS-1. Virology. 1988;163:93–103.
281. Chambers TJ, Hahn CS, Galler R, Rice CM. Flavivirus genome organization, expression, and replication. Annu Rev Microbiol. 1990;44:649–88.
282. Heinz FX, Allison SL. Structures and mechanisms in flavivirus fusion. Adv Virus Res. 2000;55:231–69.
283. Hanna SL, Pierson TC, Sanchez MD, Ahmed AA, Murtadha MM, Doms RW. *N*-linked glycosylation of west nile virus envelope proteins influences particle assembly and infectivity. J Virol. 2005;79:13262–74.
284. Bryant JE, Calvert AE, Mesesan K, Crabtree MB, Volpe KE, Silengo S, et al. Glycosylation of the dengue 2 virus E protein at N67 is critical for virus growth *in vitro* but not for growth in intrathoracically inoculated *Aedes aegypti* mosquitoes. Virology. 2007;366:415–23.
285. Mondotte JA, Lozach PY, Amara A, Gamarnik AV. Essential role of dengue virus envelope protein *N*-glycosylation at asparagine-67 during viral propagation. J Virol. 2007;81:7136–48.
286. Moudy RM, Zhang B, Shi PY, Kramer LD. West Nile virus envelope protein glycosylation is required for efficient viral transmission by *Culex* vectors. Virology. 2009;387:222–8.
287. Murata R, Eshita Y, Maeda A, Maeda J, Akita S, Tanaka T, et al. Glycosylation of the West Nile virus envelope protein increases *in vivo* and *in vitro* viral multiplication in birds. Am J Trop Med Hyg. 2010;82:696–704.
288. Hyde JA. *Borrelia burgdorferi* keeps moving and carries on: a review of borrelial dissemination and invasion. Front Immunol. 2017;8:114.
289. Hooper LV, Gordon JI. Glycans as legislators of host-microbial interactions: spanning the spectrum from symbiosis to pathogenicity. Glycobiology. 2001;11:1R–10R.
290. Nizet V, Esko JD. Bacterial and viral infections. In: Varki A, Cummings RD, Esko JD, Freeze HH, Stanley P, Bertozzi CR, et al., editors. Essentials of Glycobiology. 2nd ed. Cold Spring Harbor: Cold Spring Harbour Laboratory Press; 2009.
291. de la Fuente J, Canales M, Kocan KM. The importance of protein glycosylation in development of novel tick vaccine strategies. Parasite Immunol. 2006;28:687–8.

292. Sprong H, Trentelman J, Seemann I, Grubhoffer L, Rego RO, Hajdusek O, et al. ANTIDotE: anti-tick vaccines to prevent tick-borne diseases in Europe. Parasit Vectors. 2014;7:77.
293. Boysen A, Palmisano G, Krogh TJ, Duggin IG, Larsen MR, Moller-Jensen J. A novel mass spectrometric strategy "BEMAP" reveals extensive *O*-linked protein glycosylation in enterotoxigenic *Escherichia coli*. Sci Rep. 2016;6:32016.
294. Parveen N, Leong JM. Identification of a candidate glycosaminoglycan-binding adhesin of the Lyme disease spirochete *Borrelia burgdorferi*. Mol Microbiol. 2000;35:1220–34.
295. Guo BP, Brown EL, Dorward DW, Rosenberg LC, Hook M. Decorin-binding adhesins from *Borrelia burgdorferi*. Mol Microbiol. 1998;30:711–23.
296. Fuchs H, Wallich R, Simon MM, Kramer MD. The outer surface protein A of the spirochete *Borrelia burgdorferi* is a plasmin(ogen) receptor. Proc Natl Acad Sci USA. 1994;91:12594–8.
297. Lagal V, Portnoi D, Faure G, Postic D, Baranton G. *Borrelia burgdorferi sensu stricto* invasiveness is correlated with OspC-plasminogen affinity. Microbes Infect. 2006;8:645–52.
298. Onder O, Humphrey PT, McOmber B, Korobova F, Francella N, Greenbaum DC, et al. OspC is potent plasminogen receptor on surface of *Borrelia burgdorferi*. J Biol Chem. 2012;2870:16860–8.
299. Floden AM, Watt JA, Brissette CA. *Borrelia burgdorferi* enolase is a surface-exposed plasminogen binding protein. PLoS One. 2011;6:e27502.
300. Cinco M, Cini B, Murgia R, Presani G, Prodan M, Perticarari S. Evidence of involvement of the mannose receptor in adhesion of *Borrelia burgdorferi* to monocyte/macrophages. Infect Immun. 2001;69:2743–7.
301. Guo BP, Teneberg S, Munch R, Terunuma D, Hatano K, Matsuoka K, et al. Relapsing fever *Borrelia* binds to neolacto glycans and mediates rosetting of human erythrocytes. Proc Natl Acad Sci USA. 2009;106:19280–5.
302. Kuismanen E, Hedman K, Saraste J, Pettersson RF. Uukuniemi virus maturation: accumulation of virus particles and viral antigens in the Golgi complex. Mol Cell Biol. 1982;2:1444–58.

2

The pervasive effects of recombinant *Fasciola gigantica* Ras-related protein Rab10 on the functions of goat peripheral blood mononuclear cells

Ai-Ling Tian[1], MingMin Lu[2], Fu-Kai Zhang[1], Guillermo Calderón-Mantilla[3], Evangelia Petsalaki[3], XiaoWei Tian[2], WenJuan Wang[2], Si-Yang Huang[4,5], XiangRui Li[2], Hany M. Elsheikha[6*] and Xing-Quan Zhu[1,4,5*]

Abstract

Background: *Fasciola gigantica*-induced immunomodulation is a major hurdle faced by the host for controlling infection. Here, we elucidated the role of *F. gigantica* Ras-related protein Rab10 (FgRab10) in the modulation of key functions of peripheral blood mononuclear cells (PBMCs) of goats.

Methods: We cloned and expressed recombinant FgRab10 (rFgRab10) protein and examined its effects on several functions of goat PBMCs. Protein interactors of rFgRab10 were predicted *in silico* by querying the databases Intact, String, BioPlex and BioGrid. In addition, a total energy analysis of each of the identified interactions was also conducted. Gene Ontology (GO) enrichment analysis was carried out using FuncAssociate 3.0.

Results: The *FgRab10* gene (618 bp), encodes 205-amino-acid residues with a molecular mass of ~23 kDa, had complete nucleotide sequence homology with *F. hepatica* Ras family protein gene (PIS87503.1). The rFgRab10 protein specifically cross-reacted with anti-*Fasciola* antibodies as shown by Western blot and immunofluorescence analysis. This protein exhibited multiple effects on goat PBMCs, including increased production of cytokines [interleukin-2 (IL-2), IL-4, IL-10, transforming growth factor beta (TGF-β) and interferon gamma (IFN-γ)] and total nitric oxide (NO), enhancing apoptosis and migration of PBMCs, and promoting the phagocytic ability of monocytes. However, it significantly inhibited cell proliferation. Homology modelling revealed 63% identity between rFgRab10 and human Rab10 protein (Uniprot ID: P61026). Protein interaction network analysis revealed more stabilizing interactions between Rab proteins geranylgeranyltransferase component A 1 (CHM) and Rab proteins geranylgeranyltransferase component A 2 (CHML) and rFgRab10 protein. Gene Ontology analysis identified RabGTPase mediated signaling as the most represented pathway.

Conclusions: rFgRab10 protein exerts profound influences on various functions of goat PBMCs. This finding may help explain why *F. gigantica* is capable of provoking recognition by host immune cells, less capable of destroying this successful parasite.

Keywords: *Fasciola gigantica*, Ras-related protein Rab10, Recombinant proteins, Peripheral blood mononuclear cells, Immunomodulation

* Correspondence: hany.elsheikha@nottingham.ac.uk; xingquanzhu1@hotmail.com
[6]Faculty of Medicine and Health Sciences, School of Veterinary Medicine and Science, University of Nottingham, Sutton Bonington Campus, Loughborough LE12 5RD, UK
[1]State Key Laboratory of Veterinary Etiological Biology, Key Laboratory of Veterinary Parasitology of Gansu Province, Lanzhou Veterinary Research Institute, Chinese Academy of Agricultural Sciences, Lanzhou, Gansu Province 730046, People's Republic of China
Full list of author information is available at the end of the article

Background

Fasciola gigantica and *Fasciola hepatica* are omnipresent agents of a zoonotic parasitic disease, fascioliasis, which continues to be a major health burden on animals and humans. Fascioliasis can adversely affect the sustainability of the farm animal industry [1]. The annual global economic loss due to fascioliasis has been estimated to be in excess of three billion dollars [2]. Worldwide, at least 2.4 million people have been infected with fascioliasis, with a further 180 million people at risk of being infected [3]. Despite this high impact and investigations for decades using clinical studies as well as animal models, knowledge about host defense mechanisms against *F. gigantica* is limited. This challenge is partly due to the fact that *Fasciola* spp. are very efficient modulators of the host immune response [4]. The immunomodulatory capacity of *F. gigantica*, mediated by parasite-derived effector molecules, is believed to play important roles in the establishment of long-lasting infection in the host.

Several studies have investigated various excretory/secretory products (ESPs) and virulence effector molecules employed by *F. gigantica* flukes to ensure their survival and establishment of persistent infection [5, 6]. Rab proteins are a family of small GTP-binding proteins, part of the Ras superfamily, which regulate intracellular membrane trafficking of several pathogens; including parasites (e.g. *Plasmodium*, *Theileria*, *Cryptosporidium* and *Babesia* [7] and *Toxoplasma gondii* [8]), bacteria (e.g. *Mycobacterium* spp. [9] and *Listeria monocytogenes* [10]) and fungi [11]. Despite their crucial role as regulators of vesicular membrane traffic, the roles of Rab proteins in the pathogenesis of *F. gigantica* infection remain largely unknown. Understanding the influence of parasite-secreted proteins on the function of immune cells, such as goat peripheral blood mononuclear cells (PBMCs), is essential due to their important role in the immunopathogenesis of fascioliasis [12]. In a recent study, we cloned and expressed a recombinant *F. gigantica* 14-3-3 epsilon protein (rFg14-3-3e), and characterized its effects on specific functions of goat PBMCs [6].

In the present study, we expand our investigation of the effects of *F. gigantica* ESPs on the functions of these immune cells. Specifically, the gene encoding *F. gigantica* Rab10 (FgRab10) was cloned and expressed in *Escherichia coli*. Then, the modulatory effects of the purified recombinant FgRab10 (rFgRab10) protein on the functions of goat PBMCs; including cytokine secretion, proliferation, migration, nitric oxide (NO) production, phagocytosis and apoptosis were investigated. Our results indicate that rFgRab10 protein can significantly influence key functions of goat PBMCs, all are critical facets of the immunopathogenesis of *F. gigantica* infection.

Methods

Animals

Three crossbred goats (3–6 months-old) were obtained from the teaching and research flock at Nanjing Agricultural University. Goats were treated with triclabendazole (50 mg/kg body weight) in order to exclude the possibility of any prior infection with liver flukes. Two weeks post-treatment, a faecal specimen from each goat was examined microscopically to exclude the presence of helminth eggs. Female Sprague Dawley (SD) rats (150–200 g) were purchased from the Experimental Animal Center of Jiangsu Province, China (Certificate: SCXK 2008-0004), and used for the production of antibodies. Rats were raised under specific pathogen-free conditions, and fed with sterilized food and water *ad libitum*. All efforts were made to minimize the suffering of animals, and daily health checks were performed throughout the experiment.

Purification and culture of goat PBMCs

Venous blood samples were collected from the jugular vein of goats, with no history of *F. gigantica* infection or other parasitic infections, into Vacutainer tubes coated with ethylenediaminetetraacetic acid (EDTA). PBMCs were isolated from freshly collected blood using a PBMC isolation kit (TBD, Tianjin, China). Culturing was done by incubating the isolated PBMCs in RPMI 1640 medium containing 10% fetal bovine serum (FBS) and 1% penicillin-streptomycin (Gibco, New York, USA). Cultures were maintained in a humidified atmosphere of 5% CO_2 at 37 °C. The number of PBMCs was adjusted to 10^6 cells/ml in RPMI 1640 medium and cell viability was assessed using trypan blue dye exclusion method. The number of viable cells was counted in a haemocytometer and only cells with > 95% viability were used in the experiments. All assays were performed using freshly isolated PBMCs. For the monocyte phagocytosis experiment, adherent monocytes were obtained after incubation of PBMCs for 48 h at 37 °C in 5% CO_2, followed by removal of the non-adherent cells. In all assays performed to investigate the effects of rFgRab10 protein on certain functions of goat PBMCs and monocytes, cultured cells were exposed to rFgRab10 protein at concentrations of 10 μg/ml, 20 μg/ml, 40 μg/ml or 80 μg/ml. PBMCs treated with SUMO protein expressed in pET-SUMO expression vector and sham-treated with phosphate buffered saline (PBS, pH 7.4) were used as controls in all assays. All experiments were performed in triplicate.

Parasite strain

Adult *F. gigantica* flukes were harvested from the gall-bladder of naturally infected buffaloes at local abattoirs in Guangxi Zhuang Autonomous Region, PR China. The collected flukes were washed twice in PBS and used for RNA isolation or stored frozen at -80 °C with RNA stabilizer for later analysis. The identity of the flukes collected was ascertained to be *F. gigantica* based on PCR and sequencing analysis of the second internal transcribed spacer (ITS2) of ribosomal DNA [13]. This analysis revealed 100% ITS2 sequence homology between the flukes collected and *F. gigantica* samples examined previously from the same region (GenBank: AJ557569).

Cloning and characterization of *FgRab10* gene

Because *F. gigantica* genome sequences are not available, we searched the NCBI/BLASTx (https://blast.ncbi.nlm.nih.gov/Blast.cgi), *F. hepatica* cDNA library and liquid chromatography-tandem mass spectrometry (LC-MS/MS)-based *F. hepatica* ESPs dataset from previously unpublished proteomics studies to identify homologous Ras family protein gene sequences. This analysis identified *F. hepatica Ras* family protein gene (GenBank: PIS87503.1), which was utilized to design primers to amplify *F. gigantica* Ras-related protein *Rab10* (*FgRab10*) gene. Total RNA was isolated from adult *F. gigantica* flukes using Trizol reagent (Invitrogen, San Diego, USA), and was used to synthesize first-strand cDNA with reverse transcription polymerase chain reaction (RT-PCR) using the RevertAid First Strand cDNA Synthesis Kit [Thermo Scientific (EU), Vilnius, Lithuania]. The cDNA was used for the amplification of *FgRab10* gene using a forward primer (5'-CCG GAA TTC ATG GCT AAG AAG TCG TAC GAT G -3') and a reverse primer (5'-ATT TGC GGC CGC TGT AGG ACA CCA GGA GCA-3'). *Eco*R I and *Not* I restriction sites, which were underlined, were incorporated into the primers. The amplified *FgRab10* gene was digested with *Eco*R I and *Not* I, and ligated into the corresponding cloning sites in the T-vector pMD19 (Simple) (Takara, Dalian, Liaoning, China). The recombinant plasmid was transformed into *Trans5α* chemically competent cells (TransGen Biotech, Beijing, China). Positive clones were sequenced by GenScript (Nanjing, Jiangsu, China) in order to confirm the correct insertion/orientation of *FgRab10* gene in the vector. The *FgRab10* cDNA sequence was translated into amino acid sequences using EditSeq (DNASTAR Lasergene). The signal peptide and conserved domains of FgRab10 were predicted by SignalP 4.1 Server (http://www.cbs.dtu.dk/services/SignalP/), and (https://www.ncbi.nlm.nih.gov/Structure/cdd/wrpsb.cgi), respectively.

Expression and purification of rFgRab10 protein

Positive clones containing the *FgRab10* gene were selected. The *FgRab10* gene fragment was sub-cloned into the pET-SUMO expression vector. The pET-SUMO-*FgRab10* plasmid was transformed into *E. coli* BL2 (DE3), then induced by addition of 1 mM isopropyl-β-d-thiogalactopyranoside (IPTG) (Solarbio, Beijing, China) to a culture with an optical density at 600 nm (OD_{600}) of 0.6 at 37 °C. After 5 h, the bacterial cells were collected by centrifugation (10,000× *g*, 10 min, 4 °C), resuspended in 5 ml imidazole buffer (20 mM phosphate, 0.5 M NaCl, 10 mM imidazole), and frozen at -20 °C. The cell preparation was sonicated at 600 W for 20 min and further centrifuged at 10,000× *g* for 10 min at 4 °C, and the recombinant His-tagged protein was isolated from bacterial pellets under denaturing conditions in a solution containing 8 M urea. After a third centrifugation, the supernatant was purified using the His GaviTrap kit (GE Healthcare, Buckinghamshire, UK). The eluted protein was first dialyzed in a solution containing 0.1 M urea to be refolded and renatured in a buffer containing a linear decreased urea gradient (6 M, 4 M, 2 M and 0 M urea), and then dialyzed against PBS to remove imidazole. The non-recombinant pET-SUMO expression vector (without *FgRab10* gene) was used to produce the control His-tagged SUMO protein, which was expressed and purified using the same method used to obtain rFgRab10 protein. The lipopolysaccharide (LPS) was depleted from the rFgRab10 protein using Detoxi-Gel Affinity Pak prepacked columns (Thermo Scientific, Waltham, MA, USA). The concentration of the rFgRab10 protein was adjusted to 1 mg/ml. The endotoxin level of the sample was measured with a Limulus Amebocyte Lysate (LAL) gel clot assay using a Pyrosate® Kit (Cape Cod Inc., East Falmouth, MA, USA).

Preparation of polyclonal antibodies

Polyclonal antibodies were produced by subcutaneous immunization of SD rats with purified rFgRab10 protein. Briefly, SD rats were immunized with 300 μg of the purified protein emulsified with complete Freund's adjuvant (1:1). After each 2-week interval, SD rats were boosted four times with the same dose of the rFgRab10 protein mixed with incomplete Freund's adjuvant. One week after the last injection, rat serum was collected and stored frozen at -80 °C.

Western blot analysis of rFgRab10 protein

The purity of the protein was detected by 12% SDS-PAGE, followed by Coomassie blue staining. Also, 20 μg of the purified rFgRab10 protein were resolved on 12% SDS-PAGE and transferred onto Hybond-C extra nitrocellulose membrane (Amersham, London, UK). The membrane was washed 5 times (5 min each) in TBS-T. The membrane was then incubated with primary antibodies (serum from sheep naturally infected with *Fasciola*) for 1 h at 37 °C (1:100 in TBS-T). After washing 5 times in TBS-T, the membrane was incubated with horseradish peroxidase (HRP)-conjugated rabbit anti-goat immunoglobulin (Ig)-G antibody (Sigma, St. Louis, MO, USA) at 37 °C for 1 h (1:2000 in TBS-T). The immunoreaction was visualized using WesternBright ECL (Advansta, Menlo

Park, CA, USA) and LucentBlue X-ray film (Advansta, Menlo Park, CA, USA).

Immunofluorescence staining of rFgRab10 protein bound to goat PBMCs

PBMCs were incubated with rFgRab10 protein in a humidified atmosphere of 5% CO_2 at 37 °C for 1 h. Cells were fixed with 4% paraformaldehyde, washed 3 times in PBS and treated with blocking solution (4% BSA in PBS) for 1 h to minimize background staining. rFgRab10-treated, SUMO protein-treated, or PBS-treated PBMCs were incubated with rat anti-rFgRab10 protein antibody (1:100 in 4% BSA) for 1 h at 37 °C. Cells were stained with Cy3 conjugated goat anti-rat IgG secondary antibody (1:500 in 4% BSA) (Beyotime, Jiangsu, China) for 1 h at 37 °C. Hoechst 33342 (Invitrogen, Oregon, USA) was used to stain the nuclei. Stained cells were imaged using a confocal laser scanning microscope (LSM710, Zeiss, Jena, Germany) and digital images were analyzed using Zen 2012 imaging software.

Quantification of cytokines in goat PBMCs culture supernatant

Cytokine production was detected in the culture supernatants of PBMCs incubated with rFgRab10 protein. PBMCs were plated at a cell density of 10^6 cells/well in 24-well tissue culture plates in 1 ml culture medium with various concentrations (10, 20, 40 and 80 μg/ml) of rFgRab10 protein. The culture plates were maintained in 5% CO_2 at 37 °C for 24 h. The PBMCs supernatant was then collected and assayed for the production of interleukin (IL)-2, IL-4, IL-10, transforming growth factor beta (TGF-β) and interferon gamma (IFN-γ) using goat ELISA kit (Mlbio, Shanghai, China). Limits of detection were between 2 and 1200 pg/ml depending on the cytokine.

Assessment of nitric oxide (NO) production

PBMCs were seeded into 24-well flat-bottomed plates at 10^6 cells per well in 1 ml RPMI medium. PBMCs were allowed to adhere for 2 h in 5% CO_2 at 37 °C; cells were then stimulated by rFgRab10 protein using the same concentrations used above. The supernatant was collected after 24 h and analyzed for NO production by Total Nitric Oxide Assay Kit (Beyotime, Haimen, Jiangsu, China). A microplate reader (Bio-Rad, Hercules, CA, USA) was used to measure the optical density at 540 nm (OD_{540}). NO levels were calculated against a standard curve generated using 0-80 μM/l sodium nitrites.

Determination of apoptosis assay using Annexin V/PI staining

PBMCs were seeded into 24-well tissue culture plates at 10^6 cells/well in 1 ml RPMI medium with each of the rFgRab10 protein concentrations used above. The plate was incubated in 5% CO_2 at 37 °C for 24 h. PBMCs were then stained with Annexin V and PI using the Annexin V-FITC kit (Miltenyi Biotec, Bergisch Gladbach, Nordrhein-Westfalen, Germany). Apoptosis in PBMCs was quantified by flow cytometry. Data were analyzed using FlowJo 10. Annexin V-positive/PI-negative PBMCs were considered to be apoptotic and were analyzed as a percentage of the entire PBMCs population.

In vitro goat PBMCs migration assay

To test whether rFgRab10 protein can stimulate the *in vitro* the migration of PBMCs, we assessed the movement of untreated and rFgRab10-tretaed PBMCs from the upper chamber of a Transwell plate (Corning, Kennebunk, USA), through an 8-μm-pore polycarbonate membrane inserts toward the lower chamber. Briefly, ~10^6 cells in 100 μl RPMI medium without or with rFgRab10 at the concentrations used above were seeded into the upper chamber of the Transwell in 24-well tissue culture plates. The bottom chamber was filled with ~600 μl RPMI medium. The plate was incubated in 5% CO_2 at 37 °C for 4 h. After incubation, PBMCs were collected from the bottom chamber and the number of cells migrated through the membrane into the lower chamber was determined using an Automated Cell Counter (Countstar, Shanghai, China). The results are presented as percentages of the seeded PBMCs.

Measurement of FITC-dextran uptake

Goat monocytes were seeded into 24-well tissue culture plates at 10^6 cells/well in 1 ml RPMI medium with the various rFgRab10 protein concentrations. The plate was incubated in 5% CO_2 at 37 °C for 48 h. After centrifugation at 500× *g*, monocytes were resuspended in chilled PBS, and incubated with 1 mg/ml FITC-dextran (average molecular weight of dextran, 4000; Sigma, St. Louis, MO, USA) in RPMI 1640 Medium at 4 °C or 37 °C for 1 h in darkness. To halt phagocytosis, chilled PBS containing 2% FBS was added after incubation and goat monocytes were washed trice with PBS and resuspended in chilled PBS. FITC-dextran uptake of monocytes was analyzed using flow cytometry (BD Biosciences, San Jose, CA, USA). The data were analyzed using FlowJo 10.

Determination of goat PBMCs proliferation

PBMCs were plated in 96-well tissue culture plates at a cell density of 10^4 PBMCs/well in triplicate in 100 μl complete RPMI medium with each of the rFgRab10 protein concentrations used above. The plate was incubated in a humidified atmosphere of 5% CO_2 at 37 °C. After 48 h, 10 μl of Cell Counting Kit-8 (CCK-8) (Beyotime, Jiangsu, China) reagent was added to each well and the plate was further incubated under the same conditions in darkness. A microplate reader (Bio-Rad) was used to measure the optical density at 450 nm (OD_{450}).

Bioinformatics

We used blastx (https://blast.ncbi.nlm.nih.gov/) to obtain the protein sequence of rFgRab10 and the Fragments Library of ROBETTA (http://robetta.bakerlab.org/) [14] to obtain the 3-mer and 9-mer fragments. Using the sequence of rFgRab10, and the 3-mers and 9-mers, the *de novo* 3D protein structure was predicted using ROSETTA's AbinitioRelax function (https://www.rosettacommons.org/) [15]. The pdb result was aligned to the human Rab10 chain A protein using the Match-maker and match-align tools of UCSF Chimera (https://www.cgl.ucsf.edu/chimera/) [16]. UCSF Chimera was also used to visualize the *ab initio* structure and the alignment to the human Rab10 chain A protein.

Protein Blast [17] was used to retrieve the protein sequence of humans (taxid: 9606), most similar to the rFgRab10 protein sequence. The human Rab10 protein (Uniprot ID: P61026) was used to query interactions in the following databases: Intact [18], String [19], BioPlex [20] and BioGrid [21]. The results were summarized and filtered by P61026 (Rab10) protein using a Python script; this list of interacting pairs was the input used to obtain structure interactions using Interactome3D [22]. All experimental and modeled interactions were used to build a model using the aligned fasta recombinant Rab10 protein sequence to the P61026 (Rab10) protein. A total energy analysis was performed using FoldX Suite [23] in order to calculate the structure energy of each protein involved in the interaction. We used Cytoscape (http://www.cytoscape.org/) to build a protein interaction network. Finally, Gene Ontology (GO) enrichment analysis was performed, using as input the 13 human proteins that interacted with P61026 (Rab10), using FuncAssociate 3.0 [24].

Statistical analysis

Data values were expressed as the mean ± standard deviation (SD). Differences between the groups were examined for statistical significance using GraphPad Prism 6.0. Statistical analysis was performed using one-way analysis of variance (ANOVA). *P* values < 0.05, 0.01, 0.001 and 0.0001 were represented as *, **, *** and ****, respectively, in comparison with untreated controls. All experiments were repeated at least three independent times.

Results

Cloning of *FgRab10* gene

PCR products (~618 bp) of *FgRab10* gene were successfully cloned into T-vector pMD19. The identity of the construct (pMD19T-*FgRab10*) was verified by DNA sequence analysis. FgRab10 is a 205 amino-acid protein with a molecular mass of ~23 kDa (GenBank: MH532439). Conserved domain analysis showed that *FgRab10* protein belonged to P-loop NTPase domain superfamily. Amino

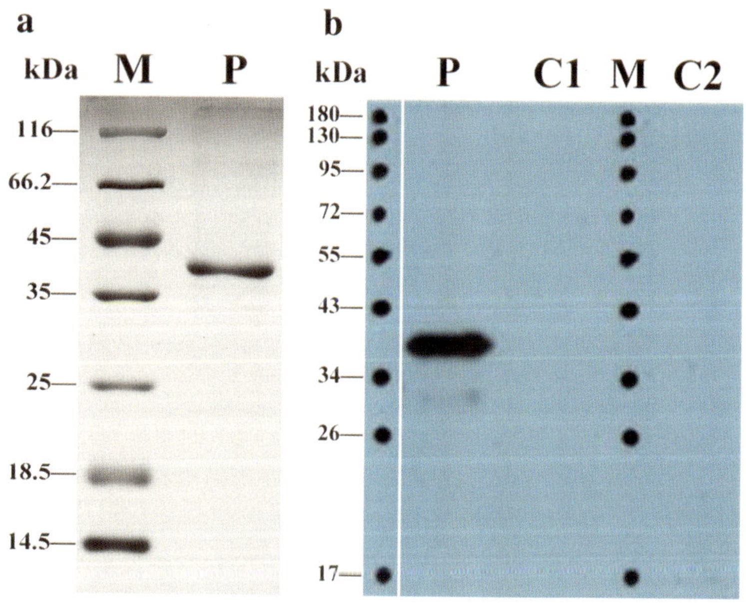

Fig. 1 SDS-PAGE and Western blot analyses of the purified rFgRab10 protein from the sonicated culture sediment of *E. coli*. **a** rFgRab10 protein was resolved on 12% acrylamide gel and stained with Coomassie blue. Lane M: prestained protein ladder in kilodaltons; Lane P: purified recombinant protein, rFgRab10, which appeared as a single band of ~39 kDa. **b** rFgRab10 protein was run under non-reducing conditions, and the immunoreaction was visualized using chemiluminescent HRP substrate and X-ray film. Lane M: prestained protein ladder; Lane P: loaded with rFgRab10 protein expressed from *E. coli*. Serum from *Fasciola*-infected sheep detected a single band of ~39 kDa; Lane C1: loaded with protein expressed from sonicated culture supernatant of *E. coli* transformed with empty pET-SUMO vector without *rFgRab10* gene insert, which did not react with goat serum containing anti-*F. gigantica* IgG antibodies; Lane C2: loaded with rFgRab-10 protein expressed from *E. coli* that did not react with the serum of healthy uninfected goats

acid sequence comparison of the *FgRab10* gene with that of *F. hepatica Ras* family protein gene (GenBank: PIS87503.1) showed 100% sequence homology.

SDS-PAGE and Western blot analysis

The *FgRab10* gene fragment was successfully sub-cloned into pET-SUMO expression vector and the positive clones, pET-SUMO-*FgRab10,* were induced by IPTG in *E. coli* BL2 (DE3). The recombinant rFgRab10 protein was successfully expressed as a soluble His-tagged fusion protein using the small ubiquitin-like modifier (SUMO). A protein with an apparent molecular mass of ~39 kDa (~23 kDa rFgRab10 protein + ~16 kDa SUMO tag protein) was detected in SDS-PAGE (Fig. 1a). The specificity of rFgRab10 protein was confirmed by Western blot analysis, wherein rFgRab10 protein specifically reacted with serum from *Fasciola*-infected sheep as indicated by the presence of a single ~39 kDa band. No bands were observed in negative controls [empty pET-SUMO vector without *rFgRab10* gene insert or in samples probed with serum from healthy sheep (Fig. 1b)].

Binding affinity of rFgRab10 protein to goat PBMCs

Binding of rFgRab10 protein to PBMCs surface was determined by immunofluorescent staining. By incubating rFgRab10-treated PBMCs with specific anti-rFgRab10 antibodies, we detected an even distribution and localization of the red Cy3 dye on the PBMCs membrane, indicating the successful binding of rFgRab10 protein to PBMCs surface (Fig. 2). No fluorescence was observed in PBMCs incubated with SUMO protein obtained from sonicated culture supernatant of *E. coli* transformed with empty pET-SUMO vector or in PBS-treated goat PBMCs.

rFgRab10 protein modulates cytokine production by goat PBMCs

rFgRab10 protein caused alteration in the levels of five cytokines, IL-2, IL-4, IL-10, IFN-γ and TGF-β. As shown in Fig. 3, when PBMCs were treated with different concentrations of rFgRab10 protein, the production of cytokines was significantly increased, when compared with PBMCs treated with SUMO protein obtained from sonicated culture of *E. coli* transformed with empty pET-SUMO vector (ANOVA tests: IL-2 (0 μg/ml: $F_{(5, 48)} = 53.63$, $P = 0.0778$; 10 μg/ml: $F_{(5, 48)} = 53.63$, $P < 0.0001$; 20 μg/ml: $F_{(5, 48)} = 53.63$, $P < 0.0001$; 40 μg/ml: $F_{(5, 48)} = 53.63$, $P < 0.0001$; 80 μg/ml: $F_{(5, 48)} = 53.63$, $P < 0.0001$), IL-4 (0 μg/ml: $F_{(5, 48)} = 47.06$, $P = 0.8419$; 10 μg/ml: $F_{(5, 48)} = 47.06$, $P = 0.0020$; 20 μg/ml: $F_{(5, 48)} = 47.06$, $P < 0.0001$; 40 μg/ml: $F_{(5, 48)} =$

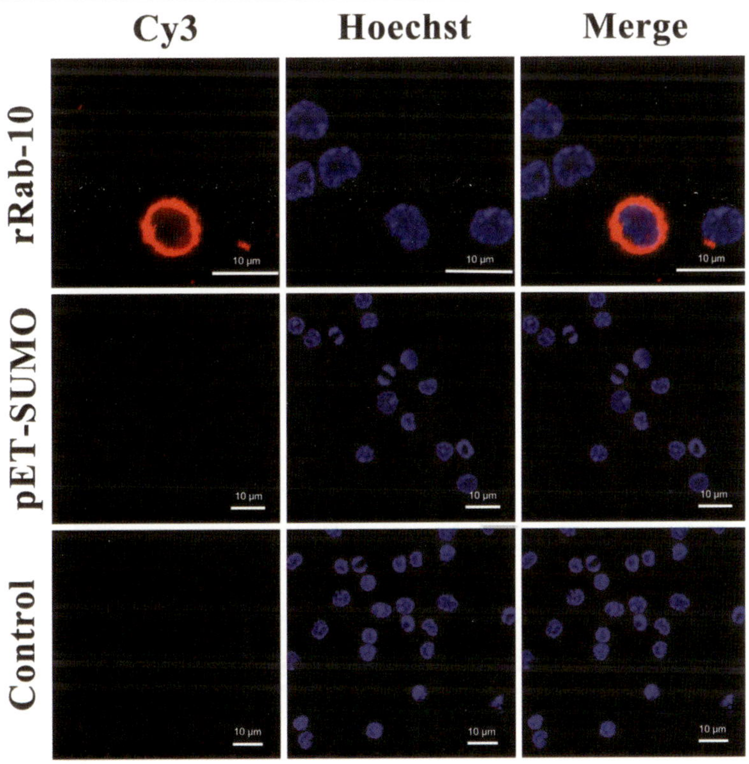

Fig. 2 Localization of *F. gigantica*-derived rFgRab10 protein to the PBMCs surface. rFgRab10 protein binding to goat PBMCs surface was determined by incubating PBMCs treated with purified rFgRab10 protein, protein from sonicated culture of *E. coli* transformed with empty pET-SUMO vector or sham-treated with PBS (control) with primary anti-rFgRab-10 protein antibody raised in rats. PBMCs' nuclei and rFgRab10 protein were stained by Hoechst 33342 (blue) and Cy3-conjugated secondary antibody (red), respectively. Surface staining was detected in rFgRab10-treated cells, but not in PBMCs incubated with SUMO protein and sham-treated PBMCs. *Scale-bars*: 10 μm

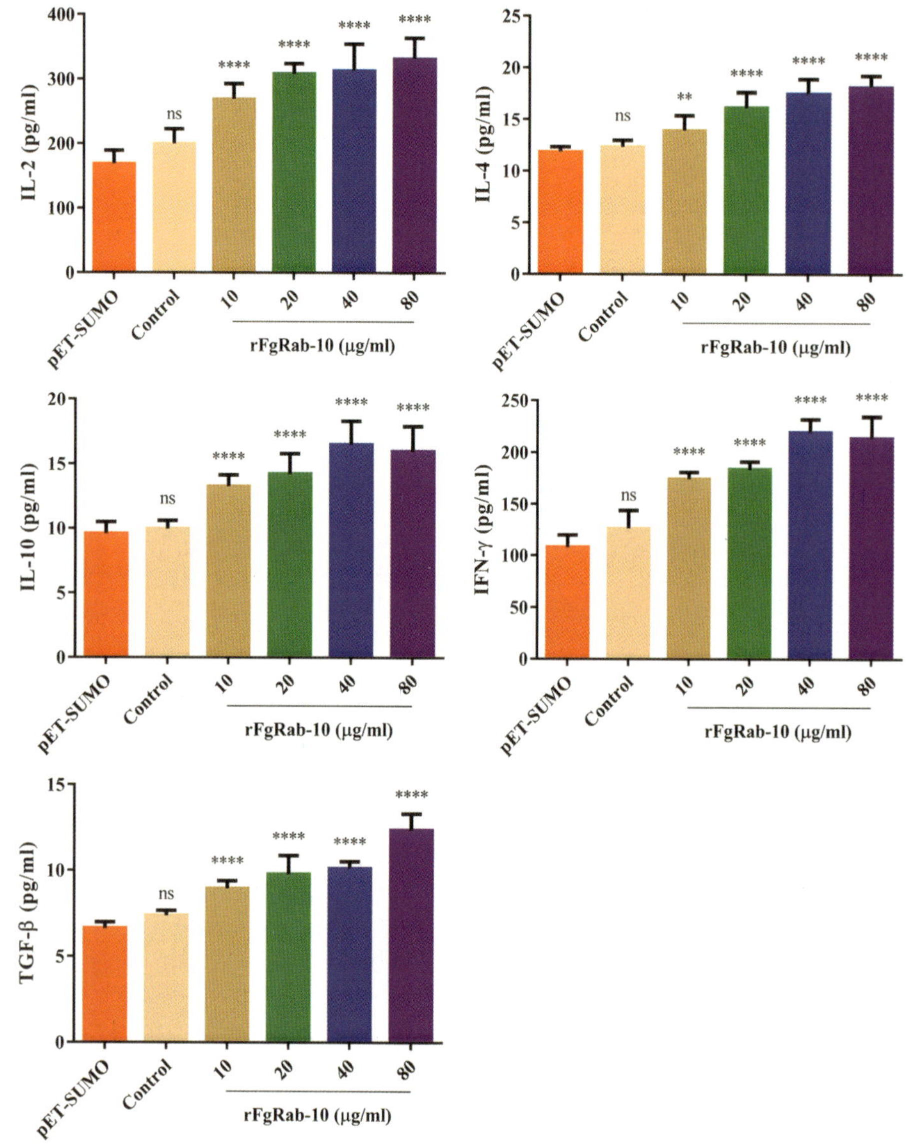

Fig. 3 rFgRab10 protein induced the cytokine secretion. Goat PBMCs were incubated for 24 h in the presence of serial concentrations of rFgRab10 protein. PBMCs incubated with SUMO protein or PBS-treated PBMCs served as controls. The levels of cytokine concentration in the supernatant of cultured PBMCs was quantified by ELISA. Graphs represent means ± SD of data from three independent biological replicates. Asterisks indicate statistical significance between the different indicated groups (**$P < 0.01$; ****$P < 0.0001$; ns, non-significant)

47.06, $P < 0.0001$; 80 μg/ml: $F_{(5, 48)} = 47.06$, $P < 0.0001$), IL-10 (0 μg/ml: $F_{(5, 48)} = 39.92$, $P = 0.9661$; 10 μg/ml: $F_{(5, 48)} = 39.92$, $P < 0.0001$; 20 μg/ml: $F_{(5, 48)} = 39.92$, $P < 0.0001$; 40 μg/ml: $F_{(5, 48)} = 39.92$, $P < 0.0001$; 80 μg/ml: $F_{(5, 48)} = 39.92$, $P < 0.0001$), TGF β (0 μg/ml: $F_{(5, 48)} = 83.54$, $P = 0.0839$; 10 μg/ml: $F_{(5, 48)} = 83.54$, $P < 0.0001$; 20 μg/ml: $F_{(5, 48)} = 83.54$, $P < 0.0001$; 40 μg/ml: $F_{(5, 48)} = 83.54$, $P < 0.0001$; 80 μg/ml: $F_{(5, 48)} = 83.54$, $P < 0.0001$), and IFN-γ (0 μg/ml: $F_{(5, 48)} = 83.54$, $P = 0.0839$; 10 μg/ml: $F_{(5, 48)} = 83.54$, $P < 0.0001$; 20 μg/ml: $F_{(5, 48)} = 83.54$, $P < 0.0001$; 40 μg/ml: $F_{(5, 48)} = 83.54$, $P < 0.0001$; 80 μg/ml: $F_{(5, 48)} = 83.54$, $P < 0.0001$).

rFgRab10 protein promotes goat PBMCs NO production

As shown in Fig. 4, NO release from PBMCs was significantly increased in the presence of rFgRab10 protein compared with controls, but not at 0 μg/ml and 10 μg/ml (ANOVA tests: 0 μg/ml: $F_{(5, 24)} = 126.2$, $P = 0.2183$; 10 μg/ml: $F_{(5, 24)} = 126.2$, $P = 0.9998$; 20 μg/ml: $F_{(5, 24)} = 126.2$, $P < 0.0001$; 40 μg/ml: $F_{(5, 24)} = 126.2$, $P < 0.0001$; 80 μg/ml: $F_{(5, 24)} = 126.2$, $P < 0.0001$).

rFgRab10 protein stimulates goat PBMCs apoptosis

We monitored the level of apoptosis in rFgRab10-treated PBMCs using the Annexin V-FITC/PI double staining

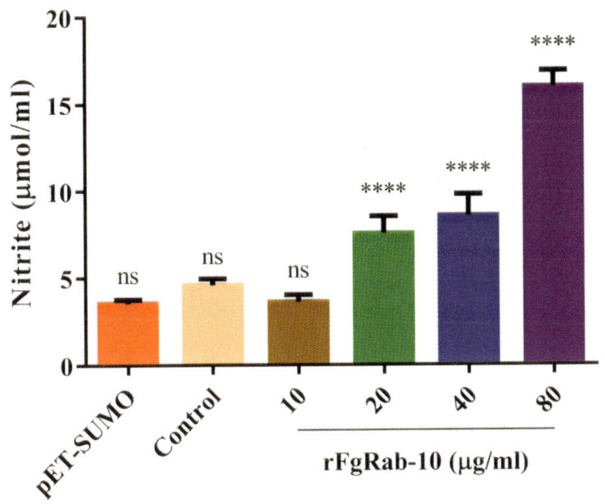

Fig. 4 Effects of rFgRab10 protein on the production of intracellular NO. PBMCs were sham-treated with PBS, SUMO protein or serial concentrations of rFgRab10 protein and incubated for 24 h at 37 °C at 5% CO_2. NO concentration in the PBMCs was measured using Griess assay. Graphs represent means ± SD of data from 3 independent biological replicates. Asterisks indicate statistical significance between the different indicated groups (****$P < 0.0001$; ns, non-significant)

apoptosis assay. rFgRab10 protein significantly induced apoptosis in PBMCs in a dose-dependent manner (ANOVA tests: 0 μg/ml: $F_{(5, 48)} = 117.6$, $P = 0.5249$; 10 μg/ml: $F_{(5, 48)} = 117.6$, $P = 0.7685$; 20 μg/ml: $F_{(5, 48)} = 117.6$, $P = 0.0531$; 40 μg/ml: $F_{(5, 48)} = 117.6$, $P < 0.0001$; 80 μg/ml: $F_{(5, 48)} = 117.6$, $P < 0.0001$) (Fig. 5).

rFgRab10 protein stimulates goat PBMCs migration

rFg14-3-3e protein significantly promoted, in a dose-dependent manner, the migration of goat PBMCs at all tested concentrations compared to control PBMCs treated with SUMO protein (10 μg/ml: $F_{(5, 12)} = 176.5$, $P = 0.0230$; 20 μg/ml: $F_{(5, 12)} = 176.5$, $P = 0.0015$; 40 μg/ml: $F_{(5, 12)} = 176.5$, $P < 0.0001$; 80 μg/ml: $F_{(5, 12)} = 176.5$, $P < 0.0001$; one-way ANOVA) (Fig. 6).

rFgRab10 protein increases goat monocyte phagocytosis

We determined whether rFgRab10 protein influences the phagocytic ability of monocytes that were cultured with PBS, SUMO protein or serial concentrations of rFgRab10 protein prior to exposure to FITC-dextran. The phagocytic capability of monocytes was examined by assessment of FITC-dextran uptake. rFgRab10 protein at 10 μg/ml, 20 μg/ml and 40 μg/ml (but not at 80 μg/ml) significantly increased the phagocytic ability of monocytes compared with cells incubated with SUMO protein (10 μg/ml: $F_{(5, 48)} = 28.37$, $P = 0.0006$; 20 μg/ml: $F_{(5, 48)} = 28.37$, $P < 0.0001$; 40 μg/ml: $F_{(5, 48)} = 28.37$, $P < 0.0001$; $F_{(5, 48)} =$ F7 495 28.37, $P = 0.4258$; oneway ANOVA) (Fig. 7).

rFgRab10 protein inhibits goat PBMCs proliferation

rFgRab10 protein at 20 μg/ml, 40 μg/ml and 80 μg/ml concentrations (but not at 10 μg/ml) significantly inhibited PBMCs proliferation compared with PBMCs treated with SUMO protein obtained from *E. coli* transformed with empty pET-SUMO vector (10 μg/ml: $F_{(5, 30)} = 140.5$, $P = 0.5720$; 20 μg/ml: $F_{(5, 30)} = 140.5$, $P < 0.0001$; 40 μg/ml: $F_{(5, 30)} = 140.5$, $P < 0.0001$; 80 μg/ml: $F_{(5, 30)} = 140.5$, $P < 0.0001$; one-way ANOVA) (Fig. 8).

3D modeling

The Protein Blast result showed that the rFgRab10 protein was very similar to Chain A, structure of Human Rab10, with an identity of 63%, an E-value of 3e-85, a Query cover of 90% and a Max score of 253. The human Rab10 protein is a 200 amino-acid protein, with a molecular mass of ~22.5 KDa and is annotated as Ras-related protein Rab10 (Uniprot ID: P61026). *De novo* rFgRab10 protein structure (Fig. 9) was similar to human Rab10 protein. Figure 10 shows the structure alignment of rFgRab10 protein to the human Rab10 protein, and Fig. 11 shows a 3D representation of both proteins at the same time: Chain A of Rab10 human protein (red) and rFgRab10 protein (blue), with the aligned region shown in yellow.

Protein interactions analysis

Interactome3D analysis detected 36 interactions between human Rab10 (P61026) and 13 other human proteins. All interactions with their respective total energy for the WildType (P61026 - human Rab10), Total Energy Mutant (rFgRab10 protein sequence aligned to P61026), and the difference of the previous values are provided in Additional file 1: Table S1. The protein interactions network (Fig. 12) showed that Rab proteins geranylgeranyltransferase component A 1 (CHM) and Rab proteins geranylgeranyltransferase component A 2 (CHML) had more stable interactions (red edges) with rFgRab10 protein compared to the human ortholog, whereas [F-actin]-monooxygenase MICAL3 (MICAL3) and guanine nucleotide exchange factor MSS4 (RABIF) had fewer stable interactions (blue edges) with rFgRab10 protein. These interacting partners were enriched in terms related to RabGTPase signalling, with Rab GDP-dissociation inhibitor activity (GO:0005093), Rab-protein geranylgeranyltransferase complex (GO:0005968) and protein geranylgeranylation (GO:0018344), being the overrepresented GO terms (Additional file 2: Table S2).

Discussion

To establish a persistent infection in their mammalian definitive host, liver flukes have developed sophisticated strategies to interfere with the host's immune response. In a recent study, we showed that rFg14-3-3e protein, another *F. gigantica* ESP, modulates several cellular and immunological functions of goat PBMCs [6]. In the

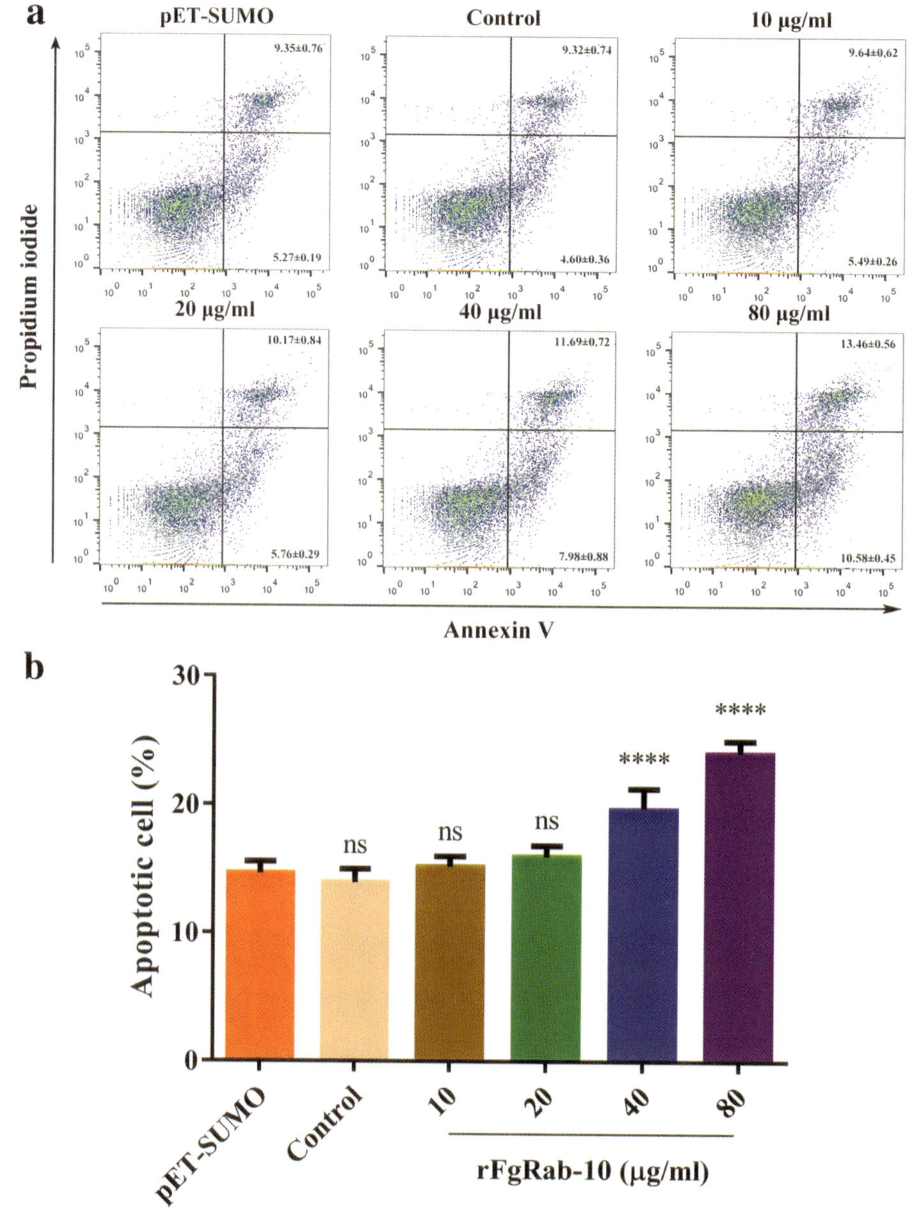

Fig. 5 rFgRab10 protein induced apoptosis in PBMCs. Annexin V/PI staining combined with flow cytometry analysis was used to count apoptotic cells. **a** Dot plots showing apoptosis of PBMCs in response to exposure to rFgRab10 protein. **b** Percentage of cell population was compared with plotted apoptotic cells (Annexin V+/PI-). Graphs represent means ± SD of data from three independent biological replicates. Asterisks indicate statistical significance between rFgRab10-treated, SUMO protein and sham-treated PBMCs (*****P* < 0.0001; ns, non-significant). The statistical significance was only achieved at the two highest concentrations (40 µg/ml and 80 µg/ml)

present study, the gene encoding Rab10 of *F. gigantica* was amplified by PCR, cloned, and expressed in a prokaryotic expression system. SDS-PAGE and Western blot analysis of the recombinant protein (rFgRab10) using sera from *Fasciola*-infected sheep revealed a molecular mass of ~23 kDa. rFgRab10 protein cross-reacted with anti-rFgRab10 antibody as indicated by specific binding of rFgRab10 protein to the surface of the PBMCs. Thus, it is reasonable to hypothesize that stimulation of goat PBMCs with rFgRab10 protein may interfere with several functions of PBMCs. Understanding the mechanisms of rFgRab10 interaction with PBMCs has important *in vivo* relevance for the definition of early events of the cellular responses to rFgRab10 released by liver flukes during infection. Therefore, we examined the influences of rFgRab10 protein on various functions of goat PBMCs. When incubated with PBMCs, rFgRab10 protein significantly (i) promoted the secretion of IL-2, IL-4, IL-10, TGF-β, and IFN-γ; (ii) increased the release of total NO from

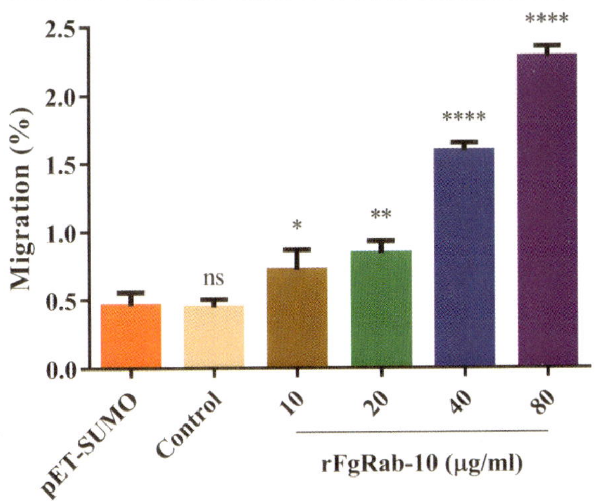

Fig. 6 rFgRab10 protein promoted goat PBMCs migration. PBMCs were treated with PBS, SUMO protein or serial concentrations of rFgRab10 protein and then the goat PBMCs migration percentage (%) was determined. Graphs represent means ± SD of data from 3 independent biological replicates. Asterisks indicate statistical significance between the different indicated groups (**P* < 0.05; ***P* < 0.01; *****P* < 0.0001; ns, non-significant)

PBMCs; (iii) stimulated goat PBMCs apoptosis and migration; and (iv) enhanced monocyte phagocytosis; but (v) inhibited PBMCs proliferation. Alterations of these functions in PBMCs may contribute to multiple aspects of *F. gigantica* pathogenesis.

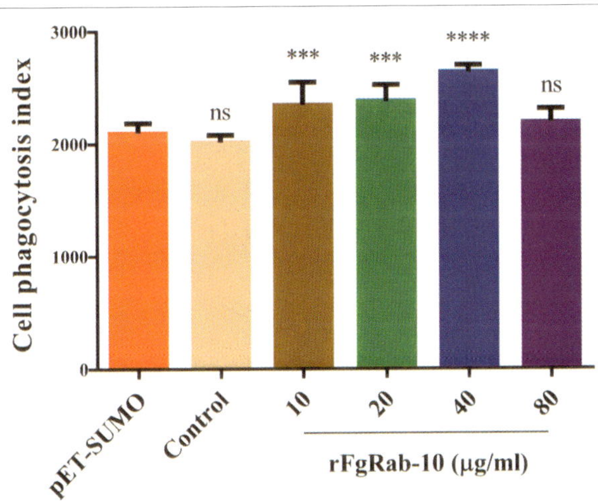

Fig. 7 rFgRab10 protein promoted phagocytosis of goat monocytes. rFgRab10 protein increased the phagocytic ability of goat monocytes as indicated by the increase in FITC-dextran uptake in goat monocytes treated with serial concentrations of rFgRab10 protein, compared with those treated with PBS or SUMO protein. Graphs represent means ± SD of data from three independent biological replicates. Asterisks indicate statistical significance between the different indicated groups (****P* < 0.001; *****P* < 0.0001; ns, non-significant)

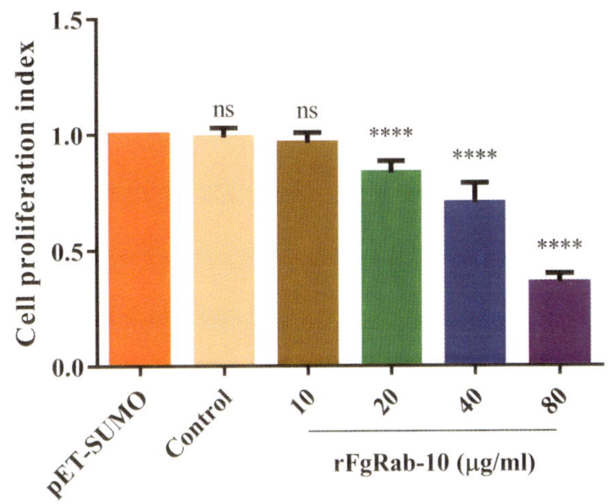

Fig. 8 rFgRab10 protein inhibited goat PBMCs proliferation. Goat PBMCs were treated with PBS, SUMO protein or serial concentrations of rFgRab10 protein and incubated for 48 h at 37 °C at 5% CO_2. Proliferation of goat PBMCs was determined using CCK-8 assay. Results indicated that rFgRab10 protein significantly inhibited PBMCs proliferation. Mean values and the respective standard deviation of three independent experiments are presented. Asterisks indicate statistical significance between the different indicated groups (*****P* < 0.0001; ns, non-significant)

Cytokines are produced by a variety of leukocytes and play many roles in maintaining immune homeostasis in the host [25, 26]. *Fasciola gigantica* infection can induce a mixed Th1/Th2 immune response [27, 28]. Our evaluation of the cytokine production [Th1 (IFN-γ and IL-2) and Th2 (IL-4, IL-10 and TGF-β)] in PBMCs culture supernatants showed that rFgRab10 protein can induce both humoral and cellular immune responses, confirming an earlier observation [27, 28]. Th1 cells secrete

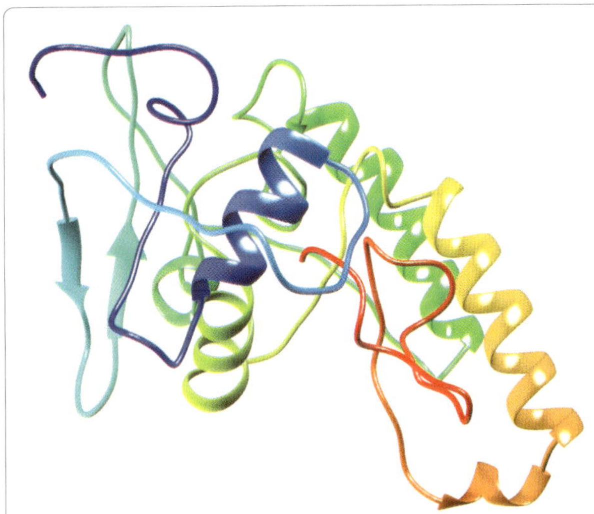

Fig. 9 *De novo* 3D *ab initio* model for rFgRab10 protein. The model was generated using Rosetta

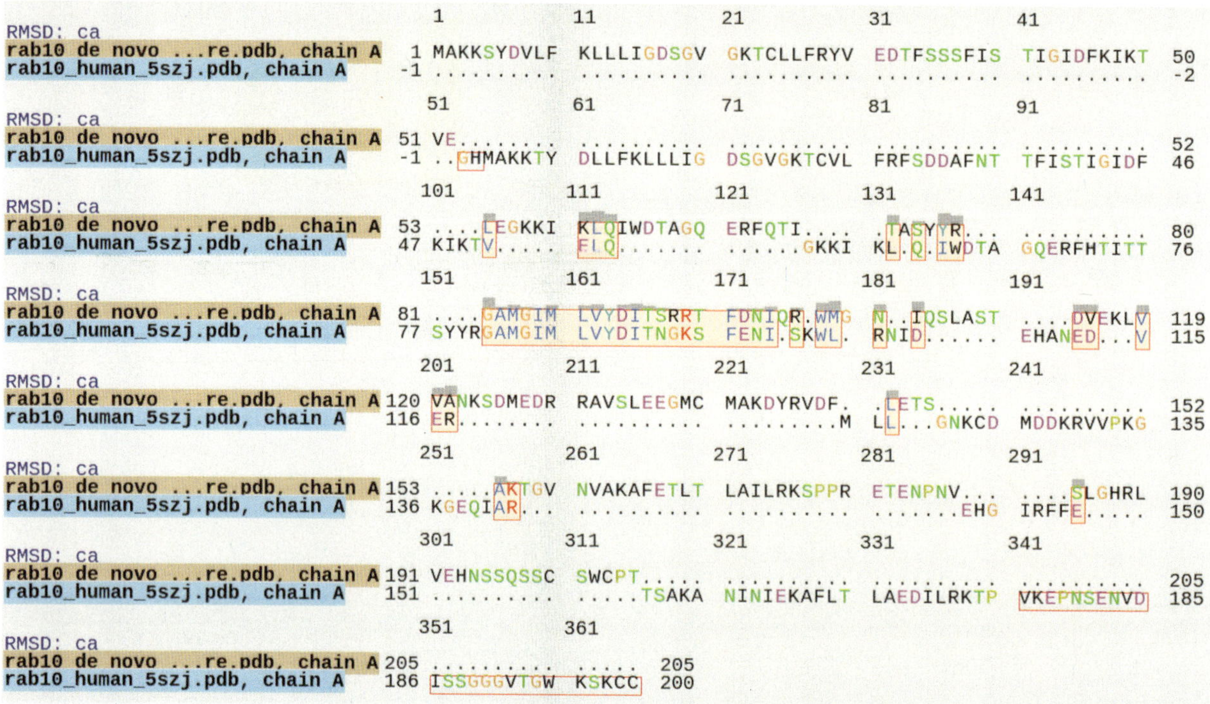

Fig. 10 The structure alignment of rFgRab10 to the human Rab10 protein. The predicted rFgRab10 model shared 63% similarity with the human Rab10 protein (Uniprot ID: P61026)

IFN-γ, which activates monocytes, thereby promoting the production of NO and phagocytosis [29], which may influence the development of the adaptive cellular immune response. Th2 cells secrete IL-4 to mediate humoral immunity and control helminthic infection [30] *via* the production of IgE by B cells, which can activate antibody-dependent killing of eosinophils, macrophages and mast cells [31–33]. Earlier studies indicated that apoptotic cells may participate in suppressing inflammatory responses through inducing the anti-inflammatory cytokines IL-10 [34, 35] and TGF-β [36, 37], which inhibit T-cell activation and differentiation [38]. Thus, reduced proliferation of rFgRab10-treated PBMCs is likely to be caused by cytokines IL-10 and TGF-β, released from apoptotic PBMCs.

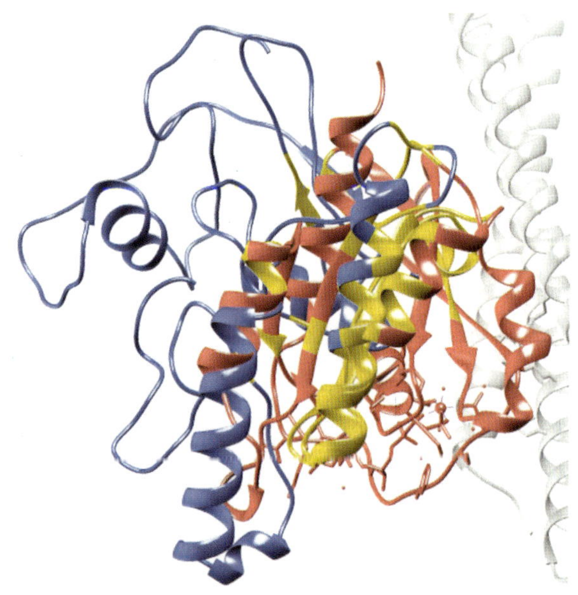

Fig. 11 3D representation of both rFgRab10 protein and human Rab10 protein: Chain A of human Rab10 protein (red) and rFgRab10 protein (blue), with the aligned region shown in yellow

Induction of apoptosis to prevent potentially harmful immune responses has been reported in macrophages and eosinophils exposed to *F. hepatica* ESPs [39, 40]. The same observation has been reported in peritoneal leucocytes of sheep experimentally infected with *F. hepatica*, and has been assumed to facilitate the juvenile flukes survival during the migration through the peritoneum to the liver [41]. *Fasciola hepatica* seemed to suppress the inflammatory response by inducing apoptosis in goat PBMCs [42]. Likewise, *F. gigantica* rFg14-3-3e protein significantly induced apoptosis in goat PBMCs [6]. In support of these findings, we have demonstrated the induction of apoptosis in goat PBMCs cultures following *in vitro* exposure to rFgRab10 protein. rFgRab10-mediated reduction in cellular proliferation and increased apoptosis of PBMCs seems to be mechanisms employed by *F. gigantica* to evade host immune defenses.

A previous study indicated that the intrinsic mitochondrial pathway and the extrinsic death receptor

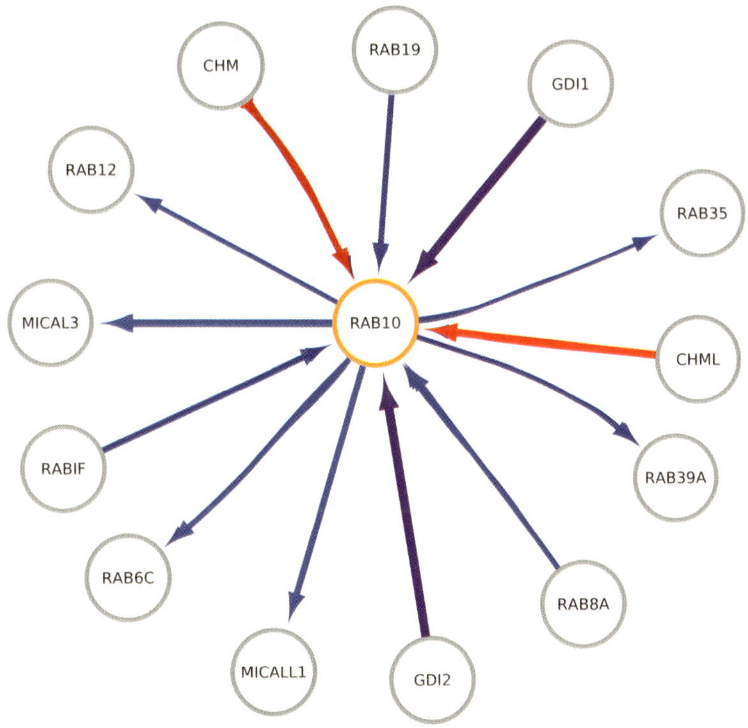

Fig. 12 The protein interaction network revealed more stable interactions, compared to the human ortholog Rab10, between Rab proteins geranylgeranyltransferase component A 1 (CHM) and Rab proteins geranylgeranyltransferase component A 2 (CHML) and rFgRab10 sequence (red edges); whereas fewer stable interactions were detected between [F-actin]-monooxygenase MICAL3 (MICAL3) and Guanine nucleotide exchange factor MSS4 (RABIF) proteins and rFgRab10 (blue edges)

pathway may impact *F. hepatica*-induced apoptosis in goat PBMCs [42]. However, apoptotic mechanisms may vary in response to different parasite effectors and the mechanism that underpins rFgRab10 protein-induced apoptosis remains unknown. The host immune system produces substances with oxidizing activities, such as NO, reactive oxygen species (ROS) and reactive nitrogen intermediates (RNI) in order to counter the parasite infection [43, 44]. NO can be released by a variety of immune cells, especially in response to IFN-γ stimulation [29, 45]. Our data show that rFgRab10 protein promoted the secretion of IFN-γ from PBMCs [46]. IFN-γ is a potent inducer of nitric oxide synthase 2 (Nos2) in a range of leukocytes, which converts l-arginine into l-citrulline and NO [47]. NO may therefore serve as a mediator of IFN-γ-induced cellular damage. Further studies are warranted to investigate the process by which rFgRab10 protein induces apoptosis in goat PBMCs.

Our bioinformatics analysis revealed 63% identity between rFgRab10 and human Rab10 protein (Uniprot ID: P61026). The diverse roles of rFgRab10 protein suggest that this protein functions through coordinated interactions with several regulatory partners. Thus, we used human Rab10 as an input to identify potential interactions of rFgRab10 protein with human proteins in major databases. Interactions identified between rFgRab10 and human proteins were of special interest. The protein interaction network revealed that Rab proteins geranylgeranyltransferase component A 1 (CHM) and Rab proteins geranylgeranyltransferase component A 2 (CHML) had more stable interactions with rFgRab10 protein, whereas [F-actin]-monooxygenase MICAL3 (MICAL3) and guanine nucleotide exchange factor MSS4 (RABIF) had fewer stable interactions with rFgRab10 protein. Host-parasite protein interactions are critical determinants in pathogenesis. Our study provides the first identification of host protein partners for rFgRab10 protein. Further understanding of the interactions existing between rFgRab10 and host proteins, and how the involved proteins interact, can advance our understanding of molecular mechanisms involved in *F. gigantica* infection and provide new opportunities for developing immunomodulatory therapies. We also performed GO enrichment analysis, which identified terms related to Rab GTPase signaling, with Rab GDP-dissociation inhibitor activity, Rab-protein geranylgeranyltransferase complex, and protein geranylgeranylation. These findings suggest that rFgRab10 can initiate signaling events to modulate various cellular immune functions that may have implications in *F. gigantica* pathogenesis.

Conclusions

To our knowledge, this is the first study to characterize the rFgRab10 protein and to illustrate that this protein, when incubated with goat PBMCs, modulates the cellular immune response, and enhances the release of NO, cell apoptosis, cell migration, and monocyte phagocytosis, but inhibits cell proliferation. The demonstration of the cross-reactivity of rFgRab10 protein with serum from infected animals, its binding to and interaction with goat PBMCs, and its influence on various cellular functions suggest that rFgRab10 protein plays various roles in the immunopathogenesis of fascioliasis. The immunomodulatory roles of rFgRab10 protein and its potential to influence the host-parasite equilibrium in the context of *F. gigantica* infection makes rFgRab10 a potentially good candidate for developing an immunomodulatory therapy for *F. gigantica* infection. Our study provided a "proof of concept" for clinical evaluation of the immunomodulatory roles of rFgRab10 protein in infected goats.

Abbreviations

BSA: Bovine serum albumin; cDNA: Complementary deoxyribonucleic acid; ELISA: Enzyme linked immunosorbent assay; ESPs: Excretory/secretory proteins; FBS: Fetal bovine serum; FITC: Fluorescein isothiocyanate; HRP: Horseradish peroxidase; IFA: Immunofluorescence assay; IFN-γ: Interferon gamma; IgG: Immunoglobulin G; IL-10: Interleukin 10; IL-2: Interleukin 2; IL-4: Interleukin 4; ITS: Internal transcribed spacer; LC-MS/MS: Liquid chromatography-tandem mass spectrometry; LPS: Lipopolysaccharide; MFI: Median fluorescence intensity; NO: Nitric oxide; PBMCs: Peripheral blood mononuclear cells; PBS: Phosphate-buffered solution; PI: Propidium iodide; PS: Penicillin-streptomycin; RNA: Ribonucleic acid; RT-PCR: Reverse transcription polymerase chain reaction; SD: Sprague Dawley; SD: Standard deviation; SDS-PAGE: Sodium dodecyl sulfate polyacrylamide gel electrophoresis; TBS-T: Tris-buffered saline containing 0.1% tween-20; TGF-β: Transforming growth factor beta

Acknowledgements

We thank Ms Rong Li for valuable technical help regarding the experiments.

Funding

The work was supported by a grant from the National Key Basic Research Program (973 Program) of China (Grant No. 2015CB150300) and by the Elite Program of Chinese Academy of Agricultural Sciences.

Authors' contributions

XQZ, XRL and HME conceived the idea, planned the experiments and critically revised the manuscript. ALT performed the experiments, analyzed the data and drafted the manuscript with the help of HME. MML, FKZ, XWT, WJW and SYH helped in the implementation of the study. GCM, EP and HME performed and interpreted the computational analysis. All authors read and approved the final manuscript.

Competing interests

The authors declare that they have no competing interests.

Author details

[1]State Key Laboratory of Veterinary Etiological Biology, Key Laboratory of Veterinary Parasitology of Gansu Province, Lanzhou Veterinary Research Institute, Chinese Academy of Agricultural Sciences, Lanzhou, Gansu Province 730046, People's Republic of China. [2]College of Veterinary Medicine, Nanjing Agricultural University, Nanjing 210095, People's Republic of China. [3]European Molecular Biology Laboratory-European Bioinformatics Institute, Wellcome Genome Campus, Hinxton CB10 1SD, UK. [4]College of Veterinary Medicine, Yangzhou University, Yangzhou, Jiangsu Province 225009, People's Republic of China. [5]Jiangsu Co-innovation Center for the Prevention and Control of Important Animal Infectious Diseases and Zoonoses, Yangzhou, Jiangsu Province 225009, People's Republic of China. [6]Faculty of Medicine and Health Sciences, School of Veterinary Medicine and Science, University of Nottingham, Sutton Bonington Campus, Loughborough LE12 5RD, UK.

References

1. Mas-Coma S, Valero MA, Bargues MD. Fascioliasis. Adv Exp Med Biol. 2014; 766:77–114.
2. Piedrafita D, Spithill TW, Smith RE, Raadsma HW. Improving animal and human health through understanding liver fluke immunology. Parasite Immunol. 2010;32:572–81.
3. Meemon K, Sobhon P. Juvenile-specific cathepsin proteases in *Fasciola* spp.: their characteristics and vaccine efficacies. Parasitol Res. 2015;114:2807–13.
4. Girones N, Valero MA, Garcia-Bodelon MA, Chico-Calero I, Punzon C, Fresno M, et al. Immune suppression in advanced chronic fascioliasis: an experimental study in a rat model. J Infect Dis. 2007;195:1504–12.
5. Khan MAH, Ullah R, Rehman A, Rehman L, Shareef APA, Abidi SMA. Immunolocalization and immunodetection of the excretory/secretory (ES) antigens of *Fasciola gigantica*. PLoS One. 2017;12:e0185870.
6. Tian AL, Lu MM, Calderón-Mantilla G, Petsalaki E, Dottorini T, Tian XW, et al. A recombinant *Fasciola gigantica* 14-3-3 epsilon protein (rFg14-3-3e) modulates various functions of goat peripheral blood mononuclear cells. Parasit Vectors. 2018;11:152.
7. Langsley G, van Noort V, Carret C, Meissner M, de Villiers EP, Bishop R, et al. Comparative genomics of the Rab protein family in Apicomplexan parasites. Microbes Infect. 2008;10:462–70.
8. Kremer K, Kamin D, Rittweger E, Wilkes J, Flammer H, Mahler S, et al. An overexpression screen of *Toxoplasma gondii* Rab-GTPases reveals distinct transport routes to the micronemes. PLoS Pathog. 2013;9:e1003213.
9. Clemens DL, Lee BY, Horwitz MA. Deviant expression of Rab5 on phagosomes containing the intracellular pathogens *Mycobacterium tuberculosis* and *Legionella pneumophila* is associated with altered phagosomal fate. Infect Immun. 2000;68:2671–84.
10. Alvarez-Dominguez C, Barbieri MA, Beron W, Wandinger-Ness A, Stahl PD. Phagocytosed live *Listeria monocytogenes* influences Rab5-regulated *in vitro* phagosome-endosome fusion. J Biol Chem. 1996;271:13834–43.
11. Okai B, Lyall N, Gow NA, Bain JM, Erwig LP. Rab14 regulates maturation of macrophage phagosomes containing the fungal pathogen *Candida albicans* and outcome of the host-pathogen interaction. Infect Immun. 2015;83:1523–35.
12. Islam MA, Große-Brinkhaus C, Pröll MJ, Uddin MJ, Aqter Rony S, Tesfaye D, et al. PBMC transcriptome profiles identifies potential candidate genes and functional networks controlling the innate and the adaptive immune response to PRRSV vaccine in Pietrain pig. PLoS One. 2017;12:e0171828.
13. Huang WY, He B, Wang CR, Zhu XQ. Characterisation of *Fasciola* species from Mainland China by ITS-2 ribosomal DNA sequence. Vet Parasitol. 2004;120:75–83.
14. Kim DE, Chivian D, Baker D. Protein structure prediction and analysis using the Robetta server. Nucleic Acids Res. 2004;32:W526–31.
15. Leaver-Fay A, Tyka M, Lewis SM, OF L, Thompson J, Jacak R, et al. ROSETTA3: an object-oriented software suite for the simulation and design of macromolecules. Methods Enzymol. 2011;487:545–74.

16. Pettersen EF, Goddard TD, Huang CC, Couch GS, Greenblatt DM, Meng EC, et al. UCSF Chimera - a visualization system for exploratory research and analysis. J Comput Chem. 2004;25:1605–12.
17. States DJ, Gish W. Combined use of sequence similarity and codon bias for coding region identification. J Comput Biol. 1994;1:39–50.
18. Orchard S, Ammari M, Aranda B, Breuza L, Briganti L, Broackes-Carter F, et al. The MIntAct project-IntAct as a common curation platform for 11 molecular interaction databases. Nucleic Acids Res. 2014;42:D358–63.
19. Szklarczyk D, Morris JH, Cook H, Kuhn M, Wyder S, Simonovic M, et al. The STRING database in 2017: quality-controlled protein-protein association networks, made broadly accessible. Nucleic Acids Res. 2017;45:D362–8.
20. Huttlin EL, Bruckner RJ, Paulo JA, Cannon JR, Ting L, Baltier K, et al. Architecture of the human interactome defines protein communities and disease networks. Nature. 2017;545:505–9.
21. Chatr-Aryamontri A, Oughtred R, Boucher L, Rust J, Chang C, Kolas NK, et al. The BioGRID interaction database: 2017 update. Nucleic Acids Res. 2017;45: D369–79.
22. Mosca R, Céol A, Aloy P. Interactome3D: adding structural details to protein networks. Nat Methods. 2013;10:47–53.
23. Schymkowitz J, Borg J, Stricher F, Nys R, Rousseau F, Serrano L. The FoldX web server: an online force field. Nucleic Acids Res. 2005;33:W382–8.
24. Berriz GF, King OD, Bryant B, Sander C, Roth FP. Characterizing gene sets with FuncAssociate. Bioinformatics. 2003;19:2502–4.
25. Sun B. T helper cell differentiation and their function. Adv Exp Med Biol. 2014;841:1–209.
26. Stenken JA, Poschenrieder AJ. Bioanalytical chemistry of cytokines - a review. Analytica Chimica Acta. 2015;853:95–115.
27. Kumar N, Raina OK, Nagar G, Prakash V, Jacob SS. Th1 and Th2 cytokine gene expression in primary infection and vaccination against *Fasciola gigantica* in buffaloes by real-time PCR. Parasitol Res. 2013;112:3561–8.
28. Changklungmoa N, Phoinok N, Yencham C, Sobhon P, Kueakhai P. Vaccine potential of recombinant cathepsinL1G against *Fasciola gigantica* in mice. Vet Parasitol. 2016;226:124–31.
29. Gazzinelli RT, Oswald IP, James SL, Sher A. IL-10 inhibits parasite killing and nitrogen oxide production by IFN-gamma-activated macrophages. J Immunol. 1992;148:1792–6.
30. Lacroux C, Nguyen TH, Andreoletti O, Prevot F, Grisez C, Bergeaud JP, et al. *Haemonchus contortus* (Nematoda: Trichostrongylidae) infection in lambs elicits an unequivocal Th2 immune response. Vet Res. 2006;37:607–22.
31. Schallig HD. Immunological responses of sheep to *Haemonchus contortus*. Parasitology. 2000;120:S63–72.
32. Moreau E, Chauvin A. Immunity against helminths: Interactions with the host and the intercurrent infections. J Biomed Biotechnol. 2010;2010:428593.
33. Alba-Hurtado F, Muñoz-Guzmán MA. Immune responses associated with resistance to haemonchosis in sheep. Biomed Res Int. 2013;2013:162158.
34. Voll RE, Herrmann M, Roth EA, Stach C, Kalden JR, Girkontaite I. Immunosuppressive effects of apoptotic cells. Nature. 1997;390:350–1.
35. Bzowska M, Guzik K, Barczyk K, Ernst M, Flad HD, Pryjma J. Increased IL-10 production during spontaneous apoptosis of monocytes. Eur J Immunol. 2002;32:2011–20.
36. Fadok VA, Bratton DL, Konowal A, Freed PW, Westcott JY, Henson PM. Macrophages that have ingested apoptotic cells *in vitro* inhibit proinflammatory cytokine production through autocrine/paracrine mechanisms involving TGF-beta, PGE2, and PAF. J Clin Invest. 1998;101:890–8.
37. Chen W, Frank ME, Jin W, Wahl SM. TGF-beta released by apoptotic T cells contributes to an immunosuppressive milieu. Immunity. 2001;14:715–25.
38. Taylor A, Verhagen J, Blaser K, Akdis M, Akdis CA. Mechanisms of immune suppression by interleukin-10 and transforming growth factor-beta: the role of T regulatory cells. Immunology. 2006;117:433–42.
39. Serradell MC, Guasconi L, Cervi L, Chiapello LS, Masih DT. Excretory-secretory products from *Fasciola hepatica* induce eosinophil apoptosis by a caspase-dependent mechanism. Vet Immunol Immunopathol. 2007;177:197–208.
40. Guasconi L, Serradell MC, Masih DT. *Fasciola hepatica* products induce apoptosis of peritoneal macrophages. Vet Immunol Immunopathol. 2012;148:359–63.
41. Escamilla A, Pérez-Caballero R, Zafra R, Bautista MJ, Pacheco IL, Ruiz MT, et al. Apoptosis of peritoneal leucocytes during early stages of *Fasciola hepatica* infections in sheep. Vet Parasitol. 2017;238:49–53.
42. Fu Y, Chryssafidis AL, Browne JA, O'Sullivan J, McGettigan PA, Mulcahy G. Transcriptomic study on ovine immune responses to *Fasciola hepatica* infection. PLoS Negl Trop Dis. 2016;10:e0005015.
43. Cervi L, Rossi G, Cejas H, Masih DT. *Fasciola hepatica*-induced immune suppression of spleen mononuclear cell proliferation: role of nitric oxide. Clin Immunol Immunopathol. 1998;87:145–54.
44. Colasanti M, Gradoni L, Mattu M, Persichini T, Salvati L, Venturini G, et al. Molecular bases for the anti-parasitic effect of NO (Review). Int J Mol Med. 2002;9:131–4.
45. Wandurska-Nowak E. The role of nitric oxide (NO) in parasitic infections. Wiad Parazytol. 2004;50:665–78.
46. Chen HY, Weng IC, Li CS, Wan L, Liu FT. Examination of galectins in phagocytosis. Methods Mol Biol. 2015;1207:201–13.
47. MacMicking J, Xie QW, Nathan C. Nitric oxide and macrophage function. Annu Rev Immunol. 1997;15:323–50.

3

Multiple paralogues of α-SNAP in *Giardia lamblia* exhibit independent subcellular localization and redistribution during encystation and stress

Shankari Prasad Datta[1], Kuladip Jana[2], Avisek Mondal[1,3], Sandipan Ganguly[4] and Srimonti Sarkar[1*]

Abstract

Background: The differently-diverged parasitic protist *Giardia lamblia* is known to have minimal machinery for vesicular transport. Yet, it has three paralogues of SNAP, a crucial component that together with NSF brings about disassembly of the *cis*-SNARE complex formed following vesicle fusion to target membranes. Given that most opisthokont hosts of this gut parasite express only one α-SNAP, this study was undertaken to determine whether these giardial SNAP proteins have undergone functional divergence.

Results: All three SNAP paralogues are expressed in trophozoites, encysting trophozoites and cysts. Even though one of them clusters with γ-SNAP sequences in a phylogenetic tree, functional complementation analysis in yeast indicates that all the three proteins are functionally orthologous to α-SNAP. Localization studies showed a mostly non-overlapping distribution of these α-SNAPs in trophozoites, encysting cells and cysts. In addition, two of the paralogues exhibit substantial subcellular redistribution during encystation, which was also seen following exposure to oxidative stress. However, the expression of the three genes remained unchanged during this redistribution process. There is also a difference in the affinity of each of these α-SNAP paralogues for GlNSF.

Conclusions: None of the genes encoding the three α-SNAPs are pseudogenes and the encoded proteins are likely to discharge non-redundant functions in the different morphological states of *G. lamblia*. Based on the difference in the interaction of individual α-SNAPs with GlNSF and their non-overlapping pattern of subcellular redistribution during encystation and under stress conditions, it may be concluded that the three giardial α-SNAP paralogues have undergone functional divergence. Presence of one of the giardial α-SNAPs at the PDRs of flagella, where neither GlNSF nor any of the SNAREs localize, indicates that this α-SNAP discharges a SNARE-independent role in this gut pathogen.

Keywords: α-SNAP, NSF, SNARE, Oxidative stress, Encystation, Functional divergence, Gene duplication

Background

Giardia lamblia is a gut pathogen that causes the diarrheal disease giardiasis. In addition, this protist serves as an excellent model to study how eukaryotic evolution has proceeded along different paths [1]. Studies show that the molecular machinery for multiple cellular processes of this protist are highly diverged compared to that present in most well-studied model eukaryotes [2]. Whether the differently-diverged cellular pathways of present-day *Giardia* results from early divergence from the main line of eukaryotic evolution or is a consequence of reductive evolution is still debatable. This divergence is particularly evident in the machinery for maintaining its endomembrane system, which is composed of fewer compartments compared to that present in most eukaryotes [2]. Besides the endoplasmic reticulum (ER), the only other identifiable endomembrane compartments are the small peripheral vesicles (PVs) that discharge both endosomal and

* Correspondence: srimonti@jcbose.ac.in
[1]Department of Biochemistry, Bose Institute, P 1/12 CIT Road Scheme VII M, Kolkata, West Bengal 700054, India
Full list of author information is available at the end of the article

lysosomal functions [3]. Thus, this parasite is an interesting model to study how vesicular trafficking proceeds in the backdrop of reduced endomembrane compartment diversity and uncovering the molecular machinery that supports this system is important to understand how life has evolved to use different approaches to address the same challenge.

The exchange of material between different endomembrane compartments takes place either through direct contact between the organellar membranes or *via* transport vesicles [4]. Such exchanges are very precise and sustained by a complex machinery whose molecular components include both proteins and lipids [5]. Vesicle-mediated exchange requires membrane deformation and vesicle budding from donor membrane, transport of these vesicles on the cytoskeletal network, followed by docking at the appropriate target membrane, and finally its fusion to the target membrane [6]. Proteins that ensure the fidelity of this process include: (i) the adapter protein (AP) complex and members of the Sar/Arf GTPases that selectively load appropriate cargo molecules into the budding vesicle and recruit the coat proteins at the donor compartment; (ii) the coat proteins (clathrin, COPI and COPII) that deform the membrane to form the vesicle; and (iii) the Rab GTPases, tether proteins and the SNAREs, which ensure that the vesicles only fuse to the appropriate acceptor compartment [7]. While tether proteins extend out from the acceptor membrane to "scout" for the correct vesicle and bring it closer, the SNAREs operate over a shorter distance and the formation of the *trans*-SNARE complex brings about the fusion between the membranes of the vesicle and acceptor compartment.

Different members of the SNARE proteins decorate the surfaces of various vesicles and also the target compartments. A *trans*-SNARE complex is formed when the SNARE on the incoming vesicle precisely pairs-up with the cognate SNAREs on the target membrane. This pairing enables the vesicle and target membranes to come close together such that they can fuse [8]. Following membrane fusion, the helical bundle of the newly-formed *cis*-SNARE complex is disassembled so that the SNAREs arriving on the incoming vesicle may be recycled back to the donor compartment. The strong intermolecular interactions within the *cis*-SNARE complexes are broken with the help of a protein complex, consisting of the AAA ATPase N-ethylmaleimide sensitive factor (NSF) and soluble NSF-attachment protein (SNAP), as the energy derived from ATP hydrolysis drives *cis*-SNARE uncoupling [9].

As previously mentioned, the machinery supporting the endomembrane system of *Giardia* is composed of fewer components. For example, instead of four, only two AP complexes have been identified in *Giardia*; in the tethering complexes, three components of both HOPS and TRAPP1, and two components of DSL1 were found to be missing [10, 11]. Only eight Rab GTPases have been identified in this protist, in contrast to the large repertoire of Rab members in other parasitic protists such as *Trichomonas* and *Entamoeba* [12–15]. Even the ESCRT machinery for endosomal sorting is composed of fewer components, with either entire complexes, such as ESCRT-I, being absent, or complexes being composed of fewer subunits, as in the case of ESCRT-II and ESCRT-III [16, 17].

Interestingly, there appear to be exceptions to this observed reduction of cellular machinery, as in the case of SNAPs. Many organisms, including mammals, have multiple paralogues of SNAPs, termed α-, β- and γ-SNAPs [18]. In mammals, while α- and β-SNAPs share a high degree of homology (> 80% identity), γ-SNAP shares only 20% identity with α-SNAP. Also, while both α- and γ-SNAPs are expressed in most tissues, expression of β-SNAP is restricted to the brain [19]. In addition, expression of α-SNAP commences in the developing embryo and continues into adulthood, but β-SNAP is expressed only after birth [19]. These SNAPs also discharge different cellular functions. α-SNAP is required for transport from ER to the Golgi, within the Golgi, homotypic vesicle fusion, store-operated calcium release and ER/endosome membrane fusion [20–22]. β-SNAP is functionally similar, except it has a different affinity for a binding partner, PICK1 [23]. γ-SNAP can stimulate the Ca^{2+}-dependent exocytosis but is unable to function in ER to Golgi transport [24, 25]. While most eukaryotes characterized thus far have only one copy of α-SNAP, two α-SNAPs have been reported in *Giardia* [26]. Here we report the presence of not two, but three SNAP genes in the *Giardia* genome. All the three genes were expressed in trophozoites, encysting trophozoites and cysts. The predicted secondary and tertiary structures of all the three proteins are similar to the yeast α-SNAP, Sec17, and all three giardial genes can rescue the growth defect of the *sec17-1* temperature-sensitive yeast mutant. Interestingly, there is a distinct difference in the subcellular distribution of all three paralogues. Apart from the anticipated localization at the cell periphery where many membranous compartments are present, two of the paralogues exhibit a dramatic change in subcellular distribution both during encystation and oxidative stress. This observed difference in subcellular distribution is indicative of the paralogues performing distinct functions in this protist.

Results

Giardia lamblia encodes three paralogues of SNAP

Given that SNAPs play pivotal roles in vesicle-mediated trafficking, we wanted to characterize the previously-reported putative giardial orthologues encoded by the

ORFs GL50803_17224 and GL50803_16521 [26]. This report also identified the ORF GL50803_10856 as a putative NSF. However, domain analysis in Pfam indicates that like the first two ORFs, the protein encoded by the last also contains a SNAP domain and consistently, GiardiaDB annotates it as an α-SNAP. To determine if the proteins encoded by these ORFs have the potential to function as SNAPs, we analyzed their sequence to determine their probable secondary structures. All characterized SNAP orthologues are small α-helical proteins, including the 292 residue-long *S. cerevisiae* orthologue, Sec17 [27]. The three putative giardial SNAPs are

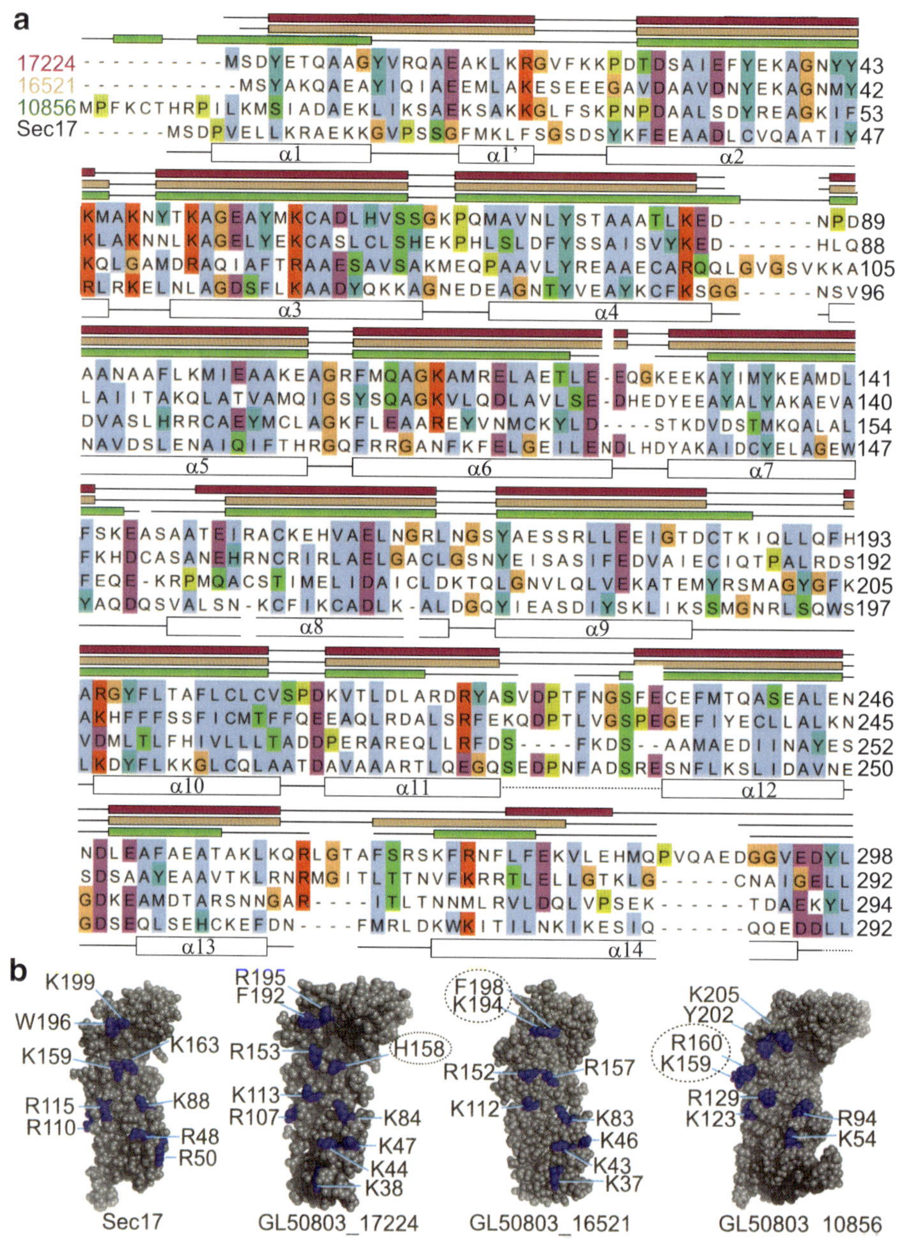

Fig. 1 Secondary structural elements and SNARE-binding residues of giardial SNAPs. **a** Sequence alignment of the putative giardial SNAPs with Sec17 of *S. cerevisiae*. α-helical regions of the Sec17 crystal structure (1QQE) have been marked with white boxes below the sequence alignment. The regions of the *Giardia* SNAPs that are predicted to be α-helical have been marked with colored boxes ($SNAP_{17224}$, cherry; $SNAP_{16521}$, fawn; $SNAP_{10856}$, green) above the alignment. Lines indicate loops regions and dashed lines denote the disordered regions in the Sec17 crystal structure. The discontinuity in boxes or lines correspond to gaps in the alignment. **b** Residues that may participate in SNARE binding. Residues, mostly carrying a positive charge (see text), which occupy positions comparable to those of the SNARE-binding residues of the *B. taurus* α-SNAP have been mapped in blue onto the concave face of the threading models of both yeast and *Giardia* SNAPs. Residues that deviate from those of the *B. taurus* α-SNAP, either in terms of charge (GL50803_17224) or position (GL50803_16521 and GL50803_10856), have been marked with dotted circles

comparable in size; while GL50803_17224 encodes 298 amino acids, GL50803_16521 and GL50803_10856 are composed of 292 and 294 amino acids, respectively. However, the three ORFs do not share extensive sequence homology; while the sequence of GL50803_17224 is 30.6 and 22.6% identical to GL50803_16521 and GL50803_10856, respectively, the remaining two ORFs share 21.6% identity. Secondary structure predictions indicate that all the three putative proteins are composed of α-helices and loops (Fig. 1a). This conclusion is independently supported by circular dichroism spectroscopy, which indicates that the percentage helicity of the three proteins is comparable to Sec17 (Additional file 1: Figure S1). Consistent with the crystal structure of Sec17, the three giardial proteins are predicted to have fourteen α-helices each (Fig. 1a) [27]. One notable difference is that while in the Sec17 crystal structure, the membrane-interacting hydrophobic patch, GFMKLF, adopts a short α turn (α-1'), the hydrophobic residues in the corresponding region of all the three putative giardial orthologues are located in an unstructured loop between helices α1 and α2 [28]. Thus, all the three giardial proteins are like Sec17 both in terms of their size and the secondary structure they are likely to adopt.

A previous report had identified residues on the SNARE-binding surface of the *Bos taurus* α-SNAP, of which all but one (Y200) were charged [29]. Perusal of the crystal structure of Sec17 showed that almost all the analogous positions are also occupied by similar residues, including W196 occupying a position comparable to Y200 (Fig. 1b). Given the low sequence identity of the three giardial proteins with known SNAP orthologues (Additional file 2: Tables S1 and S2), we wanted to determine their possible tertiary structures to see if similarly-charged amino acid residues occupy analogous positions on their surface as well. The possible tertiary structures of the three giardial proteins were determined using protein threading. While most positions on the modeled structures of the giardial SNAPs were occupied by residues analogous to those of the bovine α-SNAP, there were few exceptions: (i) in GL50803_17224, a histidine (H158) was present in place of a canonical arginine or lysine; (ii) there was an interchange of position between an aromatic (F198) and a positively charged residues (K194) in GL50803_16521; and (iii) two positively charged residues (K159 and R160) were shifted more towards the edge of the concave face in GL50803_10856 (dotted circles in Fig. 1b; Additional file 2: Table S3). Barring these minor variations, the pattern of distribution of the positively-charged residues was mostly conserved for all the three giardial proteins and Sec17, indicating that they are likely to be functionally analogous.

Existing literature documents that two of the three α-SNAP proteins, α-$SNAP_{17224}$ and α-$SNAP_{16521}$, are expressed in trophozoites and up to 14 h of encystation [30]. Reverse transcription PCR indicates that all the three identified genes are transcribed in trophozoites, encysting trophozoites (8 and 16 h following induction of encystation), and cysts (Additional file 1: Figure S2). Thus, the identified ORFs are not pseudogenes and the activity encoded by each is required in all stages of this parasite's life-cycle. Perusal of the genomes of the other *Giardia* isolates included in the GiardiaDB (assemblage A2 isolate DH, assemblage B isolate GS, assemblage B isolate GS_B and assemblage E isolate P15) indicates that each of these also encodes three putative α-SNAPs (data not shown). The presence of multiple α-SNAP paralogues in the genome of a unicellular protist that lacks diversity of endomembrane compartments is unusual given that most eukaryotic genomes encode only one orthologue of this protein; exceptions include *Arabidopsis thaliana*, which has two (Additional file 2: Tables S1 and S2) [31]. To determine if the identified sequences are α- or γ-SNAPs, we reconstructed a phylogenetic tree with known α- and γ-SNAP sequences from diverse taxonomic groups. Sequences of putative SNAP paralogues from the closely-related diplomonad, *S. salmonicida* and *Trepomonas* sp., were also included. From the tree topology, we observed that while two sets of sequences, one with GL50803_17224 and another with GL50803_16521 of the reference strain (assemblage A, isolate WB), cluster together with the α-SNAPs, the third set, with GL50803_10856, clusters closer to the γ-SNAPs (Fig. 2). *Trepomonas*, a close relative of *Giardia*, also contains three SNAP paralogues, of which two cluster with the γ-SNAPs and the third is within the α-SNAP cluster. Unlike *Giardia* and *Trepomonas*, *S. salmonicida* encodes only two putative SNAPs, of which one clusters with the α-SNAPs while the other with the γ-SNAPs. Based on this analysis, it appears that while two of the identified giardial sequences are likely to be α-SNAPs, the third may be a γ-SNAP.

It is known that α-, but not β- or γ-SNAP can substitute for Sec17 [18]. We used this criterion to evaluate if the identified giardial proteins are α- or γ-SNAP orthologues. Towards this, we used a mutant yeast strain having the temperature-sensitive *sec17-1* allele, which is functional at 30 °C but not at 37 °C [32]. We used functional complementation to assess if any of three giardial genes can functionally substitute for the *sec17-1* hypomorph. All three giardial genes were expressed in the *sec17-1* mutant under the control of a constitutive promoter. Expression of yeast's own *SEC17* gene from the same vector served as a positive control while yeast transformants containing just the vector backbone served as negative control (Fig. 3). All the five transformants exhibited equivalent growth at the permissive temperature of 30 °C. At the non-permissive temperature of 37 °C,

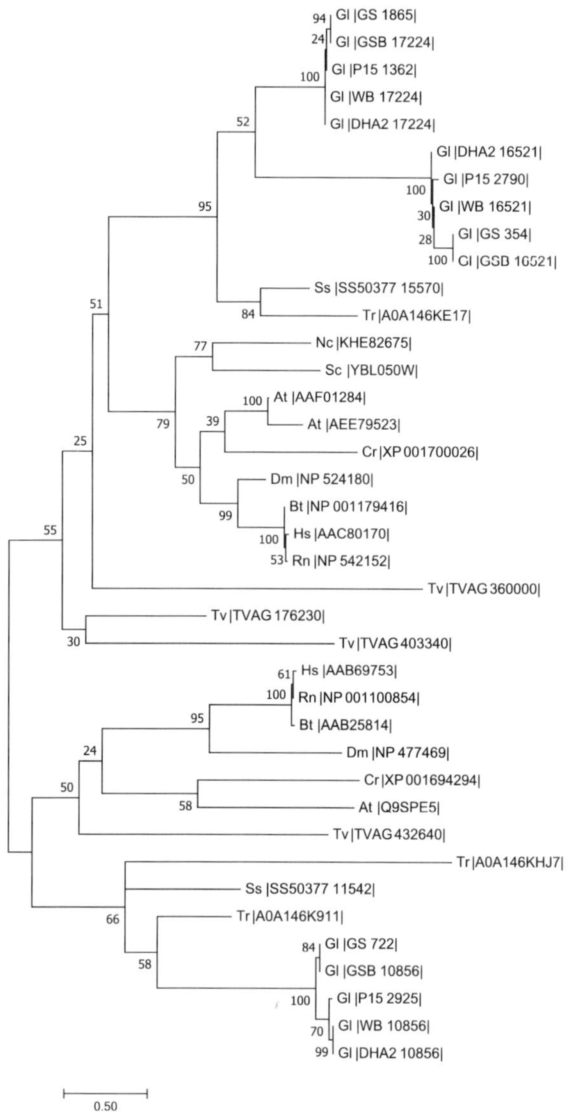

Fig. 2 Phylogenetic analysis of the putative SNAPs of *G. lamblia*. Sequences of α- and γ-SNAPs from diverse taxonomic groups, along with those from all five isolates of *G. lamblia* [assemblage A isolate WB (WB), assemblage A2 isolate DHA2 (DHA2), assemblage E isolate P15 (P15), assemblage B isolate GS (GS) and assemblage B isolate GS_B (GSB)] were used to reconstruct a phylogenetic tree using the Maximum Likelihood algorithm. The accession numbers for all homologs used in the analysis are listed next to the organism's name, while the numerical value next to each node of the phylogenetic tree indicates bootstrap values obtained from 100 replicates. The names of the organisms have been abbreviated as follows: Gl, *Giardia lamblia*; Tr, *Trepomonas* sp.; Tv, *Trichomonas vaginalis*; Ss, *Spironucleus salmonicida*; Nc, *Neurospora crassa*; Sc, *Saccharomyces cerevisiae*; At, *Arabidopsis thaliana*; Cr, *Chlamydomonas reinhardtii*; Dm, *Drosophila melanogaster*; Bt, *Bos taurus*; Hs, *Homo sapiens*; Rn, *Rattus norvegicus*. The scale-bar represents the number of amino acid substitution for each site

mutants expressing the plasmid-borne copy of *SEC17* exhibited robust growth while those transformants harboring just the vector backbone failed to grow at this non-permissive temperature (Fig. 3). Growth of yeast cells expressing any one of the three giardial genes was comparable to the positive control. Thus, the survival of the temperature sensitive *sec17-1* mutant expressing any of the three giardial genes at 37 °C indicates that even though one of the three SNAP sequences from *Giardia* clusters with γ-SNAPs, all these genes encode proteins that are functionally equivalent to Sec17 of yeast, which is an α-SNAP. Based on the results of this complementation analysis, we conclude that all the three SNAP proteins of *Giardia* are orthologous to α- and not γ-SNAP.

Unique subcellular localization of the three α-SNAPs indicate functional divergence

The presence of three putative α-SNAPs that are expressed in multiple stages of the parasite's life-cycle raises the possibility that these may have undergone functional divergence during the course of evolution. Thus, while one of them may be under strong selection pressure to discharge the essential functions of an α-SNAP, the other(s) may have been adapted to perform alternative functions. To investigate if such functional divergence has taken place, we wanted to determine the subcellular distribution of the three α-SNAPs. Towards this, we raised polyclonal antibodies against α-$SNAP_{17224}$ and α-$SNAP_{16521}$ in rabbit and against α-$SNAP_{10856}$ in mouse. Each of the polyclonal antibodies specifically detected only the corresponding protein that had been purified from *E. coli* as a band of ~34 kDa; none of them detected any of the other two α-SNAPs (Additional file 1: Figure S3a). Each antibody also detected a single band in *G. lamblia* trophozoite extract whose size corresponded to that predicted for the α-SNAPs of *Giardia* (Additional file 1: Figure S3a). Thus, in the absence of any observed cross-reactivity, it can be concluded that each antibody recognizes its target α-SNAP with a high degree of specificity. This also indicates substantial structural differences amongst these three proteins.

The polyclonal antibodies were used for immunolocalization of the three α-SNAPs in all the different stages of the parasite life-cycle in which their expression had been detected previously (Additional file 1: Figure S2). Given that all three genes can functionally complement the *sec17-1* temperature-sensitive allele (Fig. 3), it is expected that these proteins will be associated with vesicles and/or membrane compartments such as the ER. Consistently, a previous study has already reported the localization of α-$SNAP_{16521}$ to the PVs [33]. We observed that along with α-$SNAP_{16521}$, α-$SNAP_{10856}$ also localizes to the PVs as the signal for this protein colocalizes with that of the fluorescent dye Lucifer yellow, which is endocytosed and delivered to acidic compartments (Fig. 4a; Additional file

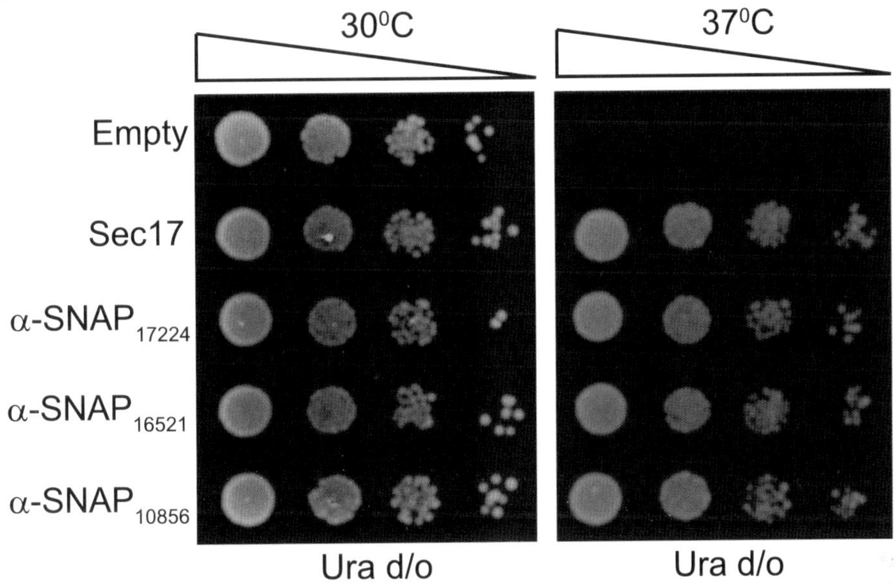

Fig. 3 Functional complementation of a temperature-sensitive α-SNAP mutant of yeast with the putative SNAPs of *Giardia*. Temperature-sensitive *sec17-1*mutant yeast strain (RSY269) was transformed with constructs expressing either *SEC17* (positive control) or each of the giardial SNAPs; transformants carrying the empty vector served as negative control. Transformants were spotted onto synthetic medium lacking uracil and incubated at either 30 °C (permissive temperature) or 37 °C (non-permissive temperature)

1: Figure S4a). α-SNAP$_{10856}$ also colocalizes with the PX domain-containing protein encoded by the ORF GL50803_16548, which is known to localize to the PVs (Additional file 1: Figure S4b) [34, 35]. Unlike the other two, α-SNAP$_{17224}$ localized to the anterior part of the cell, mostly around the two nuclei; another pool of the protein appeared to be cytoplasmic (Fig. 4a). This difference in the subcellular localization between α-SNAP$_{17224}$ and the two other α-SNAP paralogues indicates that the former performs a specific function that is different from that of the other two. Thus, there appears to be a functional divergence for at least one of the three α-SNAPs.

We observed additional evidence of such functional divergence in trophozoites undergoing encystation. While the pattern of localization of α-SNAP$_{10856}$ in trophozoites and encysting cells remained the same, that of the other two paralogues changed significantly (Fig. 4a). At 8 and 16 h after induction of encystation, α-SNAP$_{17224}$ still localized at the perinuclear regions, but its cytoplasmic distribution was no longer evident. Such a distribution persisted even after 30 h of induction (Additional file 1: Figure S5a). However, at 48 h post-induction, it was exclusively located at the PVs, with no signal at the perinuclear region (Fig. 4a; Additional file 3: Figure S9 and Additional file 2: Table S6). α-SNAP$_{16521}$ also underwent a change in cellular distribution during encystation, but this change was much more rapid compared to α-SNAP$_{17224}$. At 8 and 16 h post-induction, α-SNAP$_{16521}$ was present exclusively at the paraflagellar dense rods (PDRs), which are electron-dense structures that are associated with the anterior, caudal and posteriolateral flagella (Fig. 4a; Additional file 1: Figure S5b and c, Additional file 3: Figure S9 and Additional file 2: Table S6) [36]. This transition from the PVs to the PDRs starts as early as 1.5 h after the start of encystation as such cells exhibit both peripheral as well as distribution to the PDRs of the anterior and caudal flagella; complete redistribution of the signal appears to be completed by 4 h (Additional file 1: Figure S5b). The signal was more prominent at the PDRs of the anterior flagella, compared to that of the posteriolateral or caudal flagella. At the 48 h time-point, besides the signal at the PDRs, α-SNAP$_{16521}$ was also observed at the periphery of the ventral disc (Fig. 4a and Additional file 1: Figure S5d). This α-SNAP continued to associate with flagellar structures even in the tetranucleated cysts and also localized to cytoplasmic puncta (Fig. 4a). α-SNAP$_{17224}$ and α-SNAP$_{10856}$ also exhibited a similar punctate distribution in cysts, without any association with the flagella. These puncta are likely to be vesicles as many of these are also positive for the lipid-binding PX domain-containing protein mentioned above (Additional file 1: Figure S6). Although the change in the pattern of subcellular distribution during encystation is unique to each α-SNAP, the pattern of expression of the corresponding genes was very similar during this period. Real-time PCR indicated that the expression of all the three genes remained largely unchanged during encystation, with significant downregulation observed only in cysts (Fig. 4b, lower panel). The expression of the gene

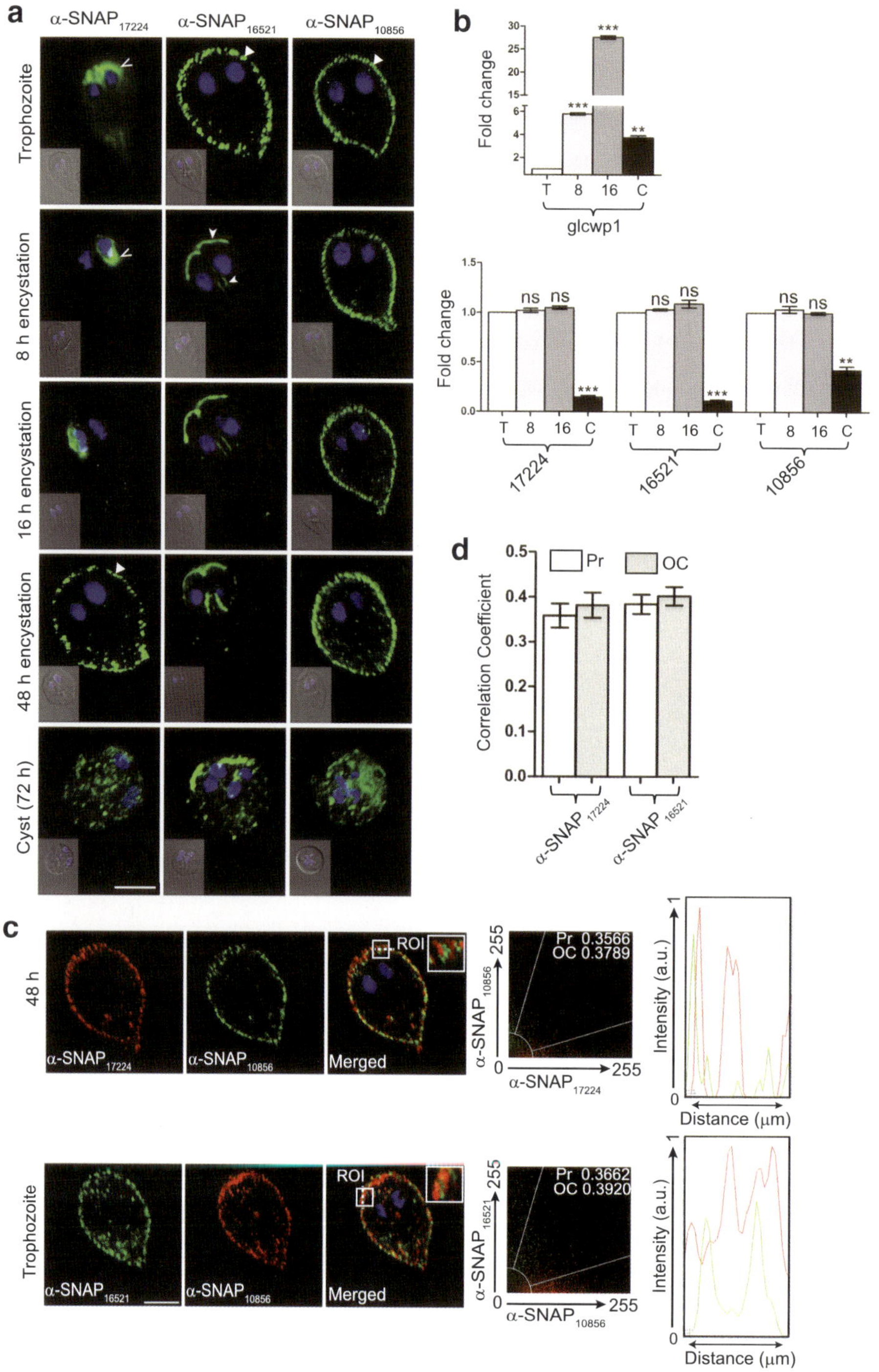

Fig. 4 (See legend on next page.)

(See figure on previous page.)
Fig. 4 Localization and expression of *Giardia* α-SNAPs in trophozoites, encysting trophozoites and cysts. **a** Immunofluorescence localization, with polyclonal antibodies, of α-$SNAP_{17224}$ (left column), α-$SNAP_{16521}$ (middle column) and α-$SNAP_{10856}$ (right column) in trophozoites, encysting trophozoites (8, 16 and 48 h post-induction of encystation) and cysts. The caret marks the perinuclear region, the arrowhead marks the PDR, and the triangle indicates PVs. To show the localization of α-$SNAP_{16521}$ at both the PDRs and the ventral disc periphery (48 h post-induction), the corresponding panel is an overlay of two z-sections (individual images of the z-stack shown in Additional file 1: Figure S5d). Inset depicts overlay of the DIC and DAPI images. **b** Expression of the α-SNAP genes in trophozoites, encysting trophozoites and cysts were determined by real-time PCR (lower panel), where the expression of CWP1 gene serves as a positive control (upper panel). The asterisks indicate the significance of the difference between the expression under a given condition with that in trophozoites (**$P < 0.01$; ***$P < 0.001$; ns, not significant). **c** Colocalization of α-$SNAP_{17224}$ and α-$SNAP_{10856}$ in 48 h encysting trophozoites (top row) or that of α-$SNAP_{16521}$ and α-$SNAP_{10856}$ in trophozoites (bottom row). Insets depict magnification of the region of interest (ROI) that has been marked with a white box. The scattergram in each row indicates the analysis of colocalization between the two fluorophores over the entire z-stack by considering all the pixels within the whole area occupied by that cell. The values for Pearson correlation coefficient (Pr) and overlap coefficient (OC) written inside the scattergrams. The intensity plots at the extreme right indicate changes in fluorescence intensity of the red and green signals across the dotted white line in the ROI. **d** Mean Pr and OC values for multiple z-stacks to determine the extent of colocalization of either α-$SNAP_{17224}$ or α-$SNAP_{16521}$ with α-$SNAP_{10856}$. *Scale-bars*: **a**, **c**, 5 μm

encoding CWP1 served as a positive control (Fig. 4b, upper panel) [37]. Such subcellular redistribution of proteins, without any change at the level of transcription, has been previously observed for other giardial proteins, such as β'COP subunit, Rab11, YiP, heavy chain of clathrin, DRP, ESCP and Rpn10 [13, 38–40]. Thus, many regulatory changes in this protist appear to be dependent on protein relocation, rather than synthesis of new proteins.

There are two situations in which two of the α-SNAPs exhibit a similar peripheral distribution in trophozoites or encysting trophozoites: (i) α-$SNAP_{16521}$ and α-$SNAP_{10856}$ in trophozoites and (ii) α-$SNAP_{17224}$ and α-$SNAP_{10856}$, 48 h post-induction of encystation (Fig. 4a). To determine if the two above-mentioned protein pairs colocalize, we carried out quantitative colocalization analysis for each pair under the conditions in which they exhibit similar cellular distribution. Scattergrams of multiple images of both the protein pairs did not indicate any substantial colocalization as the distributions of the green and red-colored pixels did not overlap significantly (Fig. 4c). Both the scattergram and the intensity plot of the two different fluorophores indicate that while there was some overlap for α-$SNAP_{16521}$ and α-$SNAP_{10856}$ in trophozoites, the same was not observed for α-$SNAP_{17224}$ and α-$SNAP_{10856}$, in encysting trophozoites (Fig. 4c). This is supported by colocalization analysis of multiple images wherein both the Pearson's correlation (Pr) and overlap coefficient (OC) values are below 0.5 for each protein pair (Fig. 4d). Incidentally, $SNAP_{16521}$ and α-$SNAP_{17224}$ never localize to the same subcellular region under any of the conditions tested (trophozoites, encysting trophozoites and cysts) (Fig. 4a). Given this lack of colocalization of the three α-SNAP paralogues, it may be concluded that there are functional differences among these three proteins.

All the α-SNAP paralogues colocalize with NSF

Even though all the three paralogues function as α-SNAP in yeast, they exhibit heterogeneity in terms of their localization in *Giardia*. This scenario may arise if one or more of these paralogues do not function as an α-SNAP. Since α-SNAP and NSF assemble into the functional 20S complex that brings about SNARE unwinding, we examined if the three paralogues colocalize with the giardial NSF (GlNSF), which is encoded by the ORF 50803_114776. Immunolocalization of GlNSF in trophozoites was performed with an antibody (raised in rat) that specifically recognized this protein in giardial protein extract (Additional file 1: Figure S3b). It was observed that GlNSF localized to the PVs and the "brush border" structures associated with the part of the anterior flagella that is proximal to the basal bodies (Fig. 5a) [41]. This distribution persisted in 48 h encysting cells, with the enhanced signal at the brush borders. While none of the α-SNAPs localized to the brush borders, all of them exhibit a peripheral distribution in either trophozoites or encysting trophozoites (Fig. 4a). Hence for colocalization of the α-SNAPs with GlNSF, conditions were chosen where each of the α-SNAPs exhibit a predominantly peripheral distribution, 48 h encysting trophozoites for α-$SNAP_{17224}$, trophozoites for α-$SNAP_{16521}$, and both trophozoites and encysting trophozoites (48 h) for α-$SNAP_{10856}$ (Fig. 5a). Under each of the conditions tested, all the three α-SNAPs showed significant colocalization with the GlNSF at the cell periphery, but not at the brush borders of the anterior flagella (Fig. 5a, Additional file 1: Figure S7). Both the Pr and the OC values indicate significant colocalization in multiple cells (Fig. 5b). Since all three α-SNAPs colocalize with GlNSF and each of them functionally complements the *sec17-1* temperature-sensitive allele (Fig. 3), it is likely that they function as α-SNAP in *Giardia*. Interestingly, barring α-$SNAP_{10856}$, the two other α-SNAPs and GlNSF localize to regions where there is no overlap of the SNAP and NSF signals. These include the perinuclear regions for α-$SNAP_{17224}$, the PDR for α-$SNAP_{16521}$, and the brush borders for GlNSF. Thus, it seems likely that in addition to functioning in the 20S complex, each of these proteins also discharges additional cellular function(s).

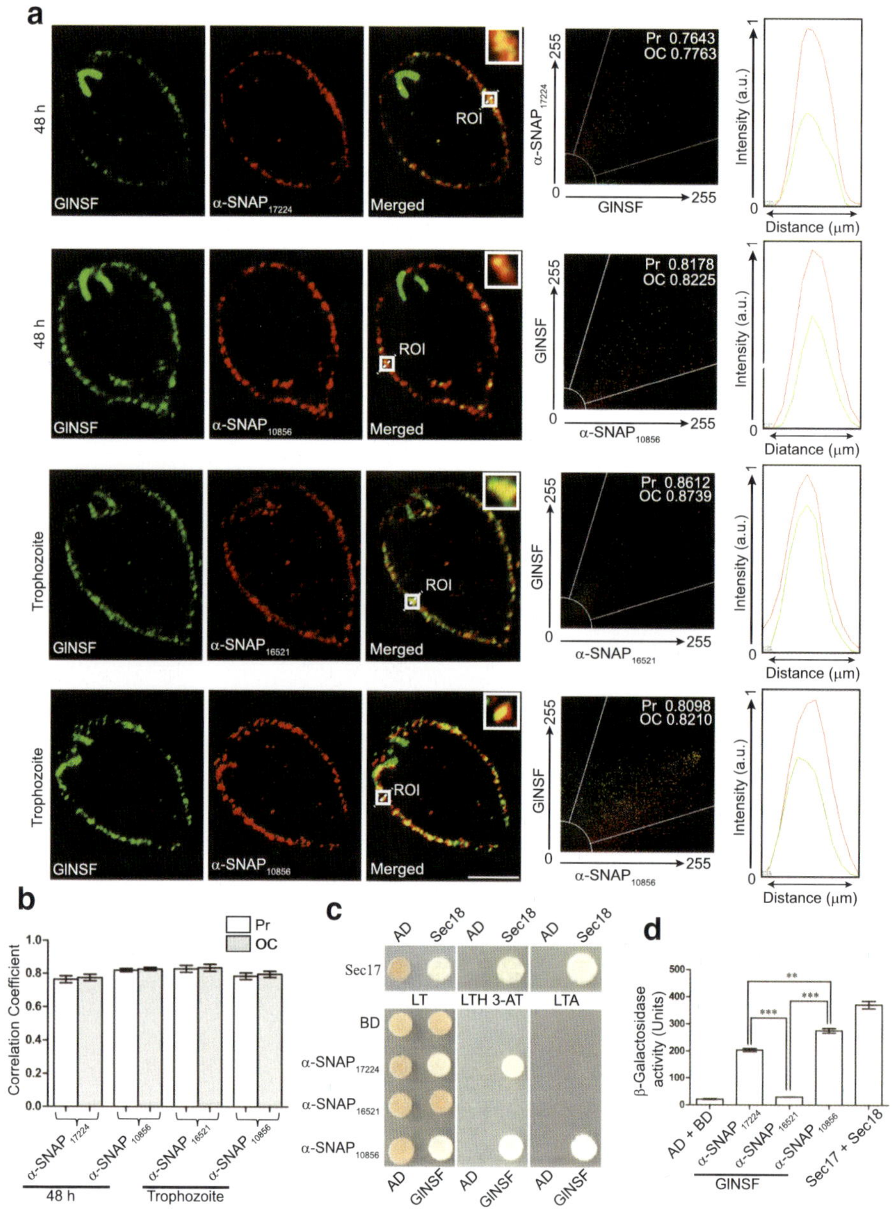

Fig. 5 Colocalization and binary interaction between GlNSF and the giardial α-SNAPs. **a** Colocalization of GlNSF with α-SNAP$_{17224}$ or α-SNAP$_{10856}$ in 48 h encysting trophozoites, and with α-SNAP$_{16521}$ or α-SNAP$_{10856}$ in trophozoites. Insets depict magnification of the ROI (marked with a white box). The scattergram in each row indicates the analysis of colocalization between the two fluorophores over the entire z-stack by considering the pixels within the entire area occupied by the particular cell. The values for Pearson correlation coefficient (Pr) and overlap coefficient (OC) are indicated inside the scattergrams. The intensity plots at the extreme right indicate changes in the intensity of the red and green fluorescence signals across the diagonal of the ROI depicted by a dotted white line. **b** The bar graph denotes the mean Pr and OC calculated from the z-stacks of six independent images. **c** PJ69-4A cells were transformed with various combinations of constructs expressing fusion proteins with either Gal4 DNA binding domain (BD) or its activation domain (AD). Expression of the BD or AD alone served as negative controls. Transformants were spotted on YCM plates lacking leucine and tryptophan (LT), or leucine, tryptophan and histidine with 2.5 mM 3-AT (LTH 3-AT), or leucine, tryptophan and adenine (LTA). **d** β galactosidase activity of the indicate transformants was quantified. Statistical significance of the difference in interaction between any two interacting pairs is indicated (**$P < 0.01$, ***$P < 0.001$). *Scale-bar*: **a**, 5 μm

Difference in the interactions between GlNSF and each of the three α-SNAPs

Given that the three α-SNAP paralogues colocalize with GlNSF, we wanted to test whether each of these three proteins is capable of directly interacting with the latter. We used yeast two-hybrid to assess this binary interaction (Fig. 5c). It is known that yeast Sec17 physically interacts with its own NSF (Sec18) [18]. Consequently, these two proteins exhibit strong interaction in our two-hybrid assay as cells co-expressing Sec17 from the bait vector (pGBT9 with *TRP1* selection marker) and Sec18 from the prey vector (pGAD424 with *LEU2* selection marker), exhibited robust growth, not only on plates lacking histidine (LTH 3-AT), but also on plates lacking adenine (LTA); in comparison to the former, the later selection medium imposes greater stringency as only cells harboring strongly interacting bait-prey pairs can grow in the absence of exogenously-added adenine [42]. Results of the spot assay indicated that the interaction between GlNSF and α-SNAP$_{10856}$ was comparable to that between Sec17 and Sec18 as yeast transformants expressing this giardial protein pair were able to grow on both LTH 3-AT and LTA plates (Fig 5c). However, estimation of the activity of the *LacZ* reporter gene, which provides a quantitative estimation of binary interaction, indicates that the interaction between the giardial proteins was weaker compared to that between the yeast proteins (Fig. 5d). Transformants expressing GlNSF and α-SNAP$_{17224}$ exhibited growth on LTH 3-AT, but not on LTA plates (Fig. 5c). Even the β-galactosidase activity indicates that this giardial α-SNAP's interaction with GlNSF was weaker compared to that between GlNSF and α-SNAP$_{10856}$ (Fig. 5d). However, there does not appear to be any interaction between GlNSF and α-SNAP$_{16521}$ as there is no growth on both LTA and LTH 3-AT plates. Even the color of the spot growing on plates lacking leucine and tryptophan (LT) is comparable to those of the negative control (Fig. 5c), as is the β-galactosidase activity of this transformant (Fig. 5d). Based on these observations there appears to be a lack of binary interaction between α-SNAP$_{16521}$ and GlNSF; however, we cannot rule out an interaction between these two proteins *in vivo* where additional cellular factors may stabilize this interacting pair. Taken together, the results of the yeast two-hybrid assay indicate that GlNSF interacts differentially with the three α-SNAPs, with the strongest interaction taking place with α-SNAP$_{10856}$, followed by that with α-SNAP$_{17224}$, and very little or no interaction with α-SNAP$_{16521}$. This observed difference in the interaction of the three paralogous proteins with GlNSF further underscores the fact that the three giardial α-SNAPs are likely to have undergone functional divergence in this protist.

Oxidative stress induced relocalization of α-SNAPs

Based on the observed relocalization of α-SNAP$_{17224}$ and α-SNAP$_{16521}$ during encystation, we hypothesize that change in subcellular distribution of these two α-SNAPs may be part of *Giardia*'s response to changes in the external environment. If this hypothesis is true, then similar changes may occur when cells encounter oxidative stress. We chose oxidative stress in particular because existing literature indicates that *Giardia* is likely to have a unique mechanism for handling this stress. Not only is *Giardia* unable to tolerate elevated oxygen levels, it lacks several key components that are used by most eukaryotes to detoxify cellular reactive oxygen species [43]. Thus, while *Giardia* lacks enzymes such as catalase, glutathione peroxidase, and superoxide dismutase, its defense against oxidative stress includes noncanonical enzymes like an NADH oxidase, an NADH peroxidase, and a flavodiiron protein, to name a few [44]. To investigate if the presence of multiple paralogues of α-SNAP may be a part of this organism's atypical mechanism to combat oxidative stress, we monitored the cellular distribution of these three proteins after inducing oxidative stress in trophozoites with two different agents, H_2O_2 (150 μM) and metronidazole (1 μg/ml) [45, 46]. Treatment with both reagents for a period of 1 h was sufficient to induce intracellular oxidative stress, as monitored by the conversion of DCFDA to the fluorescent DCF (Additional file 1: Figure S8). Following induction of oxidative stress, the relocalization of α-SNAP$_{17224}$ and α-SNAP$_{16521}$ was similar to that previously observed during the late stages of encystation (Compare Fig. 4a and Fig. 6; Additional file 3: Figure S10a and b, Additional file 2: Table S7). Thus, while α-SNAP$_{16521}$ relocalized from the cell periphery to the PDRs, the signal for α-SNAP$_{17224}$ moved from the perinuclear region to the cell periphery.

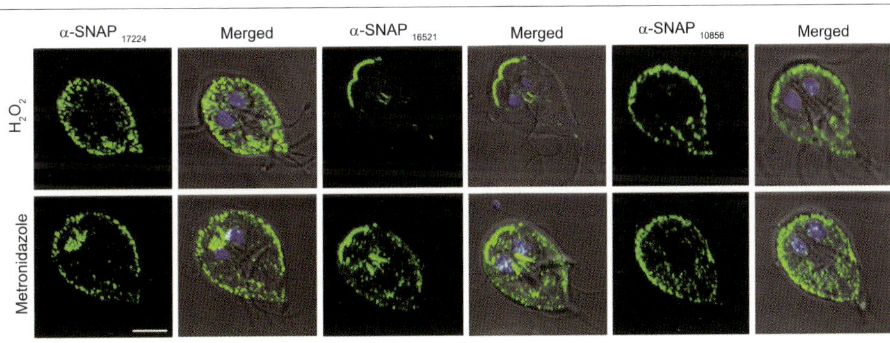

Fig. 6 Localization of giardial α-SNAPs following oxidative stress. Localization of the three α-SNAPs in trophozoites exposed for 1 h to either 150 μm H_2O_2 (top row) or 1 μg/ml metronidazole (bottom row). *Scale-bar*: 5 μm

However, unlike the change observed during encystation, a punctate cytoplasmic signal was also observed in both cases, with a cluster of puncta at the perinuclear region especially in case of α-$SNAP_{17224}$ (Fig. 6). Consistent with the observed lack of change in subcellular distribution during encystation (Fig. 4a), α-$SNAP_{10856}$ remained at the cell periphery even during oxidative stress (Fig. 6). However, like the other two α-SNAPs, cytoplasmic puncta were also observed in this case. Thus, in contrast to α-$SNAP_{10856}$, the change in the distribution of α-$SNAP_{17224}$ and α-$SNAP_{16521}$ during both encystation and oxidative stress indicates that these two paralogues may have acquired additional functions during the course of evolution.

Discussion

Although most eukaryotes encode only one α-SNAP, here we report that there are three paralogues in *Giardia*. These three genes are expressed in multiple morphological states of the parasite, thereby indicating that these three proteins are unlikely to discharge redundant functions in these different stages. Although α-$SNAP_{10856}$ clusters with γ-SNAP sequences in the reconstructed phylogenetic tree, the results of the complementation analysis clearly indicate that it is functionally orthologous to α-SNAP (Fig. 3). The presence of three functional α-SNAP paralogues in a unicellular organism appears to be in stark contrast to most multicellular eukaryotes having only one homolog. Interestingly, the presence of multiple SNAPs has been documented in 47 protist genomes, including those of *Trichomonas*, *Entamoeba*, *Naegleria*, *Trypanosoma* and *Leishmania* and *in silico* analyses indicate that some of these putative proteins may be γ-SNAPs [47] (Dirk Fasshauer, personal communication). We have identified two SNAP paralogues in *S. salmonicida* and three in *Trepomonas* (Fig. 2). Thus, the presence of multiple SNAPs seems to be the norm for protists. Given that Protista represents a paraphyletic group, it is not possible to ascertain if a single gene duplication event gave rise to the expansion of the SNAP family, or if there were multiple independent such events. However, the fact that there is a difference in the number of SNAPs in closely-related diplomonad species, two in *S. salmonicida* and three in both *Giardia* and *Trepomonas*, indicates that later duplication events have also contributed to the expansion of this family of proteins in Protista.

While the results of the complementation assay indicate that each of the three paralogues are functionally analogous to Sec17 of yeast, the distinct subcellular localization of each protein in *Giardia* indicates that they do not perform redundant functions. In addition, results of the two-hybrid assay indicate that GlNSF had varying affinity for the three α-SNAPs. Given that GlNSF binds to α-$SNAP_{10856}$ with the highest affinity, it may be hypothesized that the bulk of giardial *cis*-SNARE unpairing may be carried out by this paralogue. Its localization to the PV, where most of the SNAREs are present, lends support to this hypothesis [48]. Notably, this distribution does not change even during encystation, and after exposure to oxidative stress. Conversely, GlNSF has little or no interaction with α-$SNAP_{16521}$ and this paralogue relocalizes to PDR region where neither GlNSF nor the SNAREs are documented to be present, suggesting that NSF attachment may not be necessary for the function(s) this protein discharges at the PDR. However, since α-$SNAP_{16521}$ localizes to the PVs in trophozoites, its participation in SNARE complex disassembly cannot be ruled out.

One reason for the presence of such complexity in this unicellular protist may be the necessity to maintain *Giardia*'s asymmetric cell morphology. Unlike amoeboid protists, *Giardia* has a very unique tear-drop shape. The maintenance of this distinct asymmetric shape is likely to entail polarized vesicular trafficking to selective regions of the cell surface. However, the morphologically-simple endomembrane system of *Giardia* appears to lack key sorting stations, such as the Golgi. In the absence of readily-identifiable sorting compartments, *Giardia* may have evolved another system of determinants that allow selective targeting of vesicles to specific regions of the plasma membrane so that the shape of the cell is maintained. α-SNAP is already known to participate in such selective targeting in metazoans; it has been documented to enable polarized sorting to the apical surface of neuroepithelium as a single mutation causes missorting of apical proteins such as E-cadherin, β-catenin and F-actin [49]. The factors that play a role in giardial cell shape maintenance are difficult to trace as mutant hunts cannot be undertaken in this polyploid organism. Thus, it would be interesting to determine if there are any morphological changes following selective ablation of any one of these α-SNAPs.

The presence of α-$SNAP_{17224}$ and α-$SNAP_{16521}$ at cellular locations where NSF is not detectable is intriguing (Figs. 4a, 5a). One possibility is that α-SNAP may be performing NSF-independent functions at these locations. Existing literature indicates that α-SNAP has various NSF-independent roles [50]. An example of this is α-SNAP's involvement in regulating calcium uptake *via* calcium release activated calcium (CRAC) channels [22]. Hexameric assemblies of the Orai1 protein at the PM forms the CRAC channel pores and this assembly process is regulated by α-SNAP as its deficiency results in loss of calcium selectivity of the CRAC channels, leading to dysregulated entry of sodium into the cell [51]. In another instance, α-SNAP interacts directly with the Bcl-2 family member, BNIP1, which is known to regulate the morphology of the ER [52]. Incidentally, we have also observed enhanced α-$SNAP_{17224}$ signal at perinuclear regions, which are known to be occupied by the

ER (Fig. 4a). The distribution of α-$SNAP_{16521}$ at the PDRs is also indicative of a noncanonical role for this paralogue. Other proteins of *Giardia* with similar localization at the PDR include four proteins belonging to the Nek family of kinases (ORFs 5375, 92498, 16279 and 101534) and the catalytic subunits of protein phosphatase 2A (PP2Ac) and protein kinase A (PKAc) [53–55]. Nek proteins are documented to regulate ciliary function and assembly [56]. They also coordinate ciliary function with the cell cycle as they regulate the function of the centrioles, which serve both as basal bodies and microtubule-organizing centers [57]. Consistently, a study encompassing a large number of unikont and bikont organisms indicated that there is a direct correlation between the number of Nek genes encoded by a given genome and the presence of diving ciliated cell(s) in that particular organism [58]. *Giardia* has 56 active Neks, although its genome encodes 198; no other genome encodes such a large number of Neks and it is hypothesized that the expansion of this family of kinases is necessary to solve the challenges of coordinating the division of eight flagella with the cell cycle [58, 59]. Both PKAc and PP2Ac localize to the PDR in trophozoites [53, 54]. Since the signal for both proteins disappear simultaneously from the PDR of the anterior flagella early in encystation, it is postulated that they function in the same pathway in *Giardia* [53, 54]. PKAc is a known regulator of flagellar motility through its phosphorylation of dynein [60]. Thus, it is possible that since several other proteins that regulate flagellar function also localize to the PDRs, α-$SNAP_{16521}$ may play a similar role. The difference in the α-$SNAP_{16521}$ signal intensity at various PDRs may be because of differences in motility of each flagellar pair [61]. It may be noted that we have not detected the α-SNAPs at all the subcellular location where SNAREs of *Giardia* are known to localize [48]. For example, while gQb3 localizes to mitosomes, we have not observed similar distribution for any of the α-SNAPs. However, we cannot rule out the presence of a minor, and therefore undetectable, pool of any of the three α-SNAPs at other locations within the cell.

Conclusions

The present study has uncovered the presence of three paralogues of α-SNAPs in *G. lamblia*. Expression of these three genes during multiple morphological states of the protist indicates that the function of each of these three α-SNAPs is required by the cell. Thus, these must be performing non-redundant functions. Antibodies raised against each of these three proteins were used to determine their subcellular distribution during different stages of the parasite's life-cycle, and also upon exposure of the trophozoites to oxidative stress. These immunofluorescence experiments indicated a non-overlapping pattern of subcellular redistribution, without any accompanying change in the expression of the corresponding genes. In addition, two-hybrid assay established that these three paralogues have varying affinity for GlNSF. Taken together, it may be concluded that the three α-SNAP paralogues have undergone functional divergence in this protist. It was observed that α-$SNAP_{16521}$ localizes to the PDRs associated with the anterior, posterolateral and caudal flagellar pairs. Given that nither GlNSF nor any of the SNAREs localize to the PDRs, it is possible that this paralogue performs an NSF-independent function. Thus, following duplication of the α-SNAP genes of *Giardia*, there may have been neofunctionalization of some of the paralogues.

Methods

Sequence analyses and secondary structure predictions

The protein sequences of *Giardia* SNAPs were curated from GiardiaDB and secondary structure predictions were carried out using iterative threading assembly refinement (I-TASSER) and Protein Homology/analogY Recognition Engine (Phyre2) servers [62, 63]. By default, both approaches used the crystal structure of *S. cerevisiae* Sec17 (PDB ID: 1QQE) as a template [27]. Based on these predictions, the secondary structural elements were marked on the multiple-sequence alignment that was generated with ClustalW, with editing in Jalview [64, 65]. Three-dimensional automatic threading models were generated in I-TASSER server, with the crystal structure of Sec17 as a template. The conserved positively charged residues were marked in Pymol [66].

Phylogenetic analysis

Sequences of both α- and γ-SNAPs from organisms were curated using either NCBI (https://www.ncbi.nlm.nih.gov), UniProt (https://www.uniprot.org) or Eukaryotic Pathogen Database Resources (https://eupathdb.org) [67–69]. Domain analysis was performed with Pfam to ensure that the identified sequences contained a SNAP domain [70]. The curated sequences were used to reconstruct a maximum likelihood tree using MEGA7, with 100 bootstrap replicates [71].

Giardia lamblia culture and *in vitro* encystation

Trophozoites of Assemblage A isolate Portland-1 were grown in slanted 15 ml culture tubes containing Diamond TYI-S-33 medium (pH 6.8) and the encystation was carried out as previously described [72, 73]. In order to obtain a pure preparation of cysts, 72 h post-induction of encystation, cells were harvested and incubated in distilled water at 4 °C, for 24 h for selective lysis of trophozoites that did not undergo encystation.

Functional complementation

The temperature-sensitive strain RSY269 (MATα *ura3-52 his4-619 sec17-1*) was used for functional complementation [32]. *SEC17* and all the three *Giardia* α-SNAPs were PCR amplified with primers are listed in Additional file 2: Table S4. The PCR products were cloned under the control of a constitutive yeast promoter, in a 2 μm vector having *URA3* as a selectable marker (Additional file 2: Table S5). Each construct was individually transformed into RSY269. Resulting transformants were grown overnight in liquid YCM lacking uracil; serial dilutions of these cultures were spotted onto YCM plates lacking uracil and incubated at 30 and 37 °C.

Polyclonal antibodies against giardial α-SNAPs and NSF

Each of the three giardial α-SNAPs was expressed and purified from BL21 (DE3) as previously described, except 0.2 mM IPTG was used [17]. The N-terminal region of GlNSF was also induced with the same concentration of IPTG but was purified from the pellet fraction, as previously described [35]. The primers used for cloning in pET32a are listed in Additional file 2: Table S4. The purified proteins were used to raise antibodies against α-$SNAP_{17224}$ and α-$SNAP_{16521}$ in rabbit, against α-$SNAP_{10856}$ in mouse and against GlNSF in rat. All animal experiments adhered to the guidelines approved by the Institutional Animal Ethical Committee of Bose Institute (IAEC/BI/37/2015).

Immunofluorescence and quantitative colocalization analyses

Immunofluorescence was performed in trophozoites, encysting trophozoites (time of encystation indicated in respective figures) and cysts as previously described [40]. Briefly, cells were harvested by chilling the culture tubes on ice, followed by centrifugation at 1000× *g* for 10 min. After washing with 1× PBS, the cells were fixed with 4% formaldehyde for 20 min at room temperature (RT). Following fixation, cells were harvested by centrifugation and treated with 0.1 M glycine for 5 min at RT. Subsequently, trophozoites and encysting trophozoites were permeabilized with 0.1% Triton X-100 in 1× PBS (v/v) for 15 min, followed by blocking with 2% BSA for 2 h at RT. Cysts were permeabilized with 0.2% Triton X-100 and 0.1% SDS for 15 min, before blocking with 2% BSA. For labeling of all the four giardial proteins, the respective primary antisera were used at 1:50 dilution in 0.2% BSA and incubated for overnight at 4 °C, with shaking. The following day, cells were washed thrice with 1× PBS and incubated with 1:400 dilution of any combination of the following secondary antibodies, as per requirement: Alexa Fluor 488-conjugated goat anti-rabbit, Alexa Fluor 488-conjugated goat anti-mouse, Alexa Fluor 594-conjugated goat anti-mouse, Alexa Fluor 594-conjugated goat anti-rabbit and Alexa Fluor 488-conjugated goat anti-rat. All secondary antibodies were procured from Abcam (Cambridge, UK). Before washing away secondary antibodies, cells incubated with DAPI at 1 μg/ml concentration for 15 min. Finally, cells washed three times with 1× PBS and resuspended in antifade medium (0.1% *p*-phenylenediamine in 90% glycerol). Samples were imaged with the 63× objective of a confocal laser scanning microscope (Leica TCS SP8, Wetzlar, Germany). 3D deconvolution and colocalization analyses were performed with Leica Application Suit X and images were assembled with Adobe Photoshop CS3 and Adobe Illustrator CS3.

Statistical analysis

Statistical analyses for all the colocalization studies were performed with Leica Application Suit X (LAS X) software. The correlation coefficients, Pearson (Pr) and overlap (OC), values for each colocalization experiment were calculated on the basis of pixel-wise correlation between the signals emitted by the two fluorophores in each layer of six independent Z-stack. The Pr and OC values were plotted with GraphPad Prism 5.

Real-time PCR

cDNA preparation and real-time PCR was performed as previously described, with primers designed against unique regions of giardial α-SNAPs (Additional file 2: Table S4) [35, 40]. PCR condition was as follows: initial denaturation at 95 °C for 5 min, second denaturation at 95 °C for 30 s, and annealing for 20 s at 56, 64.5 or 65.8 °C for $SNAP_{17224}$, $SNAP_{16521}$ and $SNAP_{10856}$, respectively. The C_T values obtained for the three α-SNAP genes were normalized against the expression of ribosomal protein S5 (GL50803_12981), while the expression of the CWP1 gene served as positive control for encystation [37, 46]. Each experiment was performed in triplicate, with three technical replicates for each and data validation was done using two-tailed, paired t-test analysis in GraphPad Prism 5.

Yeast two-hybrid assay

Yeast two-hybrid assay was performed using full length NSF and α-SNAPs of both yeast and *Giardia*, which were cloned in pGAD424 (prey vector having *LEU2* marker) and pGBT9 (bait vector having *TRP1* marker), respectively (Clontech Laboratories, Mountain View, USA); the resulting fusion proteins had either the Gal4 activation domain (AD) or its DNA binding domain (BD), respectively (Additional file 2: Table S5) [74]. As per requirement, different pairs of the AD and BD constructs were co-transformed into the yeast strain PJ69-4A and the growth of each transformant, on YCM plates either lacking leucine, tryptophan and adenine

(LTA) or lacking leucine, tryptophan and histidine, but having 2.5 mM 3-AT (LTH 3-AT), was monitored following incubation at 30 °C for 2 to 3 days [75]. The binary interaction between the various NSF and α-SNAP orthologues were also measured quantitatively by assessing the β-galactosidase activity by determining the nmol of o-nitrophenol formed from the hydrolysis of ONPG per min per mg of protein [76]. For this assay, experiments were performed in triplicate with two technical replicates for each sample. Results were statistically validated using a two-tailed, paired t-test in GraphPad Prism 5 software.

Oxidative stress in *Giardia*

Trophozoites were grown to confluency. The old medium was replaced with freshly-prepared medium and cells were allowed to grow for another 2 h, prior to treatment with oxidative stress-inducing agents, either 150 μM H_2O_2 or 1 μg/ml metronidazole, for a period of 1 h, at 37 °C [45, 46]. To confirm intracellular ROS generation, cells were first harvested by chilling the tubes on ice, harvested by centrifugation at 1000× *g* for 10 min, washed thrice with warm PBS and treated with 2',7'-dichlorodihydrofluoresceine diacetate (H_2DCFDA) (Sigma D6883, St. Louis, USA) at a concentration of 1.5 μM, for 15 mins at 37 °C [45]. Finally, cells were fixed with 2% paraformaldehyde, washed thrice with PBS and observed under a confocal microscope.

Additional files

Additional file 1: Figure S1. Circular dichroism spectrum of giardial SNAPs. Far-UV circular dichroism spectra of the three giardial SNAPs, in 20 mM sodium phosphate buffer at 16°C. Predicted helicity percentage, calculated by using the BeStSel server (bestsel.elte.hu/), is indicated in each spectrum. Percent helicity of Sec17, calculated on the basis of the crystal structure of Sec17 (1QQE), is 73%. **Figure S2.** Expression of the putative SNAPs during the life cycle of *Giardia*. The expression of the three putative SNAP orthologues of *Giardia* were determined by reverse transcriptase PCR, using the cDNA prepared from trophozoites, encysting cells and cysts. The primers used for this analysis are given in Additional file 2: Table S4. PCR products were visualized on 1.2% agarose gel. The length of all the PCR products for each SNAP correspond to the expected size. **Figure S3.** Specificities of the antibodies for giardial α-SNAPs and NSF. **a** Western blot with trophozoite extract and each of the three purified giardial α-SNAPs. Expression and purification of the proteins have been described in the Experimental Procedures section. The 6xHis-tag was removed from all three proteins prior to western blotting. The upper blot was incubated with anti-α-$SNAP_{17224}$ antibody while the middle and lower blots were incubated with anti-α-$SNAP_{16521}$ and anti-α-$SNAP_{10856}$ antibodies, respectively. All antibodies were diluted 1000× prior to use. The presence of a ~34 kDa band in both the giardial extract and the corresponding overexpressed protein fraction in each blot indicates the specificity of that particular antibody. **b** Western blot with anti-GlNSF antibody using extracts of *Giardia* trophozoites and *E. coli* overexpressing GlNSF. Instead of the full-length protein, a stretch of 200-amino acids from the N-terminal segment of GlNSF was tagged with the 6xHis tag and expressed in *E. coli*. The expected size of this overexpressed protein is 39 kDa, while the size of the full-length GlNSF is 91 kDa. **Figure S4.** Localization of α-$SNAP_{10856}$ to peripheral vesicles. **a** Colocalization of α-$SNAP_{10856}$ with Lucifer yellow, a fluorescent dye that specifically stains acidic compartments, and, **b** a giardial PX domain-containing protein encoded by ORF GL50803_16548 and known to localize to the peripheral vesicles indicates that α-$SNAP_{10856}$ localizes to the peripheral vesicles of trophozoites. The scattergram in each row indicates the analysis of colocalization between the two fluorophores, over the entire z-stack, by considering all the pixels within the whole area occupied by that cell. The values for Pearson correlation coefficient (Pr) and overlap coefficient (OC) are indicated within the respective scattergrams. The intensity plot at the right in the lower panel indicates changes in fluorescence intensity of the red and green signals across the dotted white line drawn across the ROI. *Scale-bars*: **a**, **b**, 5 μm. **Figure S5.** Immunolocalization of α-$SNAP_{17224}$ and α-$SNAP_{16521}$ to various subcellular structures. **a** Localization of α-$SNAP_{17224}$ at the perinuclear region persisted after 30 h of encystation. The caret marks the perinuclear region. **b** α-$SNAP_{16521}$ is located both at the peripheral vesicles (PV) and the paraflagellar dense rods (PDRs) of different flagella at 1.5 h post induction of encystation. However, at 4 h post induction, α-$SNAP_{16521}$ is exclusively present at the PDRs, with no signal at the PVs. The triangle and arrow heads indicate PVs and the PDRs of different flagella, respectively. **c** Colocalization of α-tubulin (red) with α-$SNAP_{16521}$ (green) in 16 h encysting trophozoites. The red and green signals are juxtaposed to each other at the anterior flagella, without any significant overlap. Cells were visualized with Alexa Fluor 488 and Cy5-conjugated secondary antibodies that bind to rabbit anti-α-$SNAP_{16521}$ and mouse anti α-tubulin, respectively. **d** Two individual z-sections showing localization to the ventral disc periphery (left panel) and the PDRs (right panel). *Scale-bars*: **a**, **b**, **c**, **d**, 5 μm. **Figure S6.** Colocalization of α-$SNAP_{10856}$ and a PX-domain containing protein in cysts. Both α-$SNAP_{10856}$ and a PX-domain containing protein (GL50803_16548), a known lipid-interactor that localizes to vesicles, colocalize to cytoplasmic puncta in cysts. Carets mark some of the regions where there is considerable overlap of the red and green signals. The lower panels show regions of colocalization across the entire z-stack, with the left panel showing colocalization of the green signal (α-$SNAP_{10856}$) on red (GL50803_16548) and the right panel shows the opposite, i.e. red on green. The intensity plot at the extreme right indicates changes in fluorescence intensity of the red and green signals across the dotted white line in the ROI. The values for Pearson (Pr) and overlap (OC) coefficient are given in the scatter plot. *Scale-bar*: 5 μm. **Figure S7.** Localization of GlNSF and α-$SNAP_{16521}$. Localization of GlNSF (green) at the brush border (BB) and α-$SNAP_{16521}$ (red) at the paraflagellar dense rods (PDRs) in 48 h encysting trophozoites. Each of the two fluorescent images has been individually merged with the DIC image to show the distribution of the fluorescent signals w.r.t. the flagella. *Scale-bar*: 5 μm. **Figure S8.** Detection of intracellular reactive oxygen species (ROS) by H_2DCFDA. *Giardia* trophozoites were treated with either 150 μM H_2O_2 or 1μg/ml metronidazole for 1 h and intracellular ROS generation was monitored using H_2DCFDA. The top row shows untreated cells with no fluorescence signal of DCF. Green fluorescence signal was observed in cells exposed to oxidative stress, with either H_2O_2 (middle row) or metronidazole (bottom row) due to the formation of reactive oxygen species. *Scale-bar*: 5 μm. (PPTX 3310 kb)

Additional file 2: Table S1. α-SNAP orthologues throughout the eukaryotes. **Table S2.** γ-SNAP orthologues throughout the eukaryotes. **Table S3.** SNARE binding residues of bovine α-SNAP and residues at analogous positions on Sec17 and giardial SNAPs. **Table S4.** Primer sequences. **Table S5.** List of constructs. **Table S6.** Percentage of cells exhibiting relocalization of the various α-SNAPs in different stages of encystation. **Table S7.** Percentage of cells exhibiting relocalization of the various α-SNAPs under oxidative stress. (DOCX 43 kb)

Additional file 3: Figure S9. Total number of *Giardia* cells with desired localization of three different α-SNAPs (α-SNAP17224 and α-SNAP10856 at the PVs, and α-SNAP16521 at the PDRs of different flagella) under, (**a**) H_2O_2 (150 μM) or (**b**) metronidazole (1 μg/ml) stress were counted from five different fields. The "banned" sign indicates cells that were excluded from the final count, either due to absence of signal or because the cells were deformed. Cells where a given α-SNAP localized to the region other than the desired one, were marked with "cross" sign. *Scale-bar*: 25 μm. **Figure S10.** Total number of *Giardia* cells with desired localization of three different α-SNAPs (α-SNAP17224 and α-SNAP10856 at the PVs, and α-SNAP16521 at the PDRs of different flagella) under, (**a**) H_2O_2 (150 μM) or (**b**) metronidazole (1 μg/ml) stress were counted from five different fields. The "banned" sign indicates cells that were excluded from the final count, either due to absence of signal or because the cells were deformed. Cells where a given α-SNAP localized to the region other than the desired one, were marked with "cross" sign. *Scale-bar*: 25 μm. (PDF 14472 kb)

Abbreviations

3-AT: 3-amino-1,2,4-triazole; DAPI: 4′, 6-diamidino-2-phenylindole; DIC: Differential interference contrast; GlNSF: *Giardia lamblia* N-ethylmaleimide sensitive factor; NSF: N-ethylmaleimide sensitive factor; ONPG: Ortho-nitrophenyl-β-D-galactopyranoside; ORF: Open reading frame; PBS: Phosphate-buffered saline; PDR: Paraflagellar dense rod; PM: Plasma membrane; ROS: Reactive oxygen species; RT: Room temperature; SNAP: Soluble NSF attachment protein; SNARE: Soluble NSF attachment protein receptor; YCM: Yeast complete medium

Acknowledgments

We acknowledge Dr A. K. Sil for his valuable suggestions during the course of this study and also for critically reading the manuscript. We thank Professor Randy Schekman and Professor Peter Novick for providing yeast strains. We acknowledge the Central Instrumentation Facility of Bose Institute, Kolkata, India, for DNA sequencing and confocal imaging and thank its staff members A. Poddar and S. Ghosh-Chakraborty for imaging and S. Biswas for CD spectroscopy. We are thankful to Dr A. Ghosh for helping with database searches and Dr A. Banerjee of Leica Microsystems for providing technical assistance during image processing. We acknowledge the assistance of D. Samanta and P. P. Dey of the Centre for Translational Animal Research, Bose Institute. We thank Professor P. Chakrabarti and Dr A. K. Sil for allowing us to use their laboratory facilities. We also thank members of the Sarkar Laboratory, Bose Institute, Kolkata, India, for proofreading the manuscript and providing valuable comments.

Funding

This study was supported by funds provided by the Bose Institute, Kolkata, India. SPD received fellowship support from the INSPIRE programme of the Department of Science and Technology, Government of India (IF120153).

Authors' contributions

SPD and SS conceived the study. SPD and AM carried out the experiment. KJ raised the antibodies. SG participated in the study design, provided critical inputs and helped draft the manuscript. SPD and SS analyzed the data and drafted the manuscript. All authors read and approved the final manuscript.

Competing interests

The authors declare that they have no competing interests.

Author details

[1]Department of Biochemistry, Bose Institute, P 1/12 CIT Road Scheme VII M, Kolkata, West Bengal 700054, India. [2]Division of Molecular Medicine, Bose Institute, P 1/12 CIT Road Scheme VII M, Kolkata, West Bengal 700054, India. [3]Present Address: Section on Developmental Genetics, Eunice Kennedy Shriver National Institute of Child Health and Human Development, NIH, Bethesda, Maryland, USA. [4]Division of Parasitology, National Institute of Cholera and Enteric Diseases, P-33, CIT Road, Scheme XM, Beliaghata, Kolkata, West Bengal 700010, India.

References

1. Dacks JB, Field MC. Evolution of the eukaryotic membrane-trafficking system: origin, tempo and mode. J Cell Sci. 2007;120:2977–85.
2. Lujan HD, Svärd S. *Giardia*: A Model Organism. New York: Springer; 2011.
3. Lanfredi-Rangel A, Attias M, de Carvalho TM, Kattenbach WM, De Souza W. The peripheral vesicles of trophozoites of the primitive protozoan *Giardia lamblia* may correspond to early and late endosomes and to lysosomes. J Struct Biol. 1998;123:225–35.
4. Cooper GM, Hausman RE. The Cell - A Molecular Approach. 3rd ed. Washington DC: ASM Press; 2004.
5. Alberts B, Johnson A, Lewis J, Morgan D, Raff M, Roberts K, Walter P. Molecular Biology of the Cell. 6th ed. New York: Garland Science; 2014.
6. Bonifacino JS, Glick BS. The mechanisms of vesicle budding and fusion. Cell. 2004;116:153–66.
7. Cai H, Reinisch K, Ferro-Novick S. Coats, tethers, Rabs, and SNAREs work together to mediate the intracellular destination of a transport vesicle. Dev Cell. 2007;12:671–82.
8. Hong W. SNAREs and traffic. Biochim Biophys Acta. 1744;2005:493–517.
9. Söllner T, Whiteheart SW, Brunner M, Erdjument-Bromage H, Geromanos S, Tempst P, et al. SNAP receptors implicated in vesicle targeting and fusion. Nature. 1993;362:318–24.
10. Koumandou VL, Klute MJ, Herman EK, Nunez-Miguel R, Dacks JB, Field MC. Evolutionary reconstruction of the retromer complex and its function in *Trypanosoma brucei*. J Cell Sci. 2011;124:1496–509.
11. Touz MC, Rivero MR, Miras SL, Bonifacino JS. Lysosomal protein trafficking in *Giardia lamblia*: common and distinct features. Front Biosci Elite Ed. 2012;4: 1898–909.
12. Langford TD, Silberman JD, Weiland ME-L, Svärd SG, McCaffery JM, Sogin ML, et al. *Giardia lamblia*: identification and characterization of Rab and GDI proteins in a genome survey of the ER to Golgi endomembrane system. Exp Parasitol. 2002;101:13–24.
13. Marti M, Regös A, Li Y, Schraner EM, Wild P, Müller N, et al. An ancestral secretory apparatus in the protozoan parasite *Giardia intestinalis*. J Biol Chem. 2003;278:24837–48.
14. Saito-Nakano Y, Loftus BJ, Hall N, Nozaki T. The diversity of Rab GTPases in *Entamoeba histolytica*. Exp Parasitol. 2005;110:244–52.
15. Lal K, Field MC, Carlton JM, Warwicker J, Hirt RP. Identification of a very large Rab GTPase family in the parasitic protozoan *Trichomonas vaginalis*. Mol Biochem Parasitol. 2005;143:226–35.
16. Leung KF, Dacks JB, Field MC. Evolution of the multivesicular body ESCRT machinery; retention across the eukaryotic lineage. Traffic. 2008;9:1698–716.
17. Saha N, Dutta S, Datta SP, Sarkar S. The minimal ESCRT machinery of *Giardia lamblia* has altered inter-subunit interactions within the ESCRT-II and ESCRT-III complexes. Eur J Cell Biol. 2018;97:44–62.
18. Clary DO, Griff IC, Rothman JE. SNAPs, a family of NSF attachment proteins involved in intracellular membrane fusion in animals and yeast. Cell. 1990; 61:709–21.
19. Whiteheart SW, Griff IC, Brunner M, Clary DO, Mayer T, Buhrow SA, et al. SNAP family of NSF attachment proteins includes a brain-specific isoform. Nature. 1993;362:353–5.
20. Whiteheart SW, Kubalek EW. SNAPs and NSF: general members of the fusion apparatus. Trends Cell Biol. 1995;5:64–8.
21. Apodaca G, Cardone MH, Whiteheart SW, DasGupta BR, Mostov KE. Reconstitution of transcytosis in SLO-permeabilized MDCK cells: existence of an NSF-dependent fusion mechanism with the apical surface of MDCK cells. EMBO J. 1996;15:1471–81.
22. Miao Y, Miner C, Zhang L, Hanson PI, Dani A, Vig M. An essential and NSF independent role for α-SNAP in store-operated calcium entry. eLife. 2013;2: e00802.
23. Hanley JG, Khatri L, Hanson PI, Ziff EB. NSF ATPase and alpha-/beta-SNAPs disassemble the AMPA receptor-PICK1 complex. Neuron. 2002;34:53–67.
24. Morgan A, Burgoyne RD. A role for soluble NSF attachment proteins (SNAPs) in regulated exocytosis in adrenal chromaffin cells. EMBO J. 1995; 14(2):232–9.

25. Peter F, Wong SH, Subramaniam VN, Tang BL, Hong W. Alpha-SNAP but not gamma-SNAP is required for ER-Golgi transport after vesicle budding and the Rab1-requiring step but before the EGTA-sensitive step. J Cell Sci. 1998; 111(Pt 17):2625–33.
26. Rivero FD, Müller D, Lujan HD. Secretory events during *Giardia* encystation. In: de Souza W, editor. Structures and Organelles in Pathogenic Protists. Microbiology Monographs, vol 17. Berlin-Heidelberg: Springer; 2010. p. 195–225.
27. Rice LM, Brunger AT. Crystal structure of the vesicular transport protein Sec17: implications for SNAP function in SNARE complex disassembly. Mol Cell. 1999;4:85–95.
28. Winter U, Chen X, Fasshauer D. A conserved membrane attachment site in alpha-SNAP facilitates N-ethylmaleimide-sensitive factor (NSF)-driven SNARE complex disassembly. J Biol Chem. 2009;284:31817–26.
29. Marz KE, Lauer JM, Hanson PI. Defining the SNARE complex binding surface of alpha-SNAP: implications for SNARE complex disassembly. J Biol Chem. 2003;278:27000–8.
30. Faso C, Bischof S, Hehl AB. The proteome landscape of *Giardia lamblia* encystation. PLoS One. 2013;8:e83207.
31. Sanderfoot AA, Assaad FF, Raikhel NV. The *Arabidopsis* genome. An abundance of soluble N-ethylmaleimide-sensitive factor adaptor protein receptors. Plant Physiol. 2000;124:1558–69.
32. Kaiser CA, Schekman R. Distinct sets of SEC genes govern transport vesicle formation and fusion early in the secretory pathway. Cell. 1990;61:723–33.
33. Wampfler PB, Tosevski V, Nanni P, Spycher C, Hehl AB. Proteomics of secretory and endocytic organelles in *Giardia lamblia*. PLoS One. 2014;9:e94089.
34. Abodeely M, DuBois KN, Hehl A, Stefanic S, Sajid M, DeSouza W, et al. A contiguous compartment functions as endoplasmic reticulum and endosome/lysosome in *Giardia lamblia*. Eukaryot Cell. 2009;8:1665–76.
35. Jana A, Sinha A, Sarkar S. Phosphoinositide binding profiles of the PX domains of *Giardia lamblia*. Parasitol Int. 2017;66:606–14.
36. Elmendorf HG, Dawson SC, McCaffery JM. The cytoskeleton of *Giardia lamblia*. Int J Parasitol. 2003;33:3–28.
37. Mowatt MR, Luján HD, Cotten DB, Bowers B, Yee J, Nash TE, et al. Developmentally regulated expression of a *Giardia lamblia* cyst wall protein gene. Mol Microbiol. 1995;15:955–63.
38. Touz MC, Lujan HD, Hayes SF, Nash TE. Sorting of encystation-specific cysteine protease to lysosome-like peripheral vacuoles in *Giardia lamblia* requires a conserved tyrosine-based motif. J Biol Chem. 2003;278:6420–6.
39. Gaechter V, Schraner E, Wild P, Hehl AB. The single dynamin family protein in the primitive protozoan *Giardia lamblia* is essential for stage conversion and endocytic transport. Traffic. 2008;9:57–71.
40. Sinha A, Datta SP, Ray A, Sarkar S. A reduced VWA domain-containing proteasomal ubiquitin receptor of *Giardia lamblia* localizes to the flagellar pore regions in microtubule-dependent manner. Parasit Vectors. 2015;8:120.
41. Brown JR, Schwartz CL, Heumann JM, Dawson SC, Hoenger A. A detailed look at the cytoskeletal architecture of the *Giardia lamblia* ventral disc. J Struct Biol. 2016;194:38–48.
42. Kroetz MB, Hochstrasser M. Identification of SUMO-interacting proteins by yeast two-hybrid analysis. Methods Mol Biol. 2009;497:107–20.
43. Lloyd D, Harris JC, Maroulis S, Biagini GA, Wadley RB, Turner MP, et al. The microaerophilic flagellate *Giardia intestinalis*: oxygen and its reaction products collapse membrane potential and cause cytotoxicity. Microbiol. 2000;146(Pt 12):3109–18.
44. Brown DM, Upcroft JA, Upcroft P. Free radical detoxification in *Giardia duodenalis*. Mol Biochem Parasitol. 1995;72:47–56.
45. Raj D, Ghosh E, Mukherjee AK, Nozaki T, Ganguly S. Differential gene expression in *Giardia lamblia* under oxidative stress: significance in eukaryotic evolution. Gene. 2014;535:131–9.
46. Ma'ayeh SY, Knörr L, Svärd SG. Transcriptional profiling of *Giardia intestinalis* in response to oxidative stress. Int J Parasitol. 2015;45:925–38.
47. Kienley N. Phylogenetic studies of the vesicular fusion machinery. PhD Thesis, Georg-August-Universität, Göttingen; 2010. https://d-nb.info/1042305226/34.
48. Elias EV, Quiroga R, Gottig N, Nakanishi H, Nash TE, Neiman A, et al. Characterization of SNAREs determines the absence of a typical Golgi apparatus in the ancient eukaryote *Giardia lamblia*. J Biol Chem. 2008;283: 35996–6010.
49. Chae TH, Kim S, Marz KE, Hanson PI, Walsh CA. The hyh mutation uncovers roles for alpha Snap in apical protein localization and control of neural cell fate. Nat Genet. 2004;36:264–70.
50. Andreeva AV, Kutuzov MA, Voyno-Yasenetskaya TA. A ubiquitous membrane fusion protein alpha SNAP: a potential therapeutic target for cancer, diabetes and neurological disorders? Expert Opin Ther Targets. 2006;10:723–33.
51. Li P, Miao Y, Dani A, Vig M. α-SNAP regulates dynamic, on-site assembly and calcium selectivity of Orai1 channels. Mol Biol Cell. 2016;27:2542–53.
52. Nakajima K, Hirose H, Taniguchi M, Kurashina H, Arasaki K, Nagahama M, et al. Involvement of BNIP1 in apoptosis and endoplasmic reticulum membrane fusion. EMBO J. 2004;23:3216–26.
53. Abel ES, Davids BJ, Robles LD, Loflin CE, Gillin FD, Chakrabarti R. Possible roles of protein kinase A in cell motility and excystation of the early diverging eukaryote *Giardia lamblia*. J Biol Chem. 2001;276:10320–9.
54. Lauwaet T, Davids BJ, Torres-Escobar A, Birkeland SR, Cipriano MJ, Preheim SP, et al. Protein phosphatase 2A plays a crucial role in *Giardia lamblia* differentiation. Mol Biochem Parasitol. 2007;152:80–9.
55. Manning G, Reiner DS, Lauwaet T, Dacre M, Smith A, Zhai Y, et al. The minimal kinome of *Giardia lamblia* illuminates early kinase evolution and unique parasite biology. Genome Biol. 2011;12:R66.
56. Quarmby LM, Mahjoub MR. Caught Nek-ing: cilia and centrioles. J Cell Sci. 2005;118:5161–9.
57. Fry AM, O'Regan L, Sabir SR, Bayliss R. Cell cycle regulation by the NEK family of protein kinases. J Cell Sci. 2012;125:4423–33.
58. Parker JDK, Bradley BA, Mooers AO, Quarmby LM. Phylogenetic analysis of the Neks reveals early diversification of ciliary-cell cycle kinases. PLoS One. 2007;2:e1076.
59. Smith AJ, Lauwaet T, Davids BJ, Gillin FD. *Giardia lamblia* Nek1 and Nek2 kinases affect mitosis and excystation. Int J Parasitol. 2012;42:411–9.
60. Gaillard AR, Diener DR, Rosenbaum JL, Sale WS. Flagellar radial spoke protein 3 is an A-kinase anchoring protein (AKAP). J Cell Biol. 2001;153:443–8.
61. Lenaghan SC, Davis CA, Henson WR, Zhang Z, Zhang M. High-speed microscopic imaging of flagella motility and swimming in *Giardia lamblia* trophozoites. Proc Natl Acad Sci USA. 2011;108:E550–8.
62. Zhang Y. I-TASSER server for protein 3D structure prediction. BMC Bioinformatics. 2008;9:40.
63. Kelley LA, Mezulis S, Yates CM, Wass MN, Sternberg MJ. The Phyre2 web portal for protein modelling, prediction and analysis. Nat Protoc. 2015;10: 845–58.
64. Thompson JD, Higgins DG, Gibson TJ. CLUSTAL W: improving the sensitivity of progressive multiple sequence alignment through sequence weighting, position-specific gap penalties and weight matrix choice. Nucleic Acids Res. 1994;22:4673–80.
65. Waterhouse AM, Procter JB, Martin DMA, Clamp M, Barton GJ. Jalview Version 2 - a multiple sequence alignment editor and analysis workbench. Bioinformatics. 2009;25:1189–91.
66. DeLano WL. The PyMOL Molecular Graphics System. DeLano Scientific LLC, Palo Alto, CA, USA. 2002. https://www.pymol.org. Accessed 21 Feb 2018.
67. Wheeler DL, Barrett T, Benson DA, Bryant SH, Canese K, Chetvernin V, et al. Database resources of the National Center for Biotechnology Information. Nucleic Acids Res. 2008;36:D13–21.
68. Aurrecoechea C, Barreto A, Basenko EY, Brestelli J, Brunk BP, Cade S, et al. EuPathDB: the eukaryotic pathogen genomics database resource. Nucleic Acids Res. 2017;45:D581–91.
69. UniProt Consortium T. UniProt: the universal protein knowledgebase. Nucleic Acids Res. 2018;46:2699.
70. Punta M, Coggill PC, Eberhardt RY, Mistry J, Tate J, Boursnell C, et al. The Pfam protein families database. Nucleic Acids Res. 2012;40:D290–301.
71. Kumar S, Stecher G, Tamura K. MEGA7: Molecular Evolutionary Genetics Analysis Version 7.0 for Bigger Datasets. Mol Biol Evol. 2016;33:1870–4.
72. Diamond LS, Harlow DR, Cunnick CC. A new medium for the axenic cultivation of *Entamoeba histolytica* and other *Entamoeba*. Trans R Soc Trop Med Hyg. 1978;72:431–2.
73. Boucher SE, Gillin FD. Excystation of in vitro-derived *Giardia lamblia* cysts. Infect Immun. 1990;58:3516–22.
74. Fields S, Song O. A novel genetic system to detect protein-protein interactions. Nature. 1989;340:245–6.
75. James P, Halladay J, Craig EA. Genomic libraries and a host strain designed for highly efficient two-hybrid selection in yeast. Genetics. 1996;144:1425–36.
76. Nielsen DA, Chou J, MacKrell AJ, Casadaban MJ, Steiner DF. Expression of a preproinsulin-beta-galactosidase gene fusion in mammalian cells. Proc Natl Acad Sci USA. 1983;80:5198–202.

Echinococcus granulosus hydatid cyst location is modified by *Fasciola hepatica* infection in cattle

Caroll Stoore[1], Constanza Andrade[1], Christian Hidalgo[1], Felipe Corrêa[1], Mauricio Jiménez[1], Marcela Hernandez[2,3] and Rodolfo Paredes[1*]

Abstract

Background: Natural parasite infection occurs in wild and domestics animals with more than one parasite species at the same time, generating an infection called polyparasitism. Cystic echinococcosis reports are usually based only on infection with *Echinoccocus granulosus* leaving aside other internal parasitoses that could modulate both the immune response and pathogenesis of the natural infection. *Fasciola hepatica* is another cosmopolitan parasite in ruminants with a similar distribution to *E. granulosus* in different parts of the world, but no information of the effect of co-infection with *E. granulosus* has been described. The aims of this report were to establish *E. granulosus* prevalence and explore the association of *F. hepatica* co-infection and natural *E. granulosus* infections in cattle.

Results: From 1725 animals, the prevalence of *E. granulosus* and *F. hepatica* was 21.16 and 51.3%, respectively. Considering both infections, older cattle (> 4 years) presented higher prevalence compared to younger animals. In *E. granulosus*-infected cattle, 5.21% had fertile cysts, 71.78% infertile cysts, and in 23.01% cysts were smaller than 1 cm in diameter. Considering cyst location, 39.72% had lungs cysts, 24.72% had liver cysts and 36.94% had cysts in both organs. Cyst location significantly differed between age groups: 44.68% of younger animals had cysts only in the lungs, while older animals presented hydatid cyst in the lungs and liver simultaneously (44.15%). With *E. granulosus* infection alone, 30.26% of cysts were found in the lungs, 31.79% in the liver and 37.95% in both organs. Regarding the co-infection of *E. granulosus* with *F. hepatica*, the proportion was significantly different ($P < 0.05$) with most animals having cysts only in the lungs (49.41%) and a lower level of liver infection (15.88%). Analyzing organ cyst distribution and *F. hepatica* absence/presence ratio within each cyst type, small cysts showed the highest difference in ratio.

Conclusions: To the best of our knowledge, this is the first report indicating that *F. hepatica* co-infection in cattle could be affecting the instate of hydatid cysts in the liver, displacing toward lung localization, suggesting an antagonistic relationship.

Keywords: *Echinococcus granulosus*, *Fasciola hepatica*, Polyparasitism, Hydatid cyst localization

Background

Co-infection with different parasite species in the same host (also known as polyparasitism) is a well-documented fact in medical, veterinary and zoological literature. Most of the animals that live in the wild and humans of rural areas can be hosts of many concurrent parasite species [1]. However, the synergistic or antagonic relationship that different parasite species can have within the same host remains poorly studied [2]. Helminth parasites are a very diverse group of animals that are classified in four taxonomic groups: nematodes, trematodes, cestodes and acanthocephalans [3]. In cattle, two parasites usually represent a frequent infection: the cestode *E. granulosus* (*sensu lato*) and the trematode *F. hepatica*. *Echinococcus granulosus* (*s.l.*) has an indirect life-cycle, with ruminants as intermediate hosts, dogs and other canids as definitive hosts, and humans as dead-end

* Correspondence: rparedes@unab.cl
[1]Escuela de Medicina Veterinaria, Facultad de Ciencias de la Vida, Universidad Andres Bello, Santiago, Chile
Full list of author information is available at the end of the article

hosts [4]. The metacestode stage called hydatid cysts develops in the viscera (mainly lungs and liver) of the intermediate hosts [5], causing a disease known as cystic echinococcosis. *Fasciola hepatica* also has an indirect life-cycle; however, herbivores act as the definitive hosts, with the adult worms located in the bile ducts [6].

Echinococcus granulosus (*s.l.*) is composed of *E. granulosus* (*sensu stricto*) (genotypes G1-3), *E. equinus* (genotype G4), *E. ortleppi* (genotype G5), *E. canadensis* (genotypes G6-8/G10) and *E. felidis* ("lion strain"), with *E. granulosus* (*s.s.*) being the most commonly distributed worldwide [7].

Although *E. granulosus* (*s.l.*) is able to infect a wide range of mammalian hosts, the metacestode stage has a different capacity to produce protoscoleces, the stage infective to the definitive host. For unknown reasons, the parasite can, in some animals, produce protoscoleces inside the cyst, generating a fertile hydatid cyst, but other animals with cystic echonococcosis possess cysts without protoscoleces called infertile hydatid cysts [8, 9]. Since cyst fertility is associated with the size of the hydatid cyst [4], there is a subset of hydatid cysts that are too small to be classified as either fertile or infertile. The cellular and molecular mechanisms involved in the process of cyst fertility remain unknown [10]. In cattle, hydatid cyst fertility status ranges from 0 to 96% in different parts of the world [11–22] and infection with *F. hepatica* is common in many parts of the world. However, there are no studies on relationships between *E. granulosus* (*s.l.*) and *F. hepatica* in co-infections.

Although belonging to different higher-level flatworm taxa, both parasites exhibit common traits regarding their interaction with the mammalian host; as such, serum of animals infected experimentally with *E. granulosus* (*s.l.*) can recognize *F. gigantica* antigens in immunoassays [23] but there are no specific data on cross-reaction with *F. hepatica*. However, both parasites have the ability to uptake host glycolipids [6] which could explain the latter. Reports of polyparasitism involving *E. granulosus* (*s.l.*) are scarce. There is only one report that includes the interaction with *Schistosoma mansoni* (a trematode), where in murine models simultaneous concomitant infection lead to higher IFN-γ profiles, displaying a T_H1 response; however, adding *E. granulosus* infection seven weeks after *S. mansoni* infection led to significant lower IL-10 production, changing the immune profile to a T_H2 response [24]. Here, we provide the first report that in bovines infected with *E. granulosus* (*s.l.*), the presence of co-infection with *F. hepatica* is associated with changes in the hydatid cysts localization.

Methods

Sampling design

A total of 1725 cattle were examined for the presence of hydatid cyst and *F. hepatica* infection at *post-mortem* inspection in a Region Metropolitana slaughterhouse, Chile. In routine slaughtering, animals were individually identified, age and sex was recorded, and visceral organs of each animal, mainly the lungs and liver, were visually examined, palpated and incised along with official veterinarian inspectors for the presence of hydatid cysts and *F. hepatica*.

Fasciola hepatica diagnosis was made either by direct visualization of adult parasites in bile ducts, or by *F. hepatica* compatible lesions such as enlarged and thickened bile ducts, calcification of bile ducts, black parasitic material and black lymph nodes in the liver: signs of chronic *F. hepatica* infection.

Suspected cystic samples were removed from the infected organ, placed in separate polythene bags and transported in an isothermal container within 3 h to Universidad Andres Bello Veterinary School for further examination. For hydatid cysts confirmation and fertility determination, cysts were microscopically examined as previously described [25]. *Echinococcus granulosus* (*s.l.*) genotyping in hydatid cyst samples was determined as previously reported [26]. Briefly, DNA was extracted from fertile, infertile and small hydatid cysts from both livers and lungs. The *cox*1 mtDNA was amplified and sequenced, and a 345-nucleotide consensus sequence was used for comparison analysis.

Study groups

Animals were classified according to their age, hydatid cyst type and location. By age range, individuals were divided into two groups: 4 years-old or younger (≤ 4 years) and over 4 years of age (> 4 years). Cysts were classified into 3 types: small cysts (< 1 cm in diameter); fertile cysts (with protoscoleces); and infertile cysts (> 1 cm in diameter and without protoscoleces). Animals were also separated into 3 groups according to the location of the hydatid cysts: in lungs only; in liver only; and in both organs simultaneously. All groups were also separated by their *F. hepatica* co-infection status.

Data analysis

Data were recorded in an Excel 2010 datasheet and analyzed with RStudio IDE version 1.0.136 and R version 3.3.3 for statistical associations among variables using a Chi-square test. Logistic regressions were performed using STATA v.12 software (StataCorp, College Station, TX, USA). Statistical significance was considered when *P*-values were below the 0.05 threshold.

Results

Prevalence of *E. granulosus* and *F. hepatica*

Of the animals examined, 1217 were 4 years of age or under, and 508 were over 4 years-old. The overall prevalence of *E. granulosus* and *F. hepatica* was 21.16% (95% CI: 19.25–23.16%) and 51.3% (95% CI: 48.92–53.69%), respectively. For both parasites, older cattle (> 4 years-old) had a significantly

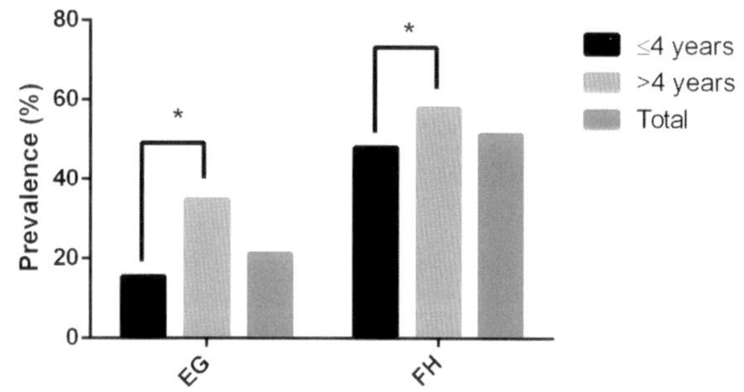

Fig. 1 *Echinococcus granulosus* (EG) and *Fasciola hepatica* (FH) overall prevalence per age group in inspected cattle (n = 1725). Data shown as percentage of infected/ total examined cattle in the respective categories. *$P < 0.05$ (Chi-square test)

higher prevalence than younger animals (≤ 4 years-old) (*E. granulosus*: χ^2 = 80.81, df = 1, $P < 0.0001$; *F. hepatica*: χ^2 = 12.56, df = 1, P = 0.0002) (Fig. 1). Separating co-infected animals, which represented 9.86% (n = 170) of the sampled population, *E. granulosus*-only infected cattle (n = 195, 11.3%) remains higher in older animals (χ^2 = 22.72, df = 1, $P < 0.0001$), as in co-infected cattle (χ^2 = 52.63, df = 1, $P < 0.0001$), but not in animals with *F. hepatica*-only infection (n = 715, 41.45%) where no significant difference between age groups was found (χ^2 = 0.4273, df = 1, P = 0.5133) (Table 1).

Hydatid cyst type, location and genotype

In *E. granulosus*-infected cattle, 5.21% (n = 19) had fertile cysts, 71.78% (n = 262) had infertile cysts, and in 23.01% (n = 84) cysts were smaller than 1 cm in diameter. Considering cyst location, 143 animals (39.72%) had cysts only in the lungs, 89 (24.72%) had cysts in the liver only and 133 (36.94%) had cysts in both organs simultaneously. A statistically significant difference was found regarding the location and type of the cysts (χ^2 = 66.32, df = 4, $P < 0.0001$). The majority of the animals with fertile cysts had these located in the lungs only (68.42%) whereas the majority of infertile cysts were located in both organs and small cysts were mainly located in the liver (Table 2). Of the recovered hydatid cyst samples, 47.95% (n = 175) were genotyped. Of these, 98.86% (n = 173) were identified as *E. granulosus* (*s.s.*) and only 1.14% (n = 2) were identified as *E. ortleppi.*

Association of hydatid cyst characteristics with animal age and co-infection with *F. hepatica*

As shown in Fig. 2a, hydatid cyst location significantly differed between age groups (χ^2 = 16.30, df = 2, P = 0.0003), where the highest percentage of younger animals had cysts only in the lungs (44.68%) while the largest portion of older animals had cysts in the liver and lungs simultaneously (44.15%). Hydatid cyst in animals lacking *F. hepatica* were present in only the lungs of 30.26% of infected cattle, 31.79% had the cysts in the liver only and 37.95% in both organs. However, in the presence of concomitant *F. hepatica* infection, the proportion was significantly different (χ^2 = 18.20, df = 2, P = 0.0001) with a higher percentage of animals with cysts only in the lungs (49.41%) and a lower percentage with hydatid cysts only in the liver (15.88%) and 34.71% of animals with both organs simultaneously affected (Fig. 2b). Within animals lacking *F. hepatica* co-infection, no association between location and age group (χ^2 = 5.065, df = 2, P = 0.0795) or significant variation within each age group was observed (≤ 4 years: χ^2 = 0.1800, df = 2, P = 0.9139; > 4 years: χ^2 = 5.070, df = 2, P = 0.0793) (Fig. 2c). However, in co-infected animals, cyst location was associated with age (χ^2 = 14.16, df = 2, P = 0.0008) and varied within each age group (≤ 4 years: χ^2 = 15.38, df = 2, P = 0.0005; > 4 years: χ^2 = 17.24, df = 2, P = 0.0002) (Fig. 2d). Specifically, in *E. granulosus* (*s.s.*)-infected animals, cyst location also significantly varied with *F. hepatica* co-infection (χ^2 = 6.841, df = 2, P = 0.0327) but not with age (χ^2 = 5.674, df = 2, P = 0.0586). Location in host varied only in animals co-infected with *F. hepatica* (χ^2 = 6.209, df = 2, P = 0.0448) (Table 3).

No general association was found between cyst type and the age range of animals (χ^2 = 1.452, df = 2, P = 0.4838) or co-infection with *F. hepatica* (χ^2 = 1.64, df = 2, P = 0.4405). Conversely, the co-infection ratio (absence/presence of *F. hepatica* co-infection) of animals with infertile cysts was significantly higher in young animals (1.14, 76/54) than in older cattle (0.81, 59/73) (χ^2 = 4.968, df = 1, P = 0.0258), while in the latter group there were fewer animals with small (< 1 cm) cysts in the presence of the co-infection than in the absence (24/12), resulting in a statistical association between cyst type and co-infection in this age group (χ^2 = 6.349, df = 2, P = 0.0418). In animals with small hydatid cysts, *E. granulosus*-affected organs significantly varied with *F. hepatica* co-infection (χ^2 = 19.45, df = 2, $P < 0.0001$),

Table 1 *Echinococcus granulosus, Fasciola hepatica* and co-infection prevalence, per age range classification of slaughtered cattle

	Examined	EG only			FH only			EG and FH co-infected		
	N	*n*	%	95% CI	*n*	%	95% CI	*n*	%	95% CI
Overall	1725	195	11.30	9.90–12.89	715	41.45	39.15–43.79	170	9.86	8.54–11.35
≤ 4 years	1217	109	8.96	7.48–10.69	507	41.66	38.92–44.45	79	6.49	5.24–8.02
> 4 years	508	86	16.93	13.92–20.44	203	39.96	35.79–44.28	91	17.91	14.82–21.48

Abbreviations: FH Fasciola hepatica, EG Echinococcus granulosus, N/n number of animals by category, %, percentage of infection(s) positive animals of the total of animals examined by category

Table 2 Frequency and percentage of organ localization according to cyst type

Cyst type	*N*	Lungs only *n* (%)	Liver only *n* (%)	Both *n* (%)
Infertile	262	107 (40.84)	40 (15.27)	115 (43.89)
Fertile	19	13 (68.42)	2 (10.53)	4 (21.05)
Small	84	23 (27.38)	47 (55.95)	14 (16.67)
Total	365	143 (39.18)	89 (24.39)	133 (36.44)

Abbreviation: *N/n* number of animals

where the ratio in lungs, liver and both organs was 0.28 (5/18), 3.27 (36/11) and 1.8 (9/5), respectively (Table 4).

Logistic regression analysis revealed a statistically significant association between the localization of the hydatid cysts and the presence of *F. hepatica* co-infection in both, bivariate and multivariate models (Table 5). In animals with *F. hepatica* co-infection, hydatid cyst were less likely to localize in the liver than lungs, while this association remained similar in the adjusted model (OR = 0.31, $P < 0.0001$, bivariate; OR = 0.36, $P = 0.027$, adjusted model).

Discussion

The prevalence of *E. granulosus* and *F. hepatica* in the present study is consistent with the official national

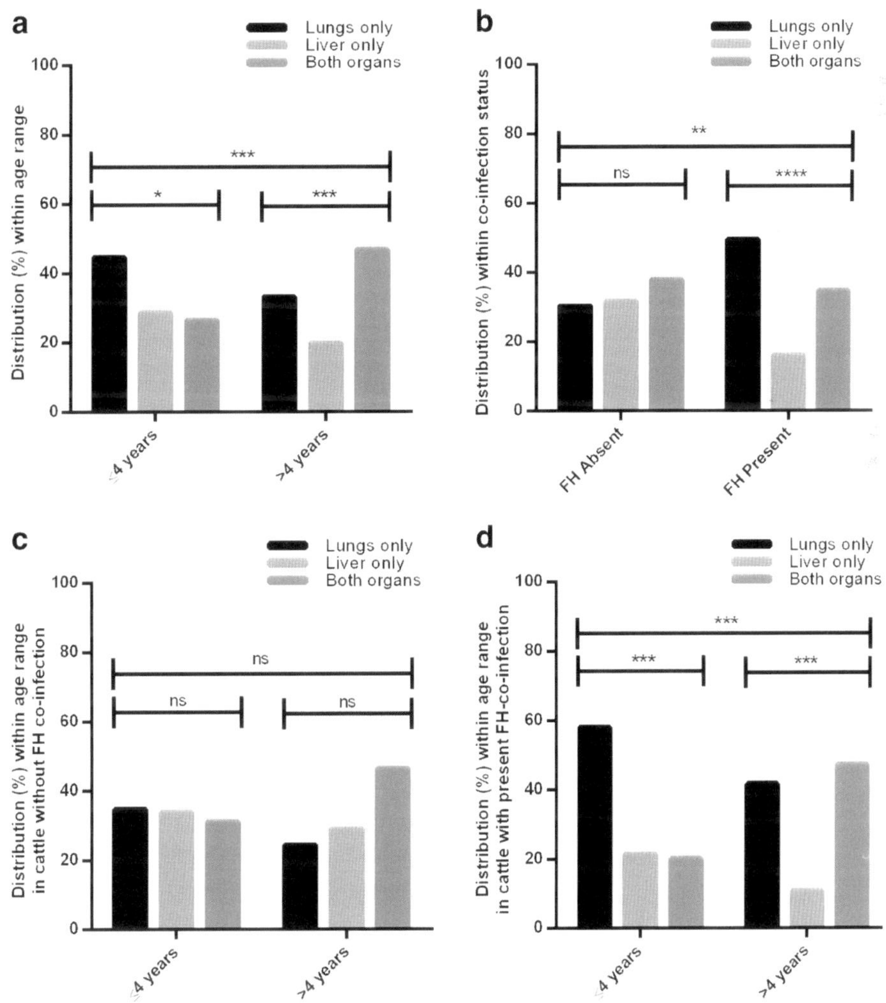

Fig. 2 Anatomical distribution of hydatid cyst in cattle within age range (**a**); *Fasciola hepatica* (FH) co-infection status (**b**); within age range in animals without FH co-infection (**c**) and with FH co-infection (**d**). In **a** cyst anatomical distribution significantly varied among young (≤ 4 years) ($\chi^2 = 7.973$, $df = 2$, $P = 0.0186$) and old animals (> 4 years) ($\chi^2 = 14.80$, $df = 2$, $P = 0.0006$) and within age groups. In **b** a significant association was found between cyst location and FH co-infection status, where a significant difference was found in animals with FH co-infection ($\chi^2 = 22.30$, $df = 2$, $P < 0.0001$), and not in animals without FH co-infection ($\chi^2 = 1.432$, $df = 2$, $P = 0.4883$). **c** No association was found between age range and cyst location in animals absent of FH co-infection, or location within each age group. **d** In cattle with FH co-infection, a significant association was identified between age range and cyst location as well as among each age group. Data are presented as percentage (%) of the number of animals/ total examined cattle in the respective categories. *$P < 0.05$, **$P < 0.01$, ***$P < 0.001$, ****$P < 0.0001$. *Abbreviation*: ns, not statistically significant

Table 3 Hydatid cyst anatomical location within age range and *Fasciola hepatica* co-infection in *E. granulosus* (s.s.)-infected animals

FH-EG co-infection	Host age range	Lungs only n (%)	Liver only n (%)	Both organs n (%)	χ^2	P
Absent	≤ 4 years	17 (32.69)	14 (26.92)	21 (40.38)	0.6903	0.7081
	> 4 years	10 (37.04)	5 (18.52)	12 (44.44)		
	Total[a]	27 (34.18)	19 (24.05)	33 (41.77)		
Present	≤ 4 years	24 (55.81)	7 (16.28)	12 (27.91)	6.209	0.0448*
	> 4 years	22 (43.14)	3 (5.88)	26 (50.98)		
	Total[a]	46 (48.94)	10 (10.64)	38 (40.43)		
Total	≤ 4 years	41 (43.16)	21 (22.11)	33 (34.74)	5.674	0.0586
	> 4 years	32 (41.03)	8 (10.26)	38 (48.72)		
	Total	73 (42.20)	29 (16.76)	71 (41.04)		

*Statistically significant difference at $P < 0.05$
[a]Statistically significant association of cyst location and co-infection ($\chi^2 = 6.841$, $P = 0.0327$)
Abbreviations: *EG E. granulosus (s.s.), FH Fasciola hepatica*

slaughter and condemnation data at abattoirs. The prevalence of *E. granulosus* infection has remained steady since 1995; however, *F. hepatica* infection has increased [27, 28]. Older animals had a higher prevalence of *E. granulosus* infection, as reported in other studies [11, 29, 30], and this prevalence in older animals remains regardless of *F. hepatica* co-infection. This could be due to an increase in time in which the animal can be exposed to *E. granulosus* [31]. For the prevalence of *F. hepatica* however, a difference was found only when *E. granulosus*-infected animals were included; no association was found between age and the proportion of animals infected. Innocent et al. [32] found an increase of liver condemnation due to *F. hepatica* in older cattle; however, the group studied had no animals over 30 months of age and disease prevalence was considerably lower [32].

The location of hydatid cysts varies among studies. In our study, most of the animals had hydatid cysts in their lungs as reported by some studies [14, 29, 33, 34]; however in others, liver was the most commonly affected organ [11, 18, 35]. A recent study in Chile, found that the proportion of organs infected with *E. granulosus* varied among geographical locations [36]. These authors have shown that of the genotyped cysts, belonging to 47.95% of *E. granulosus*-infected animals, most were identified as *E. granulosus* (*s.s.*) as has previously been reported in cattle in Chile [26]; this species is also the most common worldwide [37].

We found that hydatid cysts organ distribution varied with age, a factor not previously considered. Conversely, separating by co-infection with *F. hepatica*, a difference was found only in *F. hepatica* co-infected animals, where the proportion of animals with cysts in both liver and lungs was higher in older co-infected animals when compared with younger co-infected animals. As has been reported, older animals could have a higher number of cysts as exposure time is increased [31], which could also increase the number of organs affected.

Anatomical location was associated with co-infection status, with a decrease in liver-affected animals and an increase in lung-only-affected animals. In *E. granulosus*, portal circulation has been described as the primary route of infection by oncospheres, with a high tropism for the liver [38]. As *F. hepatica* in acute and chronic infections can damage the liver [39], it could be interfering with the establishment of *E. granulosus* in this organ. In the absence of *F. hepatica*, small hydatid cysts were

Table 4 Associations between hydatid cyst with or without *Fasciola hepatica* co-infection and host variables: age range and cyst location

Co-infection	Fertile				Infertile				< 1 cm diameter			
	(-/+)	Ratio	χ^2	P	(-/+)	Ratio	χ^2	P	(-/+)	Ratio	χ^2	P
≤ 4 years	7/3	2.33	2.554	0.11	76/54	1.41	4.968	0.0258*	26/22	1.18	13.341	0.2481
> 4 years[a]	3/6	0.5			59/73	0.81			24/12	2		
Lungs only	7/6	1.17	b		47/60	0.78	4.409	0.1103	5/18	0.28	19.45	<0.0001*
Liver only	2/0	–			24/16	1.63			36/11	3.27		
Both organs	1/3	0.33			64/51	1.25			9/5	1.8		

*Statistically significant difference at $P < 0.05$
[a]Statistically significant association between cysts type and co-infection in this group ($\chi^2 = 6.349$, $P = 0.0418$)
[b]*n* too small for statistical analyses
Abbreviations: *(-/+)* number of animals without *F. hepatica* co-infection/number of animals with *F. hepatica* co-infection

Table 5 Association between hydatid cyst location in liver and the presence of *Fasciola hepatica* co-infection

Variable	OR (95% CI)	Z	P
Co-infection[a]	0.31 (0.18–0.54)	-4.14	<0.0001
Co-infection[b]	0.36 (0.15–0.90)	-2.21	0.027

[a]Crude model (hydatid cyst location in liver *versus Fasciola hepatica* co-infection)
[b]Hydatid cyst location in liver *versus Fasciola hepatica* coinfection adjusted by age, hydatid cyst fertility and *Echinococcus granulosus* genotype
Abbreviation: *CI* confidence interval

mainly located in the liver, whereas when *F. hepatica* was present, small cysts were found in a larger proportion in the lungs only. Small cysts may represent either immature cysts that could develop into fertile or infertile cysts, or they could be non-viable cysts.

As reported in other studies, we found that cyst fertility significantly varied in different organs [11, 15, 29, 40], with more fertile cysts in the lungs than in other locations. No statistical association was found between cyst type and age or co-infection with *F. hepatica*, analyzed independently. However, in older cattle there was an association between cyst type and co-infection with *F. hepatica*. In the presence of the latter, there were more animals with infertile cysts and fewer with small cysts than in single infections.

Cattle cyst fertility reported in this study, is similar to that reported by other authors [11, 15], but noticeably lower than in other studies [13, 18, 33, 34, 41]. Literature data suggest that polyparasitism interactions can alter the site in host used by the parasites. For example, the antagonic relationship between *Moniliformis moniliformis* and *Hymenolepis diminuta*, in which when both parasites co-infect the gut of rats, *M. moniliformis* is able to displace *H. diminuta* to a less nutrient rich site in the small intestine; this antagonic relationship was host-specific [1]. The fact that there are different viscera affected when both *F. hepatica* and *E. granulosus* (*s.l.*) parasitize the same bovine host could be an example of an antagonic relationship, since the liver is the main organ or site in host that both parasites seek to establish themselves. The mechanisms that could explain how *F. hepatica* infection can affect the parasitized viscera by *E. granulosus* (*s.l.*) remains to be studied, since it could be *via* immune response modulation or merely the physical condition of the liver tissue after *F. hepatica* infection that makes it unsuitable for *E. granulosus* (*s.l.*) to establish. This could also be a factor that contributes to the low cyst fertility in cattle from Chile, since the liver is usually infected with *F. hepatica*. One of the limitations of our study is that we worked with natural infections, so we cannot determine the temporality of *F. hepatica* and *E. granulosus* infection in cattle, but here we have shown an effect of displacing the hydatid cysts toward the lungs and an increased proportion of small cysts associated with co-infection with *F. hepatica*.

Conclusions

Cattle naturally co-infected with *E. granulosus* and *F. hepatica* have a lower chance of presenting hydatid cysts in the liver with an increased chance for lung cyst localization, especially for smaller hydatid cysts, suggesting that *F. hepatica* may affect the instate of *E. granulosus* in the liver. These results suggest that in cattle natural infected with *E. granulosus* and *F. hepatica*, both parasites display an antagonistic relationship.

Funding
Funding was provided by FONDECYT-Chile No. 1161475 and the Universidad Andres Bello internal project DI-1249-16/RG. The funding bodies had no role in the design of the study, the collection, analysis and interpretation of data, or in writing the manuscript.

Authors' contributions
CS participated in the sample and data collection, analyzed the obtained data and wrote most of the initial draft of the manuscript. CA participated in the sample and data collection and initial data analysis. CH participated in data analysis, wrote part of manuscript and provided critical review of the manuscript. FC acquired samples and provided critical review of the manuscript. MJ acquired samples. MH provided assistance with the statistical analysis of the results. RP did the study design, results analysis and was a major contributor in writing the manuscript. All authors read and approved the final manuscript.

Competing interests
The authors declare that they have no competing interests.

Author details
[1]Escuela de Medicina Veterinaria, Facultad de Ciencias de la Vida, Universidad Andres Bello, Santiago, Chile. [2]Laboratorio de Biología Periodontal, Facultad de Odontología, Universidad de Chile, Santiago, Chile. [3]Facultad de Ciencias de la Salud, Universidad Autonoma de Chile, Santiago, Chile.

References
1. Behnke JM. Structure in parasite component communities in wild rodents: predictability, stability, associations and interactions .... or pure randomness? Parasitology. 2008;135:751–66.
2. Blackwell AD, Martin M, Kaplan H, Gurven M. Antagonism between two intestinal parasites in humans: the importance of co-infection for infection risk and recovery dynamics. Proc Biol Sci. 2013;280:20131671.
3. Moreau E, Chauvin A. Immunity against helminths: interactions with the host and the intercurrent infections. J Biomed Biotechnol. 2010;2010:428593.
4. Romig T, Deplazes P, Jenkins D, Giraudoux P, Massolo A, Craig PS, et al. Ecology and life cycle patterns of *Echinococcus* species. Adv Parasitol. 2017; 95:213–314.
5. Agudelo Higuita NI, Brunetti E, McCloskey C. Cystic echinococcosis. J Clin Microbiol. 2016;54:518–23.

6. Wuhrer M, Grimm C, Dennis RD, Idris MA, Geyer R. The parasitic trematode *Fasciola hepatica* exhibits mammalian-type glycolipids as well as Gal(beta1-6)Gal-terminating glycolipids that account for cestode serological cross-reactivity. Glycobiology. 2004;14:115–26.
7. Cucher MA, Macchiaroli N, Baldi G, Camicia F, Prada L, Maldonado L, et al. Cystic echinococcosis in South America: systematic review of species and genotypes of *Echinococcus granulosus sensu lato* in humans and natural domestic hosts. Trop Med Int Health. 2016;21:166–75.
8. Riesle S, Garcia MP, Hidalgo C, Galanti N, Saenz L, Paredes R. Bovine IgG subclasses and fertility of *Echinococcus granulosus* hydatid cysts. Vet Parasitol. 2014;205:125–33.
9. Paredes R, Godoy P, Rodriguez B, Garcia MP, Cabezon C, Cabrera G, et al. Bovine (*Bos taurus*) humoral immune response against *Echinococcus granulosus* and hydatid cyst infertility. J Cell Biochem. 2011;112:189–99.
10. Paredes R, Jimenez V, Cabrera G, Iraguen D, Galanti N. Apoptosis as a possible mechanism of infertility in *Echinococcus granulosus* hydatid cysts. J Cell Biochem. 2007;100:1200–9.
11. Addy F, Alakonya A, Wamae N, Magambo J, Mbae C, Mulinge E, et al. Prevalence and diversity of cystic echinococcosis in livestock in Maasailand, Kenya. Parasitol Res. 2012;111:2289–94.
12. Al Kitani FA, Al Riyami S, Al Yahyai S, Al Rawahi AH, Al Maawali M, Hussain MH. Abattoir based surveillance of cystic echinococcosis (CE) in the Sultanate of Oman during 2010–2013. Vet Parasitol. 2015;211:208–15.
13. Andresiuk MV, Gordo FP, Saarma M, Elissondo MC, Taraborelli A, Casalongue C, et al. *Echinococcus granulosus* genotype G1 dominated in cattle and sheep during 2003–2006 in Buenos Aires Province, an endemic area for cystic echinococcosis in Argentina. Acta Trop. 2013;127:136–42.
14. Balbinotti H, Santos GB, Badaraco J, Arend AC, Graichen DÂS, Haag KL, et al. *Echinococcus ortleppi* (G5) and *Echinococcus granulosus sensu stricto* (G1) loads in cattle from southern Brazil. Vet Parasitol. 2012;188:255–60.
15. Daryani A, Sharif M, Amouei A, Nasrolahei M. Fertility and viability rates of hydatid cysts in slaughtered animals in the Mazandaran Province, northern Iran. Trop Anim Health Prod. 2009;41:1701–5.
16. Founta A, Chliounakis S, Antoniadou Sotiriadou K, Koidou M, Bampidis V. Prevalence of hydatidosis and fertility of hydatid cysts in food animals in northern Greece. Vet Ital. 2016;52:123–7.
17. Kamelli M, Borji H, Naghibi A. Genetic identification of cattle hydatid cyst isolates from northeast and southwest of Iran. Ann Parasitol. 2016;62:301–5.
18. Latif AA, Tanveer A, Maqbool A, Siddiqi N, Kyaw-Tanner M, Traub RJ. Morphological and molecular characterisation of *Echinococcus granulosus* in livestock and humans in Punjab, Pakistan. Vet Parasitol. 2010;170:44–9.
19. Thapa NK, Armua-Fernandez MT, Kinzang D, Gurung RB, Wangdi P, Deplazes P. Detection of *Echinococcus granulosus* and *Echinococcus ortleppi* in Bhutan. Parasitol Int. 2017;66:139–41.
20. Gonzalez H, Plaza J, Abalos P. Fertilidad del quiste hidatídico en tres especies animales en Chile y estudio de la vitalidad de sus escólices. Bol Chil Parasitol. 1981;1-2:14–9.
21. Poglayen G, Varcasia A, Pipia AP, Tamponi C, Parigi M, Marchesi B, et al. Retrospective study on cystic echinococcosis in cattle of Italy. Infect Dev Ctries. 2017;11:719–26.
22. Scala A, Bosco A, Pipia AP, Tamponi C, Musella V, Costanzo N, et al. Cystic echinococcosis in cattle dairy farms: spatial distribution and epidemiological dynamics. Geospat Health. 2017;12:562.
23. Abdel-Rahman EH, Abdel-Megeed KN, Abuel-Ezz NM. Cross-reaction: a common trait among helminthes. J Egypt Soc Parasitol. 2003;33:457–71.
24. Talaat RM, Ali NM, Elwakil HS. Impact of *Schistosoma mansoni* and *Echinococcus granulosus* experimental coinfection on interleukin 10 and interferon gamma cytokines profile. Exp Parasitol. 2013;134:474–81.
25. Galindo M, Schadebrodt G, Galanti N. *Echinococcus granulosus*: cellular territories and morphological regions in mature protoscoleces. Exp Parasitol. 2008;119:524–33.
26. Correa F, Stoore C, Horlacher P, Jimenez M, Hidalgo C, Alvarez Rojas CA, et al. First description of *Echinococcus ortleppi* and cystic echinococcosis infection status in Chile. PLoS One. 2018;13:e0197620.
27. Morales MA, Luengo J, Vasquez J. Distribución y tendencia de la fasciolosis en ganado de abasto en Chile, 1989–1995. Parasitol Día. 2000;24:115–8.
28. Luengo J, Olivares M. Causales de decomiso en bovinos beneficiados en mataderos de Chile. Av Cien Vet. 1995;10:1.
29. Negash K, Beyene D, Kumsa B. Cystic echinococcosis in cattle slaughtered at Shashemanne Municipal Abattoir, south central Oromia, Ethiopia: prevalence, cyst distribution and fertility. Trans R Soc Trop Med Hyg. 2013;107:229–34.
30. Rinaldi L, Maurelli MP, Veneziano V, Capuano F, Perugini AG, Cringoli S. The role of cattle in the epidemiology of *Echinococcus granulosus* in an endemic area of southern Italy. Parasitol Res. 2008;103:175–9.
31. Craig PS, Hegglin D, Lightowlers MW, Torgerson PR, Wang Q. Echinococcosis: control and prevention. Adv Parasitol. 2017;96:55–158.
32. Innocent GT, Gilbert L, Jones EO, McLeod JE, Gunn G, McKendrick IJ, et al. Combining slaughterhouse surveillance data with cattle tracing scheme and environmental data to quantify environmental risk factors for liver fluke in cattle. Front Vet Sci. 2017;4:65.
33. Kebede W, Hagos A, Girma Z, Lobago F. Echinococcosis/hydatidosis: its prevalence, economic and public health significance in Tigray region, North Ethiopia. Trop Anim Health Prod. 2008;41:865–71.
34. Pednekar RP, Gatne ML, Thompson RCA, Traub RJ. Molecular and morphological characterisation of *Echinococcus* from food producing animals in India. Vet Parasitol. 2009;165:58–65.
35. Ibrahim MM. Study of cystic echinococcosis in slaughtered animals in Al Baha region, Saudi Arabia: interaction between some biotic and abiotic factors. Acta Trop. 2010;113:26–33.
36. Acosta-Jamett G, Cleaveland S, Cunningham AA. Bronsvoort BMd, Craig PS. *Echinococcus granulosus* infection in humans and livestock in the Coquimbo region, north-central Chile. Vet Parasitol. 2010;169:102–10.
37. Alvarez Rojas CA, Romig T, Lightowlers MW. *Echinococcus granulosus sensu lato* genotypes infecting humans - review of current knowledge. Int J Parasitol. 2014;44:9–18.
38. Brehm KK. U. *Echinococcus*-host interactions at cellular and molecular levels. Adv Parasitol. 2017;95:147–212.
39. Sohair IB, Eman MN. Histopathological and bacteriological studies on livers affected with fascioliasis in cattle. Egypt J Comp Path Clinic Path. 2009;22: 19–45.
40. Mitrea IL, Ionita M, Costin II, Predoi G, Avram E, Rinaldi L, et al. Occurrence and genetic characterization of *Echinococcus granulosus* in naturally infected adult sheep and cattle in Romania. Vet Parasitol. 2014;206:159–66.
41. Ernest E, Nonga HE, Kassuku AA, Kazwala RR. Hydatidosis of slaughtered animals in Ngorongoro district of Arusha region, Tanzania. Trop Anim Health Prod. 2008;41:1179–85.

Urogenital schistosomiasis elimination in Zanzibar: accuracy of urine filtration and haematuria reagent strips for diagnosing light intensity *Schistosoma haematobium* infections

Stefanie Knopp[1,2,3*], Shaali M Ame[4], Jan Hattendorf[1,2], Said M Ali[4], Iddi S Khamis[5], Faki Bakar[4], Mwanaidi A Khamis[5], Bobbie Person[6], Fatma Kabole[5] and David Rollinson[3]

Abstract

Background: Urine filtration and microhaematuria reagent strips are basic standard diagnostic methods to detect urogenital schistosomiasis. We assessed their accuracy for the diagnosis of light intensity infections with *Schistosoma haematobium* as they occur in individuals living in Zanzibar, an area targeted for interruption of transmission.

Methods: Urine samples were collected from children and adults in surveys conducted annually in Zanzibar from 2013 through 2016 and examined with the urine filtration method to count *S. haematobium* eggs and with the reagent strip test (Hemastix) to detect microhaematuria as a proxy for infection. Ten percent of the urine filtration slides were read twice. Sensitivity was calculated for reagent strips, stratified by egg counts reflecting light intensity sub-groups, and kappa statistics for the agreement of urine filtration readings.

Results: Among the 39,207 and 18,155 urine samples examined from children and adults, respectively, 5.4% and 2.7% were *S. haematobium* egg-positive. A third (34.7%) and almost half (46.7%) of the egg-positive samples from children and adults, respectively, had ultra-low counts defined as 1–5 eggs per 10 ml urine. Sensitivity of the reagent strips increased significantly for each unit log10 egg count per 10 ml urine in children (odds ratio, OR: 4.7; 95% confidence interval, CI: 4.0–5.7; $P < 0.0001$) and adults (OR: 2.6; 95% CI: 1.9–3.7, $P < 0.0001$). Sensitivity for diagnosing ultra-light intensity infections was very low in children (50.1%; 95% CI: 46.5–53.8%) and adults (58.7%; 95% CI: 51.9–65.2%). Among the 4477 and 1566 urine filtration slides read twice from children and adults, most were correctly identified as negative or positive (kappa = 0.84 for children and kappa = 0.81 for adults). However, 294 and 75 slides had discrepant results and were positive in only one of the two readings. The majority of these discrepant slides (76.9% of children and 84.0% of adults) had counts of 1–5 eggs per 10 ml urine.

Conclusions: We found that many individuals infected with *S. haematobium* in Zanzibar excrete > 5 eggs per 10 ml urine. These ultra-light infections impose a major challenge for accurate diagnosis. Next-generation diagnostic tools to be used in settings where interruption of transmission is the goal should reliably detect infections with ≤ 5 eggs per 10 ml urine.

(Continued on next page)

* Correspondence: s.knopp@swisstph.ch
[1]Swiss Tropical and Public Health Institute, Socinstrasse 57, 4002 Basel, Switzerland
[2]University of Basel, Petersplatz 1, 4001 Basel, Switzerland
Full list of author information is available at the end of the article

(Continued from previous page)

Keywords: Control, Diagnosis, Elimination, Macrohaematuria, Microhaematuria, Reagent strip, *Schistosoma haematobium*, Surveillance, Urine filtration, Urogenital schistosomiasis, Zanzibar,

Background

Urogenital schistosomiasis, caused by the blood fluke *Schistosoma haematobium*, is a common neglected tropical disease (NTD) in many countries of sub-Saharan Africa and the Middle East [1, 2]. In 2012, the World Health Organization (WHO) encouraged endemic countries to increase the coverage of preventive chemotherapy programmes for the control of morbidity due to schistosomiasis and to initiate elimination campaigns where appropriate, through strengthened health systems, intensified treatment, provision of water and sanitation, addition of health education for behaviour change and snail control to the programmes [3, 4]. As a reaction, over the past years, efforts for control and elimination of schistosomiasis have substantially increased.

The typical sign for urogenital schistosomiasis is the presence of blood in urine [5]. High-risk communities can be identified by using a simple questionnaire asking for visible blood (macrohaematuria) in urine [6, 7]. Another recommended proxy for a *S. haematobium* infection is the detection of microhaematuria using reagent strips [8–10]. The standard method for urogenital schistosomiasis diagnosis in endemic areas is the microscopic quantification of *S. haematobium* eggs in urine using polycarbonate filters [7, 11]. However, after praziquantel treatment and repeated preventive chemotherapy, macro- and microhaematuria decrease, as well as intensities of infection and the overall prevalence [12–15]. Hence, in areas that have achieved morbidity control (prevalence of heavy-intensity infection < 5% across sentinel sites) and move towards elimination of urogenital schistosomiasis as public health problem (prevalence of heavy-intensity infections < 1% in all sentinel sites) and finally interruption of transmission (reduction of incidence of infection to zero) according to WHO thresholds [4], macro- and microhaematuria and the number of eggs excreted in urine will be extremely low and eventually zero. These light intensity infections impose a challenge for accurate diagnosis.

A large dataset with *S. haematobium* diagnostic results was derived from a 5-year cluster randomized trial assessing different interventions against urogenital schistosomiasis in Zanzibar funded by the Schistosomiasis Consortium for Operational Research and Evaluation (SCORE) [16]. Zanzibar is one of the first areas in sub-Saharan Africa that is targeted for urogenital schistosomiasis elimination as public health problem and interruption of transmission. Using these data, we aimed to assess whether the sensitivity of microhaematuria testing using reagent strips increases with increasing egg counts measured with the standard urine filtration method. In addition, we aimed to determine the diagnostic test sensitivity at different light intensity infection sub-groups.

Methods

Study area

The Zanzibar islands, Unguja and Pemba, are part of the United Republic of Tanzania. The population size is estimated at 1.3 million. Historically, urogenital schistosomiasis has been a considerable public health problem on both islands [17–19]. Over the past decades, regular mass drug administration (MDA) with praziquantel, improved access to safe water, better socio-economic conditions and likely also climatic changes have lowered the disease prevalence and reduced morbidity [20, 21]. Efforts to eliminate urogenital schistosomiasis as public health problem on Pemba and to interrupt transmission on Unguja started in 2011 by the Zanzibar Elimination of Schistosomiasis Transmission (ZEST) alliance [16, 22]. These efforts were fostered by a three-arm multi-year cluster randomized trial implemented from 2011 to 2017 to assess the effect of biannual MDA, snail control and behaviour change interventions [16]. To date, with the exception of some areas where transmission is still considerably high [21], the prevalence of *S. haematobium* infections is well below 10% and infection intensities are light in most administrative areas (shehias).

Sample size calculation

The sample size calculations for the cluster randomized trial and annual cross-sectional surveys in schools and communities are provided elsewhere [16]. The results of all individuals with a complete urine examination, by urine filtration and reagent strip methods, in 2013, 2014, 2015 and 2016, were included into the analyses presented here.

Field procedures

The cross-sectional surveys in schools and communities were conducted annually, in both Unguja and Pemba, between February and June in 2013, 2014, 2015 and 2016. Children aged 9–12 years attending the study primary schools and adults aged 20–55 years living in the study communities were included. In each primary school, the headmaster and teachers were informed about the aims of the study and in each community the community leader was consulted. The participant selection procedure in schools and communities has been described elsewhere in detail [16]. In brief, in public primary schools, classes of grades 3 and 4 were visited by the field teams of the NTD Programme and the Public Health Laboratory-Ivo de Carneri (PHL-IdC) on Unguja and Pemba, respectively. The purpose of the study was explained in lay terms to the children. The name, age, sex, and additional demographic information of the selected children were recorded. The children registered for participation received an information sheet and a consent form to bring to their parents. The following day, each child returning the consent form signed by its parent or legal guardian received a urine collection container and was asked to fill the container with its own urine (urine collection occurred between 10:00 and 12:00 hours) and to give the filled container to the field team. In each shehia, households were randomly selected and an adult household member, present at the time, was invited to participate in the study [16]. After consenting and replying to a brief questionnaire concerning demographic characteristics, the adult received a container for collection of his/her own urine. All urine samples from adults were collected between 10:00 and 14:00 hours. The urine samples collected in Unguja were examined in the laboratory of the NTD Programme of the Ministry of Health in Zanzibar Town, Unguja. The urine samples collected in Pemba were examined in the PHL-IdC in Chake Chake, Pemba.

Laboratory procedures

On the day of collection, all urine samples (i.e. one single sample per person) were examined by trained laboratory technicians for macrohaematuria using a colour chart and for microhaematuria using reagent strips (Hemastix; Siemens Healthcare Diagnostics GmbH, Eschborn, Germany). Macrohaematuria was graded with numbers from 1 to 6 from transparent to dark red urine using a pretested colour chart [23, 24]. Microhaematuria in urine was coded semi-quantitatively according to the Hemastix manufacturer's instructions (negative; trace; +; ++; and +++). Additionally, all urine samples of sufficient quantity were rigorously shaken and 10 ml of each sample pressed through a polycarbonate filter with a pore size of 20 μm (Sterlitech, Kent, WA, USA) using a standard 10 ml plastic syringe. All urine filters were put on a microscope slide, covered with a piece of hydrophilic cellophane soaked in glycerol solution, and examined by trained laboratory technicians under the microscope using some drops of Lugol's iodine to stain *S. haematobium* eggs after cellophane coverage. The presence and number of *S. haematobium* eggs was recorded. After microscopy, the slides were stored at room temperature for a potential second reading for quality control. Quality control was performed on 10% of the stored urine filtration slides several months after the initial reading. For the selection of quality control urine filtration (QCUF) slides, 10% of the slides of each technician were included, prioritizing slides from microhaematuria-positive urine samples and adding computer randomized microhaematuria-negative slides until the number representing 10% of the total number of slides read by the technician was reached. The QCUF slides were read by trained external microscopists who were blinded to the reagent strip and initial urine filtration results.

Data management and analysis

The macrohaematuria, microhaematuria, urine filtration, and QCUF results were recorded on paper laboratory forms and subsequently entered into a Microsoft Excel 2010 electronic database (Microsoft Corporation 2010) and cleaned. Data were analysed using STATA version 14.0 (StataCorp., College Station, TX, USA). Only data from urine samples with complete examination (i.e. microhaematuria, microhaematuria and urine filtration result available) and from children aged 9-12 years or adults aged 20-55 years were included in the analyses.

Microhaematuria-positive was defined as a urine sample that had a trace or positive reagent strip colour reaction. *S. haematobium*-positive was defined as a urine filtration slide that contained at least one *S. haematobium* egg. The WHO differentiates *S. haematobium* infections into light (1–49 eggs per 10 ml urine) and heavy (≥ 50 eggs per 10 ml urine) intensity [25]. In our study we further stratified egg counts into the following sub-classes: "negative" (0 eggs/10 ml), "ultra-light" (1–5 eggs/10 ml), "very light" (6–10 eggs/10 ml), "light" (11–49 eggs/10 ml) and "heavy" (≥ 50 eggs/10 ml) infections. Association between *S. haematobium* infection (binary outcome variable or categorical explanatory variable) and microhaematuria (binary outcome variable or categorical explanatory variable) was assessed by multivariable logistic regression analyses, adjusted by sex (binary variable), age (continuous variable), study year (categorical variable) and school or shehia as a sampling unit (categorical variable) and expressed as odds ratios (OR) plus 95% confidence intervals (95% CI).

For both children and adults separately, the sensitivity and specificity of the reagent strip method was calculated overall and stratified by the egg count thresholds chosen for ultra-light, very light, light, and heavy infections as described above. The original urine filtration was considered as the diagnostic reference test. The sensitivity of a reagent strip result was calculated as the proportion of positives that were correctly identified

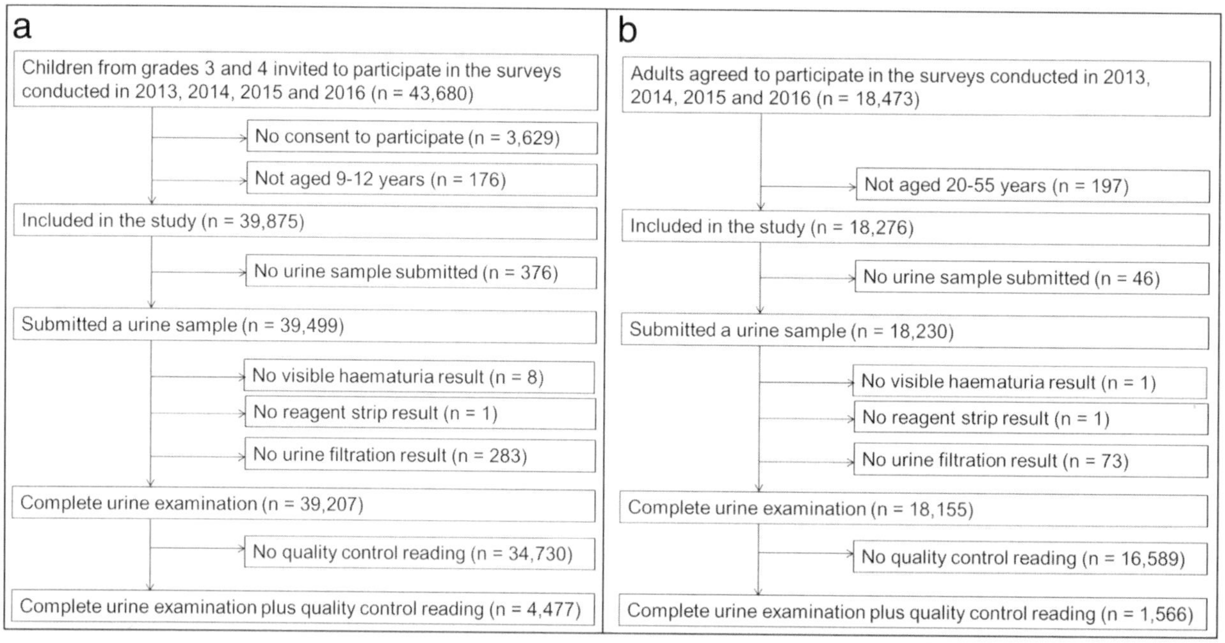

Fig. 1 Flowchart detailing study participation and urine sampling procedures. **a** Children sampled in public primary schools. **b** Adults sampled in communities in Unguja and Pemba islands, United Republic of Tanzania

when compared to the reference test. The specificity of a reagent strip result was calculated as the proportion of negatives that were correctly identified when compared to the reference test. We used 95% CIs to indicate the contrast between groups. In addition, we used logistic regression to assess whether the sensitivity of the reagent strip method is increasing with increasing egg counts determined by the urine filtration method. For this purpose we used the decimal logarithm of the egg counts of the filtration-positive samples as predictor.

Table 1 Multivariate frequency distribution of *S. haematobium* infection and egg counts and haematuria presence and grading

Urine filtration original reading			Microhaematuria			Microhaematuria grading				Macrohaematuria grading					
	n	%	*n* negative	*n* positive including trace	% positive	Trace	+	++	+++	1	2	3	4	5	6
Total children examined	39,207		36,675	2532	6.5										
S. haematobium egg-negative	37,077	94.6	36,070	1007	2.7	430	264	205	108	19,070	14,265	3508	223	11	0
S. haematobium egg-positive	2130	5.4	605	1525	71.6	292	290	468	475	801	1030	279	18	2	0
S. haematobium egg counts															
1–5 eggs	740	34.7	369	371	50.1	102	91	116	62	332	216	89	30	0	0
6–10 eggs	284	13.3	85	199	70.1	52	41	62	44	117	137	28	2	0	0
11–49 eggs	646	30.3	119	527	81.6	103	113	167	144	234	325	81	6	0	0
50+ eggs	460	21.6	32	428	93.0	35	45	123	225	118	252	81	7	2	0
Total adults examined	18,155		16,131	2024	11.1										
S. haematobium egg-negative	17,673	97.3	15,985	1688	9.6	541	475	383	289	7275	7972	2250	170	5	1
S. haematobium egg-positive	482	2.7	146	336	69.7	65	62	99	110	157	245	67	11	2	0
S. haematobium egg counts															
1–5 eggs	225	46.7	93	132	58.7	28	40	29	35	80	109	31	5	0	0
6–10 eggs	64	13.3	18	46	71.9	11	5	19	11	25	27	9	2	1	0
11–49 eggs	124	25.7	27	97	78.2	17	14	32	34	38	71	13	1	1	0
50+ eggs	69	14.3	8	61	88.4	9	3	19	30	14	38	14	3	0	0

The graphical representation of the predicted values is shown in Additional file 1.

The agreement between the positive and negative readings of the original urine filtration *versus* the QCUF reading was determined using kappa (κ)-statistics. The κ-statistics were interpreted as follows: < 0.00 indicating no agreement; 0.00–0.20 indicating slight agreement; 0.21–0.40 indicating fair agreement; 0.41–0.60 indicating moderate agreement; 0.61–0.80 indicating substantial agreement; 0.81–0.99 indicating almost perfect agreement; and 1.00 indicating perfect agreement [26].

Results

Study participation and operational results

As shown in Fig. 1a, a total of 43,680 children were invited to participate in the cross-sectional surveys conducted in 2013, 2014, 2015 and 2016. Among them, 39,875 were aged 9–12 years and submitted a signed form from their parents consenting to their participation. Complete urine sample examinations including results on macrohaematuria, microhaematuria and *S. haematobium* egg counts were available for 39,207 children. Among them, 20,680 (52.7%) were girls and 18,527 (47.3%) were boys. A QCUF reading was performed for 4477 slides.

Figure 1b indicates that a total of 18,473 adults participated in the study. Among them, 18,276 were aged 20–55 years and included in the study. Complete urine sample examinations were available for 18,155 adults. Among them, 10,573 (58.2%) were female and 7582 (41.8%) were male. A QCUF reading was performed for 1566 slides.

Association between infection intensity and haematuria in children

As shown in Table 1, among the 39,207 urine filtration slides examined for *S. haematobium* infection in children, 2130 (5.4%) were found to be egg-positive. Among the *S. haematobium*-positive slides, ultra-light infections with 1–5 eggs/10 ml urine were most common (34.7%). Very light infections with 6–10 eggs/10 ml were found in 13.3%, light infections with 11–49 eggs/10 ml were found in 30.3%, and heavy infections with ≥ 50 eggs/10 ml urine were found in 21.6% of the *S. haematobium*--positive slides. Among all urine samples examined, 1.2% were identified with heavy infection intensities.

Table 1 indicates that the majority of urines were lightly coloured and only very few children and adults had visible haematuria. A total of 2532 (6.5%) urine samples from children were microhaematuria-positive. Among the 2130 *S. haematobium* egg-positive urine samples, 605 (71.6%) were microhaematuria-positive and among the 37,077 *S. haematobium* egg-negative urine samples, 1007 (2.7%) were microhaematuria-positive.

Table 2 Association between *S. haematobium* egg counts and microhaematuria

Variable type	Variable name	*n*	OR	95% CI
Children aged 9–12 years		39,207		
Outcome	*S. haematobium* egg-positive			
Explanatory	Microhaematuria-positive		86.6	75.6–99.1
	Trace		42.8	35.0–52.3
	+		66.8	53.4–83.2
	++		129.6	104.2–161.2
	+++		188.8	146.5–243.3
	Boys		1.9	1.67–2.17
Outcome	Microhaematuria-positive			
Explanatory	*S. haematobium* egg-positive		85.7	74.9–98.1
	1-5 eggs		45	37.6–53.9
	6-10 eggs		96.1	72.8–126.9
	11-49 eggs		208.7	166.0–262.5
	50+ eggs		604.2	414.5–880.8
	Boys		0.83	0.74–0.93
Adults aged 20–55 years		18,155		
Outcome	*S. haematobium* egg-positive			
Explanatory	Microhaematuria-positive		29.6	23.6–37.2
	Trace		19.3	13.7–27.1
	+		21.6	15.3–27.1
	++		34.6	25.3–47.3
	+++		50.2	36.4–69.3
	Men		2.5	2.0–3.1
Outcome	Microhaematuria-positive			
Explanatory	*S. haematobium* egg-positive		29.5	23.6–36.8
	1–5 eggs		19.9	15.0–26.3
	6–10 eggs		42.3	24.2–74.0
	11–49 eggs		50.6	32.0–79.9
	50+ eggs		129.1	60.6–274.8
	Men		0.5	0.44–0.55

Abbreviations: *OR* odds ratio; *95% CI* 95% confidence interval

Compared with *S. haematobium* egg-negative children, egg-positive children had significantly higher odds to present with microhaematuria (OR: 85.7; 95% CI: 74.9–98.1). The odds increased with increasing egg counts and were highest for heavy (OR: 604.2; 95% CI: 414.5–880.8), followed by light (OR: 208.7; 95% CI: 166.0–265.5), very light (OR: 96.1; 95% CI: 72.8–126.9), and ultra-light (OR: 45.0; 95% CI: 37.6–53.9) infections. Boys had higher odds to be *S. haematobium*-positive (OR: 1.9; 95% CI: 1.7–2.2) but lower odds to be microhaematuria-positive (OR: 0.9; 95% CI: 0.7–0.9) than girls. More details about the associations between *S. haematobium* infection intensity and microhaematuria are presented in Table 2 and Fig. 2a.

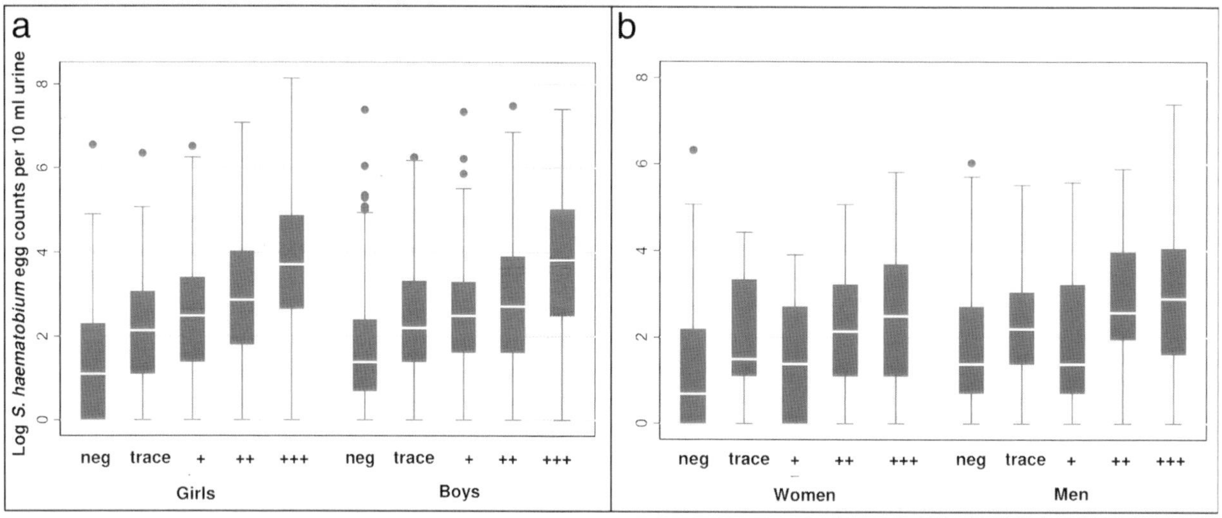

Fig. 2 Boxplots of *S. haematobium* log egg counts of egg-positive urine samples from Zanzibar, United Republic of Tanzania, stratified by microhaematuria grading, sex and age category. **a** log *S. haematobium* egg-counts by microhaematuria grading for female and male children. **b** log *S. haematobium* egg-counts by microhaematuria grading for female and male adults. Correlation between positive egg counts and microhaematuria grading (data pooled over both sexes): Spearman's rho in children= 0.65, P < 0.001 (n = 39,207), Spearman's rho in adults = 0.32; P < 0.001 (n = 18,155). In contrast to the boxplots, the correlation coefficients were calculated using egg counts from positive and negative urine samples

Association between infection intensity and haematuria in adults

As shown in Table 1, among the 18,155 urine filtration slides examined for *S. haematobium* infection in adults, 482 (2.7%) were egg positive. Ultra-light infections were most common (46.7%), followed by light (25.7%), heavy (14.3%) and very light (13.3%) infections. Among all examined urine samples, 0.4% were identified with heavy infection intensities. Among the *S. haematobium* egg-positive samples, 336 (69.7%) were microhaematuria-positive and among the egg-negative urine samples, 1688 (9.6%) were microhaematuria-positive.

Adults had higher odds to be microhaematuria-positive if *S. haematobium* eggs were found in their urine (OR: 29.5; 95% CI: 23.6–36.8). The odds increased with increasing egg counts (Table 2). They were highest for heavy (OR: 129.1; 95% CI: 60.6–274.8), followed by light (OR: 50.6; 95% CI: 32.0–79.9), very light (OR: 42.3; 95% CI: 24.2–74.0), and ultra-light (OR: 19.9; 95% CI: 15.0–26.3) infections. Men had higher odds to be *S. haematobium*-positive (OR: 2.5; 95% CI: 2.0–3.1) but lower odds to be microhaematuria-positive (OR: 0.50; 95% CI: 0.4–0.6) than women.

Specificity and sensitivity of the reagent strip method

As shown in Table 3, in children, the specificity of the reagent strip method was 97.3% (97.1–97.4%). The overall sensitivity was 71.6% (95% CI: 69.6–73.5%). When considering intensity subgroups, the sensitivity was lowest for ultra-light infections (50.1%; 95% CI: 46.5–53.8%), followed by very light (70.1%; 95% CI: 64.4–75.3%), light (81.6%; 95% CI: 78.4–84.5%), and heavy (93.0%; 95% CI: 90.3–95.2%) infections.

As indicated in Table 4 among adults, the specificity of the reagent strip method was 90.4% (95% CI: 90.0–90.9%). The overall sensitivity was 69.7% (95% CI: 65.4–73.8%). Stratified by intensity, the sensitivity was 58.7% (95% CI: 51.9–65.2%) for ultra-light, 71.9% (95% CI: 59.2–82.4%) for very light, 77.9% (95% CI: 69.5–84.9%) for light and 88.7% (95% CI: 79.0–95.0%) for heavy infections.

Additional file 1 shows that the sensitivity of the reagent strip method increased significantly for each unit $\log_{10}$ egg count per 10 ml urine in children (OR: 4.7; 95% CI: 4.0–5.7, $P < 0.0001$) and adults (OR: 2.6; 95% CI: 1.9–3.7, $P < 0.0001$). The difference of the test sensitivity between children and adults ($P = 0.001$) as well as the population-egg-count interaction ($P = 0.002$) were statistically significant.

Urine filter microscopy

Table 5 shows that among the 4477 urine filtration slides from children that were subjected to QCUF, 3087 slides were negative and 1096 slides were recorded as egg-positive in both the original and the QCUF reading. The kappa-agreement was almost perfect (κ = 0.84). However, 163 slides were only positive in the original and 131 slides were only positive in the QCUF reading. As presented in Table 5, among the 294 slides that were only positive in one or the

Table 3 Sensitivity and specificity of the reagent strip method for *S. haematobium* diagnosis in children when urine filtration results are considered as reference test

Reference test: urine filtration		Microhaematuria		
All individuals included		Positive	Negative	Total
	Positive	1525	605	2130
	Negative	1007	36,070	37,077
	Total	2532	36,675	39,207
Sensitivity of reagent strips		71.6% (69.6–73.5%)		
Specificity of reagent strips		97.3% (97.1–97.4%)		
Subgroup: 1–5 eggs/10 ml		Positive	Negative	Total
	Positive	371	369	740
	Negative	1007	36,070	37,077
	Total	1378	36,439	37,817
Sensitivity of reagent strips		50.1% (46.5–53.8%)		
Subgroup: 6–10 eggs/10 ml		Positive	Negative	Total
	Positive	199	85	284
	Negative	1007	36,070	37,077
	Total	1206	36,155	37,361
Sensitivity of reagent strips		70.1% (64.4–75.3%)		
Subgroup: 11–49 eggs/10 ml		Positive	Negative	Total
	Positive	527	119	646
	Negative	1007	36,070	37,077
	Total	1534	36,189	37,723
Sensitivity of reagent strips		81.6% (78.4–84.5%)		
Subgroup: 50+ eggs/10 m		Positive	Negative	Total
	Positive	428	32	460
	Negative	1007	36,070	37,077
	Total	1435	36,102	37,537
Sensitivity of reagent strips		93.0% (90.3–95.2%)		

other microscopy reading, 93 slides had an egg count of 1 (31.6%). The vast majority of the discrepant slides had egg counts between 1 and 5 (76.9%), followed by egg counts between 6 and 10 (12.2%), egg counts between 11 and 49 (7.5%), and 50 and above (3.4%).

A total of 1566 urine filtration slides from adults were subjected to QCUF. Among them, 1292 were negative and 199 were recorded as egg-positive in both the original and the QCUF reading. Hence, the kappa-agreement was almost perfect (κ = 0.81). However, 35 slides were only positive in the original reading and 40 slides were only positive in the QCUF reading. For adults, among the 75 slides that had discrepant results, almost half (45.3%) had an egg count of 1. The majority of the discrepant slides, had egg counts between 1 and 5 (84.0%), followed by egg counts between 6 and 10 (13.3%), egg counts between 11 and 49 (1.3%), and 50 and above (1.3%).

Discussion

Reagent strips and urine filtration are basic standard diagnostic methods to detect urogenital schistosomiasis [7, 27–29]. Their sensitivity is, however, reduced in low prevalence settings, treated populations, or subgroups with light intensity infections [27, 30, 31]. Moving towards the goal of interruption of *Schistosoma* transmission, it is important to assess at what level of egg counts the diagnostic methods start to lose their accuracy. Here, we evaluated the performance of urine filtration readings and microhaematuria assessment for diagnosing *S. haematobium* infections in several thousand urine samples from children and adults living in Zanzibar, an area targeted for interruption of transmission of urogenital schistosomiasis.

Our study clearly showed that both reagent strip and urine filtration method have a particularly low diagnostic accuracy for the detection of ultra-light infections with egg counts of 1–5 eggs per 10 ml of urine. In line with a

Table 4 Sensitivity and specificity of the reagent strip method for *S. haematobium* diagnosis in adults when urine filtration results are considered as reference test

Reference test: urine filtration		Microhaematuria		
All individuals included		Positive	Negative	Total
	Positive	336	146	482
	Negative	1688	15,985	17,673
	Total	2024	16,131	18,155
Sensitivity of reagent strips		69.7% (65.4–73.8%)		
Specificity of reagent strips		90.4% (90.0–90.9%)		
Subgroup: 1–5 eggs/10 ml		Positive	Negative	Total
	Positive	132	93	225
	Negative	1688	15,985	17,673
	Total	1820	16,078	17,898
Sensitivity of reagent strips		58.7% (51.9–65.2%)		
Subgroup: 6–10 eggs/10 ml		Positive	Negative	Total
	Positive	46	18	64
	Negative	1688	15,985	17,673
	Total	1734	16,003	17,737
Sensitivity of reagent strips		71.9% (59.2–82.4%)		
Subgroup: 11–49 eggs/10 ml		Positive	Negative	Total
	Positive	95	27	122
	Negative	1688	15,985	17,673
	Total	1783	16,012	17,795
Sensitivity of reagent strips		77.9% (69.5–84.9%)		
Subgroup: 50+ eggs/10 ml		Positive	Negative	Total
	Positive	63	8	71
	Negative	1688	15,985	17,673
	Total	1751	15,993	17,744
Sensitivity		88.7% (79.0–95.0%)		

recent meta-analysis, indicating sensitivities of reagent strips of 65% for light intensity infection and 72% for post-treatment groups [30], the overall sensitivity to detect *S. haematobium* infections with reagent strips in children and adults in our study was 71.6% and 69.7%, respectively. However, the sensitivity of reagent strips to detect ultra-light infections was considerably lower (50.1% in children and 58.7% in adults). Comparing the results of urine filtration microscopy, we found that the overall agreement when slides were read twice was almost perfect. However, false-negative diagnosis by one of the two readings occurred and particularly when egg counts were between 1 and 5 eggs per 10 ml urine.

In Zanzibar, only a small portion of the samples examined by urine filtration were *S. haematobium* egg-positive (5.4% of children and 2.7% of adults) and more than a third of these egg-positive slides showed ultra-light infections with 1–5 eggs per 10 ml urine (34.7% of children and 46.7% of adults). Only about half of these ultra-lightly infected individuals (50.1% of children and 58.7% of adults) presented with detectable microhaematuria. Our results highlight that a large proportion of individuals living in elimination settings such as Zanzibar that are targeted by regular interventions harbour ultra-light infections. These cases may be missed when reagent strips or single urine filtration readings are applied as diagnostic approach. Hence, in settings where interruption of transmission is the goal and already the excretion of a single egg into a water body with intermediate host snails can result in resurgence of transmission and (re-)infection of a whole community, more sensitive diagnostic methods are needed to identify and subsequently treat infected individuals. These next-generation diagnostic tools should be able to reliably detect infections with ≤ 5 eggs per 10 ml urine.

In line with other studies, the performance of both reagent strips and urine filtration improved significantly when egg counts increased [12, 18, 27]. The odds of

Table 5 *Schistosoma haematobium* egg counts on discrepant slides when examined by original or quality control urine filtration (QCUF) microscopy

Microscopic examination		*n*	%
Children	Slides with original and QCUF reading	4477	
	Slides with positive results in both readings	1096	
	Slides with negative results in both readings	3087	
	Slides with discrepant results (one reading positive, one reading negative)	294	
	S. haematobium egg counts on discrepant slides		
	1 egg	93	31.6
	2 eggs	57	19.4
	3 eggs	39	13.3
	4 eggs	23	7.8
	5 eggs	14	4.8
	1–5 eggs	226	76.9
	6–10 eggs	36	12.2
	11–49 eggs	22	7.5
	50+ eggs	10	3.4
Adults	Slides with original and QCUF reading	1566	
	Slides with positive results in both readings	199	
	Slides with negative results in both readings	1292	
	Slides with discrepant results (one reading positive, one reading negative)	75	
	S. haematobium egg counts on discrepant slides		
	1 egg	34	45.3
	2 eggs	12	16.0
	3 eggs	6	8.0
	4 eggs	7	9.3
	5 eggs	4	5.3
	1–5 eggs	63	84.0
	6–10 eggs	10	13.3
	11–50 eggs	1	1.3
	51+ eggs	1	1.3

urine samples being microhaematuria-positive increased significantly from ultra-light to very light to light to heavy infection egg outputs. Also, the number of false-negative or false-positive urine filtration slide readings decreased considerably with increasing egg counts. Only very few slides were wrong-negative or wrong-positive at counts of ≥ 50 eggs per 10 ml urine, errors that might be attributed to wrong labelling.

Hence, urine filtration and reagent strip methods are valid means to detect *S. haematobium* infections in epidemiological surveys and outpatient centres in areas where infection intensities are reasonably high [30, 32]. In areas identified to have high prevalences and infection intensities, preventive chemotherapy without individual diagnosis will be the key intervention to control morbidity [7]. Urine filtration and reagent strips might also be suitable tools for monitoring progress in areas where preventive chemotherapy plus complementary interventions are used to achieve elimination as a public health problem. However, only urine filtration allows classification of *S. haematobium* infections into light and heavy intensities as defined by the WHO [25]. Where interruption of transmission is the goal, novel intervention strategies need to be considered and tested. The sensitive and specific identification of infected individuals excreting *S. haematobium* eggs, including ultra-lightly infected individuals, will gain importance. Hence, next-generation diagnostic tools that are reliably working below a level of 5 eggs per 10 ml urine are urgently needed.

A first step into improved diagnosis of *S. haematobium* infections in population groups excreting low numbers of eggs was done with the development and evaluation of the up-converting phosphor-lateral flow circulating anodic antigen (UCP-CAA) assay and the detection of parasite specific DNA *Dra*1 fragments in urine using PCR-based methods, respectively [29, 31, 33–35]. However, these tests need a considerable amount of equipment, material and training of technicians and will hence mostly be of use in well-equipped central laboratories. For monitoring and surveillance at the peripheral level, e.g. in local schools and health facilities, a simple rapid diagnostic test with high sensitivity such as the point-of-care circulating cathodic antigen test available for *S. mansoni* [36, 37] is needed also for *S. haematobium* diagnosis. Such a sensitive rapid diagnostic test would facilitate focal screen-and-treat and other tailored surveillance-response scenarios that could become part of a strategy for interrupting *S. haematobium* transmission.

A clear limitation of our study is that no third and highly sensitive diagnostic method such as the UCP-CAA or PCR was used to validate results derived with the urine filtration and reagent strip methods. Also the collection of multiple urine samples from the same individuals would have allowed to assess more thoroughly the relationship between low egg intensity and macro- or microhaematuria while accounting for variation between individuals as well as changes in egg excretion during the day. Nevertheless, the analysis of our large dataset allows for the following conclusions and considerations.

Conclusions

We found that ultra-light *S. haematobium* infections are most common in Zanzibar and impose a major challenge for accurate diagnosis using basic parasitological methods. Next-generation diagnostic tools to be used in settings where interruption of transmission is the goal should reliably detect infections ≤ 5 eggs per 10 ml urine. These new tests should not only be highly sensitive, but also rapid and easy to apply so that they can be used for surveillance at the central and peripheral level, triggering an effective and focused intervention response.

Acknowledgements
We are grateful to the Schistosomiasis Consortium for Operational Research and Evaluation (SCORE) secretariat for advisory support. We thank the staff of the parasitology teams in Unguja and Pemba who helped with the collection and examination of urine samples, subjected to haematuria testing and urine filtration. We acknowledge Colin Cercamondi for helping with the quality control of urine filtration slides in 2013. Last but not least, we acknowledge the children and adults participating in our study.

Funding
This study received financial support from the University of Georgia Research Foundation Inc., which is funded by the Bill & Melinda Gates Foundation for these Schistosomiasis Consortium for Operational Research and Evaluation (SCORE) projects (prime award no. 50816, sub-award no. RR374-053/4893206). SK is financially supported by sub-award no. RR374-053/4893196. SK is also financially supported by a direct grant from the Bill & Melinda Gates Foundation (Investment ID: OPP1191423). The funders had no role in study design, data collection and analysis, decision to publish, or preparation of the manuscript.

Authors' contributions
Conception and design of the study: SK and DR. Acquisition of data: SK, SMAm, SMAI, FB, MAK, ISK and FK. Analysis and interpretation of data: SK, JH and DR. Drafting the article: SK. Revising the article critically for important intellectual content: SMAm, JH, SMAI, FB, MAK, ISK, BP, FK and DR. All authors read and approved the final manuscript.

Ethics approval and consent to participate
Our study protocol was approved by the Zanzibar Medical Research Ethics Committee (ZAMREC) in Zanzibar, United Republic of Tanzania (reference no. ZAMREC 0003/Sept/011), the Ethics Committee of Basel, Switzerland (reference no. EKBB 236/11), and the Institutional Review Board of the University of Georgia in the USA (project no. 2012-10138-0) [16]. The study is registered with the International Standard Randomized Controlled Trial Number register (ISRCTN48837681). All children and adults invited to participate in the study received a participant information sheet and a consent sheet. The study was explained in lay terms to the children in school and to the adults in the communities using the local language Kiswahili. Only individuals, who submitted a written informed consent for their participation, were included in the study. In the case of children, parents or their legal guardians were asked to provide their written consent for the child's participation. All study participants were offered praziquantel (40 mg/kg) against schistosomiasis and albendazole (400 mg) against soil-transmitted helminthiasis free of charge *via* the biannual island-wide mass drug administration conducted as part of the elimination interventions by the Zanzibar Neglected Diseases Programme in 2013, 2014, 2015 and 2016.

Competing interests
The authors declare that they have no competing interests.

Author details
[1]Swiss Tropical and Public Health Institute, Socinstrasse 57, 4002 Basel, Switzerland. [2]University of Basel, Petersplatz 1, 4001 Basel, Switzerland. [3]Wolfson Wellcome Biomedical Laboratories, Department of Life Sciences, Natural History Museum, Cromwell Road, London SW7 5BD, UK. [4]Public Health Laboratory Ivo-de Carneri, P.O. Box 122, Chake-Chake, Pemba, United Republic of Tanzania. [5]Neglected Diseases Programme, Ministry of Health, P.O. Box 236, Unguja, United Republic of Tanzania. [6]Schistosomiasis Consortium for Operational Research and Evaluation, 145 Coverdell Center, The University of Georgia, 500 D.W. Brooks Drive, Athens, Georgia 30602, USA.

References

1. Gryseels B. Schistosomiasis. Infect Dis Clin North Am. 2012;26:383–97.
2. Colley DG, Bustinduy AL, Secor WE, King CH. Human schistosomiasis. Lancet. 2014;383:2253–64.
3. WHO. WHA65.21. Elimination of schistosomiasis. Sixty-fifth World Health Assembly Geneva 21–26 May 2012 Resolutions, decisions and annexes. Geneva: World Health Organization; 2012. p. 36–7.
4. WHO. Schistosomiasis: progress report 2001–2011 and strategic plan 2012–2020. Geneva: World Health Organization; 2013. p. 1–80.
5. Gryseels B, Polman K, Clerinx J, Kestens L. Human schistosomiasis. Lancet. 2006;368:1106–18.
6. The Red Urine Study Group. Identification of high-risk communities for schistosomiasis in Africa: a multicountry study. Geneva: World Health Organization; 1995. p. 1–103.
7. WHO. Preventive chemotherapy in human helminthiasis: coordinated use of anthelminthic drugs in control interventions: a manual for health professionals and programme managers. Geneva: World Health Organization; 2006. p. 1–74.
8. Briggs M, Chadfield M, Mummery D, Briggs M. Screening with reagent strips. Br Med J. 1971;3:433–4.
9. Wilkins HA, Goll P, Marshall TF, Moore P. The significance of proteinuria and haematuria in *Schistosoma haematobium* infection. Trans R Soc Trop Med Hyg. 1979;73:74–80.
10. King CH, Sutherland LJ, Bertsch D. Systematic review and meta-analysis of the impact of chemical-based mollusciciding for control of *Schistosoma mansoni* and *S. haematobium* transmission. PLoS Negl Trop Dis. 2015;9: e0004290.
11. Peters PA, Warren KS, Mahmoud AA. Rapid, accurate quantification of schistosome eggs *via* nuclepore filters. J Parasitol. 1976;62:154–5.
12. Emukah E, Gutman J, Eguagie J, Miri ES, Yinkore P, Okocha N, et al. Urine heme dipsticks are useful in monitoring the impact of praziquantel treatment on *Schistosoma haematobium* in sentinel communities of Delta State, Nigeria. Acta Trop. 2012;122:126–31.
13. Stete K, Krauth SJ, Coulibaly JT, Knopp S, Hattendorf J, Müller I, et al. Dynamics of *Schistosoma haematobium* egg output and associated infection parameters following treatment with praziquantel in school-aged children. Parasit Vectors. 2012;5:298.
14. Karanja DMS, Awino EK, Wiegand RE, Okoth E, Abudho BO, Mwinzi PNM, et al. Cluster randomized trial comparing school-based mass drug administration schedules in areas of western Kenya with moderate initial prevalence of *Schistosoma mansoni* infections. PLoS Negl Trop Dis. 2017;11: e0006033.
15. Phillips AE, Gazzinelli-Guimaraes PH, Aurelio HO, Ferro J, Nala R, Clements M, et al. Assessing the benefits of five years of different approaches to treatment of urogenital schistosomiasis: a SCORE project in northern Mozambique. PLoS Negl Trop Dis. 2017;11:e0006061.
16. Knopp S, Mohammed KA, Ali SM, Khamis IS, Ame SM, Albonico M, et al. Study and implementation of urogenital schistosomiasis elimination in Zanzibar (Unguja and Pemba islands) using an integrated multidisciplinary approach. BMC Public Health. 2012;12:930.
17. FS MC, Krafft JG. Schistosomiasis in Zanzibar and Pemba. Report on a mission 1 April - 7 June 1975. Geneva: World Health Organization; 1976.
18. Savioli L, Dixon H, Kisumku UM, Mott KE. Control of morbidity due to *Schistosoma haematobium* on Pemba Island; selective population chemotherapy of schoolchildren with haematuria to identify high-risk localities. Trans R Soc Trop Med Hyg. 1989;83:805–10.
19. Mgeni AF, Kisumku UM, McCullough FS, Dixon H, Yoon SS, Mott KE. Metrifonate in the control of urinary schistosomiasis in Zanzibar. Bull World Health Organ. 1990;68:721–30.
20. Knopp S, Stothard JR, Rollinson D, Mohammed KA, Khamis IS, Marti H, et al. From morbidity control to transmission control: time to change tactics against helminths on Unguja Island, Zanzibar. Acta Trop. 2013; 128:412–22.
21. Pennance T, Person B, Muhsin MA, Khamis AN, Muhsin J, Khamis IS, et al. Urogenital schistosomiasis transmission on Unguja Island, Zanzibar: characterisation of persistent hot-spots. Parasit Vectors. 2016;9:646.
22. Knopp S, Person B, Ame SM, Mohammed KA, Ali SM, Khamis IS, et al. Elimination of schistosomiasis transmission in Zanzibar: baseline findings before the onset of a randomized intervention trial. PLoS Negl Trop Dis. 2013;7:e2474.
23. Rollinson D, Klinger EV, Mgeni AF, Khamis IS, Stothard JR. Urinary schistosomiasis on Zanzibar: application of two novel assays for the detection of excreted albumin and haemoglobin in urine. J Helminthol. 2005;79:199–206.
24. Stothard JR, Sousa-Figueiredo JC, Standley C, Van Dam GJ, Knopp S, Utzinger J, et al. An evaluation of urine-CCA strip test and fingerprick blood SEA-ELISA for detection of urinary schistosomiasis in schoolchildren in Zanzibar. Acta Trop. 2009;111:64–70.
25. Montresor A, Crompton DWT, Hall A, Bundy DAP, Savioli L. Guidelines for the evaluation of soil-transmitted helminthiasis and schistosomiasis at community level. Geneva: World Health Organization; 1998.
26. Landis JR, Koch GG. The measurement of observer agreement for categorical data. Biometrics. 1977;33:159–74.
27. Taylor P, Chandiwana SK, Matanhire D. Evaluation of the reagent strip test for haematuria in the control of *Schistosoma haematobium* infection in schoolchildren. Acta Trop. 1990;47:91–100.
28. Feldmeier H, Poggensee G. Diagnostic techniques in schistosomiasis control. A review. Acta Trop. 1993;52:205–20.
29. Knopp S, Becker S, Ingram K, Keiser J, Utzinger J. Diagnosis and treatment of schistosomiasis in children in the era of intensified control. Expert Rev Anti Infect Ther. 2013;11:1237–58.
30. King CH, Bertsch D. Meta-analysis of urine heme dipstick diagnosis of *Schistosoma haematobium* infection, including low-prevalence and previously-treated populations. PLoS Negl Trop Dis. 2013;7:e2431.
31. Knopp S, Corstjens PL, Koukounari A, Cercamondi CI, Ame SM, Ali SM, et al. Sensitivity and specificity of a urine circulating anodic antigen test for the diagnosis of *Schistosoma haematobium* in low endemic settings. PLoS Negl Trop Dis. 2015;9:e0003752.
32. Ephraim RK, Abongo CK, Sakyi SA, Brenyah RC, Diabor E, Bogoch II. Microhaematuria as a diagnostic marker of *Schistosoma haematobium* in an outpatient clinical setting: results from a cross-sectional study in rural Ghana. Trop Doct. 2015;45:194–6.
33. Ibironke OA, Phillips AE, Garba A, Lamine SM, Shiff C. Diagnosis of *Schistosoma haematobium* by detection of specific DNA fragments from filtered urine samples. Am J Trop Med Hyg. 2011;84:998–1001.
34. Ibironke O, Koukounari A, Asaolu S, Moustaki I, Shiff C. Validation of a new test for *Schistosoma haematobium* based on detection of Dra1 DNA fragments in urine: evaluation through latent class analysis. PLoS Negl Trop Dis. 2012;6:e1464.
35. Corstjens PLAM, Nyakundi RK, de Dood CJ, Kariuki TM, Ochola E, Karanja DM, et al. Improved sensitivity of the urine CAA lateral-flow assay for diagnosing active *Schistosoma* infections by using larger sample volumes. Parasit Vectors. 2015;8:241.
36. Colley DG, Binder S, Campbell C, King CH, Tchuem Tchuenté LA, N'Goran EK, et al. A five-country evaluation of a point-of-care circulating cathodic antigen urine assay for the prevalence of *Schistosoma mansoni*. Am J Trop Med Hyg. 2013;88:426–32.
37. Utzinger J, Becker SL, van Lieshout L, van Dam GJ, Knopp S. New diagnostic tools in schistosomiasis. Clin Microbiol Infect. 2015;21:529–42.

6

Species distribution and seasonal dynamics of equine tick infestation in two Mediterranean climate niches in Israel

Sharon Tirosh-Levy[1], Yuval Gottlieb[1*], Dmitry A. Apanaskevich[2], Kosta Y. Mumcuoglu[3] and Amir Steinman[1]

Abstract

Background: Ticks are important ectoparasites of horses that can affect animal welfare and vector several infectious, including zoonotic, diseases. In order to investigate the species distribution, epidemiology and seasonal dynamics of ticks infesting horses in Israel, 3267 ticks were collected from 396 horses in 24 farms across the country from July 2014 to June 2015.

Results: Ticks were found on 50% of the farms and on 25% of the horses, with *Hyalomma* being the most prevalent genus (70% of ticks). Pasture was the most prominent risk factor for tick infestation (99% of ticks, $P < 0.001$), and is represented here by two areas with a Mediterranean climate that differ in their environmental characteristics: the Golan Heights (GH, 74% of ticks); and the Carmel mountain ridge (CMR, 24%). Although these two sites are less than 100 km apart, the composition of the tick populations infesting horses differed significantly between them. In GH the most abundant tick species was *Hyalomma excavatum* ($P < 0.001$), while in CMR it was *Hyalomma marginatum* ($P < 0.001$). The GH also hosted a more diverse tick fauna than the CMR, including *Haemaphysalis parva* (peaking in the autumn, $P < 0.001$) and *Rhipicephalus turanicus* (peaking in the spring, $P < 0.001$), which were not found at the other sites. A few *Rhipicephalus bursa*, *Hyalomma rufipes* and *Hyalomma turanicum* were also found on horses.

Conclusions: The current findings can be used in epidemiological studies assessing the risk of tick-borne equine diseases in the area. Further analysis is needed to determine the specific distribution and habitat preferences of each tick species.

Keywords: *Hyalomma*, *Rhipicephalus*, *Haemaphysalis*, Horse, Epidemiology, Israel

Background

Ticks are important ectoparasites of horses that can affect animal welfare and vector several infectious, including zoonotic, diseases. In recent years there has been a growing interest in assessing the climate niches of different tick species in order to better understand the relationship between pathogens, vectors and hosts [1]. The survival of different life stages of ticks, as well as their successful reproduction, is dependent on a combination of environmental and biotic factors, including climate, vegetation and host availability. Some ticks also exhibit ecological plasticity and may easily adapt to changing climate and new habitats [2, 3]. Climate changes in recent years have led to changes in the distribution of several tick species and introduction of certain tick species and infectious agents into previously unaffected areas [2, 4–6].

Israel is situated in the Mediterranean region, with a climate ranging from Mediterranean to extreme arid (Fig. 1) and provides a habitat for a variety of ixodid tick species. As a result, Israel has many endemic tick-borne diseases that affect humans and other animals, including pets and livestock (www.gideononline.com/ebooks/country/infectious-diseases-of-israel/). Equine piroplasmosis (EP) is highly prevalent in Israel [7–9], and zoonotic diseases such as Crimean Congo hemorrhagic fever (CCHF) and Mediterranean spotted fever (MSF) have been reported in the country and can be transmitted from ticks to horses [10–13]. Several tick species have been reported to infest horses in Israel. The ticks

* Correspondence: gottlieb.yuval@mail.huji.ac.il
[1]Koret School of Veterinary Medicine, The Robert H. Smith Faculty of Agriculture, Food and Environment, The Hebrew University of Jerusalem, Rehovot, Israel
Full list of author information is available at the end of the article

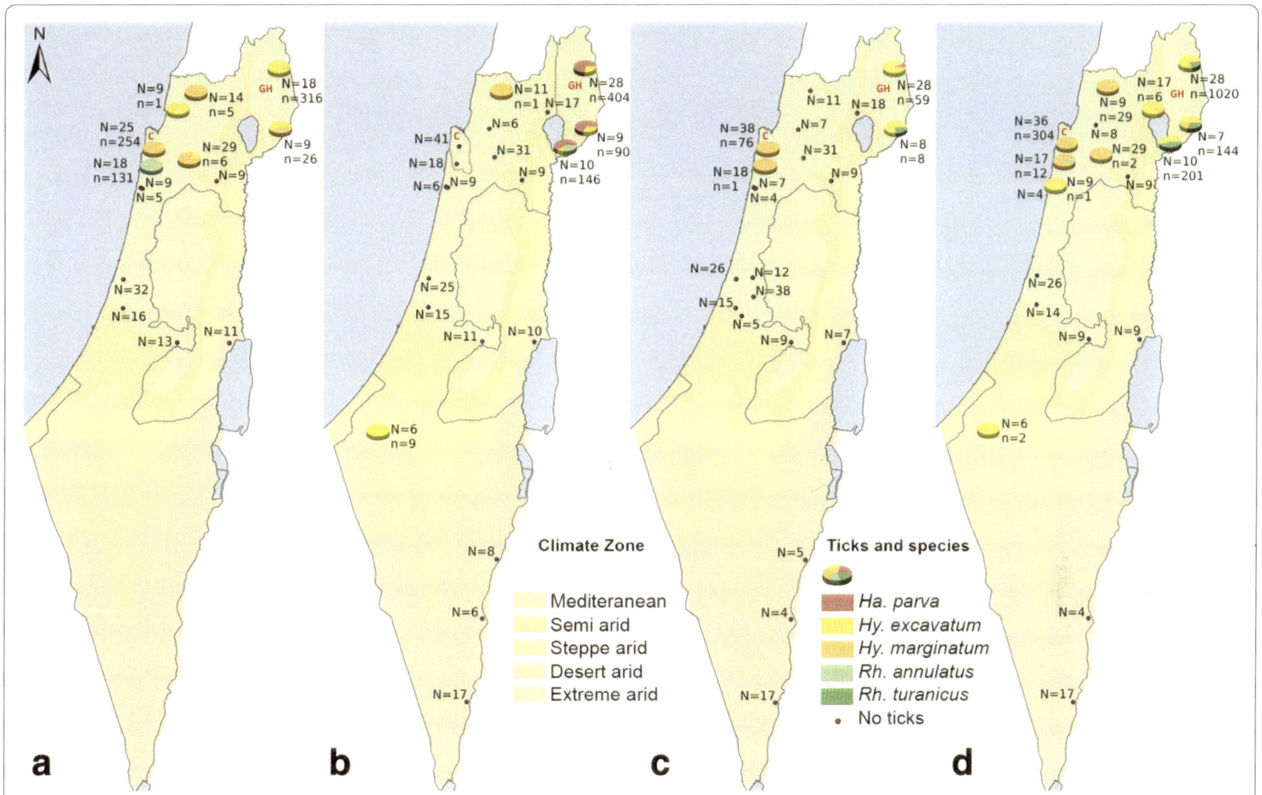

Fig. 1 Geographical and seasonal distribution of equine ticks in Israel. Tick species distribution in each farm is depicted in a pie chart. **a** Summer (July-August 2014). **b** Autumn (November-December 2014). **c** Winter (February-March 2015). **d** Spring (May-June 2015). *Abbreviations*: N, number of horses scanned; n, number of ticks collected, C- Carmel mountain ridge, CG- Golan Heights

are mainly of the genus *Hyalomma*, including several possible vectors of EP and CCHF. However, none of the previous studies focused on horses as a host, and all were performed more than four decades ago [14–16].

The present study was designed as a large-scale survey of the horse population in Israel in order to describe equine tick infestation, identify risk factors, and explore the environmental and climatic factors associated with different tick species.

Methods

Tick collection and identification

Ticks were collected from horses at 24 farms selected to represent different geographical and climatic areas in Israel. Collections were performed every three months to represent all seasons: summer, July-August 2014; autumn, November-December 2014; winter, February-March 2015; and spring, May-June 2015. On each occasion 14–21 farms were visited, all available horses were inspected thoroughly, and all ticks were removed manually and stored in absolute ethanol until processing. During sampling, data were collected regarding the characteristics of each horse, the management of the farm (housing in stalls, paddocks or pasture), and the site of the body of the horse from which ticks were removed.

The sex, stage and species of each tick were determined according to its morphological characteristics [16–19].

Environmental data

Geographical and environmental characteristics of each farm were analyzed using the geographical information system (GIS). Data obtained using remote sensing MODIS (moderate resolution imaging spectroradiometer satellite) technology comprised altitude, average salinity of soil, two vegetation indices (normalized difference vegetation index (NDVI) and enhanced vegetation index (EVI), and minimum, maximum and mean land surface temperature during the day (LSTD) and night (LSTN) [20]. Data obtained from the Israel meteorological service website (https://ims.data.gov.il/) for each sampling period comprised average rainfall, number of rainy days, and maximum daily rainfall, as well as minimum, maximum and mean ambient temperature, average moist temperature, average dew-point temperature, average humidity and average wind speed. Data of the soil type were obtained from the Israel government agency for mapping website (http://www.govmap.gov.il/).

Statistical analysis

Data were analyzed in three ways: (i) Data for each individual tick were used to determine tick species and sex distribution, and its association with factors such as season and location on the horse. Associations between categorical parameters and each specific tick species were analyzed using χ^2 or Fisher's exact test, as appropriate. Relative abundance of each tick species was calculated as the seasonal percentage of the species collected throughout the year. (ii) Data pertaining to each farm, the average number of total ticks and specific tick species per horse (total number of ticks collected/number of examined horses), in each season were used to determine associations between tick infestation and farm location, geographical area and housing of the horses. Associations with climatic parameters were analyzed only for farms with pasture. Associations between categorical parameters and tick load were determined by Student's t-test or analysis of variance (ANOVA), as appropriate. Correlations with climatic quantitative parameters were calculated using Spearman's rho (ρ). (iii) Data presenting the tick load of each of the examined horses housed on pasture were used to analyze associations between tick burden and horse age, sex, breed and color. Associations between categorical parameters and tick load were determined by Student's t-test or ANOVA, as appropriate, and odds ratios (OR) were calculated with their 95% confidence intervals (CI). All parameters that significantly correlated with total tick load were included in a multivariable forward stepwise logistic regression model, as well as a Generalized Estimating Equation (GEE), with the farm as a random variable. Statistical significance was set at $P < 0.05$. The analyses were performed using SPSS 22.0® and WinPepi 11.43® statistical software.

Table 1 The prevalence of horses' tick infestation on different farms during different seasons in Israel. The number of infested horses per the number on examined horses (%) are specified for each farm

Farm	Location	Summer (Jul-Aug 2014)	Autumn (Nov-Dec 2014)	Winter (Feb-Mar 2015)	Spring (May-Jun 2015)	Mean (%)
A[a,b]	33°13'25.8"N, 35°77'70.7"E	15/18 (83.3)	0/18 (0)	1/18 (5.5)	5/17 (29.4)	29.6
B	32°51'44.8"N, 34°94'99.9"E	0/9 (0)	0/9 (0)	0/7 (0)	1/9 (11.1)	2.9
C	32°52'95"N, 34°92'67.3"E	0/5 (0)	0/6 (0)	0/4 (0)	0/4 (0)	0
D[a,b]	32°73'16"N, 35°00'63.1"E	24/25 (96)	0/41 (0)	23/38 (60.5)	36/36 (100)	59.3
E	32°95'91.2"N, 35°80'30.7"E	0/33 (0)	0/25 (0)	0/26 (0)	0/26 (0)	0
F	29°94'16.1"N, 35°06'46.9"E	0/16 (0)	0/15 (0)	0/15 (0)	0/14 (0)	0
G	32°90'48.1"N, 35°54'97"E	0/13 (0)	0/11 (0)	0/9 (0)	0/9 (0)	0
H	33°01'64.6"N, 35°26'38.8"E	2/11 (18.2)	1/10 (10)	0/7 (0)	0/9 (0)	8.1
I	32°92'95.9"N, 35°15'08"E	4/29 (13.8)	0/31 (0)	0/31 (0)	1/29 (3.4)	4.2
J	31°92'27.8"N, 34°82'11.9"E	11/9 (11.1)	–	–	–	11.1
K[a]	32°83'28.5"N, 35°78'35.7"E	3/14 (21.4)	1/11 (9.1)	0/11 (0)	7/9 (77.8)	24.4
L[a,c]	30°36'26.4"N, 35°15'51.4"E	7/9 (77.8)	7/9 (77.8)	5/8 (62.5)	7/7 (100)	78.8
M[a,c]	31°75'21"N, 35°15'01.6"E	18/18 (100)	28/28 (100)	19/28 (67.9)	28/28 (100)	91.2
N	32°55'68"N, 35°39'29.9"E	0/10 (10)	0/9 (0)	0/9 (0)	0/9 (0)	0
O	31°75'25.5"N, 35°46'62.9"E	–	0/17 (0)	0/17 (0)	0/17 (0)	0
P	32°82'17.9"N, 35°19'01.1"E	–	0/6 (0)	0/4 (0)	0/4 (0)	0
Q	32°67'58.5"N, 35°22'39.8"E	–	0/8 (0)	0/5 (0)	–	0
R[a]	31°88'32"N, 34°85'92.3"E	–	0/17 (0)	0/18 (0)	5/17 (29.4)	9.6
S	32°61'13.2"N, 34°99'14.4"E	–	0/6 (0)	0/7 (0)	0/8 (0)	0
T[a,c]	32°06'84.2"N, 34°82'47.8"E	–	9/10 (90)	–	10/10 (100)	95
U	32°07'66.8"N, 34°92'27.6"E	–	4/6 (66.7)		2/6 (33.3)	50
V	31°98'04.9"N, 34°92'76.9"E	–	–	0/38 (0)	–	0
W	31°30'40.9"N, 34°52'48.6"E	–	–	0/12 (0)	–	0
X	30°65'87.5"N, 35°23'96.5"E	–	–	0/5 (0)	–	0
Mean (%)		33.8	17.1	15.1	38	25

[a]Farms in which horses are kept on pasture
[b]Farms located in the CMR
[c]Farms located in the GH

Results

Host study population

For the study, 396 horses were sampled on 24 farms: 218 horses on 14 farms during the summer; 293 horses on 20 farms during the autumn; 317 horses on 21 farms during the winter; and 268 horses on 19 farms during the spring. Of these, 156 horses were sampled for all four seasons, 93 horses were sampled for three seasons, 47 horses were sampled for two seasons, and 100 horses were sampled only once, making a total of 1096 samples (Additional file 1: Table S1).

Of the 396 horses, 191 (49%) were mares, 193 (48%) were geldings, and 12 (3%) were stallions. Most of the horses (251, 63%) were mixed-breed, while the rest were pure-bred, comprising 68 (17%) Quarter horses; 10 (2.5%) Paint horses; 13 (3%) Ponies; 10 (2.5%) Arabians; and several other breeds (fewer than 10 horses of each). Horses were of various colors: 54% were dark (124 chestnut, 73 bay, 9 black and 8 brown), 29% were light (61 gray, 32 palomino, 10 buckskin, 9 dun, 2 roan and one perlino), and 17% were spotted (36 pinto and 30 appaloosa).

Spatio-temporal distribution of the tick species infesting horses

A total of 3267 ticks were collected during the study period. Ticks were found on 50% (12/24) of farms and on 25% (274/1096) of horses (Additional file 1: Table S1). The vast majority (99%) of ticks (3238) were collected from horses on pasture ($F_{(2,71)} = 8.408$, $P < 0.001$). Seven of the 24 examined farms kept horses on pasture and were located in three geographical regions: two in the Galilee, two on the Carmel mountain ridge (CMR) and three on the Golan Heights (GH) (Fig. 1). The majority of ticks (98%) were collected from five of these farms: 74% (2417 ticks) in the GH and 24% (782 ticks) in the CMR ($F_{(4,69)} = 8.598$, $P < 0.001$). The number of infested horses at each farm is provided in Table 1.

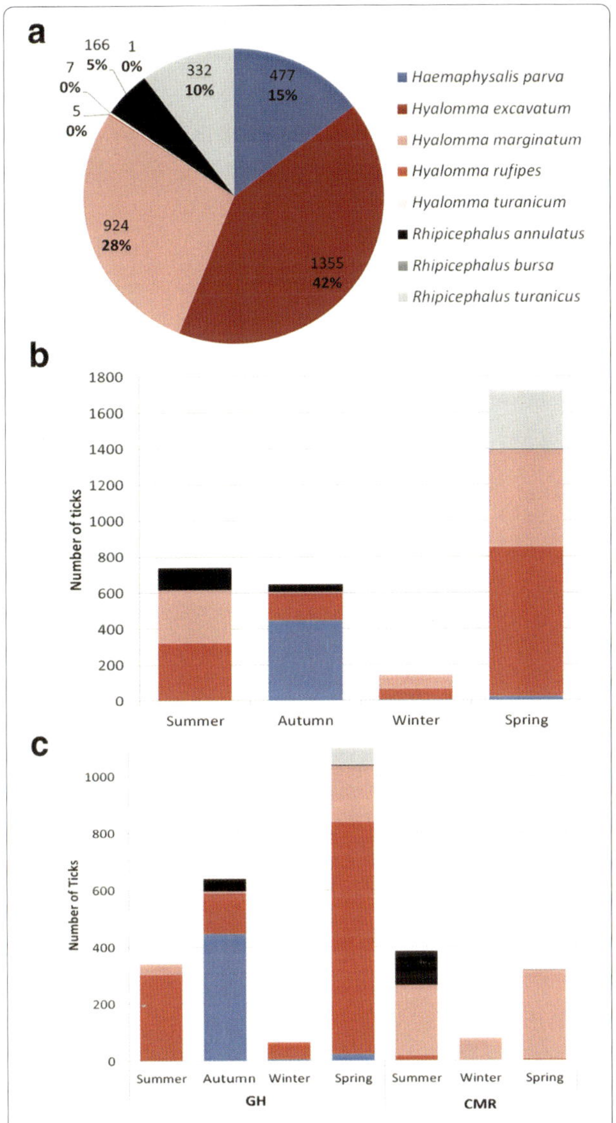

Fig. 2 The distribution of tick species found on horses in Israel during a one-year period. **a** The number of ticks collected of each species and its percentage of the total ticks collected. **b** Seasonal distribution of equine tick infestation. **c** Tick species distribution in different seasons in the Golan Heights (GH) and in the Carmel Mountain Ridge (CMR)

Eight species of ticks were found to infest horses and the total number of ticks and species distribution varied among farms and seasons (Fig. 2). *Hyalomma* was the major tick genus, peaking in the spring and summer ($\chi^2 = 826$, $df = 3$, $P < 0.001$), with *Hy. excavatum* being the most prevalent species in the GH ($\chi^2 = 665$, $df = 3$, $P < 0.001$) and *Hy. marginatum* the most prevalent in the CMR ($P < 0.001$, two-sided). *Haemaphysalis parva* and *Rhipicephalus turanicus* ticks were found only in the GH, with *Ha. parva* peaking in the autumn ($P < 0.001$, two-sided) and *Rh. turanicus* peaking in the spring ($\chi^2 = 311$, $df = 3$, $P < 0.001$). *Rhipicephalus* (*Boophilus*) *annulatus* was found mainly on two farms (one in the CMR and the other in the GH), in which the horses were used for herding cattle ($\chi^2 = 542$, $df = 1$, $P < 0.001$). *Hyalomma turanicum* was rarely found, and was almost exclusive (6/7 ticks) on one farm located in the Great Rift Valley, near the Dead Sea.

Almost all ticks found were adults (99.9%, 4 nymphs, 1 larva), 59% male (1940 ticks) and 41% female (1322) (Fig. 3). Female *Hyalomma* spp. and *Ha. parva* were more abundant than males in this tick's peak season (spring: $\chi^2 = 113$, $df = 3$, $P < 0.001$; autumn: $\chi^2 = 77$, $df = 2$, $P < 0.001$, respectively).

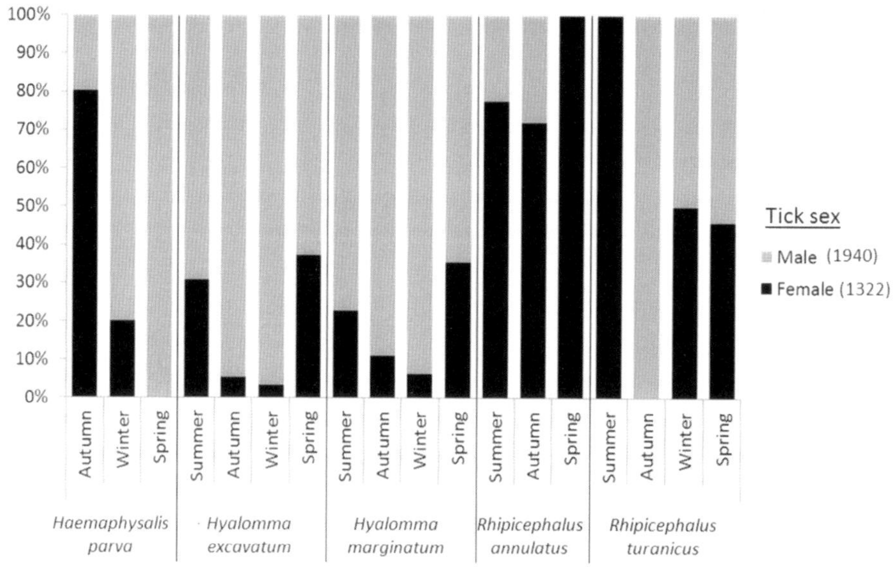

Fig. 3 Percentage of male (gray) and female (black) ticks found on horses in Israel in different seasons

Association between host parameters and tick infestation

The host parameters significantly associated with tick infestation in the univariable analysis are summarized in Table 2. Mixed-breed horses displayed a higher tick burden than pure-bred horses, with similar association for all tick species. All tick species, except *Rh.* (*B.*) *annulatus*, infested mares more than male horses (stallions and geldings). Spotted horses (pintos or appaloosas) had lower tick burdens than solid colored horses, but this burden was not different for *Hy. marginatum* and *Rh.* (*B.*) *annulatus* infestation. Horse age was not associated with tick infestation. Both breed (OR = 6.43, 95% CI: 2.05–10.82, $df = 1$, $P = 0.004$) and sex (OR = 5.34, 95% CI: 1.51–9.16, $df = 1$, $P = 0.006$) of the horse were found to be significant predictors of tick infestation in the multivariable GEE model.

The distribution of ticks on different body parts of the horse varied among tick species (Fig. 4). *Hyalomma* ticks were found mainly on the rear parts of the horse: under the tail, in the inguinal area and hidden in the prepuce or between the udders ($\chi^2 = 1312$, $df = 3$, $P < 0.001$); *Haemaphysalis parva* ticks were found mostly on the proximal parts of the horse, including the neck, chest and trunk ($\chi^2 = 1330$, $df = 8$, $P < 0.001$); and *Rh. turanicus* ticks were found in both the ears and inguinal areas ($\chi^2 = 300$, $df = 8$, $P < 0.001$), but mainly on the rear (inguinal and under the tail) part of the horse ($\chi^2 = 10$, $df = 3$, $P = 0.018$).

Table 2 Host parameters significantly associated with tick infestation in univariable analysis. Tick were collected from 396 horses on 24 farms in Israel during one year

		Mean	SD	*t*-value	*df*	*P*-value
Breed	Mixed	7.41	12.16	12.389	446	<0.001
	Pure	0.15	0.36	–	–	–
Sex	Female	10.02	14.77	4.763	307	<0.001
	Male	4.55	8.24	–	–	–
Color	Spotted	3.52	7.44	-4.332	252	<0.001
	Solid	7.89	12.68	–	–	–

Abbreviations: df degrees of freedom, *SD* standard deviation

Environmental and climatic characteristics of the inspected farms

Farms were selected to represent the distribution of the equine population in Israel, with more farms in the north and center of the country and fewer in the south. Most of the farms were located in areas of Mediterranean climate (15 farms), and the rest in areas ranging from semi arid to extreme arid (Fig. 1). Three of the five farms at which the majority of ticks were collected were located in the GH, and the remaining two in the CMR.

The GH is a volcanic plateau located between 300–1100 meters above sea level, with climate ranging from Mediterranean in the north to semi-arid in the south. The soil type is grumusol and basaltic protogrumusol. Most ticks were collected at one farm with 30 horses, located in the north of the GH, at an altitude of 980 m and with an average annual rainfall of 850 mm. The other two farms (10 horses each) were located further south, at an altitude of approximately 420 m and with an average rainfall of 625 mm.

The Carmel is a limestone mountain ridge located near the Mediterranean Sea. It peaks at 546 m, and features a Mediterranean climate and vegetation. The soil

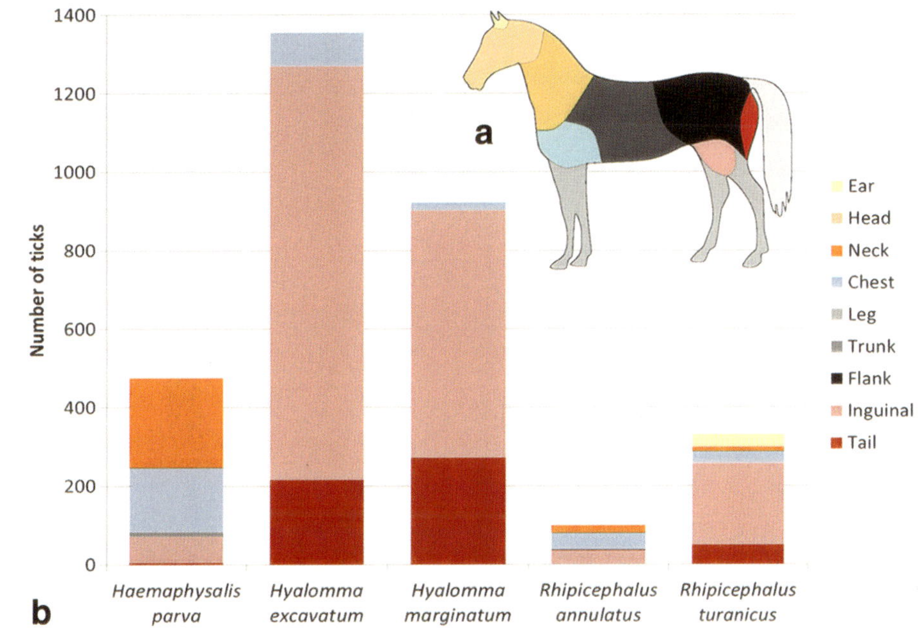

Fig. 4 Tick species and the body site of the horse from which they were removed. **a** A schematic illustration of the different body sites of the horse, as referred to in this analysis. **b** The number of ticks of the different species collected from each body site of the horse

there is mainly terra-rossa and rendzina. One of the farms had 47 horses and was located 320 m above sea level, while the other had 18 horses and was located at an altitude of 119 m. The environmental characteristics of both areas are provided in Table 3.

Associations between environmental parameters and tick infestation

Rainfall per season, number of rainy days, and maximum daily rain had a strong positive correlation ($\rho > 0.86$ and $P < 0.001$ for all associations), while maximum, minimum, and average ambient temperature, as well as moist temperature and dew point, positively correlated together ($\rho > 0.61$ and $P < 0.007$ for all, and $\rho > 0.95$ and $P < 0.001$ for all but the maximum ambient temperature) and negatively correlated with the rain parameters ($\rho < -0.69$ and $P < 0.002$).

The relative abundance of each tick species in the different seasons is provided in Table 4, and the association between tick infestation and environmental parameters is presented in Table 5. The average number of ticks per horse was moderately negatively correlated with the number of rainy days per season, mean NDVI (normalized difference vegetation index), and mean EVI (enhanced vegetation index), and showed a moderate positive correlation with maximum EVI and altitude. All these factors were also found to be statistically significant in the multivariable logistic regression model (all $P < 0.001$).

Specifically, *Ha. parva* infestation moderately and negatively correlated with all ambient temperature parameters. *Hyalomma excavatum* infestation moderately and negatively correlated with mean and minimum NDVI and EVI, mean and minimum LSTN (land surface temperature in the night), minimum LSTD (land surface temperature in the day) and soil salinity and moderately and positively correlated with mean and maximum LSTD, altitude, and wind speed. *Hyalomma marginatum* infestation negatively correlated with all rain parameters, and positively correlated with all temperature parameters, except the minimum ambient temperature. *Rhipicephalus (B.) annulatus* demonstrated a moderate negative correlation with multi-annual average rainfall and maximum LSTD and altitude, and a moderate positive correlation with the minimum LSTN.

Rhipicephalus turanicus infestation had a moderate negative correlation with mean and minimum NDVI and EVI and soil salinity, and a moderate positive correlation with maximum EVI and mean LSTD.

Discussion

The tick species infesting horses found in this survey represent species that are prevalent on livestock throughout the Mediterranean area [21–25], and differ from tick species found on horses elsewhere [26–28]. Almost all ticks found were adults, which suggests that the immature stages infest other host species. All the four nymphs and one larva that we found belonged to the species *Rh. annulatus*, which is a one-host tick, and thus all stages are expected to be found on the same host. The seasonal abundance of each species concurs with previous data on

Table 3 Environmental characteristics of the two Israeli Mediterranean climate regions examined in the current study: The Golan Heights (GH) and the Carmel mountain ridge (CMR)

	GH	CMR
Farms	3	2
Horses	49	65
Ticks	2417	782
Altitude (m)	420–980	119–320
Soil	Grumusol	Terra rosa
	Basaltic protogrumusol	Rendzina
Climate	Mediterranean to Semi-arid	Mediterranean
Annual rainfall (mm)	625–850	987
Average NVDI	0.04	0.06
Average EVI	0.024	0.03
LSTD (°C)	2–51	9–45
LSTN (°C)	-3–28	1–26
Average humidity (%)	66	69
Rainfall July-August	0	0
Ambient temperature July-August (°C)	14–37 (avg. 25)	19–34 (avg. 26)
Average rainfall November-December (mm)	90	86
Rainy days November-December	17–24	20–22
Ambient temperature November-December (°C)	-2–28.5 (avg. 13)	8–29 (avg. 17)
Average rainfall February-March (mm)	97	115
Rainy days February-March	20–28	20–22
Ambient temperature February-March (°C)	-5–29 (avg. 12)	3–29 (avg. 15)
Average rainfall May-June (mm)	1.3	2
Rainy days May-June	1	4
Ambient temperature May-June (°C)	6–40 (avg. 21)	11–39 (avg. 22)

Abbreviations: *avg* average, *NDVI* normalized difference vegetation index, *EVI* enhanced vegetation index, *LSTD* land surface temperature in the day, *LSTN* land surface temperature in the night

its peak season [24]. Tick sex ratio varied between seasons, with more females than males being found in the peak season of each species.

The vast majority of ticks were recovered from horses on pasture, which is the most prominent risk factor for tick infestation. Naturally, the chance of tick-host encounter increases on pasture environment, and most of the other studies of equine ectoparasites have focused on horses on pasture [26, 28]. Although the present study was designed to represent most of Israel's geographical and climatic areas, the pasture factor obscured most of the other examined factors and, therefore, we focused only on the population of horses on pasture for most analyses. Specifically, we focused on two pasture areas in northern Israel under Mediterranean climate: the CMR and the GH regions, which are less than 100 km apart. These geographical regions differ in rock and soil composition, vegetation type, and many environmental parameters, and form different habitats for equine infesting ticks, as demonstrated in this study.

Table 4 Seasonal relative abundance of the different tick species infesting horses in Israel. Bold represents peak season of each species

	Summer	Autumn	Winter	Spring
Haemaphysalis parva	0	**0.94**	0.01	0.05
Hyalomma excavatum	**0.24**	0.11	0.04	**0.61**
Hyalomma marginatum	**0.32**	0.01	0.08	**0.58**
Hyalomma rufipes	**0.8**	0.2	0	0
Hyalomma turanicum	**0.71**	0.14	0	0.14
Rhipicephalus annulatus	**0.72**	0.26	0	0.02
Rhipicephalus bursa	0	0	0	**1**
Rhipicephalus turanicus	0.01	0.00	0.01	**0.98**
Total	0.23	0.20	0.04	0.53

The predominant species in the CMR area was *Hy. marginatum* and the predominant species in the GH was *Hy. excavatum*. Although a similar number of horses was examined in both areas, the number of ticks found in the GH was 3-fold higher than that in the CMR, and the tick species found in the GH were more diverse. While all species found in the CMR were also found in the GH, *Rh. turanicus* and *Ha. parva* were found only in the GH (Fig. 2c). This difference in species diversity may reflect environmental or climatic preferences of different tick species or related to available hosts suitable for the tick immature stages.

Hyalomma is the most abundant tick genus infesting livestock in Mediterranean, semi-arid, and arid climates of Asia, Europe and Africa [24], and was the most abundant genus found on horses in this study (70%). *Hyalomma excavatum* was the most prevalent species, found in all examined parts of the country, but mostly in the GH. It is a two- or three-host tick species, whose adults feed mainly on ungulates, and it is the most prevalent tick species infesting cattle in Israel and Turkey [21, 24, 29, 30]. *Hyalomma marginatum* has been previously documented in Israel on cattle and horses [16], as well as on roe deer (*Capreolus capreolus*) in the CMR area [31]. This tick species is less tolerant to a dry climate [24], which may explain its presence in the more humid and arboreal environment typical of the CMR. The species is of growing significance since it is considered an important vector of CCHF, as well as of the equine

Table 5 Spearman's coefficient (ρ) and its significance (*P*) between environmental parameters and tick abundance on horses in Israel. Bold represents significant correlations

	Ticks		*Ha. parva*		*Hy. excavatum*		*Hy. marginatum*		*Rh. annulatus*		*Rh. turanicus*	
	ρ	*P*	ρ	*P*	ρ	*P*	ρ	*P*	ρ	*P*	ρ	*P*
Multiannual avg. rainfall	-0.01	0.98	0.15	0.55	0.08	0.74	0.29	0.24	**-0.51**	**0.03**	-0.03	0.92
Avg. NDVI	**-0.50**	**0.03**	-0.40	0.10	**-0.65**	**0.00**	0.25	0.33	-0.25	0.31	**-0.52**	**0.03**
Max. NDVI	0.21	0.40	0.11	0.65	0.04	0.89	0.05	0.85	0.19	0.45	-0.02	0.93
Min. NDVI	-0.42	0.08	-0.34	0.16	**-0.63**	**0.00**	0.16	0.51	-0.09	0.71	**-0.49**	**0.04**
Avg. EVI	**-0.50**	**0.03**	-0.40	0.10	**-0.65**	**0.00**	0.25	0.33	-0.25	0.31	**-0.52**	**0.03**
Max. EVI	**0.50**	**0.03**	0.40	0.10	**0.65**	**0.00**	-0.25	0.33	0.25	0.31	**0.52**	**0.03**
Min. EVI	-0.42	0.08	-0.34	0.16	**-0.63**	**0.00**	0.16	0.51	-0.09	0.71	**-0.49**	**0.04**
Max. LSTD	0.37	0.13	0.36	0.15	**0.56**	**0.02**	0.38	0.12	**-0.51**	**0.03**	0.27	0.28
Avg. LSTD	0.42	0.08	0.34	0.16	**0.63**	**0.00**	-0.16	0.51	0.09	0.71	**0.49**	**0.04**
Min. LSTD	-0.45	0.06	-0.41	0.09	**-0.58**	**0.01**	-0.30	0.23	0.35	0.16	-0.30	0.23
Max. LSTN	0.28	0.26	0.42	0.08	0.29	0.25	-0.15	0.55	0.05	0.84	0.23	0.36
Avg. LSTN	-0.19	0.46	-0.34	0.16	**-0.49**	**0.04**	-0.10	0.70	0.47	0.05	-0.34	0.17
Min. LSTN	-0.29	0.24	-0.34	0.16	**-0.60**	**0.01**	-0.30	0.22	**0.59**	**0.01**	-0.34	0.17
Altitude	**0.47**	**0.05**	0.45	0.06	**0.77**	**0.00**	0.28	0.26	**-0.49**	**0.04**	0.45	0.06
Soil salinity	-0.39	0.11	-0.41	0.09	**-0.72**	**0.00**	-0.13	0.61	0.40	0.10	**-0.48**	**0.05**
Avg. rainfall	-0.38	0.12	0.34	0.17	-0.20	0.42	**-0.52**	**0.03**	-0.29	0.24	-0.19	0.45
Rainy days	**-0.50**	**0.03**	0.35	0.15	-0.25	0.32	**-0.60**	**0.01**	-0.37	0.13	-0.21	0.40
Max. daily rain	-0.35	0.15	0.38	0.12	-0.16	0.53	**-0.53**	**0.02**	-0.24	0.33	-0.18	0.46
Max. temperature	0.34	0.17	**-0.50**	**0.04**	0.14	0.57	**0.49**	**0.04**	0.17	0.49	0.34	0.16
Min. temperature	0.07	0.79	**-0.59**	**0.01**	-0.21	0.41	0.44	0.07	0.28	0.27	-0.16	0.52
Avg. temperature	0.21	0.41	**-0.58**	**0.01**	-0.07	0.79	**0.50**	**0.04**	0.30	0.22	0.02	0.95
Moist temperature	0.17	0.51	**-0.58**	**0.01**	-0.14	0.58	**0.53**	**0.03**	0.31	0.20	-0.05	0.83
Dew point	0.15	0.56	**-0.61**	**0.01**	-0.14	0.57	**0.58**	**0.01**	0.26	0.30	-0.06	0.82
Avg. humidity	-0.19	0.45	0.15	0.54	-0.20	0.43	-0.02	0.94	0.14	0.58	-0.33	0.18
Avg. wind speed	0.37	0.19	0.05	0.86	**0.54**	**0.05**	0.29	0.32	-0.50	0.07	0.27	0.35

Abbreviations: *Min* minimum, *Max* maximum, *Avg* verage, *NDVI* normalized difference vegetation index, *EVI* enhanced vegetation index, *LSTD* land surface temperature in the day, *LSTN* land surface temperature in the night

piroplams, *Theileria* and *Babesia* species. Moreover, climate change have led to the spread of *Hy. marginatum* to new niches in Europe [2, 5, 6, 24]. Both *Hy. excavatum* and *Hy. marginatum* are established vectors of EP [32], which is endemic in Israel [7, 8].

Hyalomma turanicum and *Hy. rufipes* are closely related to *Hy. marginatum* [17, 24]. Only seven *Hy. turanicum* ticks were found in this study, six of which were on one farm located near the Dead Sea, in the Great Rift Valley area, which is characterized by a desert arid to extreme arid climate and low altitude (361 m below sea level). This species prefers steppe and desert climates [24], which may explain its restriction to this specific farm. *Hyalomma rufipes* vectors CCHF and several *Rickettsia* and *Babesia* species, and has been found on migratory birds in Israel and elsewhere [4, 24, 33]. Only five *Hy. rufipes* ticks were found in this survey in both the CMR and the GH. This number seems to be somewhat low considering that Israel is a major path for migratory birds between Africa, Asia, and Europe, and features a suitable climate for this species, although its adults are rarely found outside the Afrotropical region.

About 15% of the recovered ticks were of the genus *Rhipicephalus*. *Rhipicephalus turanicus* was the most prevalent species of this genus, and was found only in the GH and in the spring. It is found on a large variety of hosts and of climates [13, 16, 24, 29, 31, 34] and its restriction here to one geographical area was unexpected. *Rhipicephalus* (*B.*) *annulatus* was found only on horses working and grazing with cattle. It is a one-host tick with a clear preference for cattle, but can occasionally be found on horses [14, 24, 29]. It is also an important vector of several cattle hemoparasites [24, 35], but since it is mainly adapted to cattle, its role in vectoring equine pathogens is unknown.

Almost 15% of the ticks were *Ha. parva,* and were found only in the GH in the autumn and winter. This species was documented in Israel to infest mostly sheep and goats, but was also reported in horses and is found mostly in the cold season [16, 25, 29, 36].

Different tick species were found in specific places on the horse: *Hyalomma* spp. were collected mostly from the hindquarters; *Ha. parva* was found mostly on the neck and chest; while *Rhipicephalus* spp. were found on both the hindquarters and ears. These preferences have been previously documented [24, 25], and may reflect different tactics in protection against host defense, or simply different niches on the host of competing species.

Host parameters, such as sex, breed, and color that were found to be associated with tick infestation, mainly reflect the horse populations found on farms with access to pasture. Most pure-bred horses, as well as stallions, are kept in stalls and one of the farms with pasture mainly raises mixed-breed appaloosas.

Several environmental factors, including rain, temperature and vegetation, have been described to affect tick activity and life-cycle, with species-specific and also sub-population preferences [2, 5]. This may partly explain the different abundance of several *Hyalomma* species in the two niches studied. The climate niches in the CMR and the GH differ in many of the inspected parameters, including altitude, soil, the range of both ambient and land surface temperature and rainfall. While many of these parameters correlated with the abundance of different tick species, since data were collected only at four time points, many climatic factors correlated together; and since most ticks were collected in one season, the information we can deduct from these correlations is limited. A more elaborate study or a comparison with high-resolution data from other regions is needed in order to better identify the major climatic and geographical components that influence the preferences of the different species.

Conclusions

This study is the first large-scale survey of ticks infesting horses in Israel, and provides an annual picture of horse-tick interactions. Pasture was found to be the main factor influencing exposure to ticks. Consequently, horse owners as well as veterinarians should consider a practice of parasite control, especially during the peak seasons of spring and summer. The CMR and the GH areas were shown to be distinct habitats in regard both to equine tick abundance and diversity. *Hyalomma* genus was the most prevalent tick observed to affect horses, and the two dominant species are known vectors of EP. *Haemaphysalis parva* and *Rh.* (*B.*) *annulatus* are not known as vectors of equine diseases, and their potential to transmit infectious agents between horses and other hosts should be further explored.

Abbreviations

CCHF: Crimean Congo hemorrhagic fever; CMR: Carmel mountain ridge; EP: Equine piroplasmosis; EVI: Enhanced vegetation index; GH: Golan heights; *Ha.*: *Haemaphysalis*; *Hy.*: *Hyalomma*; LSTD: Land surface temperature during the day; LSTN: Land surface temperature during the night; NDVI: Normalized difference vegetation index; *Rh.* (*B.*): *Rhipicephalus* (*Boophilus*); *Rh.*: *Rhipicephalus*

Acknowledgments

The authors wish to thank the horse owners for their willingness to participate in this study. We also thank to Professor Itamar Lensky, Department of Geography and Environment, Bar-Ilan University, Israel for retrieving the satellite data, and Dr Gila A. Sutton, Professor Eyal Klement, and Wiessam Abu Ahmad, for their advice regarding data interpretation and statistical analysis.

Funding

Not applicable.

Authors' contributions

YG and AS conceived, designed, and supervised the study. DAA and KYM identified the ticks. STL designed the study, collected the ticks, analyzed the data, and drafted the manuscript. All authors read and approved the final manuscript.

Competing interests

The authors declare that they have no competing interests.

Author details

[1]Koret School of Veterinary Medicine, The Robert H. Smith Faculty of Agriculture, Food and Environment, The Hebrew University of Jerusalem, Rehovot, Israel. [2]United States National Tick Collection, James H. Oliver, Jr., Institute of Coastal Plain Sciences, Georgia Southern University, Statesboro, Georgia, USA. [3]Parasitology Unit, Department of Microbiology and Molecular Genetic, The Kuvin Centre for the Study of Infectious and Tropical Diseases, Hebrew University-Hadassah Medical School, Jerusalem, Israel.

References

1. Estrada-Pena A, Ayllon N, de la Fuente J. Impact of climate trends on tick-borne pathogen transmission. Front Physiol. 2012;3:64.
2. Estrada-Pena A. Climate, niche, ticks, and models: what they are and how we should interpret them. Parasitol Res. 2008;103(Suppl. 1):87–95.
3. Sonenshine DE. Biology of Ticks. Vol. 1. New York: Oxford University Press; 2014.
4. Chitimia-Dobler L, Nava S, Bestehorn M, Dobler G, Wolfel S. First detection of *Hyalomma rufipes* in Germany. Ticks Tick Borne Dis. 2016;7:1135–8.

5. Estrada-Pena A, Venzal JM. Climate niches of tick species in the Mediterranean region: modeling of occurrence data, distributional constraints, and impact of climate change. J Med Entomol. 2007;44:1130–8.
6. Vial L, Stachurski F, Leblond A, Huber K, Vourc'h G, Rene-Martellet M, et al. Strong evidence for the presence of the tick *Hyalomma marginatum* Koch, 1844 in southern continental France. Ticks Tick Borne Dis. 2016;7:1162–7.
7. Aharonson-Raz K, Rapoport A, Hawari IM, Lensky IM, Berlin D, Zivotofsky D, et al. Novel description of force of infection and risk factors associated with *Theileria equi* in horses in Israel and in The Palestinian Authority. Ticks Tick Borne Dis. 2014;5:366–72.
8. Rapoport A, Aharonson-Raz K, Berlin D, Tal S, Gottlieb Y, Klement E, Steinman A. Molecular characterization of the *Babesia caballi* rap-1 gene and epidemiological survey in horses in Israel. Infect Genet Evol. 2014;23:115–20.
9. Steinman A, Zimmerman T, Klement E, Lensky IM, Berlin D, Gottlieb Y, et al. Demographic and environmental risk factors for infection by *Theileria equi* in 590 horses in Israel. Vet Parasitol. 2012;187:558–62.
10. Appannanavar SB, Mishra B. An update on crimean congo hemorrhagic fever. J Glob Infect Dis. 2011;3:285–92.
11. Keysary A, Massung RF, Inbar M, Wallach AD, Shanas U, Mumcuoglu KY, et al. Molecular evidence for *Anaplasma phagocytophilum* in Israel. Emerg Infect Dis. 2007;13:1411–2.
12. Stuen S, Granquist EG, Silaghi C. *Anaplasma phagocytophilum* - a widespread multi-host pathogen with highly adaptive strategies. Front Cell Infect Microbiol. 2013;3:31.
13. Mumcuoglu KY, Frish K, Sarov B, Manor E, Gross E, Gat Z, et al. Ecological studies on the brown dog tick *Rhipicephalus sanguineus* (Acari: Ixodidae) in southern Israel and its relationship to spotted fever group rickettsiae. J Med Entomol. 1993;30:114–21.
14. Feldman-Muhsam B. On two rare genera of ticks of domestic stock in Israel. Bull Res Counc Israel. 1953;5B:193.
15. Feldman-Muhsam B, Shechter R. Some notes on the genus *Boophilus* (Ixodidae), with special reference to species found in Israel. J Med Entomol. 1970;7:677–86.16.
16. Theodor O, Costa MA. Survey of the Parasites of Wild Mammals and Birds in Israel. Part I. Ectoparasites. Jerusalem: The Israel Academy of Sciences and Humanities; 1967.
17. Apanaskevich DA, Horak IG. The genus *Hyalomma* Koch, 1844: V. Re-evaluation of the taxonomic rank of taxa comprising the *H.* (*Euhyalomma*) *marginatum* Koch complex of species (Acari: Ixodidae) with redescription of all parasitic stages and notes on biology. Int J Acarol. 2008;34:13–42.
18. Apanaskevich DA, Horak IG. The genus *Hyalomma* Koch, 1844. II. Taxonomic status of *Hyalomma* (*Euhyalomma*) *anatolicum* Koch, 1844 and *H.* (*E.*) *excavatum* Koch, 1844 (Acari, Ixodidae) with redescription of all stages. Acarina. 2005;13:181–97.
19. Filippova NA. Ixodid ticks of subfamily Amblyomminae. Fauna of Russia and Neighbouring Countries. Volume 4. St. Petersburg: Nauka Publishing House; 1997.
20. Morag N, Klement E, Saroya Y, Lensky I, Gottlieb Y. Prevalence of the symbiont *Cardinium* in *Culicoides* (Diptera: Ceratopogonidae) vector species is associated with land surface temperature. FASEB J. 2012;26:4025–34.
21. Bakirci S, Sarali H, Aydin L, Eren H, Karagenc T. Distribution and seasonal activity of tick species on cattle in the West Aegean region of Turkey. Exp Appl Acarol. 2012;56:165–78.
22. Colebrook E, Wall R. Ectoparasites of livestock in Europe and the Mediterranean region. Vet Parasitol. 2004;120:251–74.
23. Dantas-Torres F, Otranto D. Species diversity and abundance of ticks in three habitats in southern Italy. Ticks Tick Borne Dis. 2013;4:251–5.
24. Estrada-Peña A, Bouattour A, Camicas J, Walker A. Ticks of Domestic Animals in the Mediterranean Region: A Guide to Identification of Species. Spain: University of Zaragoza; 2004.
25. Feldman-Muhsam B. A note on East Mediterranean species of the genus *Haemaphysalis*. Bull Res Counc Israel. 1951;1:96–107.
26. Duell JR, Carmichael R, Herrin BH, Holbrook TC, Talley J, Little SE. Prevalence and species of ticks on horses in central Oklahoma. J Med Entomol. 2013;50:1330–3.
27. Kumsa B, Tamrat H, Tadesse G, Aklilu N, Cassini R. Prevalence and species composition of ixodid ticks infesting horses in three agroecologies in central Oromia, Ethiopia. Trop Anim Health Prod. 2012;44:119–24.
28. Payne VK, Mbafor FL, Pone JW, Tchoumboue J. Preliminary study of ectoparasites of horses in the western highlands of Cameroon. Vet Med Sci. 2017;3:63–70.
29. Feldman-Muhsam B, Saturen IM. Notes on the ecology of ixodid ticks of domestic stock in Israel. Bull Res Counc Israel. 1961;10B:53.
30. Hoogstraal H, Kaiser MN. Observations on Egyptian *Hyalomma* ticks (Ixodoidea, Ixodidae). 5. Biological notes and differences in identity of *H. anatolicum* and its subspecies *anatolicum* Koch and *excavatum* Koch among Russian and other workers. Identity of *H. lusitanicum* Koch. Ann Entomol Soc Am. 1959;52:243–61.
31. Keysary A, Eremeeva ME, Leitner M, Din AB, Wikswo ME, Mumcuoglu KY, et al. Spotted fever group rickettsiae in ticks collected from wild animals in Israel. Am J Trop Med Hyg. 2011;85:919–23.
32. Scoles GA, Ueti MW. Vector ecology of equine piroplasmosis. Annu Rev Entomol. 2015;60:561–80.
33. Azagi T, Klement E, Perlman G, Lustig Y, Mumcuoglu KY, Apanaskevich DA, et al. Francisella-like endosymbionts and *Rickettsia* species in local and imported *Hyalomma* ticks. Appl Environ Microbiol. 2017;83:18.
34. Ioffe-Uspensky I, Mumcuoglu KY, Uspensky I, Galun R. *Rhipicephalus sanguineus* and *R-turanicus* (Acari: Ixodidae): Closely related species with different biological characteristics. J Med Entomol. 1997;34:74–81.
35. Samish M, Pipano E, Hadani A. Intrastadial and interstadial transmission of *Anaplasma marginale* by *Boophilus annulatus* ticks in cattle. Am J Vet Res. 1993;54:411–4.
36. Feldman-Muhsam B, Borut S. Some ecological observations on two East-Mediterranean species of *Haemaphysalis* ticks parasitizing domestic stock. Vet Parasitol. 1983;13:171–81.

Effect of environmental variables and *kdr* resistance genotype on survival probability and infection rates in *Anopheles gambiae* (s.s.)

Mojca Kristan[1*], Tarekegn A. Abeku[2] and Jo Lines[1]

Abstract

Background: Environmental factors, especially ambient temperature and relative humidity affect both mosquitoes and malaria parasites. The early part of sporogony is most sensitive and is affected by high temperatures and temperature fluctuation immediately following ingestion of an infectious blood meal. The aim of this study was to explore whether environmental variables such as temperature, together with the presence of the *kdr* insecticide resistance mutations, have an impact on survival probability and infection rates in wild *Anopheles gambiae* (s.s.) exposed and unexposed to a pyrethroid insecticide.

Methods: *Anopheles gambiae* (s.s.) were collected as larvae, reared to adults, and fed on blood samples from 42 *Plasmodium falciparum*-infected local patients at a health facility in mid-western Uganda, then exposed either to nets treated with sub-lethal doses of deltamethrin or to untreated nets. After seven days, surviving mosquitoes were dissected and their midguts examined for oocysts. Prevalence (proportion infected) and intensity of infection (number of oocysts per infected mosquito) were recorded for each group. Mosquito mortality was recorded daily. Temperature and humidity were recorded every 30 minutes throughout the experiments.

Results: Our findings indicate that apart from the effect of deltamethrin exposure, mean daily temperature during the incubation period, temperature range during the first 24 hours and on day 4 post-infectious feed had a highly significant effect on the risk of infection. Deltamethrin exposure still significantly impaired survival of *kdr* homozygous mosquitoes, while mean daily temperature and relative humidity during the incubation period independently affected mosquito mortality. Significant differences in survival of resistant genotypes were detected, with the lowest survival recorded in mosquitoes with heterozygote *L1014S/L1014F* genotype.

Conclusions: This study confirmed that the early part of sporogony is most affected by temperature fluctuations, while environmental factors affect mosquito survival. The impact of insecticide resistance on malaria infection and vector survival needs to be assessed separately for mosquitoes with different resistance mechanisms to fully understand its implications for currently available vector control tools and malaria transmission.

Keywords: Malaria, *Anopheles gambiae*, Insecticide resistance, Pyrethroids, *Plasmodium falciparum*, Oocyst, Sporogony, Environmental factors, Temperature

* Correspondence: mojca.kristan@lshtm.ac.uk
[1]Department of Disease Control, London School of Hygiene & Tropical Medicine, London, UK
Full list of author information is available at the end of the article

Background

An increasing number of people in malaria endemic countries in sub-Saharan Africa have been protected by insecticide-treated nets (ITNs) or indoor residual spraying (IRS) [1]. Although the expansion of insecticide resistance in mosquitoes might endanger this progress [2, 3], there has not been a conclusive evidence of a complete failure of ITNs so far [4–8].

Longevity of vectors is one of the most important factors affecting malaria transmission [9, 10]. Vector mosquitoes must survive long enough to become infectious and transmit the disease to a new host. Environmental factors, especially ambient temperature and relative humidity affect *Anopheles* mosquitoes and parasite development. Temperature affects mosquito biting rates, blood meal digestion, duration of the gonotrophic cycle, fecundity, development of larval stages, and survival of larvae and adults [11]. It can also affect the immune system of mosquitoes [12–14] and consequently parasite development.

Duration of the sporogonic cycle is also temperature-dependent, with permissive range for *P. falciparum* sporogony being between 16 °C and 35 °C [15, 16]. Very high temperatures are lethal to parasites, while sporogony at low temperatures is lengthened to an extent that mosquitoes may not survive long enough to be able to transmit the parasites [17, 18]. The early part of sporogony is thought to be the most sensitive to temperature [12, 13, 18–24]. Ookinetes are the key transitional stage affecting the probability of vector infectivity, and also define thermal limits for parasite development. Once the parasites complete early sporogony and oocysts are formed, the effect of temperature is thought to be less damaging [19]. Both high and low temperatures have an effect, but the parasites are especially sensitive to high temperatures above 30 °C [19], and to temperature fluctuation immediately following the infectious blood meal [22].

Some studies have shown that the efficacy of insecticides against mosquitoes is to some extent temperature-dependent [25–28]. Furthermore, environmental factors such as temperature [25, 26, 29], larval food sources and availability of blood meals [30–34], infection by various parasites [35, 36], and insect microflora [37, 38] can all influence susceptibility to insecticides or expression of resistance.

When vectors are exposed to treated nets or sprayed surfaces, genetically resistant insects may survive doses that would have killed susceptible ones but might still be affected by the insecticide. Sub-lethal doses of pyrethroids were shown to reduce vector longevity and spontaneous flight activity, and to affect host seeking and probing responses [39, 40]. Such doses could potentially also affect mosquito physiology or trigger the immune response of mosquitoes [41]. Furthermore, sub-lethal doses of pyrethroids were shown to affect sporogonic development of *Plasmodium* parasites in laboratory conditions [39, 42–44], and also in the field [45]. The observed effects on parasite development could be caused by direct or indirect effect of insecticides, or through differential insecticidal killing of infected mosquitoes, as might be seen if infection restored phenotypic susceptibility in genotypically resistant mosquitoes.

Our aim in this study was to explore whether environmental variables such as temperature, together with the presence of the *kdr-L1014S* mutation, have an impact on survival probability and infection rates in wild *An. gambiae* (*s.s.*) exposed and unexposed to a pyrethroid insecticide.

Methods

Study area and participants

The study was conducted in Butemba, Kyankwanzi District, mid-western Uganda, between August 2013 and June 2014. Butemba is located at an altitude of 1000–1200 m above sea level in a moist savannah zone, with annual rainfall exceeding 1200 mm with two peaks (April-May and September-October). The area is highly endemic with two peaks of malaria transmission in May-July and October-December.

Forty-two gametocyte carriers were recruited among outpatients at Butemba Health Centre III. Volunteer patients who fulfilled the inclusion criteria (2 years or older, *P. falciparum*-positive with microscopically detectable gametocytes, no sign of severe illness, non-pregnant if adult female, and with a haemoglobin level of > 9.9 g/dl) were recruited. Gametocytes were counted against 200 leucocytes in thick blood smears. Density was calculated assuming a standard leukocyte count of 8000/μl of blood [46].

The experiments were carried out over three rounds (September-October 2013, November-December 2013, and May-June 2014).

Mosquito collection and rearing

A non-air-conditioned field laboratory was established within the health centre for mosquito rearing and experiments. *Anopheles gambiae* (*s.l.*) larvae were collected from breeding sites in villages around the Health Centre and reared at the Health Centre at ambient temperature and humidity, in water from the breeding sites. The emerging adult mosquitoes were given 10% glucose solution until they were fed on infected blood.

Experimental nets

Untreated polyester nets (Vestergaard Frandsen, Lausanne, Switzerland) were treated with a range of concentrations (2.5–16.7mg/m^2) of deltamethrin (K-Othrine SC 10B G, concentration 9.7g/l; Bayer CropScience Ltd, Cambridge, United Kingdom) to ensure they were sub-lethal and constant across experiments. The doses were chosen in an attempt to mimic the concentrations found on nets as they get older in domestic use [47, 48], and were much lower than those used on LLINs. Sub-lethal doses were required to ensure sufficient survival of mosquitoes during the 7-day incubation period following an infectious blood meal and insecticide exposure to allow detection of any effects of deltamethrin, environmental variables and *kdr* resistance genotypes on parasite development.

Procedures

Standard membrane feeding experiments were carried out as previously described [45]. Briefly, blood samples collected from gametocytaemic volunteers by venipuncture were transferred to pre-warmed membrane feeders (Hemotek Membrane Feeding System, Hemotek Ltd, Blackburn, UK) held at 37.5 °C. Approximately 40 female mosquitoes were placed in each paper cup and allowed to feed through an artificial Parafilm membrane for up to 2 h. Within 1–3 h following the feed, some of the blood-fed mosquitoes were exposed to a net treated with a sub-lethal dose of deltamethrin for 5 min using a wire ball frame, while others were exposed to an untreated net as control. After exposure, mosquitoes were kept in paper cups with access to 10% glucose solution. Seven days after infection, midguts of surviving females were dissected in 0.25% mercurochrome in phosphate buffered saline solution and examined for oocysts. Daily mortality of control and insecticide exposed mosquitoes was recorded.

Mosquito processing

All mosquitoes were stored dry on silica gel in individual microtubes for molecular analysis. Real-time polymerase chain reaction (qPCR) using TaqMan assays was used for *Anopheles* sibling species identification [49], and for detection of *kdr-L1014F* or *kdr-L1014S* mutations [50]. A further assay to detect the presence of *G119S* mutation in the gene *ace-1* which encodes the acetylcholinesterase enzyme was also used [51].

Temperature and relative humidity

Temperature and humidity were recorded every 30 min throughout the experiments, using EL-USB-2 data loggers (Lascar Electronics, Whiteparish, United Kingdom) placed next to the mosquito cages and pots in the laboratory.

Statistical analysis

Software

Statistical analysis was carried out using Stata version 14 (StataCorp LP, College Station, Texas 77845, USA). Excel 2016 (Microsoft Corp) and Prism 7 (GraphPad Software Inc., La Jolla, CA 92037 USA) were used for data management and presentation of graphics.

Analysis of temperature and relative humidity variations between study rounds

One-way ANOVA with Tukey-Kramer's *post-hoc* test [52] was used to compare temperature and relative humidity parameters between the three study rounds.

Effects of temperature and insecticide exposure on infection prevalence

Average daily temperatures, daily maximum and minimum temperatures, and daily temperature ranges (i.e. daily maximum minus minimum, indicating variation within a day) for each feed were obtained from the temperature records. Based on these, averages were also calculated for the period following the first 24 h post-infective blood meal until dissection day (i.e. day 7).

The effect on oocyst infection rates of temperature in the first 24 h post-feeding compared with subsequent days, together with deltamethrin exposure, was studied using mixed-effects logistic regression with backward elimination. Prevalence of oocyst infection among *An. gambiae* (*s.s.*) mosquitoes with *kdr-L1014S* homozygous genotype (692 mosquitoes) was studied as an outcome variable. Deltamethrin dosage group was entered as a categorical variable with three levels: control (untreated nets), low dose (2.5–5.0 mg/m^2 deltamethrin) and high dose (10.0–16.7 mg/m^2 deltamethrin). In addition, temperature-related variables were entered, including average daily temperature, daily maximum and minimum temperature, and daily temperature range on day 1 and during the period following the first 24 h post-feeding on infective blood meal until day 7. To account for the correlation of mosquitoes fed on the same blood sample within each experiment, gametocyte donor volunteers were included as a random (or group) variable.

Mosquito survival

Mosquito survival following the transmission experiments and insecticide exposure was studied among the *An. gambiae* (*s.s.*) with *kdr-L1014S* homozygous genotype, including the 692 mosquitoes which survived following the transmission experiments until day 7 and were successfully dissected, 53 mosquitoes which survived the period but were not successfully dissected, and 187 mosquitoes that died before day 7.

The influence of insecticide exposure and environmental variables on mosquito survival was studied using Kaplan-Meier survival curves and Log-Rank test.

The effect of temperature, relative humidity and deltamethrin exposure on mosquito survival through the seven days of incubation was studied using mixed-effects logistic regression with backward elimination. Mosquito mortality among *An. gambiae* (*s.s.*) mosquitoes with *kdr-L1014S* homozygous genotype was studied as an

Table 1 Oocyst prevalence and mean oocyst intensity (number of oocysts/midgut in infected mosquitoes) variation between the study rounds and doses of deltamethrin the mosquitoes were exposed to after infective feeds

Deltamethrin dose[a]	Study round[b]	Oocyst prevalence (%) (95% CI)	Comparison of prevalence between rounds	Mean number of oocysts/ midgut (95% CI)	Analysis of variance
Control	1	92.7 (84.2–96.8)	$\chi^2 = 94.14$; $P < 0.0001$	12.45 (10.00–14.89)	$F_{(2, 252)} = 12.32$; $P < 0.0001$
	2	41.2 (23.3–61.8)		2.96 (2.33–3.59)	
	3	82.7 (67.3–91.8)		8.78 (6.75–10.80)	
Low dose	1	79.5 (44.8–94.9)	$\chi^2 = 29.05$ $P = 0.0020$	8.48 (5.95–11.01)	$F_{(2, 67)} = 6.42$; $P = 0.0028$
	2	25.8 (18.2–35.2)		1.00 (1.00–1.00)	
	3	81.6 (72.8–87.9)		5.03 (3.18–6.88)	
High dose	1	71.4 (52.9–84.7)	$\chi^2 = 43.23$ $P = 0.0069$	8.55 (6.58–10.51)	$F_{(2, 111)} = 11.93$; $P < 0.0001$
	2	23.7 (7.0–56.1)		2.17 (1.37–2.97)	
	3	60.0 (64.5–82.9)		4.86 (3.55–6.17)	

[a]Deltamethrin dose: Low dose, 2.5–5.0 mg/m^2; high dose, 10.0–16.7 mg/m^2
[b]Study rounds: 1, September-October 2013; 2, November-December 2013; 3, May-June 2014

outcome variable. Gametocyte donor volunteers were included in the model as a random (or group) variable to account for the correlation of mosquitoes fed on the same blood sample within each experiment.

In addition, mosquito survival during the transmission experiments was studied among different *kdr* genotypes of *An. gambiae* (*s.s.*) present in the area, including 852 mosquitoes which survived following the transmission experiments until day 7, and 241 mosquitoes that died before day 7. Mortality of different *kdr* genotypes in *An. gambiae* (*s.s.*) mosquitoes used in transmission experiments was also compared using the Log-Rank test.

Results

PCR identification of *Anopheles gambiae* (*s.l.*) species

A total of 1196 *An. gambiae* (*s.l.*) were identified using PCR: 90.4% were found to be *An. gambiae* (*s.s.*), and the rest were *An. arabiensis*. Further attempts to discriminate *An. coluzzii* were not made as this species was not expected to occur in the study area.

Oocyst prevalence and intensity variations between study rounds

Significant variation in oocyst prevalence and oocyst intensity was observed between the rounds (Table 1). The lowest infection prevalence and intensity values were recorded in round 2 in all three insecticide dose categories. Within each round, both values were higher in mosquitoes that were not exposed to insecticides compared to those exposed.

Temperature and relative humidity variations between study rounds

There was significant variation in mean daily temperature (T) ($F_{(2, 21)} = 47.003$, $P < 0.0001$) and maximum daily T ($F_{(2, 21)} = 21.587$, $P < 0.0001$) during the 7-day incubation period, and in daily T range during the same period ($F_{(2, 21)} = 26.746$, $P < 0.0001$). However, the mean minimum T during the incubation period was not significantly different between the three rounds ($F_{(2, 21)} = 1.558$, $P = 0.234$). Round 2 was on average the warmest, with the largest daily T variations. Rounds 1 and 3 were similar, but round 3 had slightly higher mean daily T during the incubation period (Table 2).

There was also significant variation in all the relative humidity (RH) parameters: mean daily RH ($F_{(2, 21)} = 216.85$, $P < 0.0001$), minimum daily RH ($F_{(2, 21)} = 97.334$, $P < 0.0001$), maximum daily RH ($F_{(2, 21)} = 132.1$, $P < 0.0001$) and daily RH range ($F_{(2, 21)} = 15.005$, $P < 0.0001$) during the incubation period between the three rounds. The highest mean daily RH during the incubation period was measured in round 1, while RH in round 2 was the lowest.

Temperature variations during first 24 hours post-infectious feed

Because the early part of sporogony, especially transition from zygotes into ookinetes and their passage through the midgut wall, is thought to be sensitive to temperature, the effects of temperature variables during the first 24 h post-infectious feed in each study round were studied in comparison with values in subsequent days (Fig. 1). There was significant variation in all the temperature parameters

Table 2 Means of daily temperature (T), maximum and minimum temperature and daily temperature variation during the seven day incubation period, recorded during the three study rounds

	Mean daily T (°C)	Max T (°C)	Min T (°C)	T range (°C)
Round 1	25.2	27.8	23.4	4.3
Round 2	26.4	28.9	23.2	5.7
Round 3	25.4	28.0	23.4	4.6

Study rounds: 1, September-October 2013; 2, November-December 2013; 3, May-June 2014

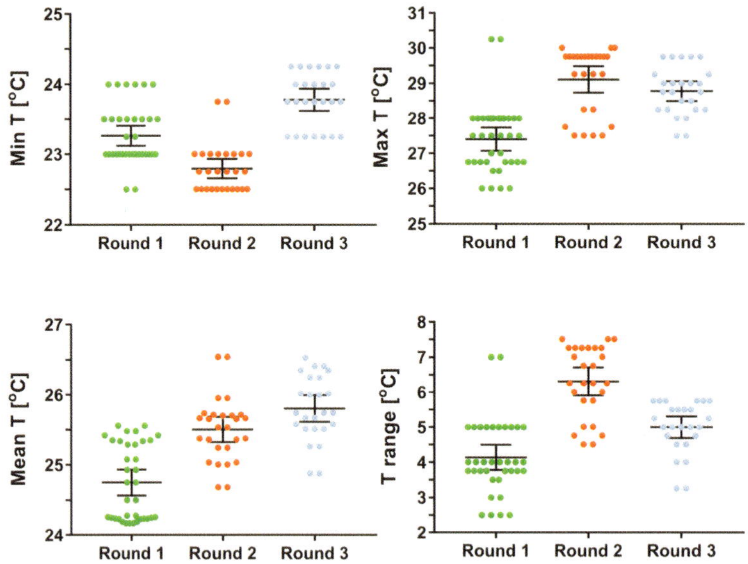

Fig. 1 Temperature measurements during the first 24 h post-infectious feed recorded in each transmission experiment, in the three study rounds. There was significant variation in all temperature parameters during the first 24 h post-infectious feed between the three rounds: mean temperature ($F_{(2, 85)} = 39.328$, $P < 0.0001$), minimum temperature ($F_{(2, 85)} = 41.749$, $P < 0.0001$), maximum temperature ($F_{(2, 85)} = 32.861$, $P < 0.0001$) and the temperature range ($F_{(2, 85)} = 36.57$, $P < 0.0001$). Error bars show 95% confidence intervals of the means

during the first 24 h post-infectious feed between the three rounds.

Effect of temperature on oocyst prevalence

The effect of different temperature variables during the first 24 h post-infective feed and deltamethrin exposure on oocyst prevalence was investigated using mixed-effects logistic regression. A total of 692 *An. gambiae* (*s.s.*) homozygous for *kdr-L1014S* genotype from experiments that used blood samples from 42 gametocyte volunteers were included in the analysis. *Ace-1* mutation was not detected in any of the samples. The results showed that apart from the effect of deltamethrin on infection rates, temperature range during the first 24 h post-infectious feed (i.e. the difference between maximum and minimum temperature on day 1) which varied between 2.50 °C and 7.50 °C between different feeds, and temperature range on day 4 post-infectious feed which varied between 2.75 °C and 7.25 °C, had a highly significant effect on risk of infection (Table 3). The results indicate that an increase in temperature range was associated with lower infection, after controlling for the effects of insecticide exposure.

Mosquito survival in relation to temperature and humidity

Following the standard membrane feeds and insecticide exposure, fed mosquitoes were kept for seven days until dissection for the presence of oocysts. Mosquito mortality was recorded daily.

Figure 2 shows Kaplan-Meier survival curves for the three insecticide exposure groups within each study round. The survival curves showed the influence of insecticide exposure on mosquito survival, together with

Table 3 Mixed-effects logistic regression analysis of *P. falciparum* oocyst prevalence rates

		OR	SE	*Z*	*P*	95% CI
Dose category	Control	1.000	–	–	–	–
	Low dose	0.423	0.139	-2.61	0.009	0.221–0.807
	High dose	0.190	0.048	-6.51	<0.0001	0.115–0.313
Temperature range day 1 (°C)		0.631	0.133	-2.18	0.029	0.417–0.954
Temperature range day 4 (°C)		0.606	0.137	-2.21	0.027	0.389–0.944
Variance of random intercept		2.092	0.729			1.057–4.143

Model $\chi^2 = 54.33$, $df = 3$, $P < 0.001$; $n = 692$; number of groups (gametocyte donors) = 42
Note: The dependent variable is oocyst infection coded as 0 (negative) and 1 (positive)
Abbreviations: *OR* odds ratio, *SE* standard error, *95% CI* 95% confidence interval

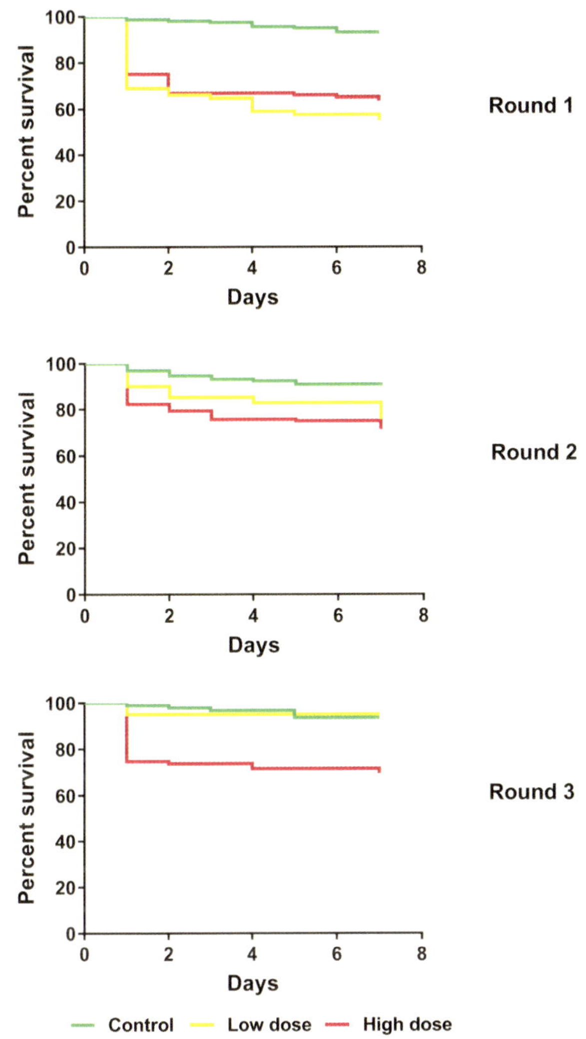

Fig. 2 The Kaplan-Meier survival curves and estimates for mosquito survival in each of the three experimental rounds per each insecticide exposure dose. Survival distributions were significantly different between the insecticide exposure groups within each study round (Round 1 Log-Rank statistic, $\chi^2 = 53.85$, $df = 2$, $P < 0.0001$; Round 2 Log-Rank statistic, $\chi^2 = 15.73$, $df = 2$, $P = 0.0004$; Round 3 Log-Rank statistic, $\chi^2 = 25.42$, $df = 2$, $P < 0.0001$). Only *An. gambiae* (*s.s.*) mosquitoes homozygous for *kdr-L1014S* mutation were included in the analysis (control, untreated netting; low dose, 2.5–5.0 mg/m^2 deltamethrin; high dose, 10.0–16.7 mg/m^2 deltamethrin)

the influence of environmental variables. The survival distributions were significantly different between the insecticide exposure groups within each study round, showing that insecticide exposure impaired survival of *kdr* homozygous mosquitoes.

Mixed-effects regression analysis showed that apart from the effect of deltamethrin, average daily temperature and average daily relative humidity during the seven day incubation period had an independent and highly significant effect on mosquito mortality (Table 4).

Interactions of temperature, relative humidity and insecticide exposure and their effect on mosquito survival are shown in Fig. 3. Increased temperature and relative humidity resulted in increased mortality of deltamethrin-exposed mosquitoes compared with unexposed mosquitoes.

Mosquito survival in relation to different *kdr* genotypes

Survival of mosquitoes with different *kdr* genotypes was compared following the membrane feeds and insecticide exposure (Fig. 4). No wild type susceptible mosquitoes or wild type/*L1014S* heterozygotes survived exposure to high doses of deltamethrin, although these two genotypes were present among the tested mosquitoes; low numbers of these samples did not allow for a more detailed analysis. Statistical tests of the effect of genotype on mortality did not provide a clear or consistent pattern among the three insecticide exposure groups. Survival of resistant homozygote *kdr-L1014S, kdr-L1014F* and heterozygote *L1014S/L1014F* genotypes was significantly different in control (Fisher's exact test, $P = 0.001$), and high dose groups (Fisher's exact test, $P = 0.007$), but not in a low dose group (Fisher's exact test, $P = 0.084$). In all three insecticide exposure groups, a higher proportion of *L1014F/L1014F* genotype mosquitoes survived than of *L1014S/L1014S* mosquitoes, whereas the resistant heterozygote *L1014S/L1014F* genotype had the lowest survival of the three genotypes.

Discussion

In order to determine whether environmental variables such as temperature and relative humidity, together with the presence of *kdr-L1014S* mutation, have an impact on survival probability and malaria infection, we compared daily survival and *Plasmodium* infection rates in wild insecticide-resistant *An. gambiae* (*s.s.*) fed on infective blood from gametocytaemic volunteers and exposed to untreated or deltamethrin-treated nets.

We have previously shown that average ambient temperature during the seven days of incubation, together with insecticide exposure, had a highly significant effect on the risk of infection in mosquitoes and on the parasite load [45]. In the present study, we wanted to further explore any possible effects of different environmental variables on parasite development and vector survival, in the presence or absence of insecticide exposure and in different *kdr* genotypes. Apart from insecticide dose, temperature range on day 1 (i.e. within the first 24 hours) and on day 4 post-infective blood meal had significant effects on parasite development.

The period of the first 24 hours following the infective feed is the time of blood meal digestion and early sporogony, with ookinete densities reaching peak numbers [20] while the peritrophic matrix, which the ookinetes must traverse, reaches its maximal thickness [53]. This

Table 4 Mixed-effects logistic regression analysis of mortality rates of *An. gambiae* (*s.s.*) homozygous for *kdr-L1014S*

		OR	SE	Z	P	95% CI
Dose category	Control	1.000	–	–	–	–
	Low dose	5.144	1.588	5.31	<0.0001	2.809–9.422
	High dose	5.069	1.299	6.34	<0.0001	3.068–8.376
Average temperature (°C)		8.472	5.133	3.53	<0.0001	2.583–27.780
Average relative humidity (%)		1.248	0.073	3.80	<0.0001	1.113–1.399
Variance of random intercept		0.105	0.122			0.011–1.029

Model $\chi^2 = 57.97$, $df = 3$, $P < 0.0001$; $n = 837$; number of groups (gametocyte donors) = 42
Note: The dependent variable dead is mosquito death coded as 0 (alive) and 1 (dead)
Abbreviations: *OR* odds ratio, *SE* standard error, *95% CI* 95% confidence interval

part of sporogony is particularly sensitive to both temperature [12, 13, 18–24] and exposure of infected mosquitoes to sub-lethal doses of pyrethroids [39]. Blood meal digestion in mosquitoes is temperature-dependent [54], while the speed of digestion also affects the sporogony, especially formation of ookinetes and their migration through the peritrophic matrix and the midgut wall [55]. During study round 2, temperature variations in the first 24 hours post-feed were significantly larger than in rounds 1 or 3, whereas parasite prevalence and intensity of infection were significantly lower, regardless of insecticide exposure.

Young oocysts can be seen from day 2 post-infection [56]. During this period, mitotic divisions start taking place, forming a multinucleate oocyst, and circumsporozoite protein (CSP) must be produced for formation and budding of the sporozoites [57, 58]. Although it is possible that some of the processes taking place during sporozoite development in the oocysts are temperature-sensitive, previous studies show that oocysts, once formed, are no longer sensitive to changes in ambient temperature [19]. A recent study shows that not all mosquitoes are equally infectious as those with lower sporozoite burdens have a lower chance of successfully spreading the infection [59]. Further work will be required to assess the impact of sub-lethal doses of pyrethroids, of environmental variables and insecticide resistance on sporozoite development and infectivity.

Exposure to insecticides, ambient temperature and relative humidity, malaria infection and insecticide resistance all interact in nature and can affect vector competence in differing ways, but their combined effect on mosquito survival is not well understood. Increase in environmental temperature has been shown to be associated with reduced adult survival [60, 61]. Temperature also affects the extent to which insecticides kill mosquitoes [25, 26], possibly because mosquito immune responses [12], nervous-system sensitivity [62], and metabolic activity [63] are all temperature-dependent. Apart from its effect on mosquito survival in combination with ambient temperature [11], humidity was shown to have a strong impact on insecticide resistance phenotype [64].

Insecticide resistance mechanisms can also exert a wide range of effects on vector longevity, competence and behavior and could in principle affect malaria

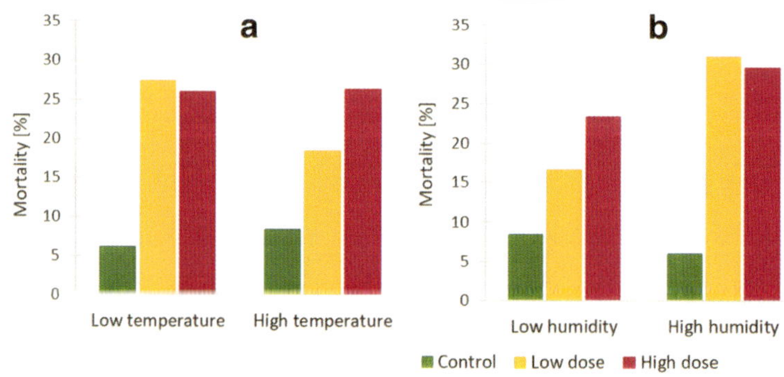

Fig. 3 Effects of deltamethrin exposure on mosquito mortality in *kdr-L1014S* homozygous resistant *An. gambiae* (*s.s.*) mosquitoes. Mortality is shown (**a**) under low (< 25.3 °C) and high temperature (≥ 25.3 °C) conditions; (**b**) under low (< 69.7%) and high relative humidity (≥ 69.7%) conditions. Mosquitoes were exposed to control untreated nets, nets treated with low dose (2.5–5.0 mg/m^2 deltamethrin) or high dose (10.0–16.7 mg/m^2 deltamethrin) after feeding on blood samples from gametocytaemic volunteers. The median of ambient temperature recorded during the experiments (25.3 °C) and ambient relative humidity (69.7%) was used as a cut-off to plot mosquito mortality charts

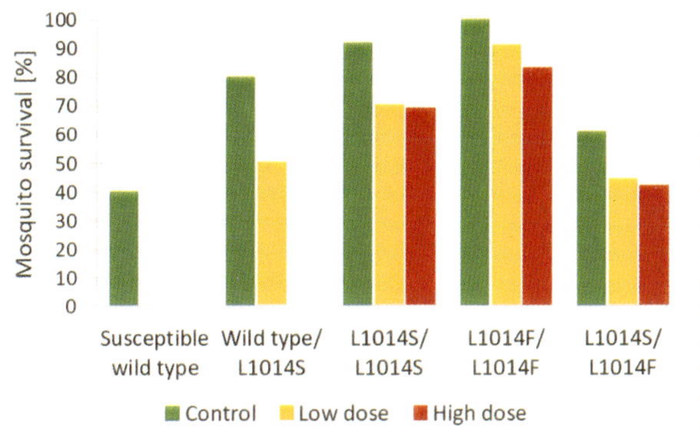

Fig. 4 Survival of mosquitoes with different *kdr* genotypes following the membrane feeds and exposure to treated or untreated nets, was determined at the end of the seven day incubation period and compared per each exposure dose. Mosquitoes were exposed for 5 minutes using a wire ball frame to control untreated nets, nets treated with low dose (2.5–5.0 mg/m^2 deltamethrin) or high dose (10.0–16.7 mg/m^2 deltamethrin) after feeding on blood samples from gametocytaemic volunteers

transmission in either a positive or negative manner [65]. Moreover, different resistance alleles can interact to influence the fitness of mosquitoes [66]. Extensive comparison of survival between different *kdr* genotypes and the wild type was not possible due to low numbers of mosquitoes with a wild type allele. However, survival over the seven day incubation period (during which the oocysts developed) of mosquitoes with resistant genotypes (i.e. with at least one resistant allele, *L1014S* or *L1014F*) was higher than survival of the wild susceptible type. There were also significant differences in survival over the incubation period of resistant *L1014S/L1014S*, *L1014F/L1014F* and *L1014S/L1014F* genotypes in control and high dose groups; in both instances, survival was the lowest in mosquitoes with *L1014S/L1014F* genotype, which could be due to combination of resistant alleles exerting a fitness cost on mosquitoes. Several properties of infected blood can impair mosquito fitness, even in the absence of actual mosquito infection, while survival of infected mosquitoes is also affected by environmental stress [67]. Furthermore, survival of uninfected *kdr* resistant mosquitoes was shown to be higher than that of the susceptible strain, while their survival was similar when exposed to *P. falciparum* infection [68].

Conclusions

This study allowed us to examine the relationships between environmental variables and insecticide exposure on survival probability and infection rates in wild *An. gambiae* (*s.s.*) in the presence of *kdr-L1014S* mutation. As previously observed, early sporogony was most sensitive to temperature, especially to temperature variation, regardless of the insecticide exposure. We also show that temperature and relative humidity, together with insecticide exposure, impact mosquito survival following infected feeds. From a vector control perspective, it was encouraging to find that deltamethrin exposure still significantly impaired survival of *kdr* homozygous mosquitoes. The impact of insecticide resistance on malaria infection and vector survival needs to be assessed separately for mosquitoes carrying target site or metabolic resistance mechanisms before we will be able to fully understand the impact of resistance on currently available vector control tools and on malaria transmission.

Acknowledgements

We would like to thank Kyankwanzi District Health Office and Butemba Health Centre III (Ministry of Health) for their cooperation and for facilitating the study; our field entomology, laboratory, and survey staff for their technical assistance; and Malaria Consortium Uganda office - Anthony Nuwa in particular - for facilitating the research. Our special thanks to Charles Ntege for assistance with training of field staff, field staff supervision and field study coordination; to Juliet Nambatya and Rebecca Nakiyingi for assistance in mosquito dissections and general laboratory work. We thank the staff of the PAMVERC Malaria Research Laboratory in Moshi, Tanzania, and Thomas Walker and James Orsborne at LSHTM for carrying out all molecular analyses of the mosquito samples. We are grateful to the study volunteers and residents of Butemba, Kyankwanzi District in Uganda for their cooperation.

Funding

The research was funded by UK aid (through the Programme Partnership Arrangement grant to Malaria Consortium) and the London School of Hygiene & Tropical Medicine. The funders had no role in study design, data collection and analysis, decision to publish, or preparation of the manuscript.

Authors' contributions

MK and TAA conceived the study and developed the study design with contributions of JL. TAA and MK trained field staff. MK carried out all field experiments and coordinated the study. TAA supervised field experiments and coordinated the study. MK carried out the statistical analyses with assistance from TAA. MK wrote the manuscript with inputs of TAA and JL who reviewed the manuscript and provided comments. All authors read and approved the final manuscript.

Competing interests

The authors declare that they have no competing interests.

Author details

[1]Department of Disease Control, London School of Hygiene & Tropical Medicine, London, UK. [2]Malaria Consortium, London, UK.

References

1. Bhatt S, Weiss DJ, Cameron E, Bisanzio D, Mappin B, Dalrymple U, et al. The effect of malaria control on *Plasmodium falciparum* in Africa between 2000 and 2015. Nature. 2015;526:207–11.
2. Ranson H, Lissenden N. Insecticide resistance in African *Anopheles* mosquitoes: a worsening situation that needs urgent action to maintain malaria control. Trends Parasitol. 2016;32:187–96.
3. Churcher TS, Lissenden N, Griffin JT, Worrall E, Ranson H. The impact of pyrethroid resistance on the efficacy and effectiveness of bednets for malaria control in Africa. eLife. 2016;5:e16090.
4. Strode C, Donegan S, Garner P, Enayati AA, Hemingway J. The impact of pyrethroid resistance on the efficacy of insecticide-treated bed nets against African anopheline mosquitoes: systematic review and meta-analysis. PLoS Med. 2014;11:e1001619.
5. Lindblade KA, Mwandama D, Mzilahowa T, Steinhardt L, Gimnig J, Shah M, et al. A cohort study of the effectiveness of insecticide-treated bed nets to prevent malaria in an area of moderate pyrethroid resistance, Malawi. Malar J. 2015;14:31.
6. WHO. Implications of insecticide resistance for malaria vector control. Geneva: World Health Organization; 2016.
7. Ochomo E, Chahilu M, Cook J, Kinyari T, Bayoh NM, West P, et al. Insecticide-treated nets and protection against insecticide-resistant malaria vectors in western Kenya. Emerg Infect Dis. 2017;23:758–64.
8. WHO. World Malaria Report 2017. Geneva: World Health Organization; 2017.
9. Garrett-Jones C, Shidrawi GR. Malaria vectorial capacity of a population of *Anopheles gambiae*: an exercise in epidemiological entomology. Bull World Health Organ. 1969;40:531–45.
10. Macdonald G. Epidemiological basis of malaria control. Bull World Health Organ. 1956;15:613–26.
11. Afrane YA, Githeko AK, Yan G. The ecology of *Anopheles* mosquitoes under climate change: case studies from the effects of deforestation in East African highlands. Ann N Y Acad Sci. 2012;1249:204–10.
12. Murdock CC, Paaijmans KP, Bell AS, King JG, Hillyer JF, Read AF, et al. Complex effects of temperature on mosquito immune function. Proc Biol Sci. 2012;279:3357–66.
13. Murdock CC, Paaijmans KP, Cox-Foster D, Read AF, Thomas MB. Rethinking vector immunology: the role of environmental temperature in shaping resistance. Nat Rev Microbiol. 2012;10:869–76.
14. Murdock CC, Moller-Jacobs LL, Thomas MB. Complex environmental drivers of immunity and resistance in malaria mosquitoes. Proc Biol Sci. 2013;280: 20132030.
15. Detinova TS. Age-grouping methods in Diptera of medical importance with special reference to some vectors of malaria. Monogr Ser World Health Organ. 1962;47:13–191.
16. Ohm JR, Baldini F, Barreaux P, Lefevre T, Lynch PA, Suh E, et al. Rethinking the extrinsic incubation period of malaria parasites. Parasit Vectors. 2018;11:178.
17. Macdonald G. The analysis of the sporozoite rate. Trop Dis Bull. 1952;49: 569–86.
18. Boyd MF. Malariology: A Comprehensive Survey of All Aspects of this Group of Diseases from a Global Standpoint. Philadelphia and London: W. B. Saunders & Co.; 1949.
19. Eling W, Hooghof J, van de Vegte-Bolmer M, Sauerwein R, van Gemert G-J. Tropical temperatures can inhibit development of the human malaria parasite *Plasmodium falciparum* in the mosquito. Proc Exper Appl Entomol. 2001;12:151–6.
20. Noden BH, Kent MD, Beier JC. The impact of variations in temperature on early *Plasmodium falciparum* development in *Anopheles stephensi*. Parasitology. 1995;111:539–45.
21. Okech BA, Gouagna LC, Kabiru EW, Walczak E, Beier JC, Yan G, et al. Resistance of early midgut stages of natural *Plasmodium falciparum* parasites to high temperatures in experimentally infected *Anopheles gambiae* (Diptera: Culicidae). J Parasitol. 2004;90:764–8.
22. Paaijmans KP, Blanford S, Bell AS, Blanford JI, Read AF, Thomas MB. Influence of climate on malaria transmission depends on daily temperature variation. Proc Natl Acad Sci USA. 2010;107:15135–9.
23. Rastogi M, Pal NL, Sen AB. Effect of variation in temperature on development of *Plasmodium berghei* (NK 65 strain) in *Anopheles stephensi*. Folia Parasitol. 1987;34:289–97.
24. Vanderberg JP, Yoeli M. Effects of temperature on sporogonic development of *Plasmodium berghei*. J Parasitol. 1966;52:559–64.
25. Glunt KD, Paaijmans KP, Read AF, Thomas MB. Environmental temperatures significantly change the impact of insecticides measured using WHOPES protocols. Malar J. 2014;13:350.
26. Hodjati MH, Curtis CF. Effects of permethrin at different temperatures on pyrethroid-resistant and susceptible strains of *Anopheles*. Med Vet Entomol. 1999;13:415–22.
27. Cutkomp LK, Subramanyam B. Toxicity of pyrethroids to *Aedes aegypti* larvae in relation to temperature. J Am Mosq Control Assoc. 1986;2:347–9.
28. Harwood AD, You J, Lydy MJ. Temperature as a toxicity identification evaluation tool for pyrethroid insecticides: toxicokinetic confirmation. Environ Toxicol Chem. 2009;28:1051–8.
29. Polson KA, Brogdon WG, Rawlins SC, Chadee DD. Impact of environmental temperatures on resistance to organophosphate insecticides in *Aedes aegypti* from Trinidad. Rev Panam Salud Publica. 2012;32:1–8.
30. Bourguet D, Guillemaud T, Chevillon C, Raymond M. Fitness costs of insecticide resistance in natural breeding sites of the mosquito *Culex pipiens*. Evolution. 2004;58:128–35.
31. Oliver SV, Brooke BD. The effect of larval nutritional deprivation on the life history and DDT resistance phenotype in laboratory strains of the malaria vector *Anopheles arabiensis*. Malar J. 2013;12:44.
32. Oliver SV, Brooke BD. The effect of multiple blood-feeding on the longevity and insecticide resistant phenotype in the major malaria vector *Anopheles arabiensis* (Diptera: Culicidae). Parasit Vectors. 2014;7:390.
33. Kulma K, Saddler A, Koella JC. Effects of age and larval nutrition on phenotypic expression of insecticide-resistance in *Anopheles* mosquitoes. PLoS One. 2013;8:e58322.
34. Owusu HF, Chitnis N, Muller P. Insecticide susceptibility of *Anopheles* mosquitoes changes in response to variations in the larval environment. Sci Rep. 2017;7:3667.
35. Farenhorst M, Mouatcho JC, Kikankie CK, Brooke BD, Hunt RH, Thomas MB, et al. Fungal infection counters insecticide resistance in African malaria mosquitoes. Proc Natl Acad Sci USA. 2009;106:17443–7.
36. Koella JC, Saddler A, Karacs TP. Blocking the evolution of insecticide-resistant malaria vectors with a microsporidian. Evol Appl. 2012;5:283–92.
37. Kikuchi Y, Hayatsu M, Hosokawa T, Nagayama A, Tago K, Fukatsu T. Symbiont-mediated insecticide resistance. Proc Natl Acad Sci USA. 2012;109: 8618–22.
38. Patil CD, Borase HP, Salunke BK, Patil SV. Alteration in *Bacillus thuringiensis* toxicity by curing gut flora: novel approach for mosquito resistance management. Parasitol Res. 2013;112:3283–8.
39. Hill N. Effects of sublethal doses of pyrethroids on malaria vectors. PhD Thesis. London: London School of Hygiene & Tropical Medicine, University of London; 2002.
40. Glunt KD, Coetzee M, Huijben S, Koffi AA, Lynch PA, N'Guessan R, et al. Empirical and theoretical investigation into the potential impacts of insecticide resistance on the effectiveness of insecticide-treated bed nets. Evol Appl. 2017;11:431–41.
41. James RR, Xu J. Mechanisms by which pesticides affect insect immunity. J Invertebr Pathol. 2012;109:175–82.
42. Carle PR, Coz J, Elissa N, Gasquet M, Sannier C, Richard A, et al. Intravector anti-*Plasmodium* activity of a pyrethrinoid: deltamethrin. C R Acad Sci III. 1986;303:565–8.
43. Elissa N, Sannier C, Coz J. Étude de la réceptivité à *Plasmodium yoelii yoelii* d'*Anopheles stephensi* soumis au stade adulte à des doses toxiques de différents pyréthrinoïdes. Cah ORSTOM, Ser Ent Méd Parasitol. 1987;25: 187–92.
44. Elissa N, Sannier C, Richard A. La receptivite a *Plasmodium yoelii yoelii* d'*Anopheles* soumis a des subletales de deltamethrine. In: IVe Congres sur la Protection de la Sante Humaine et des Cultures en Milieu Tropical. Marseille: ORSTOM; 1986;599–604.
45. Kristan M, Lines J, Nuwa A, Ntege C, Meek SR, Abeku TA. Exposure to deltamethrin affects development of *Plasmodium falciparum* inside wild pyrethroid resistant *Anopheles gambiae s.s.* mosquitoes in Uganda. Parasit Vectors. 2016;9:100.
46. WHO. Malaria parasite counting. Malaria microscopy standard operating procedure - MM-SOP-09. Geneva: World Health Organization; 2016.
47. Kilian A, Byamukama W, Pigeon O, Gimnig J, Atieli F, Koekemoer L, et al. Evidence for a useful life of more than three years for a polyester-based long-lasting insecticidal mosquito net in western Uganda. Malar J. 2011;10:299.
48. Anshebo GY, Graves PM, Smith SC, Wills AB, Damte M, Endeshaw T, et al. Estimation of insecticide persistence, biological activity and mosquito resistance to PermaNet® 2 long-lasting insecticidal nets over three to 32 months of use in Ethiopia. Malar J. 2014;13:80.
49. Bass C, Williamson MS, Field LM. Development of a multiplex real-time PCR assay for identification of members of the *Anopheles gambiae* species complex. Acta Trop 2008;107:50 3.

50. Bass C, Nikou D, Donnelly MJ, Williamson MS, Ranson H, Ball A, et al. Detection of knockdown resistance (*kdr*) mutations in *Anopheles gambiae*: a comparison of two new high-throughput assays with existing methods. Malar J. 2007;6:111.
51. Bass C, Nikou D, Vontas J, Williamson MS, Field LM. Development of high-throughput real-time PCR assays for the identification of insensitive acetylcholinesterase (*ace-1*^{R}) in *Anopheles gambiae*. Pestic Biochem Phys. 2010;96:80–5.
52. McDonald JH. Handbook of Biological Statistics, 3rd edn. Baltimore, Maryland: Sparky House Publishing; 2014.
53. Dinglasan RR, Devenport M, Florens L, Johnson JR, McHugh CA, Donnelly-Doman M, et al. The *Anopheles gambiae* adult midgut peritrophic matrix proteome. Insect Biochem Mol Biol. 2009;39:125–34.
54. O'Gower AK. The rate of digestion of human blood by certain species of mosquitoes. Aust J Biol Sci. 1956;9:125–9.
55. Feldmann AM, Billingsley PF, Savelkoul E. Bloodmeal digestion by strains of *Anopheles stephensi* Liston (Diptera: Culicidae) of differing susceptibility to *Plasmodium falciparum*. Parasitology. 1990;101:193–200.
56. Lensen AH, Van Gemert GJ, Bolmer MG, Meis JF, Kaslow D, Meuwissen JH, et al. Transmission blocking antibody of the *Plasmodium falciparum* zygote/ookinete surface protein Pfs25 also influences sporozoite development. Parasite Immunol. 1992;14:471–9.
57. Aly AS, Vaughan AM, Kappe SH. Malaria parasite development in the mosquito and infection of the mammalian host. Annu Rev Microbiol. 2009; 63:195–221.
58. Thathy V, Fujioka H, Gantt S, Nussenzweig R, Nussenzweig V, Menard R. Levels of circumsporozoite protein in the *Plasmodium* oocyst determine sporozoite morphology. EMBO J. 2002;21:1586–96.
59. Churcher TS, Sinden RE, Edwards NJ, Poulton ID, Rampling TW, Brock PM, et al. Probability of transmission of malaria from mosquito to human is regulated by mosquito parasite density in naive and vaccinated hosts. PLOS Pathog. 2017;13:e1006108.
60. Afrane YA, Zhou G, Lawson BW, Githeko AK, Yan G. Effects of microclimatic changes caused by deforestation on the survivorship and reproductive fitness of *Anopheles gambiae* in western Kenya highlands. Am J Trop Med Hyg. 2006;74:772–8.
61. Christiansen-Jucht C, Parham PE, Saddler A, Koella JC, Basanez MG. Temperature during larval development and adult maintenance influences the survival of *Anopheles gambiae s.s.* Parasit Vectors. 2014;7:489.
62. Montgomery JC, Macdonald JA. Effects of temperature on nervous system: implications for behavioral performance. Am J Physiol. 1990;259:R191–6.
63. Gillooly JF, Brown JH, West GB, Savage VM, Charnov EL. Effects of size and temperature on metabolic rate. Science. 2001;293:2248–51.
64. Weetman D, Wilding CS, Neafsey DE, Muller P, Ochomo E, Isaacs AT, et al. Candidate-gene based GWAS identifies reproducible DNA markers for metabolic pyrethroid resistance from standing genetic variation in East African *Anopheles gambiae*. Sci Rep. 2018;8:2920.
65. Rivero A, Vezilier J, Weill M, Read AF, Gandon S. Insecticide control of vector-borne diseases: when is insecticide resistance a problem? PLoS Pathog. 2010;6:e1001000.
66. Berticat C, Bonnet J, Duchon S, Agnew P, Weill M, Corbel V. Costs and benefits of multiple resistance to insecticides for *Culex quinquefasciatus* mosquitoes. BMC Evol Biol. 2008;8:104.
67. Ferguson HM, Mackinnon MJ, Chan BH, Read AF. Mosquito mortality and the evolution of malaria virulence. Evolution. 2003;57:2792–804.
68. Alout H, Dabire RK, Djogbenou LS, Abate L, Corbel V, Chandre F, et al. Interactive cost of *Plasmodium* infection and insecticide resistance in the malaria vector *Anopheles gambiae*. Sci Rep. 2016;6:29755.

8

Editing the genome of *Aphanomyces invadans* using CRISPR/Cas9

Muhammad Majeed, Hatem Soliman, Gokhlesh Kumar, Mansour El-Matbouli* and Mona Saleh

Abstract

Background: The clustered regularly interspaced short palindromic repeats (CRISPR)/CRISPR-associated protein 9 (Cas9) system is increasingly being used for genome editing experiments. It is a system to add, delete and/or replace parts of a gene *in situ* in a time- and cost-efficient manner. The genome of many organisms has been edited using this system. We tested the CRISPR/Cas9 system in *Aphanomyces invadans*, an oomycete, which is the causative agent of epizootic ulcerative syndrome (EUS) in many fish species. Extracellular proteases produced by this oomycete are believed to play a role in EUS virulence.

Methods: We designed three single guide-RNAs (gRNA) to target *A. invadans* serine protease gene. These gRNAs were individually combined with the Cas9 to form ribo-nucleo-protein (RNP) complex. *A. invadans* protoplasts were then transfected with RNP complexes. After the transfection, the target gene was amplified and subjected to sequencing. Zoospores of *A. invadans* were also transfected with the RNP complex. Three groups of dwarf gourami (*Trichogaster lalius*) were then experimentally inoculated with (i) non-treated *A. invadans* zoospores; (ii) RNP-treated *A. invadans* zoospores; and (iii) autoclaved pond water as negative control, to investigate the effect of edited serine protease gene on the virulence of *A. invadans in vivo*.

Results: Fluorescence microscopy showed sub-cellular localization of RNP complex in *A. invadans* protoplasts and zoospores. Sequencing results from the protoplast DNA revealed a point mutation in the target gene. A matching mutation was also detected in zoospores after similar treatment with the same RNP complex. *In vivo* results showed that the CRISPR/Cas9-treated *A. invadans* zoospores did not produce EUS clinical signs in the fish. These results were then confirmed by histopathological staining of the muscle sections using Gomori's methenamine silver nitrate and hematoxylin and eosin stains.

Conclusions: Results obtained in this study indicate that the RNP complex caused effective mutation in the target gene. This hindered the production of serine protease, which ultimately impeded the manifestation of EUS in the fish. Our methods thus establish a promising approach for functional genomics studies in *A. invadans* and provide novel avenues to develop effective strategies to control this pathogen.

Keywords: CRISPR/Cas9, Dwarf gourami, Epizootic ulcerative syndrome, Oomycetes, Point mutation, Proteases, Virulence

Background

Oomycetes are a group of parasites that are widespread and have the ability to invade a wide range of hosts [1]. Three oomycete genera, namely *Achlya*, *Aphanomyces* and *Saprolegnia*, have been described as the most devastating pathogens of aquatic organisms [2–4]. *Aphanomyces* alone contains approximately 35–40 species, some of which are specialized pathogens of plants and animals while others are saprotrophic or opportunistic pathogens growing on animals and plant debris [5, 6].

The species *Aphanomyces invadans* has been identified as the primary cause for epizootic ulcerative syndrome (EUS), which is an important seasonal condition implicated in mass-mortalities of cultured and wild fish in many countries [7, 8]. As soon as the free-swimming zoospore, the infective stage of *A. invadans*, finds a fish host, it germinates into vegetative non-septate hyphae,

* Correspondence: Mansour.El-Matbouli@vetmeduni.ac.at
Clinical Division of Fish Medicine, University of Veterinary Medicine, Vienna, Austria

which invade the fish skin and muscular tissue and may also reach the internal organs [9, 10]. Then, the primary zoospores develop in the sporangium in fish tissues and are released at its tip where they form a spore cluster [11]. The primary spores transform into motile, biflagellate secondary zoospores. The life-cycle is completed once they find new fish to invade [12].

In addition to the distinctive mycotic granulomas in internal tissues, infected fish display distinct dermal lesions appearing as red spots, blackish burn-like marks or deeper ulcers with red centers and white rims [7, 13–15]. More than 125 fish species have been reported to be affected by *A. invadans* [16]. Because of its epizootic nature, broad fish host range and potential impact on cultured and wild fisheries, EUS is officially recognized as a reportable disease by the World Organization for Animal Health [17].

Although a large amount of data on the gross and microscopic clinical lesions of EUS and the involvement of different pathogens during the course of the disease already exist [9, 16–18], there still is a paucity of information regarding pathogenicity, host-parasite interactions, molecular mechanisms of the disease and the functional genomics of *A. invadans*. Similar to many pathogenic microorganisms, proteases secreted by *A. invadans* are key in the pathogenesis of EUS [19]. Different extracellular proteins, most of which are proteases, secreted by *A. invadans*, have recently been identified and at least one of these proteases (serine protease belonging to peptidase_S8 domain) is believed to be involved in the degradation of the fish immunoglobulin M [20]. Serine proteases have long been thought of as the virulence factors in many of the true bacteria and fungi [21]. A serine protease secreted by the fish-pathogenic oomycete *S. parasitica* has been reported as able to degrade the fish IgM [22]. Accordingly, these genes were our target for gene editing to investigate their role in *A. invadans* pathogenesis.

Genome editing is a group of technologies that allow the scientists to make precise changes by adding, removing and/or altering genetic material at particular locations in the genomes of eukaryotic cells [23–25]. In addition to the currently used techniques for genome editing, such as zinc finger nucleases (ZFN) and transcription activator-like effector nucleases (TALEN), a relatively recent technique known as clustered regularly interspaced short palindromic repeats (CRISPR)/CRISPR-associated protein (CRISPR/Cas) system is already revolutionizing our ability to interrogate gene functions and can potentially be used clinically to correct or introduce genetic mutations [24, 26–28].

According to the current classification of CRISPR-*cas* loci the CRISPR/Cas system has been grouped into six distinct types (I-VI). Each type employs a unique set of Cas proteins along with CRISPR RNA (crRNA) for CRISPR interference [29]. The Type II CRISPR system employs a single DNA endonuclease, Cas9, to recognize double-stranded DNA (dsDNA) substrates and cleave each strand with a distinct nuclease domain [30–33]. The use of CRISPR/Cas9 as an RNA-programmable DNA targeting and editing platform is simplified by a synthetic single guide RNA (gRNA) mimicking the natural dual trans-activating CRISPR RNA (tracrRNA)-crRNA structure [34].

Because of its simplicity, specificity and versatility, the CRISPR/Cas system has recently emerged as a powerful tool for genome engineering in various species [35–38] including fungi [39–41] and bacteria [42–45]. In oomycetes, CRISPR/Cas9-mediated gene disruption and gene replacement were performed to test the function of specific genes in *Phytophthora sojae*, the causative agent of stem and root rot of soybeans [46–48].

The aim of the present study was to use CRISPR/Cas9 system to edit the genome of *A. invadans* by targeting the serine protease gene *in vitro* and study the effect of this genome editing on the virulence and pathogenicity of the *A. invadans in vivo*.

Methods

Aphanomyces invadans growth and zoospore production

Aphanomyces invadans strain 9701 was used in this study. It is routinely grown on glucose-peptone-yeast (GPY) agar and maintained on glucose-peptone (GP) agar at 25 °C according to Lilley et al. [9]. For zoospore production, agar plugs (4 mm) were aseptically transferred from stock cultures to GPY agar and grown for 4–5 days at 25 °C. A piece of agar containing hyphae from the growing edge of a colony was then aseptically transferred to GP broth supplemented with oxolinic acid (100 µg/ml) and incubated at 25 °C for 3–4 days. The resulting mycelial wads were then aseptically removed from the broth, rinsed four times with sterile distilled water and transferred into Petri dishes containing 20 ml filtered autoclaved pond water (APW) (one part filtered river water combined with one part distilled water) for 24 h. The production of secondary zoospores was microscopically monitored. The produced zoospores were counted using a hemocytometer.

Design of gRNAs and the formation of ribo-nucleoprotein (RNP) complexes

The Eukaryotic Pathogen CRISPR Guide RNA Design Tool (EuPaGDT) [49] was used to design the gRNAs for serine type protease of *A. invadans* (gene ID: 20088162). Secondary structures were checked using RNAstructure, a web server tool for RNA secondary structure prediction [50], while off-targets were checked using FungiDB as per Fang & Tyler [48]. Sequences of chosen gRNAs were submitted to Integrated DNA Technologies, Skokie, USA, for *in vitro* synthesis of crRNA. tracrRNA labeled with a fluorescent dye ATTO^{TM} 550 and Alt-R^{TM} (*Streptococcus pyogenes*) S.p. Cas9 nuclease 3NLS were purchased from Integrated DNA Technologies. crRNA and tracrRNA were separately resuspended in nuclease-free duplex buffer (Integrated DNA Technologies) to produce 100 µM stock solution. Subsequently, 30 µl from each were mixed and annealed at 95 °C, according to manufacturer's instructions, and then cooled at room temperature (RT). Each gRNA (1 µM) was combined with Cas9 (1 µM) in Opti-MEM media supplemented with GlutaMax (Thermo Fisher, Vienna, Austria) to form the RNP complexes. After incubation of the mixture for 5 min at RT, the complex was ready for transfection.

PCR primers

Three PCR primer sets (product sizes 211, 214 and 209 bp) corresponding to each gRNA were designed (Table 1) based on the *A. invadans* target gene (GenBank: XM_008877667) to amplify the target fragment and observe the genomic DNA mutation caused by Cas9 and gRNAs in the target gene *via* sequencing of the amplified products. Possible homology of the selected oligonucleotides was excluded using BLASTn analysis.

Protoplast isolation

Aphanomyces invadans protoplasts were isolated following the method described by Fang et al. [47] with minor modifications. Briefly, *A. invadans* mycelia were peeled off of the GPY plates (or the plug of germinated zoospores was isolated from the broth), rinsed first in water and then in 0.8 M mannitol (Sigma-Aldrich, Vienna, Austria) for 10 min each. Plasmolysis was carried out using 0.8 M mannitol for 20 min. Subsequently, the digestion process was completed using 20 ml enzyme solution [0.4 M mannitol, 20 mM KCl, 20 mM 2-(N-morpholino) ethanesulfonic acid (MES) (pH 5.7), 10 mM $CaCl_2$, 0.5% lysing enzymes from *Trichoderma harzianum* and 0.5% CELLULYSIN® Cellulase (Sigma-Aldrich)] for 45 min on a 50× *rpm* shaker. Digestion efficiency for the release of protoplasts in the solution was checked under a light microscope (Olympus BX53, Tokyo, Japan). The digestion product was then filtered through 70 µm Corning® cell strainers (Sigma-Aldrich) to remove mycelial debris. The flow-through was collected and centrifuged at 1200× *g* for 2 min. The supernatant was then discarded and the pellet washed by slowly adding up to 5 ml of W5 solution (5 mM KCl, 125 mM $CaCl_2$, 154 mM NaCl and 177 mM glucose). Excess W5 solution was discarded after spinning the tube at 1200× *g* for 2 min. W5 solution (2 ml) was added and protoplasts were placed on ice for 20 min. Protoplasts were spun again at RT and excess W5 solution was removed. Protoplasts were then resuspended by gently adding 2 ml of MMG solution [0.4 M mannitol, 15 mM $MgCl_2$ and 4 mM MES (pH 5.7)] at RT for 10 min. The protoplasts were counted and optimized to 10^5 per ml.

Transfection of *A. invadans* protoplasts

Polyethylene glycol (PEG)-mediated RNP delivery into the protoplasts was carried out following the protocol described by Malnoy et al. [51] with minor modifications. Briefly, 200 µl of resuspended *A. invadans* protoplasts (20,000 protoplasts) were mixed with 12 µl RNP and incubated at RT for 10 min. Another 200 µl protoplast suspension was mixed with 12 µl opti-MEM medium and incubated for 10 min at RT to be used as a control. An equal volume of PEG 4000 (Sigma-Aldrich) was added, gently mixed and incubated at RT for a further 20 min. W5 solution (400 µl) was then added, mixed and kept at RT for 10 min, followed by the addition of 800 µl W5 solution. After another 10 min of incubation at RT, the protoplasts were centrifuged at 50× *g* for 5 min. The supernatant was discarded and the pellet was washed with 500 µl W5 solution and incubated at RT overnight. To observe the efficient delivery of RNP into the protoplasts, 15 µl of each transformation mixture including control was sampled and examined by fluorescence microscopy. Regeneration media (double strength GPY broth) was then added and the mixture was divided into two parts; one part was used for DNA extraction and the other incubated for 3–4 days at 25 °C to ensure that the RNP did not affect the viability of the protoplasts.

Transfection of *A. invadans* zoospores

Aphanomyces invadans zoospores (4000 zoospores in 400 µl suspension) were transfected by adding 24 µl of RNPs and incubated at RT for 60 min. Non-treated zoospores were used as control. Both treated and non-treated zoospores (200 µl) were then subjected to DNA extraction, PCR and sequencing to observe the mutation. The other 200 µl of zoospores were added to GYP medium and incubated at 25 °C for 4–5 days to demonstrate the effect of RNP complex on the viability and growth of the treated zoospores.

Detection of targeted mutation

DNA from RNP-treated and non-treated *A. invadans* protoplasts and zoospores were isolated using Qiagen DNeasy Blood & Tissue Kit (Qiagen, Vienna, Austria) according to the manufacturer's instructions. To exclude the possibility of mutations caused during PCR amplification, Platinum SuperFi Green PCR Master Mix (Invitrogen, Vienna, Austria) was used in all PCR reactions. The amplification reaction mixture consisted of 12.5 µl Platinum SuperFi Green PCR Master Mix, 15 pmol of each sense and antisense primers, 2.5 µl DNA template and PCR grade water to a final volume of 25 µl. The reaction mixture was subjected to 35 amplification cycles comprising: denaturing at 98 °C for 10 s, annealing at 57 °C for 10 s and extension at 72 °C for 30 s. The amplification cycles were preceded by an initial denaturing step of 98 °C for 30 s followed by an extended elongation step of 72 °C for 5 min. Amplified products were analyzed on 1.5% agarose gel.

For sequencing, PCR products were purified using MinElute gel extraction kit (Qiagen) as per the manufacturer's instructions. The purified products were either directly sequenced or incubated with Taq polymerase buffer, dATP and Taq polymerase enzyme at 72 °C for 20 min to add 3' adenines to the blunt-end fragments for TA cloning. For TA cloning, PCR products were cloned into the pCR® 4-TOPO® vector using TOPO TA cloning® kit (Invitrogen) according to the manufacturer's instructions. The purified PCR products and recombinant plasmids were subjected to sequencing in a commercial sequencing laboratory (LGC Genomics, Berlin, Germany). Sequences were subjected to BLASTn analysis for sequence identity and then compared with the *A. invadans* target gene (GenBank: XM_008877667) to detect the mutation.

In vivo investigation of the effect of CRISPR/Cas9-treated *A. invadans* zoospores on dwarf gourami fish

Dwarf gourami (*Trichogaster lalius*) were purchased from a local pet shop in Austria. Five random fish were taken for bacteriological and parasitological analyses to rule out the possibility of other infections prior to the *in vivo* experiment. Furthermore, muscle samples were taken from these 5 fish for PCR to rule out the possibility of prior infection with *A. invadans* according to Vandersea et al. [52]. Fish (n = 180, mean total length 4.5 ± 0.5 cm and mean weight 5 ± 0.5 g) were kept in aquaria containing de-chlorinated water and equipped with air stones and aquarium heaters to provide aeration and maintain the temperature at 24 ± 1 °C. Water was changed (25%) weekly to maintain water quality. After 3 weeks of acclimatization, fish were divided into three groups. Each group had three replicates and each replicate contained 20 fish. The fish were anaesthetized using MS-222 (Sigma-Aldrich) 150 ppm prior to zoospore injection. After transfection of *A. invadans*' zoospores with RNP complex for 60 min, each fish in the RNP-2-treated group was intramuscularly injected with 0.1 ml of 10,000 zoospores/ml spore suspension (1000 zoospores/fish). Similarly, in the positive control group, each fish received 0.1 ml of 10,000 zoospores/ml non-treated *A. invadans* zoospores intramuscularly. The negative control group was inoculated with an equal volume of APW. All fish were monitored daily for characteristic EUS clinical signs for 30 days. Fish with clinical signs were collected as appropriate. Similarly, fish were sampled from both RNP-2-treated and negative control groups. Collected fish were euthanized and subjected to histological and PCR examinations for confirmation of *A. invadans*. Skin and muscle tissues were excised from lesion area and divided into two parts. One part was subjected to DNA extraction and the second part was fixed in 10% phosphate-buffered formalin for histology.

Histopathology

Tissue samples were processed through an automatic tissue processor and embedded in paraffin. The paraffin blocks were then sectioned at 4 μm thickness and stained with Gomori's methenamine silvernitrate (GMS) and hematoxylin and eosin (H&E) stains [53]. Stained sections were viewed under a light microscope (Olympus BX53). Photomicrographs were taken with a camera (Olympus DP73) attached to the microscope and processed using CellSens Standard software of Olympus.

Results

Design of *A. invadans* specific gRNAs

Targeting a serine type protease of *A. invadans* [20], gRNA candidates were suggested by the gRNA design tool and further filtered for secondary structure and off-targets. Based on their high total and efficiency scores and zero off-target hits, three gRNA candidates were selected (Table 2), synthesized and used for the formation of 3 separate RNP complexes.

Transfection of protoplasts and zoospores with RNP complexes

After the formation of RNP complexes, they were used separately to transfect the isolated *A. invadans* protoplasts. Examination of the successful transfection by fluorescence microscope revealed clear signals within the protoplasts (Fig. 1) and no signal in non-treated control samples. After regeneration of the RNP-treated protoplasts in GPY medium for 3–4 days, the protoplasts treated with the RNP-2 complex demonstrated a different growth pattern than those treated with RNP-1, RNP-3 and the non-treated control protoplasts (Fig. 2). Correspondingly, the RNP-treated zoospores demonstrated slow growth behavior in GYP medium compared with the non-treated controls.

Detection of targeted mutation

The expected *A. invadans* DNA fragments were successfully amplified from RNP-treated and non-treated protoplasts and zoospores (Fig. 3). Sequencing results revealed a mutation located at the 5th nt from the PAM site in sequences of the targeted fragments amplified from protoplasts and zoospores treated with RNP-2 complex (Fig. 4). Comparatively, no mutation was detected in the sequences of protoplasts and zoospores treated either with RNP-1 or RNP-3.

Table 1 PCR primers designed for each guide RNA. Three PCR primer sets corresponding to each gRNA were designed based on the *A. invadans* target gene (GenBank: XM_008877667) to detect the genomic DNA mutation, caused by CRISPR/Cas9

	Name	Position	Expected product size (bp)	Sequence (5'- 3')
Primer set 1	AiCr1F	35–54	211	GACTCCGACCTTGACGATGC
	AiCr1R	227–246		AAAGAGGAATGAGGCGGAGG
Primer set 2	AiCr2F	884–904	214	CCCACACCATGGGAACGATTG
	AiCr2R	1080–1098		TTGAGACGAGCCCCACGAG
Primer set 3	AiCr3R	1572–1591	209	GTTCGGCCGTATTAACGCCA
	AiCr3F	1763–1781		CTTGGTACATGGCTGCCCA

In vivo experiments

At 3 days post-infection (dpi), fish within the positive control group inoculated with non-treated zoospores demonstrated swelling, reddening of skin and loss of scales; red ulceration underlying musculature was observed at 5 dpi. The ulceration further developed into deep ulceration with cotton-like threads at 7 dpi (Fig. 5a, b). Swimming behavior of the fish was affected and the fish showed weakness at 10 dpi. The presence of *A. invadans* DNA in the sampled fish tissues was confirmed by PCR and sequencing. Fish inoculated with the RNP-2-treated zoospores (Fig. 5c) and fish within the negative control group inoculated with APW (Fig. 5d) did not show any clinical signs during the 30 days of the experiment. PCR did not amplify the *A. invadans* DNA from the fish samples taken from these two groups. Negative control fish did not show any illness throughout the experiment.

Histological investigation

GMS-stained muscle sections of the fish from positive control group sampled at 7 dpi showed the presence of oomycete hyphae embedded into the fish musculature, with muscle tissues appearing necrotic around the hyphae in positive control group sampled at 7 dpi (Fig. 6a, b). No such fungal structure was found in the RNP-2-treated (Fig. 6c, d) or negative control groups (Fig. 6e, f). Sections of the fish muscles stained with H&E showed infiltration of macrophages and other inflammatory cells at the site of infection in positive control group (Fig. 7a, b). No such infiltration or necrosis of muscle tissues was found in the RNP-2-treated (Fig. 7c, d) or negative control groups (Fig. 7e, f).

Discussion

Production of extracellular proteins from *A. invadans* has been reported by Majeed et al. [20]. These proteins mainly consist of proteases that are believed to be the major virulence factors that contribute to EUS infection. One of the identified proteins contains the peptidase_S8 domain which is a subtilisin or subtilase family, the second-largest family of serine proteases. Serine proteases are present in every life form including viruses and play major roles in protein metabolism, digestion, development, host invasion and immune evasion [54]. These proteases have been reported to be the virulence factors in different pathogenic species including fungi [55–57], parasites [58, 59] and bacteria [60–62]. Accordingly, in this study, this gene was selected for gene editing using CRISPR/Cas9 system in a trial to investigate its role in EUS. Currently, ZFNs and TALENs are used for genome editing experiments but the focus has been shifted to CRISPR/Cas system for such purposes. In the present study, the phenotype of germinating *A. invadans* protoplasts treated with three different RNP complexes demonstrated a different growth patterns. The PEG-mediated RNP delivery system is the most widely used system for delivering the gRNA and Cas9 into the protoplasts of oomycete and fungi. Based on fluorescence microscopy, the transfection resulted in bright and strong fluorescence signal which confirmed the efficiency of the transfection (Fig. 1). Nevertheless, obtained

Table 2 Guide RNAs used in this study. The Eukaryotic Pathogen CRISPR Guide RNA Design Tool was used to design the gRNAs for serine type protease of *A. invadans* (gene ID: 20088162). Based on their high total and efficiency scores and zero off-target hits, three gRNAs were selected for genome modification experiment

gRNA id	gRNA sequence (PAM "NGG")	Total score	Efficiency score	On-target hits in the genome (perfect-match | non-perfect-but PAM match)	Off-target hits (perfect-match | nonperfect-match)
1. Aphanomyces-invadans_106	GCT TAC CAG ATG GAA TGA CG | TGG	0.69	0.65	2 | 0	0 | 0
2. Aphanomyces-invadans_923	GTG TAG CCC CAG AAG CCC AA | TGG	0.56	0.57	1 | 1	0 | 0
3. Aphanomyces-invadans_1730	GAT GGA ACC CAA CAA CTG TG | TGG	0.53	0.65	1 | 0	0 | 0

Abbreviation: *PAM* protospacer adjacent motif

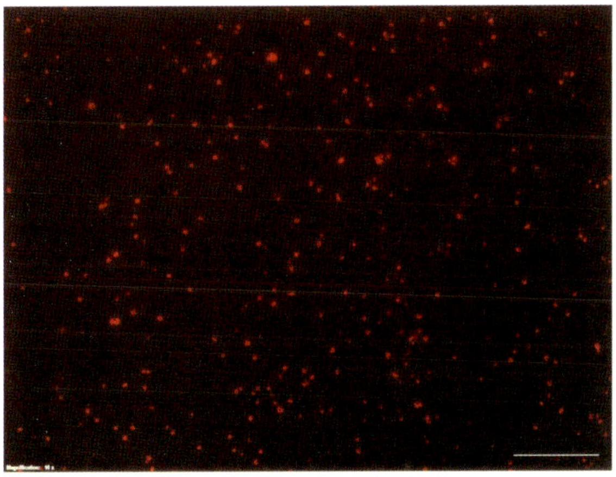

Fig. 1 Fluorescence microscope image of the protoplasts of *Aphanomyces invadans*. Protoplasts were transfected with RNPs carrying ATTO™ 550. Successful transfection shows clear RNP-complex signals within the protoplasts after overnight incubation. *Scale-bar*: 100 μm

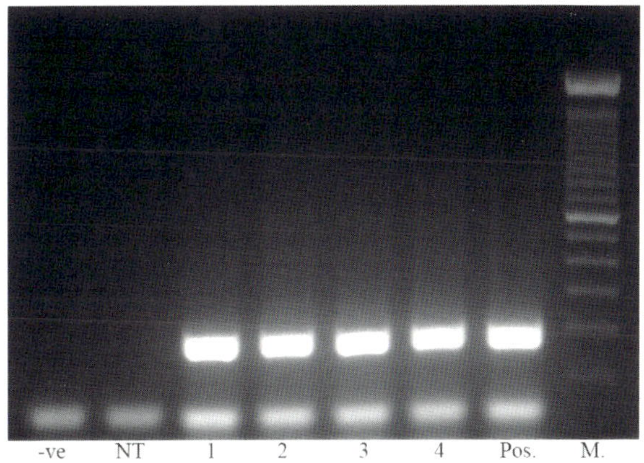

Fig. 3 PCR result (214 bp) of RNP-2-treated and non-treated protoplasts and zoospores using primer set 2. Lane -ve: negative extraction; Lane NT: non-template; Lane 1: protoplasts transfected with RNP-2; Lane 2: non-treated protoplasts; Lane 3: zoospores transfected with RNP-2. Lane 4: non-treated zoospores. Lane Pos.: positive control. Lane M: marker (100 bp)

populations are expected to carry a mixture of mutated and non-mutated protease genes.

Sequence analysis of DNA of these protoplasts revealed the presence of point mutation in amplified fragments of the target gene caused by only one out of the selected three gRNAs. The same mutation was also detected in the zoospores treated with the same RNP complex (Fig. 4). These results confirm that only RNP-2 caused the mutation, while the RNP-1 and RNP-3 failed to perform similarly. The failure of the RNP-1 and RNP-3 to cause mutation may be attributed to the self-complementarity which likely hindered their binding to the target DNA sequence and affected their functionality [47]. The different growth pattern was only observed in the protoplasts that were treated with RNP-2 while the control and RNP-1- and RNP-3-treated protoplasts demonstrated a conventional growth pattern (Fig. 2). Furthermore, the observed slow growth pattern of the treated zoospores was likely because of the point mutation in the target gene. This indicates that the target gene may also play an important role in the growth of the *A. invadans*. This is supported by the fact that the target gene is a serine protease and serine proteases play major roles in regulation of development and host invasion [54]. Thus, any effective mutation in these genes will likely affect other cellular functions as well.

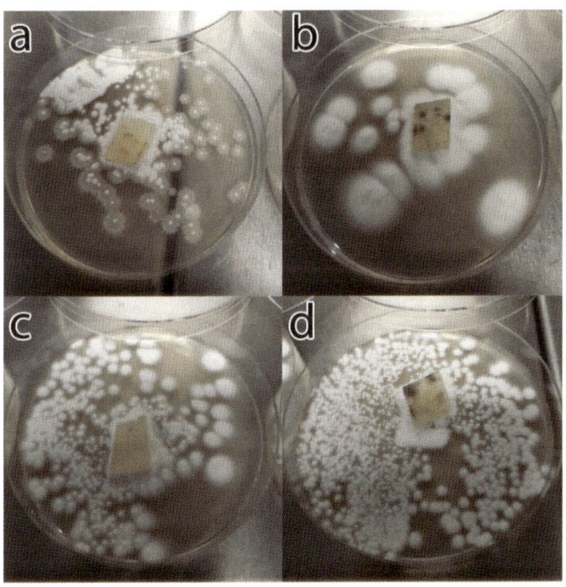

Fig. 2 Growth of RNP-transfected *Aphanomyces invadans* protoplasts after being transfected with RNP-1 (**a**), RNP-2 (**b**) and RNP-3 (**c**). **d** Growth of non-treated control protoplasts

It seems that the target gene likely plays an important role in the virulence of the *A. invadans*. Dwarf guorami that were inoculated with non-treated zoospores demonstrated characteristic EUS clinical signs such as reddening, swelling, deep ulcers in skin and muscles, and visible fungal growth at the site of infection (Fig. 5a, b). On the other hand, fish that were inoculated with the RNP-2-treated zoospores did not demonstrate any clinical signs during the 30 days of the *in vivo* experiment (Fig. 5c). Mutation was confirmed *via* sequencing and all sequenced samples have this mutation. It was, however, confirmed by the *in vivo* experiments when the edited zoospores did not produce the EUS clinical signs. This shows that the zoospores carry the mutation.

GMS staining is the standard approach for the visualization of fungal agents in granulomatous inflammation [63, 64]. It stains the walls of the fungus and gives them dark/black coloration [53, 63]. GMS-stained histopathological sections of muscle tissues of the positive control fish at 7 dpi clearly showed the stained

ATGGTCCGCATTGCCTCCATCGCATCCCTCGCCGCGTCGGCCACCGCGACCATTTCCCAGCGTACCCTTCGCG

CACTCGAAACGCAAAAGGCCATCGATATCTTGGTCACCTACAAGGCCGGCCCTGGCCTCACCAAGCTCAATA

CCGAGTCGTTGTCGCGTGAAGCCCGCGCCCAAGAAGTGTTCAACATCTTGACGACTGAAAACTTCGCCATCAC

CGCGTCCGCCGTGGAAGTCGCCAAAGCTGCCGGAGTGAAGTACACGCAGTACTGGATCGACTCCGTTGTCGC

GATTGAAGGTGCCAACGCGGAGCTCGTCGCCAAGTTGGATGCCCTTCCCAACGTCGTCAGAGTCGCCCAAGT

GGAAGTGTACGAGTTGCCGGCCTTCCTCGAATCCAACCTCGTCGCGGCCAACTCCACCAACGAATGGGGTGTT

GAGATGATCAGCGCCCCAGTTGCCTGGGCCCGCGGCAACAAGGGCAAGGGCATCGTCGTGGCCAATATCGAC

ACCGGTGTGCGCGGCACGCATGAAGCGCTCAAGGGCAACTTCCGCGCTCAGAATGGCTGGTACGAACCCTCC

Forward primer 2

ACGAAGTCCCCTGCCCCCAACGATCGACACGGCCACGGTA*CCCACACCATGGGAACGATTG*CCGGTGCCAACG

gRNA **PAM**

GCATCG*GTGTAGCCCCAGAAGCCCAATGG*ATTGCGTGTGTCGGGTGCCCGGCCGGGTCATGTCCCCAAACCGA

TTTATTGGCATGCGCCCAATTCATCCTATGCCCAACCGACACGAACGGCCAGAACCCCAACTGCAAGATGGC

Reverse primer 2

CCCTAGTGTCGTTAACAA*CTCGTGGGGCTCGTCTCAA*AGCGGCAGCACGTGGTATGAAGCATCGATCCTTGCC

TGGCGCAAGGCCGGCATCGTTCCCGTGTTTCGAACGGGAACTCCGGCCCCAGCTGCGGCACCGTAGGCTCCC

CTGGTGACTCCCCCTCGGTCATTGCTGTCGGTGCTACTGATATGACTGATGCATTGGCCAGCTTCAGCTCGAA

AGGTCCTGAGCCCCTACAAAAGCGCATCAAGCCTGATGTGTCGGCCCCCGGTAAGGGCATTCGCTCCGCTGG

TTATGCCGGCGATAGCTCGTACGTCTCGATGTCTGGTACGTCTATGGCCGCCCCCCACACCACCGGCACCGTC

GCGTTGATGTTAAATGCCAACCCCGGTGCCACCTATGAAACCGTGTACAAGTTGATCACCGGTTCGGTCGATA

CGGCCACGTTGAAGCCATCCACTGCCAACTGCGGTGGTGTGGACAACTCCAAGTACCCCAACAACGACTTCG

GGTTCGGCCGTATTAACGCCAACAAGGCGTCCGCCTCGGGTTCGTCCACCCCCGCTCCTACCTCCGCCAATCC

CGCGTGCTAA

Fig. 4 Coding sequence (mRNA sequence) of *Aphanomyces invadans'* hypothetical protein (GenBank: XM_008877667) contains 1388 nucleotides. The designed gRNA2 site is highlighted in green and the PAM site in grey. Forward and reverse primer 2 (product size 214 bp) sites are highlighted in yellow. The point mutation (deletion) located at the 5th nt from the PAM site is shown in red within the gRNA2 sequence

oomycete hyphae (Fig. 6a, b). Necrosis of muscle tissues were observed around the area of the hyphae, likely because of the intense inflammatory response [65]. Accumulation of macrophages and other inflammatory cells at the site of infection were also observed in H&E stained sections (Fig. 7a, b). Presence of *A. invadans* hyphae in fish musculature during EUS infection has been reported [14, 65] and our findings are in accordance with these results. Muscle sections of RNP-2-treated and negative control fish did not show any hyphae in GMS

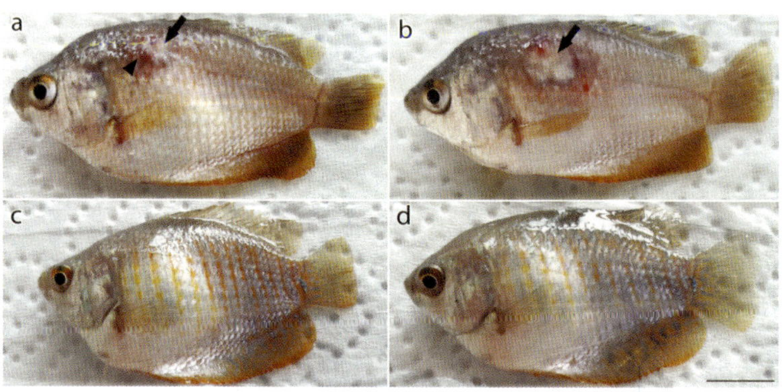

Fig. 5 Dwarf gourami showing necrotic ulceration after infection with the zoospores of *A. invadans*. Zoospore suspension (0.1 ml) coniatining 10,000 zoospores/ml of *A. invadans* was injected intramuscularly. **a** Positive control fish showing the reddening of the infected area (arrowhead) and the beginning of ulcer formation (arrow) at the site of infection at 3 dpi. **b** Positive control fish showing clear oomycete growth and necrotic ulceration (arrow) at the site of infection at 7 dpi. **c** Fish injected with RNP-2-treated *A. invadans* zoospores showing no clinical signs at 7 dpi. **d** Negative control fish at 7 dpi. *Scale-bar*: 1 cm

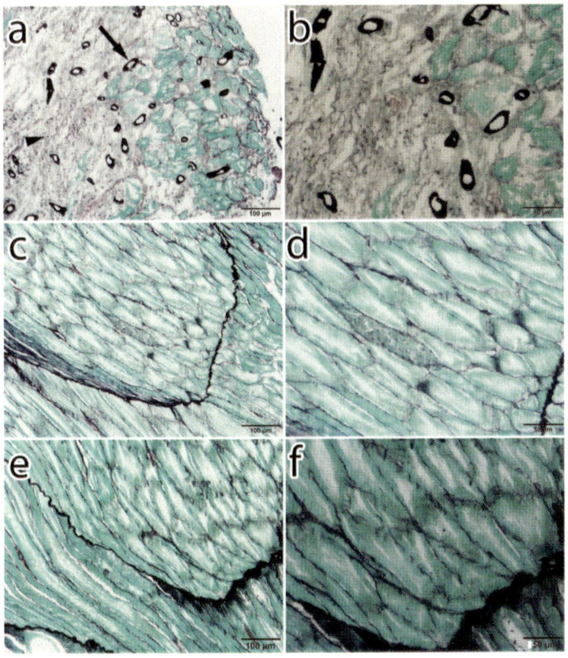

Fig. 6 Gomori's methenamine silver-stained muscle sections of dwarf gourami. **a** Muscle section of positive control fish showing presence of *A. invadans* as a black hollow structure (arrow) and muscle necrosis (arrowhead) in the gray area. **b** Higher magnification of **a**. **c** Muscle section of the fish inoculated with RNP-2-treated zoospores showing intact muscle with no oomycete hyphae. **d** Higher magnification of **c**. **e** Muscle section of negative control fish showing intact muscle with no oomycete hyphae. **f** Higher magnification of **e**. *Scale-bars*: **a**, **c**, **e**, 100 µm; **b**, **d**, **f**, 50 µm

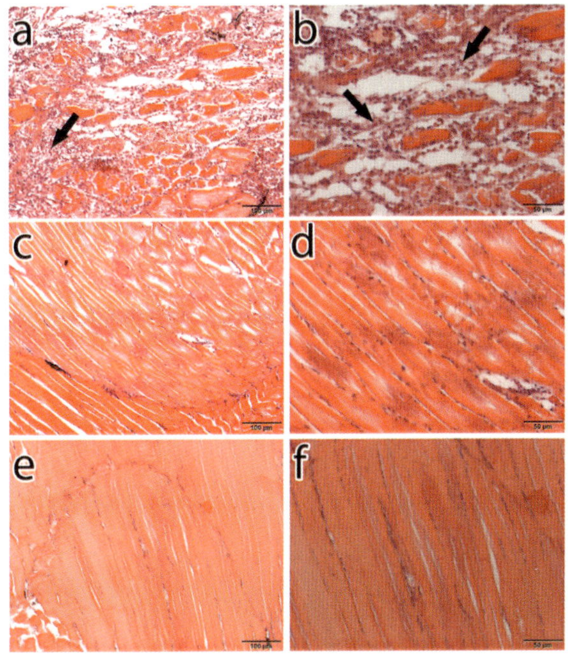

Fig. 7 Hematoxylin and eosin-stained muscle sections of dwarf gourami. **a** Muscle section of positive control fish showing muscle necrosis (arrow). **b** Muscle section of positive control fish showing high infiltration of macrophages and other inflammatory cells (arrows). **c** Muscle section of the fish inoculated with RNP-2-treated zoospores showing no necrosis or infiltration of macrophages. **d** Higher magnification of **c**. **e** Muscle section of negative control fish showing no necrosis or infiltration of macrophages. **f** Higher magnification of **e**. *Scale-bars*: **a**, **c**, **e**, 100 µm; **b**, **d**, **f**, 50 µm

staining and no infiltration of inflammatory cells was seen in H&E stained sections of these fish at 7 dpi.

During CRISPR/Cas9-mediated genome editing, the suppression of the target gene by gRNA-complex apparently affects oomycete development and virulence, resulting in the cessation of *A. invadans* pathogenesis. The results obtained from this study hint on the fact that the serine proteases are definitely required by the oomycete in order to invade the fish and penetrate into the muscles. Protease production was likely affected in RNP-2-treated *A. invadans*, which might have hindered the production of other essential proteins as well. Thus, the oomycete was left unable to invade the fish musculature.

Conclusions

In this study, despite lacking prerequisite information on molecular mechanisms of pathogenicity and interactions of *A. invadans* with the fish host, the CRISPR/Cas9 system was successfully applied to edit the serine protease gene of *A. invadans*. Our study establishes that CRISPR/Cas9 is a promising tool and offers a great opportunity to plan more advanced genomic studies on oomycetes to understand the role of different secreted proteases, their virulence mechanisms, and their interactions with their hosts. In addition, our study provides a basis for further investigations of molecular mechanisms previously suggested to be involved in EUS and may help the development of novel drugs and control methods to combat their deleterious effects in fish.

Abbreviations

APW: Autoclaved pond water; Cas9: CRISPR-associated protein 9; CRISPR: Clustered regularly interspaced short palindromic repeats; crRNA: CRISPR RNA; dpi: Days post-infection; EuPaGDT: Eukaryotic Pathogen CRISPR Guide RNA Design Tool; EUS: Epizootic ulcerative syndrome; GMS: Grocott's methenamine silver nitrate stain; GP: Glucose peptone; GPY: Glucose peptone yeast; gRNA: Guide RNA; H&E: Hematoxylin and eosin; MES: 2-(N-morpholino)ethanesulfonic acid; PEG: Polyethylene glycol; RNP: Ribo-nucleo-protein; RT: Room temperature; TALEN: Transcription activator-like effector nuclease(s); ZFN: Zinc finger nuclease(s)

Acknowledgements

MM thanks the Higher Education Commission of Pakistan for providing the scholarship to study abroad and Österreichische Austauschdienst for their institutional support and guidance.

Funding

This study was funded by the University of Veterinary Medicine, Vienna (PP291-ELM), and the Austrian Science Fund (FWF) Project No. P29294-B25.

Authors' contributions

MEM and MS conceived the study. MM and HS performed the experiments. MM, HS, GK and MS were involved in data acquisition and analyses. MM wrote the manuscript and HS, GK, MEM and MS revised it. All authors read and approved the final manuscript.

Competing interests

The authors declare that they have no competing interests.

References

1. Carris LM, Little CR, Stiles CM. Introduction to Fungi. The Plant Health Instructor. 2018. http://www.apsnet.org/edcenter/intropp/PathogenGroups/Pages/IntroFungi.aspx. Accessed 04 Jul 2018.
2. Willoughby LG, Pickering AD. Viable Saprolegniaceae spores on the epidermis of the salmonid fish *Salmo trutta* and *Salvelinus alpinus*. Trans Br Mycol Soc. 1977;68:91–5.
3. Blazer VS, Wolke RE. An exopholia-like fungus as the cause of a systematic mycosis of marine fish. J Fish Dis. 1979;2:145–52.
4. Gozlan RE, Marshall WL, Lilje O, Jessop CN, Gleason FH, Andreou D. Current ecological understanding of fungal-like pathogens of fish: what lies beneath? Front Microbiol. 2014;5:1–16.
5. Scott WW. A monograph of the genus *Aphanomyces*. Virginia Agr Exp Sta Tech Bull. 1961;151:1–95.
6. Diéguez-Uribeondo J, García MA, Cerenius L, Kozubíková E, Ballesteros I, Windels C, et al. Phylogenetic relationships among plant and animal parasites, and saprotrophs in *Aphanomyces* (Oomycetes). Fungal Genet Biol. 2009;46:365–76.
7. Roberts RJ, Willoughby LG, Chinabut S. Mycotic aspects of epizootic ulcerative syndrome (EUS) of Asian fishes. J Fish Dis. 1993;16:169–83.
8. Blazer VS, Vogelbein WK, Densmore CL, May EB, Lilley JH, Zwerner DE. *Aphanomyces* as a cause of ulcerative skin lesions of menhaden from Chesapeake Bay tributaries. J Aquat Anim Health. 1999;11:340–9.
9. Lilley JH, Callinan RB, Chinabut S, Kanchanakhan S, MacRae RH, Phillips MJ. Epizootic ulcerative syndrome (EUS) technical handbook. Bangkok: Aquatic Animal Health Research Institute; 1998.
10. Kiryu Y, Shields JD, Vogelbein WK, Kator H, Blazer VS. Infectivity and pathogenicity of the oomycete *Aphanomyces invadans* in Atlantic menhaden *Brevoortia tyrannus*. Dis Aquat Org. 2003;54:135–46.
11. Willoughby LG, Roberts RJ, Chinabut S. *Aphanomyces invaderis* sp. nov., the fungal pathogen of freshwater tropical fishes affected by epizootic ulcerative syndrome (EUS). J Fish Dis. 1995;18:273–5.
12. Oidtmann B. Review of biological factors relevant to import risk assessments for epizootic ulcerative syndrome (*Aphanomyces invadans*). Transbound Emerg Dis. 2012;59:26–39.
13. Pathiratne A, Widanapathirana GS, Chandrakanthi WHS. Association of *Aeromonas hydrophila* with epizootic ulcerative syndrome (EUS) of freshwater fish in Sri Lanka. J Appl Ichthyol. 1994;10:204–8.
14. Lilley JH, Roberts RJ. Pathogenicity and culture studies comparing the *Aphanomyces* involved in epizootic ulcerative syndrome (EUS) with other similar fungi. J Fish Dis. 1997;20:135–44.
15. Vishwanath TS, Mohan CV, Shankar KM. Epizootic Ulcerative Syndrome (EUS), associated with a fungal pathogen, in Indian fishes: histopathology - 'a cause for invasiveness'. Aquaculture. 1998;165:1–9.
16. Kamilya D, Baruah A. Epizootic ulcerative syndrome (EUS) in fish: history and current status of understanding. Rev Fish Biol Fish. 2014;24:369–80.
17. OIE. OIE-listed diseases, infections and infestations. 2018. http://www.oie.int/en/animal-health-in-the-world/oie-listed-diseases-2018/. Accessed 10 Jul 2018.
18. OIE. Infection with *Aphanomyces invadans* (epizootic ulcerative syndrome). In: Manual of diagnostic tests for aquatic animals. World Organisation for Animal Health; 2018. http://www.oie.int/standard-setting/aquatic-manual/access-online/. Accessed 10 Jul 2018.
19. Yadav MK, Pradhan PK, Sood N, Chaudhary DK, Verma DK, Debnath C, et al. Innate immune response of Indian major carp, *Labeo rohita* infected with oomycete pathogen *Aphanomyces invadans*. Fish Shellfish Immunol. 2014; 39:524–31.
20. Majeed M, Kumar G, Schlosser S, El-Matbouli M, Saleh M. *In vitro* investigations on extracellular proteins secreted by *Aphanomyces invadans*, the causative agent of epizootic ulcerative syndrome. Acta Vet Scand. 2017;59:78.
21. Minor KL, Anderson VL, Davis KS, van den Berg AH, Christie JS, Lobach L, et al. A putative serine protease, SpSsp1, from *Saprolegnia parasitica* is recognised by sera of rainbow trout, *Oncorhynchus mykiss*. Fungal Biol. 2014;118:630–9.
22. Jiang RHY, de Bruijn I, Haas BJ, Belmonte R, Lobach L, Christie J, et al. Distinctive expansion of potential virulence genes in the genome of the oomycete fish pathogen *Saprolegnia parasitica*. PLoS Genet. 2013;9: e1003272.
23. Gaj T, Gersbach CA, Barbas CF 3rd. ZFN, TALEN, and CRISPR/Cas-based methods for genome engineering. Trends Biotechnol. 2013;3:397–405.
24. Urnov FD, Rebar EJ, Holmes MC, Zhang HS, Gregory PD. Genome editing with engineered zinc finger nucleases. Nat Rev Genet. 2010;11:636–46.
25. Carroll D. Genome engineering with zinc-finger nucleases. Genetics. 2011; 188:773–82.
26. Sun N, Zhao H. Transcription activator-like effector nucleases (TALENs): A highly efficient and versatile tool for genome editing. Biotechnol Bioeng. 2013;110:1811–21.
27. Doudna JA, editing CEG. The new frontier of genome engineering with CRISPR-Cas9. Science. 2014;346:1258096.
28. Barrangou R. The roles of CRISPR-Cas systems in adaptive immunity and beyond. Curr Opin Immunol. 2015;32:36–41.
29. Wright AV, Nuñez JK, Doudna JA. Biology and applications of CRISPR Systems: harnessing nature's toolbox for genome engineering. Cell. 2016;164:29–44.
30. Garneau JE, Dupuis MÈ, Villion M, Romero DA, Barrangou R, Boyaval P, et al. The CRISPR/Cas bacterial immune system cleaves bacteriophage and plasmid DNA. Nature. 2010;468:67–71.
31. Gasiunas G, Barrangou R, Horvath P, Siksnys V. Cas9-crRNA ribonucleoprotein complex mediates specific DNA cleavage for adaptive immunity in bacteria. Proc Natl Acad Sci USA. 2012;109:E2579–86.
32. Jinek M, Chylinski K, Fonfara I, Hauer M, Doudna JA, Charpentier E. A programmable dual-RNA-guided DNA endonuclease in adaptive bacterial immunity. Science. 2012;337:816–21.
33. Rath D, Amlinger L, Rath A, Lundgren M. The CRISPR-Cas immune system: Biology, mechanisms and applications. Biochimie. 2015;117:119–28.
34. Jiang F, Doudna JA. CRISPR-Cas9 Structures and Mechanisms. Annu Rev Biophys. 2017;46:505–29.
35. Pellagatti A, Dolatshad H, Valletta S, Boultwood J. Application of CRISPR/Cas9 genome editing to the study and treatment of disease. Arch Toxicol. 2015;89:1023–34.
36. Oishi I, Yoshii K, Miyahara D, Kagami H, Tagami T. Targeted mutagenesis in chicken using CRISPR/Cas9 system. Sci Rep. 2016;6:23980.
37. Wang X, Cai B, Zhou J, Zhu H, Niu Y, Ma B, et al. Disruption of *FGF5* in Cashmere goats using CRISPR/Cas9 results in more secondary hair follicles and longer fibers. PLoS One. 2016;11:e0164640.
38. Wu M, Wei C, Lian Z, Liu R, Zhu C, Wang H, Cao J, et al. *Rosa26*-targeted sheep gene knock-in via CRISPR-Cas9 system. Sci Rep. 2016;6:24360.
39. Liu Q, Gao R, Li J, Lin L, Zhao J, Sun W, et al. Development of a genome-editing CRISPR/Cas9 system in thermophilic fungal *Myceliophthora* species and its application to hyper-cellulase production strain engineering. Biotechnol Biofuels. 2017;10:1.
40. Pohl C, Kiel JA, Driessen AJ, Bovenberg RA, Nygård Y. CRISPR/Cas9 based genome editing of *Penicillium chrysogenum*. ACS Synth Biol. 2016;5:754–64.
41. Katayama T, Tanaka Y, Okabe T, Nakamura H, Fujii W, Kitamoto K, et al. Development of a genome editing technique using the CRISPR/Cas9 system in the industrial filamentous fungus *Aspergillus oryzae*. Biotechnol Lett. 2016;38:637–42.
42. Zhang H, Cheng QX, Liu AM, Zhao GP, Wang J. A novel and efficient method for bacteria genome editing employing both CRISPR/Cas9 and an antibiotic resistance cassette. Front Microbiol. 2017;8:812.
43. Altenbuchner J. Editing of the *Bacillus subtilis* genome by the CRISPR-Cas9 system. Appl Environ Microbiol. 2016;82:5421–7.
44. Wang Y, Zhang ZT, Seo SO, Lynn P, Lu T, Jin YS, et al. Bacterial genome editing with CRISPR-Cas9: deletion, integration, single nucleotide modification, and desirable "clean" mutant selection in *Clostridium beijerinckii* as an example. ACS Synth Biol. 2016;5:721–32.
45. Jiang W, Bikard D, Cox D, Zhang F, Marraffini LA. RNA-guided editing of bacterial genomes using CRISPR-Cas systems. Nat Biotechnol. 2013;31:233–9.

46. Tyler BM. *Phytophthora sojae*: root rot pathogen of soybean and model oomycete. Mol Plant Pathol. 2007;8:1–8.
47. Fang Y, Cui L, Gu B, Arredondo F, Tyler BM. Efficient genome editing in the oomycete *Phytophthora sojae* using CRISPR/Cas9. Curr Protoc Microbiol. 2017;44:21A 1.1–21A.1.26.
48. Fang Y, Tyler BM. Efficient disruption and replacement of an effector gene in the oomycete *Phytophthora sojae* using CRISPR/Cas9. Mol Plant Pathol. 2016;17:127–39.
49. Peng D, Tarleton R. EuPaGDT: a web tool tailored to design CRISPR guide RNAs for eukaryotic pathogens. Microb Genom. 2015;1:e000033.
50. Bellaousov S, Reuter JS, Seetin MG, Mathews DH. RNAstructure: Web Servers for RNA secondary structure prediction and analysis. Nucleic Acids Res. 2013;41:W471-4.
51. Malnoy M, Viola R, Jung MH, Koo OJ, Kim S, Kim JS, et al. DNA-free genetically edited grapevine and apple protoplast using CRISPR/Cas9 ribonucleoproteins. Front Plant Sci. 2016;7:1904.
52. Vandersea MW, Litaker RW, Yonnish B, Sosa E, Landsberg JH, Pullinger C, et al. Molecular assays for detecting *Aphanomyces invadans* in ulcerative mycotic fish lesions. Appl Environ Microbiol. 2006;72:1551–7.
53. Haque A. Special stains use in fungal infections. In: Kumar GL, Kiernan JA, editors. Special Stains and H & E. 2nd Ed. California: Dako; 2010. p. 230-40.
54. Di Cera E. Serine proteases. IUBMB Life. 2009;61:510–5.
55. Pannkuk EL, Risch TS, Savary BJ. Isolation and identification of an extracellular subtilisin-like serine protease secreted by the bat pathogen *Pseudogymnoascus destructans*. PLoS One. 2015;10:e0120508.
56. Valueva TA, Kudryavtseva NN, Sofyin AV, Zaitchik BT, Pobedinskaya MA, Kokaeva LY, et al. Serine exoproteinases secreted by the pathogenic fungi of *Alternaria* genus. J Plant Pathol Microbiol. 2015;6:272.
57. Xu J, Baldwin D, Kindrachuk C, Hegedus DD. Serine proteases and metalloproteases associated with pathogenesis but not host specificity in the entomophthoralean fungus *Zoophthora radicans*. Can J Microbiol. 2006;52:550–9.
58. Yang Y, Wen YJ, Cai YN, Vallée I, Boireau P, Liu MY, et al. Serine proteases of parasitic helminths. Korean J Parasitol. 2015;53:1–11.
59. Toubarro D, Lucena-Robles M, Nascimento G, Santos R, Montiel R, Veríssimo P, et al. Serine protease-mediated host invasion by the parasitic nematode *Steinernema carpocapsae*. J Biol Chem. 2010;285:30666–75.
60. Wessler S, Schneider G, Backert S. Bacterial serine protease HtrA as a promising new target for antimicrobial therapy? Cell Commun Signal. 2017;15:4.
61. Ruiz-Perez F, Nataro JP. Bacterial serine proteases secreted by the autotransporter pathway: classification, specificity, and role in virulence. Cell Mol Life Sci. 2014;71:745–70.
62. Nissinen R, Xia Y, Mattinen L, Ishimaru CA, Knudson DL, Knudson SE, et al. The putative secreted serine protease Chp-7 is required for full virulence and induction of a nonhost hypersensitive response by *Clavibacter michiganensis* subsp. *sepedonicus*. Mol Plant Microbe Interact. 2009;22:809–19.
63. Guo C, Ghadersohi S, Kephart GM, Laine RA, Sherris DA, Kita H, et al. Improving the detection of fungi in eosinophilic mucin: seeing what we could not see before. Otolaryngol Head Neck Surg. 2012;147:943–9.
64. Grocott RG. A stain for fungi in tissue sections and smears using Gomori's methenamine-silver nitrate technic. Am J Clin Pathol. 1955;25:975–9.
65. Huchzermeyer KD, van der Waal BC. Epizootic ulcerative syndrome: exotic fish disease threatens Africa's aquatic ecosystems. J S Afr Vet Assoc. 2012;83:204.

9

Epidemiology of taeniosis/cysticercosis

Chiara Trevisan[1,2*†], Smaragda Sotiraki[3†], Minerva Laranjo-González[4], Veronique Dermauw[1], Ziqi Wang[5], Age Kärssin[6,7], Aleksandar Cvetkovikj[8], Andrea S. Winkler[9,10], Annette Abraham[9,10], Branko Bobić[11], Brian Lassen[2,7], Carmen Michaela Cretu[12], Cozma Vasile[13], Dimitris Arvanitis[14], Gunita Deksne[15,16], Ilievski Boro[17], István Kucsera[18], Jacek Karamon[19], Jovana Stefanovska[8], Břetislav Koudela[20,21], Maja Jurhar Pavlova[22], Marian Varady[23], Marina Pavlak[24], Mindaugas Šarkūnas[25], Miriam Kaminski[26], Olgica Djurković-Djaković[11], Pikka Jokelainen[7,27,28], Dagny Stojčević Jan[29], Veronika Schmidt[9,10], Zorica Dakić[30], Sarah Gabriël[31], Pierre Dorny[1,32] and Brecht Devleesschauwer[31,33]

Abstract

Background: *Taenia solium* and *Taenia saginata* are food-borne parasites of global importance. In eastern Europe only fragmented information is available on the epidemiology of these zoonotic parasites in humans and animal populations. In particular for *T. solium*, on-going transmission is suspected. The aim of this systematic review was to collect the available data and describe the current knowledge on the epidemiology of *T. solium* and *T. saginata* in eastern Europe.

Methods: Literature published in international databases from 1990 to 2017 was systematically reviewed. Furthermore, local sources and unpublished data from national databases were retrieved from local eastern European experts. The study area included 22 countries.

Results: Researchers from 18 out of the 22 countries provided data from local and unpublished sources, while no contacts could be established with researchers from Belarus, Kosovo, Malta and Ukraine. Taeniosis and human cysticercosis cases were reported in 14 and 15 out of the 22 countries, respectively. Estonia, the Former Yugoslav Republic of Macedonia, Lithuania, Moldova, Poland, Romania, Serbia, and Slovakia reported cases of porcine cysticercosis. Croatia, Czech Republic, Estonia, Former Yugoslav Republic of Macedonia, Moldova, Poland, Romania, Serbia, Slovakia, and Ukraine reported bovine cysticercosis.

Conclusions: There is indication that taeniosis and cysticercosis are present across eastern Europe but information on the occurrence of *T. solium* and *T. saginata* across the region remains incomplete. Available data are scarce and species identification is in most cases absent. Given the public health impact of *T. solium* and the potential economic and trade implications due to *T. saginata,* notification of taeniosis and human cysticercosis should be implemented and surveillance and notification systems in animals should be improved.

Keywords: *Taenia solium*, *Taenia saginata*, Epidemiology, Bovine, Porcine, Neurocysticercosis, Eastern Europe

* Correspondence: ctrevisan@itg.be
†Chiara Trevisan and Smaragda Sotiraki contributed equally to this work
[1]Department of Biomedical Sciences, Institute of Tropical Medicine, Nationalestraat 155, 2000 Antwerp, Belgium
[2]Department of Veterinary and Animal Sciences, Faculty of Health and Medical Sciences, University of Copenhagen, Dyrlægevej, 100 Frederiksberg, Denmark
Full list of author information is available at the end of the article

Background

Taenia solium and *Taenia saginata*, also referred to as the pork and beef tapeworm, respectively, are food-borne parasites of global importance. In 2014, *T. solium*, for which humans act as final hosts after consumption of undercooked pork, was ranked by an international panel of experts as the food-borne parasite of greatest global concern, affecting millions of individuals every year and causing a substantial economic impact [1]. In 2016, during a similar exercise carried out by a group of experts at the European level, *T. solium* was ranked tenth among 27 parasites as the number of human cysticercosis cases is not as high when Europe is considered as a whole. If individual regions were taken into account, the parasite was ranked higher in eastern Europe than in other parts of Europe [2]. Human cysticercosis is a condition that may arise when humans ingest eggs of *T. solium*. When the parasite migrates to the central nervous system, the neurological condition is referred to as neurocysticercosis (NCC), which may lead to a number of potentially debilitating neurological manifestations including epilepsy and severe progressive headache [3]. NCC is a major global public health concern. Recently, *T. solium* was identified as the number one food-borne parasite contributing to the global burden of disease leading to approximately 28,000 deaths per year and around 2.8 million disability-adjusted life years (DALYs) [4].

Taenia saginata ranked lower in the multicriteria-based ranking, as symptoms of taeniosis are mild or even absent and generally the disease is not of substantial public health concern [1, 2]. Nevertheless, the parasite can pose major obstacles for trade and causes a substantial financial burden due to carcass condemnation, freezing and devaluation [5–8].

Taenia solium is highly endemic in pork-consuming poor communities of Asia, Africa and Latin America, while *T. saginata* is distributed worldwide. Little is known about the situation of *T. solium* in eastern Europe, and the suspicion of on-going transmission persists [9]. For *T. saginata* a recent review on the epidemiology of bovine cysticercosis revealed the presence of the parasite in a large number of countries in western Europe; however, for eastern Europe data were scarce and of poor quality [10].

In eastern Europe, various socioeconomic and political developments such as the collapse of the Soviet Union and the dissolution of the Socialict Federal Republic of Yugoslavia in 1991 following the wars, led to political and demographic changes. As a result a number of sectors, including the veterinary and public health sectors, were negatively affected. Large numbers of veterinary control officers were replaced by a cheaper working force leading to deteriorated veterinary control systems [11]. The change to small-scale farms with reduced rearing standards and biosecurity and to small abattoirs with insufficient meat inspection and reduced government and veterinary oversight possibly contributed to an increased prevalence of zoonotic parasites such as *T. solium*, *T. saginata*, *Trichinella* spp. and *Toxoplasma gondii* [11]. Backyard slaughtering without meat inspection has also become popular, possibly leading to the perpetuation of zoonotic diseases in parts of the region [12].

Meat inspection is obligatory at slaughterhouses in the European Union (EU), according to European Regulation 854/2004 [13]. Eastern Europe consists of "old" and "new" EU Members States as well as states which are still in the pre-accession phase as candidate EU countries. Therefore, adaptation of the national legislation and/or development of implementing regulations which integrate the main principles and features of the EU legislation and institutional structures towards more modern approaches to achieve better surveillance are ongoing [11, 14].

In the past decade, the number of diagnosed autochthonous NCC cases was increasing in eastern Europe [15–17], leading to the suspicion of on-going *T. solium* transmission occurring in the area; however, according to experts the numbers have gone down in the last few years.

Changes in eating habits might further contribute to the current transmission patterns of the parasite, while imported *T. solium* tapeworm carriers and increased migration and travels further contribute to the risk [18]. More recently, increasingly, European integration and introduction of regulatory legislation have influenced the region and, e.g. made it mandatory to have modern sanitation [11].

Both *T. solium* and *T. saginata* have been considered endemic in eastern Europe. Results reported from the region in the past should however be evaluated critically for their representativeness and for the laboratory procedures applied [14]. In the World Health Organization *T. solium* endemicity map, updated in 2015, uncertainty on the epidemiological situation in eastern Europe persists [19].

In order to advance our knowledge on the occurrence of these zoonotic parasites and assess the potential needs for surveillance, we performed a systematic review on the epidemiology of taeniosis/cysticercosis in eastern Europe. This review is part of a series of two systematic reviews: the first one covered western Europe [10] and the current one covers eastern Europe.

Methods

We conducted a systematic review following the Preferred Reporting Items for Systematic Reviews and Meta-Analyses (PRISMA) guidelines [20] (Additional file 1). To search for information on the epidemiology of *T. saginata* and *T. solium* in eastern Europe we used international databases and local, unpublished sources. Epidemiology was defined as the occurrence, prevalence, incidence and geographical distribution of human/porcine/bovine cysticercosis and taeniosis. Eastern Europe was defined based on regional proximity and on gross domestic product/gross national income and included 22 countries: Albania, Belarus, Bosnia and Herzegovina, Bulgaria, Croatia, Cyprus, Czech Republic, Estonia, Former Yugoslav Republic of Macedonia, Greece, Hungary, Kosovo, Latvia, Lithuania, Malta, Moldova, Montenegro, Poland, Romania, Serbia, Slovakia and Ukraine [10].

International databases

The online international bibliographical databases PubMed, ISI Web of Knowledge, CABDirect, OAIster, and OpenGrey were searched for all published data on taeniosis and (neuro)cysticercosis using the following search phrase: (cysticerc* OR cisticerc* OR neurocysticerc* OR neurocisticerc* OR "C. bovis" OR "C. cellulosae" OR taenia* OR tenia* OR saginata OR solium OR taeniosis OR teniosis OR ténia OR taeniid OR cysticerque) AND (Albania OR Belarus OR Bosnia OR Herzegovina OR Bulgaria OR Croatia OR Cyprus OR Czech Republic OR Estonia OR Former Yugoslav Republic of Macedonia OR Greece OR Hungary OR Kosovo OR Latvia OR Lithuania OR Malta OR Moldova OR Montenegro OR Poland OR Romania OR Serbia OR Slovakia OR Ukraine). The databases were searched for papers published from January 1st 1990 up to January 31st 2017. No language restriction was applied.

Papers were excluded when fulfilling one or more of the following criteria: (i) studies concerning a different parasite than *T. saginata* and/or *T. solium*; (ii) studies reporting data from outside the specified countries; (iii) studies reporting results out of the scope of the review questions; (iv) duplicates. Papers were first screened for eligibility based upon title and abstract, and in the case of doubt, the full paper was assessed. For each eligible document, a narrative synthesis was made, which were then further digested into a qualitative review.

Local sources

To identify additional, locally published and unpublished data sources, we distributed country sheets (Additional file 2) to members of the European Network on Taeniosis/Cysticercosis (CYSTINET) COST Action TD1302 and other non-member experts, asking to specify relevant national journals or epidemiological bulletins, MSc/PhD dissertations, national Institutes, or registries, and to translate relevant search terms. Due to ethical constraints, unpublished hospital or laboratory data were only presented at an aggregated level. In addition, we searched for information in the proceedings of the CYSTINET (European Network for taeniosis/cysticercosis, COST Action TD1302) and European Network for Foodborne Parasites (COST Action FA1408, Euro-FBP) meetings. Finally, we explored the reference lists of recent topic-specific reviews [15–17] to find additional eligible papers. We applied the same inclusion and exclusion criteria to these additional sources and developed narrative syntheses for all eligible documents.

Data collection and analyses

The data collection was performed by three independent reviewers (CT, BD and SS). For data analysis, we followed the methodology described in [10]. Briefly, cases reported as case reports providing information on individual characteristics of the patient were defined as individual cases and when no individual information was given, these cases were defined as aggregated. Tables summarizing individual cases included year of diagnosis, age, gender, nationality, and reported risk factors, while for aggregated cases or prevalence, the tables included country, level of data collection, timeframe, number of cases (or prevalence or incidence), *Taenia* species, risk factors (e.g. immigration/travel history) if available, and reference (i.e. authors and publication year).

The following definitions were applied for the description of risk factors: endemic region (Asia, Africa and South and Central America, including Caribbean islands); immigrant from endemic region (any person born in or native from endemic region, or reported to have moved from endemic region); travelled/stayed in endemic region (having travelled, stayed, or resided in endemic region); no history of travels to endemic areas or immigration (autochthonous) (no history of travel/immigration reported).

Cases in which the existence of duplicates was probable (e.g. cases included in two retrospective studies on the same area/hospital, covering overlapping time periods, cases diagnosed in the same hospital in the same time-frame but reported in different sources etc.) were included only once, by selecting the one that was published first.

Descriptive analyses and maps were performed using the software environment for statistical computing R 3.5.0 and graphs were made in both R and Microsoft Excel [21].

Results

Search results

The initial search resulted in 1179 peer reviewed papers identified though international databases. After the screening process, 69 relevant references were identified and included in the review (Additional file 3: Table S1). In addition to this, researchers of 18 out of 22 eastern European countries were contacted from which additional data (92 relevant sources) from local and unpublished sources were obtained (Additional file 4: Table S2). Contacts of researchers working within the field from Belarus, Kosovo, Malta and Ukraine were not available; hence local, unpublished data for these countries are missing. The flow diagram of the search strategy steps is presented in Fig. 1. The countries for which data on *T. solium* or *T. saginata* in humans and/or animals were found are presented in Fig. 2.

Taeniosis

In total, 58 unique sources were identified providing information on taeniosis in eastern Europe. Individual (8 records) and/or aggregated cases/prevalence (50 records) of taeniosis were reported in 14 out of 22 eastern European countries (Fig. 2).

No cases of taeniosis were reported in Cyprus, and for 7 countries (Belarus, Bosnia and Herzegovina, Kosovo, Malta, Moldova, Montenegro and Ukraine), no reports on taeniosis could be retrieved for the years between 1990 and 2017. Poland was the country recording most data on taeniosis.

Taeniosis case reports

In total only 17 individual cases reported in case reports from Croatia, Greece, Lithuania and Serbia, were available (Additional file 5: Table S3). Out of the 17 cases, 13 were reported as *Taenia* spp., three reported as confirmed and one suspected *T. saginata* using microscopy.

No case reports describing *T. solium* taeniosis cases were identified through the search of published and other unpublished grey literature. Moreover none of all the case reports reported possible risk factors or how the parasite infection was acquired.

Aggregated taeniosis cases

Data on aggregated taeniosis cases were obtained from scientific publications, authorities' reports, national registries, epidemiological bulletins, and from hospitals/laboratories (Additional file 5: Table S4). Aggregated taeniosis cases were reported in 14 eastern European countries and covered different years. Data were obtained from publications ranging from the 1990 up to 2017 (Fig. 3). The largest proportion of cases was reported as *Taenia* spp. and at species level the majority of cases were reported as *T. saginata*. *Taenia solium* taeniosis cases were a rare finding, reported only in Albania, Estonia, Latvia and Poland. No indication was given on how species identification was performed. For Latvia, the two suspected cases probably originated from abroad (probably Russia) (Deksne, personal communication, 2016). No additional information on the source of infection, potential risk factors or nationality was given for the other reported cases.

The annual number of cases reported for each country varied, with Poland and Romania reporting the highest

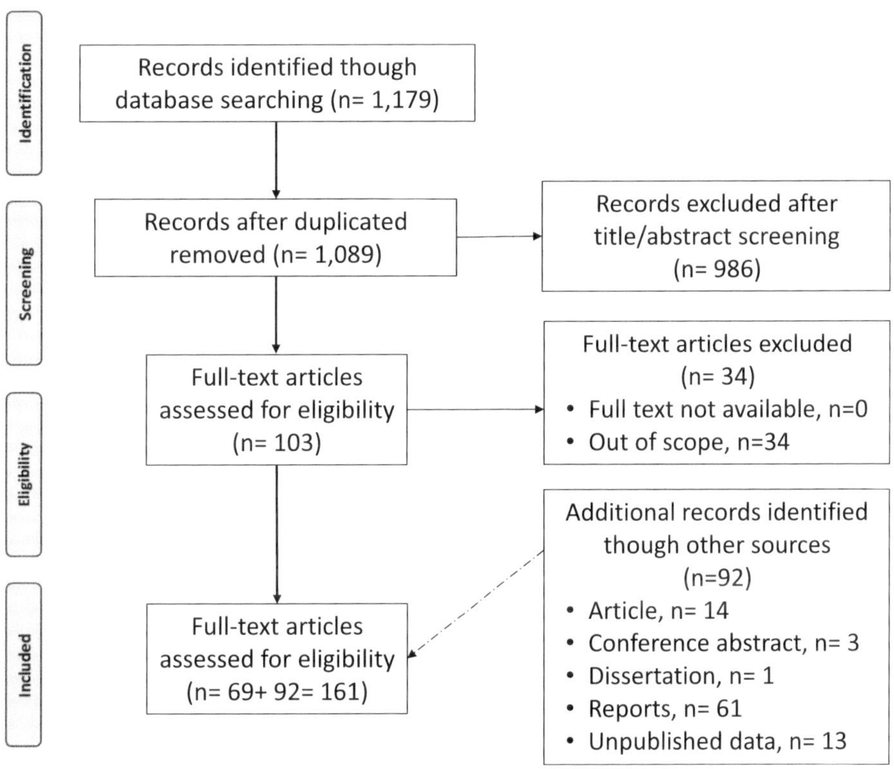

Fig. 1 Flow diagram of the search strategy steps

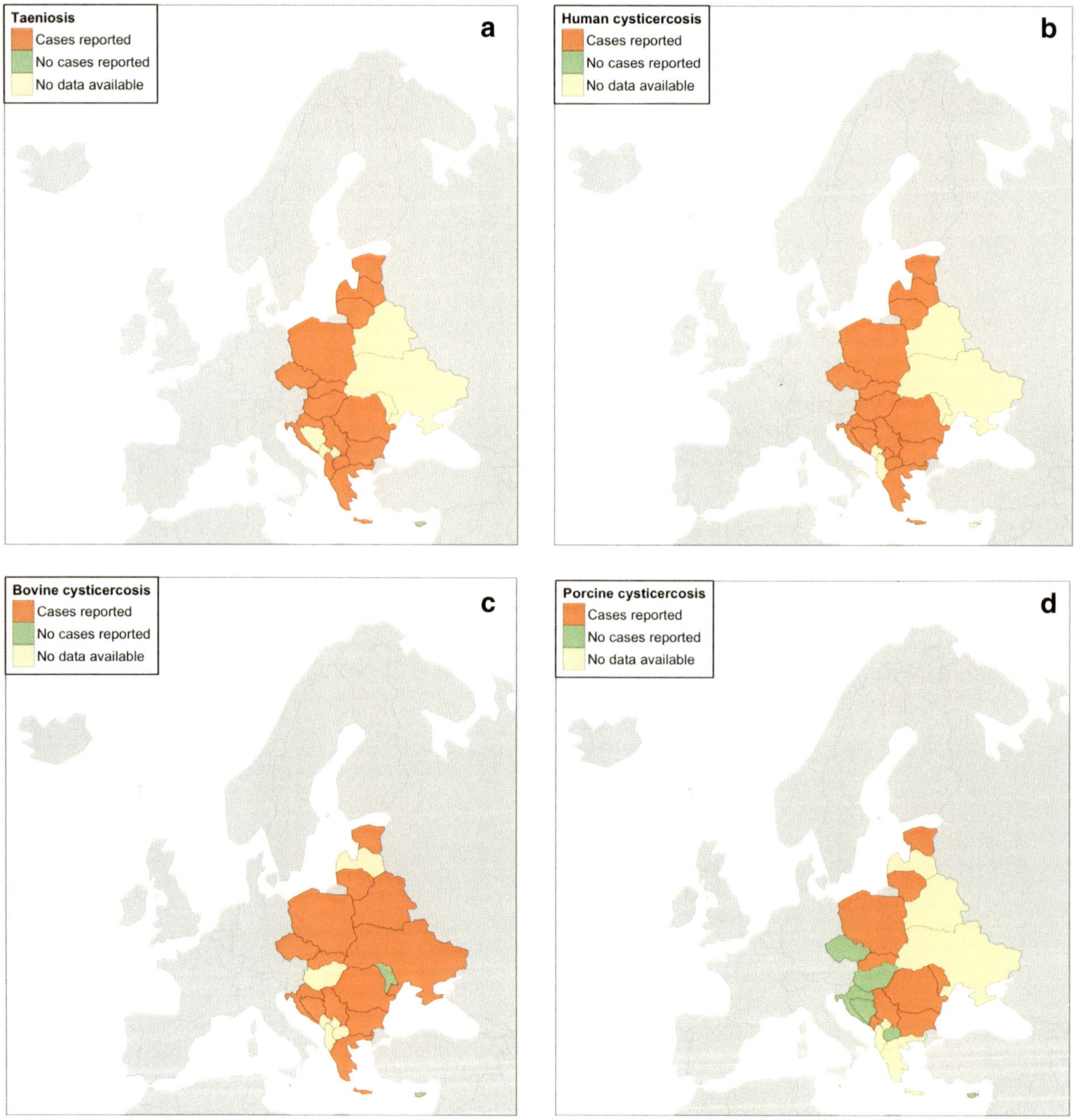

Fig. 2 Summary of identified data on taeniosis and cysticercosis (in humans and animals) in eastern Europe (1990–2017): taeniosis (**a**); human cysticercosis (**b**); bovine cysticercosis (**c**); and porcine cysticercosis (**d**)

annual number of aggregated cases. In particular for Poland, a large number of data was available as epidemiological reviews published quarterly in the journal of the National Institute of Public Health - National Institute of Hygiene and the Polish Society of Epidemiology and Infectious Diseases.

Taeniosis incidence data

Incidence data were available for seven counties (Bulgaria, Estonia, Lithuania, Poland, Romania, Serbia and Slovakia) and ranged from 0/100,000 people for Bulgaria in the year 2000 to 8.5/100,000 people in Poland in 1991 (Fig. 4).

Taeniosis prevalence data

In total, five epidemiological studies reporting taeniosis prevalence data published between 1990–2017 were identified (Additional file 5: Table S5). Within eastern Europe the prevalence of taeniosis ranged between 0–4.9%, with the highest prevalence reported in a study conducted in

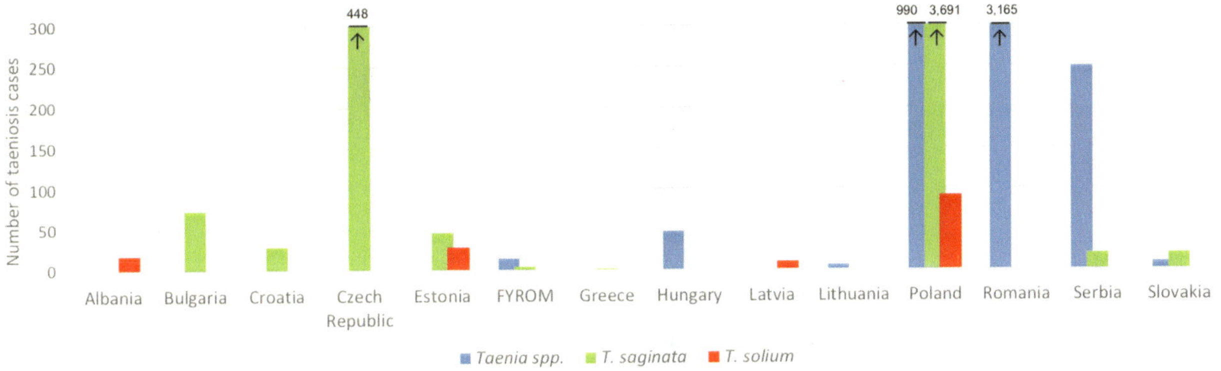

Fig. 3 Taeniosis cases reported in scientific publications, authority reports, epidemiologial bulletins, and laboratories in eastern Europe (published/reported between 1990–2017). Arrow pointing at the number, larger than 300 taeniosis cases. *Abbreviation*: FYROM, Former Yugoslav Republic of Macedonia

children of the Roma settlements of Košice and Prešov regions in Slovakia [22]. A study carried out in Estonia reported a seroprevalence of *T. solium* of 0.7% (95% confidence interval, CI: 0.3–1.4%) using a commercial NovaLisa IgG enzyme immunoassay ELISA [NovaTec Immunodiagnostica GmbH, Dietzenbach, Germany (Sp > 95%, Se 94%)], and 0.0% (95% CI: 0–0.3%) using the ELISA and a Western Blot IgG (LDBIO DIAGNOSTICS, Lyon, France) in series [23], while the other four studies used microscopy as a diagnostic tool.

Human cysticercosis

Relevant information on human cysticercosis was obtained from 63 sources. In total, 40 reports reported individual, and 23 reports reported aggregated cysticercosis cases. Information on human cysticercosis cases was available for 15 out of 22 eastern European countries (Fig. 2), while no data could be retrieved from Albania, Belarus, Cyprus, Malta, Moldova, Montenegro and Ukraine in the form of either published or unpublished sources.

Human cysticercosis case reports

In total, 58 individual cases of cysticercosis were identified in authorities' reports, from hospital/laboratories or published case reports (Table 1). Out of 58 cases, 45 were diagnosed in 7 eastern European countries, while 13 cases (22%) were originally from eastern Europe but were diagnosed abroad. The average age was 49 years and 49% of the cases were male, 42% female and for 9% the sex was not known (Additional file 5: Table S6). Of all the individual case reports, 17% were reportedly suspected to be autochthonous cases, in 14% the infection was considered aquired in endemic countries while travelling or living abroad, whereas for the majority of cases

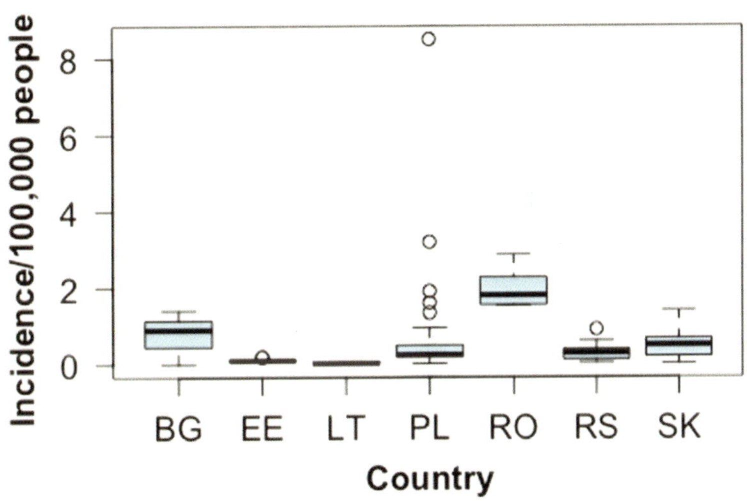

Fig. 4 Taeniosis incidence data reported between the years 1990–2017 in authorities' reports, epidemiological bulletins and national registries in eastern Europe. *Abbreviations*: BG, Bulgaria (1998 and 2000); EE, Estonia (1990–1999); PL, Poland (1991–2009); RO, Romania (2007–2014); RS, Serbia (1997–2005); SK, Slovakia (1990–2014)

Table 1 Number of human cysticercosis cases per country and most likely place of infection (Data from published and unpublished sources between 1990 and 2017)

Country	Most likely place of infection			Total no. of cases
	Eastern Europe	Endemic country	Unknown	
Croatia			10	10
Czech Republic	6	4		10
Greece	3	3	6	12
Hungary			2	2
Latvia		1	1	2
Lithuania			5	5
Serbia	1		5	6
Cyprus			1	1
Czechoslovakia			2	2
Former Yugoslav Republic of Macedonia			3	3
Bosnia and Herzegovina			5	5

(69%) the place of infection was unknown or not recorded. For Lithuania, the cases were possibly connected with travels to Argentina and South Africa (S. Petkevičius, personal communication, 2015).

Aggregated human cysticercosis cases

The number of aggregated human cysticercosis cases varied largely across countries, with over 300 cases (most of them reported as autochthonous) reported from Romania. Figure 5 shows the number of human cysticercosis cases identified in eastern Europe in documents published from 1990 to 2017. Information on risk factors and place where the disease might have been acquired were absent for most cases (Additional file 5: Table S7).

Only two serological studies using ELISA and/or western blot techniques were identified. One of the studies was in Croatia, where a prevalence of 1.5% was recorded among people with epilepsy [24]. The other study was in Estonia, where a western-blot-confirmed *T. solium* cysticercosis prevalence (commercial ELISA and commercial western blot in series) was of 0.0% in samples from the general Estonian population, children, veterinarians and hunters [23].

Porcine cysticercosis

Relevant information on porcine cysticercosis was obtained from 53 sources, which reported the occurrence of the infection in 8 countries. In Poland the causative agent was specified as being *"cysticercus cellulosae"* (name used for *T. solium* cysticercus) in two publications (Additional file 5: Table S8). The highest number of porcine cysticercosis cases (4487 cases) was recorded in Poland in 2003; however, in the report species were not specified and porcine cysticercosis could refer to

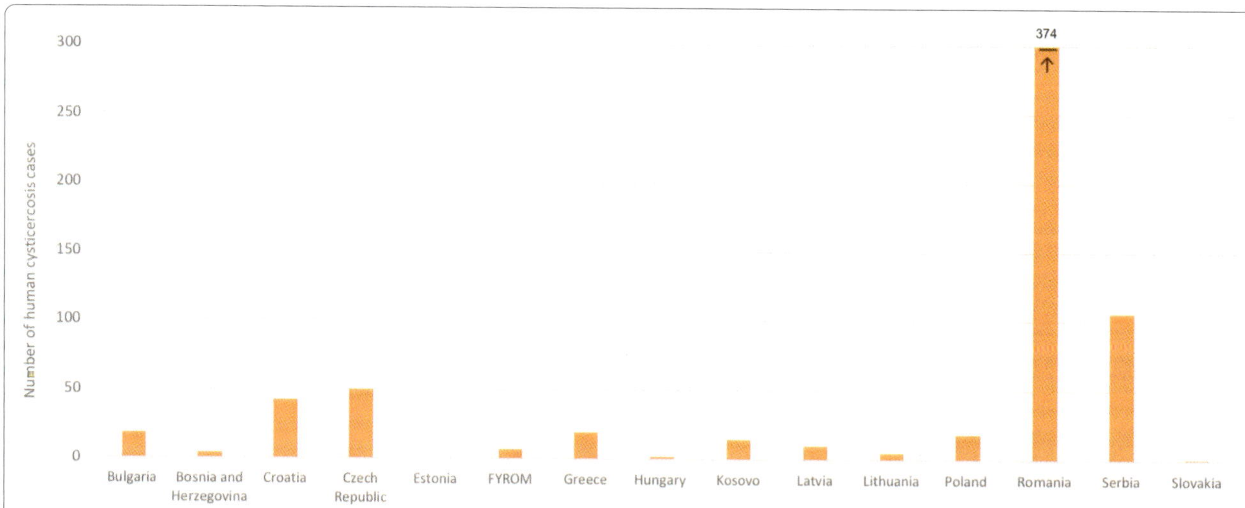

Fig. 5 Number of identified human cysticercosis cases in eastern Europe - data sources published and unpublished between 1990–2017. Arrow pointing at the number, larger than 300 human cycsticercosis cases. *Abbreviation*: FYROM, Former Yugoslav Republic of Macedonia

"*cysticercus cellulosae*" or cysticerci of other species like "*cysticercus tenuicollis*" (name used for *Taenia hydatigena* cysticercus). Of the porcine cysticercosis cases reported, a molecular method was reportedly used only in Estonia, and *T. solium* could not be confirmed [25]. No cases of porcine cysticercosis in pigs were reported from Bosnia and Herzegovina, Croatia, Cyprus, Czech Republic, Former Yugoslav Republic of Macedonia and Hungary, and no information was found for Albania, Belarus, Greece, Kosovo, Malta and Ukraine. Based on routine meat inspection, reported prevalence ranged from 0% to 0.18% in Bulgaria [9] and varied within and between countries. A single serological study was identified: in Romania, an ELISA-based prevalence of active porcine cysticercosis was reported to be 6.4% [26].

In Latvia, according to the Food and Veterinary Service, the main slaughtering monitoring authority, in the last 10 years no suspicious cysts have been found in pigs (Food and Veterinary Service Latvia, personal communication, 2015).

Bovine cysticercosis

Relevant information on bovine cysticercosis was obtained from 41 sources reporting data for 15 out of 22 countries (Additional file 5: Table S9). Only for Cyprus, no cases were recorded since 1990. For Albania, Hungary, Kosovo, Latvia, Malta and Montenegro, no data were retrieved. Based on routine meat inspection, reported prevalence ranged from 0.0% up to 1.7% and varied within and between countries (Fig. 6). No studies were found applying more sensitive methods to detect bovine cysticercosis. For Poland in particular, a large amount of data were available, in which the highest annual number of bovine cysticercosis cases (4718 cases) in the country was reported in 1994. The number of reported cases has decreased consistently over the years.

Discussion

Published and unpublished data sources were searched, and contacts with researchers of eastern European countries were established to obtain all possible information on the epidemiology of *T. solium* and *T. saginata* in eastern Europe.

Individual case reports for taeniosis were only retrieved from four countries, while reports on aggregated cases were available for nearly all the eastern European countries. At a species level, most data were reported as *Taenia* spp. or *T. saginata*, leading to uncertainty regarding the true disease epidemiology. In a few countries, *T. solium* was reported as aggregated taeniosis cases. Given the risk of having *T. solium* carriers it is essential to improve on differential diagnosis and reporting. A similar scenario was also observed in western Europe, suggesting that diagnosis and case management is not performed adequately [10]. Moreover, the laboratory procedures and the reporting seem unstandardized and often only a small part of the population is examined; therefore, the data from most countries are incomplete [14]. Hence, the reported prevalence of human

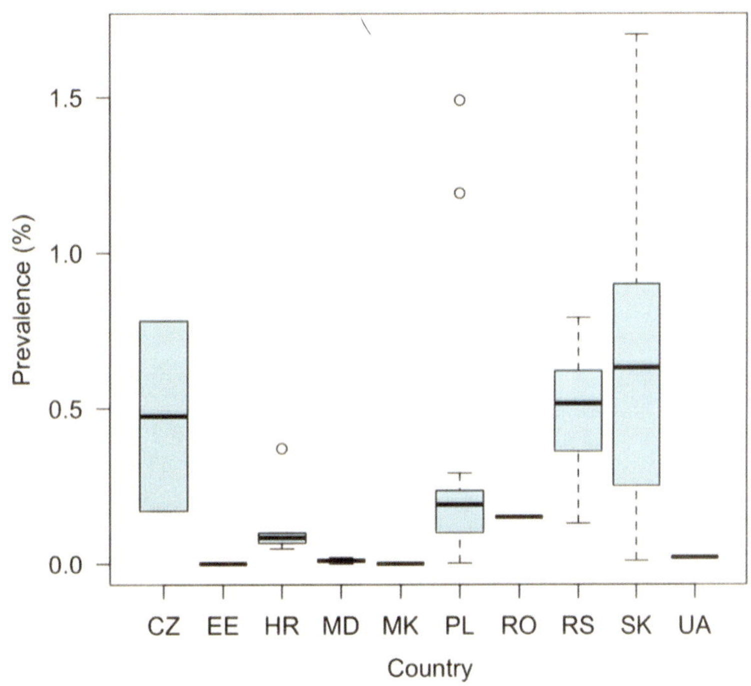

Fig. 6 Prevalence of bovine cysticercosis based on routine meat inspection detected in eastern Europe (1990–2017). *Abbreviations*: CZ, Czech Republic; EE, Estonia; HR, Croatia; MD, Moldova; MK, Former Yugoslav Republic of Macedonia; PL, Poland; RO, Romania; RS, Serbia; SK, Slovakia; UA, Ukraine

taeniosis from *T. saginata* and *T. solium* should be evaluated critically. Also, the origin of infection and risk factors were not reported, leading to continued uncertainty on the real endemic status of eastern Europe.

Human cysticercosis reports of individual and aggregated cases were available from nearly one third of the 22 eastern European countries, while for western Europe, information was available from all 18 countries [10]. Romania and Serbia reported the largest number of diagnosed human cysticercosis cases, highlighting both the reporting and possibly also the epidemiological differences among eastern European countries. Observing the difference in reported cases at a hospital level between countries, either an underestimation or an overestimation might be suspected for eastern Europe. However, several factors such as lack of knowledge, diagnostic capacity and compensation for the farmers, unwillingness or inability to report and logistic difficulties may contribute to the vicious cycle of underreporting and underdiagnosis [27, 28]. Of all cases, 14% were suspected to have travelled abroad, 17% to be autochthonous cases, while for the majority (69%) it was not specified. This lack of additional information does not allow us to unravel the question of an existing parasite transmission in eastern Europe. The results show that even if the assumption that the infection can be acquired abroad would be correct, then the same happens in Europe as frequently. The automatic assumption that brief visits abroad automatically outrule looking for answers locally, can lead to a barrier for dealing with the actual epidemiological situation.

Nearly one quarter of the cases were diagnosed abroad, possibly indicating that either the local health system is not equipped to detect these cases, or that people are actively seeking medical attention elsewhere.

For two thirds of the human cases the origin of infection was not given, further contributing to the persisting knowledge and underreporting gap. However, it should be noted that a lowering trend is registered. For instance in Serbia, no new cases were recorded after 2010.

Cases of porcine cysticercosis were reported in a number of countries, and as for the human cases, the number of cases and reports per country varied significantly. Notably, in Poland over 4000 cases of porcine cysticercosis were recorded by the veterinary inspection services in 2003; however, no information on the *Taenia* spp. involved was given and the possibility of (some of) the cases being *T. hydatigena* cannot be excluded. Also, for most other porcine cysticercosis cases reported in eastern Europe, species identification was never performed, nor molecularly confirmed. Only in one study from Estonia, molecular techniques were applied to confirm a false positive case [25]. Lack of differential diagnosis highlights the presence of poor meat inspection, due to the possible lack of: qualified meat inspectors, sensitive and specific diagnostic tools, awareness, funding and adequate mandatory reporting systems. Moreover the trend towards smaller-scale pig farming, with outdoor access and home slaughtering (without meat inspection) increases the risk of infection and therefore the need for monitoring.

Bovine cysticercosis was reported in over two thirds of the countries in the region. The highest number of cases was reported in Poland, where 4718 bovine cysticercosis cases were recorded in 1994. General meat inspection has a very low sensitivity, hence slaughterhouse figures, even when well-recorded will always underestimate the prevalence [29]. False positives, e.g. eosinophilic myositis as a consequence of sarcocystis infection or abscessess, can also occur although they usually contribute only a small (negligible) proportion of bovine cysticercosis records.

Better, cost-effective and more sensitive diagnostic tools should be developed, and data recording systems should be improved to assure that data from individual slaughterhouses are centralised. Increased availability of data will further allow estimating the overall economic impact of *T. saginata* which has been shown to be significant in Belgium (858 €/heavily infected carcass and 586 €/lightly infected carcass) [7], but less so in Catalonia [northeastern Spain (1140 €/heavily infected carcass and 509 €/lightly infected carcass)] [8]. Without reliable data from the surveillance the default assumption should be that the parasite is present, not absent. To overcome case uncertainty and to be able to have more accurate data that will improve our knowledge on the epidemiological situation of *T. saginata* and *T. solium*, the possibility to molecularly confirm *T. solium* findings should be available. Recently, the laboratories across Europe that are running tests for the larval and adult stages of the parasites have been summarised and mapped, facilitating the process when suspected lesions are detected [27].

The early species-level identification of the tapeworm and subsequent adapted management are crucial to avoid not only human-to-human transmission, but also human-to-pig/cattle transmission.

Finally, for nearly all the countries, at least some data and research on the topic could be retrieved and both published and unpublished data sources were available. Particularly the unpublished sources were of added value and contributed to an improved picture of the epidemiological situation in eastern Europe, highlighting the importance of data access and collaborations through networks such as CYSTINET. Nevertheless, for Belarus, Kosovo, Malta and Ukraine a contact could not be established and no information could be retrieved leaving information gaps. In the absence of data the presence of *T. saginata* and *T. solium* in these countries cannot be excluded. For western Europe information and a contact was established with all counties of the region, and the amount of published and unpublished literature was more than double that of eastern Europe, which helped to provide a better and more complete overview of the epidemiological situation [10]. The two zoonotic parasites would merit more attention and research in eastern Europe.

Conclusions

There is indication that taeniosis and cysticercosis are present across eastern Europe but information on the occurrence of *T. solium* and *T. saginata* across the region remains fragmented. For a number of countries, no information was available and for some, establishing a contact with experts within the field proved challenging. Species identification is not performed in most countries and the findings are not confirmed using molecular methods (especially for taeniosis and porcine cysticercosis), making the endemicity status in the region still unclear. Attention should be paid to: (i) suspected autochthonous human cysticercosis cases to rule out ongoing transmission; (ii) notification of taeniosis and human cysticercosis as these should be implemented to get better data and a clearer overview of the epidemiological situation; (iii) surveillance and reporting systems in animals; and (iv) methods for confirming findings.

Additional files

Additional file 1: PRISMA checklist. (PDF 68 kb)

Additional file 2: Country sheets template. (PDF 81 kb)

Additional file 3: Table S1. List of references included in the review retrieved through online international databases. (XLSX 24 kb)

Additional file 4: Table S2. List of references included in the review made available through local sources. (XLSX 71 kb)

Additional file 5: Table S3. Individual taeniosis cases identified in case reports in eastern Europe available from 1990 to 2017. **Table S4.** Aggregated taeniosis cases reported in documents (authorities' reports, epidemiological bulletins, national registries and publications) identified in eastern Europe available from 1990 to 2017. **Table S5.** Taeniosis prevalence data reported in epidemiological studies published between 1990–2017. **Table S6.** Individual human cysticercosis cases identified in case reports in eastern Europe (1990–2017). **Table S7.** Aggregated human cysticercosis cases identified in case reports and publications in eastern Europe (1990–2017). **Table S8.** Porcine cysticercosis cases identified and reported during meat inspection in case reports and publications in eastern Europe (1990–2017). **Table S9.** Bovine cysticercosis cases identified and reported during meat inspection in case reports and publications in eastern Europe (1990–2017). (DOCX 207 kb)

Abbreviations

CYSTINET: European Network on Taeniosis/Cysticercosis; EFSA: European Food Safety Authority; GDP/GNI: gross domestic product/gross national income; ICD: International Classification of Diseases; NCC: neurocysticercosis; OIE: World Organization for Animal Health/Office International des Epizooties

Acknowledgments

This work is a collaboration within the framework of CYSTINET, the European network on taeniasis/cysticercosis, COST ACTION TD1302. We acknowledge Dr G. Petrusevska and Dr I. Kuzmanovski, for the unpublished data about NCC in Former Yugoslav Republic of Macedonia, and Prim. Dr E. Miloskoska Blagoeska and Dr G. Kuzmanovska, Former Yugoslav Republic of Macedonia, for their valuable input for the conduction of this work. We also acknowledge Professor Olga Dulović, Clinic for Infectious and Tropical Diseases, Clinical Center of Serbia, Belgrade, Serbia, and School of Medicine, University of Belgrade, Belgrade, Serbia, for the assistance in providing medical records for Serbia.

Funding

This work is a collaboration within the framework of CYSTINET, the European network on taeniasis/cysticercosis, COST ACTION TD1302.

Authors' contributions

CT, BD and SS conducted the systematic review of the literature and extracted data. CT and BD analysed data and drafted the first version of the manuscript. AA, BD, CT, MLG, SS and VD contributed to the design of the study, interpretation of data and writing of the first draft. The remain co-authors (ZW, AK, AC, ASW, AA, BB, BL, CMC, CV, DA, GD, IB, IK, JK, JS, BK, MJP, MV, MP, MS, MK, OD, PJ, DSJ, VS, ZD, SG and PD) contributed to data collection and writing of the paper. All authors read and approved the final manuscript.

Competing interests

The authors declare that they have no competing interests.

Author details

[1]Department of Biomedical Sciences, Institute of Tropical Medicine, Nationalestraat 155, 2000 Antwerp, Belgium. [2]Department of Veterinary and Animal Sciences, Faculty of Health and Medical Sciences, University of Copenhagen, Dyrlægevej, 100 Frederiksberg, Denmark. [3]Veterinary Research Institute, HAO-DEMETER, Campus Thermi, 57001 Thessaloniki, Greece. [4]IRTA, Centre de Recerca en Sanitat Animal (CReSA, IRTA-UAB), Campus de la Universitat Autònoma de Barcelona, 08193 Bellaterra, Spain. [5]University of Florida College of Medicine, Gainesville, Florida, USA. [6]Veterinary and Food laboratory, Kreutzwaldi 30, 51006 Tartu, Estonia. [7]Institute of Veterinary Medicine and Animal Sciences, Estonian University of Life Sciences, Kreutzwaldi 1, 51006 Tartu, Estonia. [8]Department of Parasitology and Parasitic Diseases, Faculty of Veterinary Medicine, Ss. Cyril and Methodius University in Skopje, Lazar Pop Trajkov 5-7, 1000 Skopje, Former Yugoslav Republic of Macedonia. [9]Centre for Global Health, Department of Neurology, Technical University Munich, Ismaninger Strasse 22, 81675 Munich, Germany. [10]Centre for Global Health, Department of Community Medicine and Global Health, Institute of Health and Society, University of Oslo, Kirkeveien 166, 0450 Oslo, Norway. [11]Centre of Excellence for Food- and Vector-borne Zoonoses, Institute for Medical Research, University of Belgrade, Belgrade, Serbia. [12]Department of Parasitology, Carol Davila University of Medicine and Pharmacy, Colentina Clinical Hospital, Bucharest, Romania. [13]Department of Parasitology, University of Agricultural Sciences and Veterinary Medicine Cluj-Napoca, Cluj-Napoca, Romania. [14]Department of Microbiology, 424 Military General Hospital, Thessaloniki, Greece. [15]Institute of Food Safety, Health and Environment, Riga, Latvia. [16]Faculty of Biology, University of Latvia, Riga, Latvia. [17]Institute for Pathology, Medical Faculty, University "Ss. Cyril and Methodius", Skopje, Former Yugoslav Republic of Macedonia. [18]Department of Parasitology, National Institute for Public Health, Budapest, Hungary. [19]Department of Parasitology and Invasive Diseases, National Veterinary Research Institute in Pulawy, Pulawy, Poland. [20]Department of Pathology and Parasitology, Faculty of Veterinary Medicine, University of Veterinary and Pharmaceutical Sciences Brno, Palackého tř. 1946/1, 61242 Brno, Czech Republic. [21]Central European Institute of Technology, University

of Veterinary and Pharmaceutical Sciences Brno, Palackého tř. 1946/1, 61242 Brno, Czech Republic. [22]Institute for Microbiology and Parasitology, Medical faculty, University "Ss. Cyril and Methodius", Skopje, Former Yugoslav Republic of Macedonia. [23]Institute of Parasitology, Slovak Academy of Sciences, Košice, Slovakia. [24]Department of Veterinary Economics and Epidemiology, Faculty of Veterinary Medicine, University of Zagreb, Zagreb, Croatia. [25]Lithuanian University of Health Sciences, Kaunas, Lithuania. [26]Department of Neurology, Klinikum rechts der Isar, Technical University Munich, Ismaninger Straße 22, 81675 Munich, Germany. [27]Laboratory of Parasitology, Department of Bacteria, Parasites and Fungi, Infectious Disease Preparedness, Statens Serum Institute, Copenhagen, Denmark. [28]Faculty of Veterinary Medicine, University of Helsinki, Helsinki, Finland. [29]Department of Parasitology and Parasitic Diseases with Clinic, Faculty of Veterinary Medicine, University of Zagreb, Zagreb, Croatia. [30]Parasitological Laboratory, Department of Microbiology, Clinical Center of Serbia, Belgrade, Serbia. [31]Department of Veterinary Public Health and Food Safety, Faculty of Veterinary Medicine, Ghent University, Salisburylaan 133, 9820 Merelbeke, Belgium. [32]Laboratory of Parasitology, Faculty of Veterinary Medicine, Ghent University, Salisburylaan 133, B-9820 Merelbeke, Belgium. [33]Department of Epidemiology and Public Health, Sciensano, Brussels, Belgium.

References

1. FAO/WHO. Multicriteria-based ranking for risk management of food-borne parasites. Microbiologial Risk Assessment Series No. 23. Rome: FAO/WHO; 2014.
2. Bouwknegt M, Devleesschauwer B, Graham H, Robertson LJ, van der Giessen JWB, Akkari H, et al. Prioritisation of food-borne parasites in Europe, 2016. Euro Surveil. 2018;23:17–00161.
3. García HH, Gonzalez AE, Evans CAW, Gilman RH. *Taenia solium* cysticercosis. Lancet. 2003;362:547–56.
4. Torgerson PR, Devleesschauwer B, Praet N, Speybroeck N, Willingham AL, Kasuga F, et al. World Health Organization estimates of the global and regional disease burden of 11 foodborne parasitic diseases, 2010: a data synthesis. PLoS Med. 2015;12:e1001920.
5. Torgerson PR. One world health: socioeconomic burden and parasitic disease control priorities. Vet Parasitol. 2013;195:223–32.
6. Blagojevic B, Robertson LJ, Vieira-Pinto M, Johansen MV, Laranjo-González M, Gabriël S. Bovine cysticercosis in the European Union: impact and current regulations, and an approach towards risk-based control. Food Control. 2017;78:64–71.
7. Jansen F, Dorny P, Trevisan C, Dermauw V, Laranjo-González M, Allepuz A, et al. Economic impact of bovine cysticercosis and taeniosis caused by *Taenia saginata* in Belgium. Parasit Vectors. 2018;11:241.
8. Laranjo-Gonzalez M, Devleesschauwer B, Jansen F, Dorny P, Dupuy C, Requena-Mendez A, et al. Epidemiology and economic impact of bovine cysticercosis and taeniosis caused by *Taenia saginata* in northeastern Spain (Catalonia). Parasit Vectors. 2018;11:376.
9. Devleesschauwer B, Allepuz A, Dermauw V, Johansen MV, Laranjo-González M, Smit GSA, et al. *Taenia solium* in Europe: Still endemic? Acta Trop. 2017; 165:96–9.
10. Laranjo-González M, Devleesschauwer B, Trevisan C, Allepuz A, Sotiraki S, Abraham A, et al. Epidemiology of taeniosis/cysticercosis in Europe, a systematic review: western Europe. Parasit Vectors. 2017;10:349.
11. Djordjevic AM, Bacic M, Petricevic M, Cuperlovic K, Malakauskas A, Kapel CMO, Murrell KD. Social, political, and economic factors responsible for the reemergence of trichinellosis in Serbia: a case study. J Parasitol. 2003;89: 226–31.
12. Bružinskaite R, Šarkunas M, Torgerson PR, Mathis A, Deplazes P. Echinococcosis in pigs and intestinal infection with *Echinococcus* spp. in dogs in southwestern Lithuania. Vet Parasitol. 2009;160:237–41.
13. European-Commission. Regulation (EC) No. 854/2004 of the European Parliament and of the Council laying down specific rules for the organisation of official controls on products of animal origin intended for human consumption. Off J Eur Union. 2004; L 226/83. https://eur-lex.europa.eu/LexUriServ/LexUriServ.do?uri=OJ:L:2004:226:0083:0127:EN:PDF.
14. Cuperlovic K. Current status of food-borne parasitic zoonoses - eastern Europe. Southeast Asian J Trop Med Public Health. 1991;22:72–7.
15. Del Brutto OH. Neurocysticercosis in Western Europe: a re-emerging disease? Acta Neurol Belg. 2012;112:335–43.
16. Fabiani S, Bruschi F. Neurocysticercosis in Europe: still a public health concern not only for imported cases. Acta Trop. 2013;128:18–26.
17. Zammarchi L, Strohmeyer M, Bartalesi F, Bruno E, Muñoz J, Buonfrate D, et al. Epidemiology and management of cysticercosis and *Taenia solium* taeniasis in Europe, systematic review 1990–2011. PLoS One. 2013;8:e69537.
18. Gabriël S, Johansen MV, Pozio E, Smit GSA, Devleesschauwer B, Allepuz A, et al. Human migration and pig/pork import in the European Union: what are the implications for *Taenia solium* infections? Vet Parasitol. 2015;213:38–45.
19. Donadeu M, Lightowlers MW, Fahrion AS, Kessels J, Abela-Ridder B. *Taenia solium*: WHO endemicity map update. Relev Epidemiol Hebd. 2016;91:595–9.
20. Liberati A, Altman DG, Tetzlaff J, Mulrow C, Gøtzsche PC, Ioannidis JPA, et al. The PRISMA statement for reporting systematic reviews and meta-analyses of studies that evaluate health care interventions: explanation and elaboration. PLoS Med. 2009;6:e1000100.
21. R Core Team. A language and environment for statistical computing. Vienna: R Foundation of Statistical Computing; 2018. https://www.r-project.org/.
22. Rudohradská P, Halánová M, Ravaszová P, Goldová M, Valenčáková A, Halán M, et al. Prevalence of intestinal parasites in children from minority group with low hygienic standards in Slovakia. Helminthologia. 2012;49:63–6.
23. Lassen B, Janson M, Viltrop A, Neare K, Hütt P, Golovljova I, et al. Serological evidence of exposure to globally relevant zoonotic parasites in the Estonian population. PLoS One. 2016;11:e0164142.
24. Mestrovic T, Sviben M, Vilibic-Cavlek T, Ljubin-Sternak S, Tabain I, Mlinaric-Galinovic G. Seroprevalence of *Taenia solium* infections in Croatian patients presenting with epilepsy. J Helminthol. 2012;86:259–62.
25. Dorbek-Kolin E, Ahlberg T, Tummeleht L, Tappe D, Johansen MV, Lassen B. Prevalence of cysticercosis in Estonian pigs and cattle. Parasitol Res. 2018; 117:591–5.
26. Oleleu AM, Gherman CM, Blaga R, Györke A, Cozma V. Seroprevalence of porcine cysticercosis and influence of some associated risk factors in northwestern Romania. Acta Vet Brno. 2016;85:121–6.
27. Gomez-Morales MA, Garate T, Blocher J, Devleesschauwer B, Smit GSA, Schmidt V, et al. Present status of laboratory diagnosis of human taeniosis/ cysticercosis in Europe. Eur J Clin Microbiol Infect Dis. 2017;36:2029–40.
28. Halliday J, Daborn C, Auty H, Mtema Z, Lembo T, Bronsvoort BMD, et al. Bringing together emerging and endemic zoonoses surveillance: shared challenges and a common solution. Philos Trans R Soc Lond B Biol Sci. 2012;367:2872–80.
29. Jansen F, Dorny P, Berkvens D, Van Hul A, Van den Broeck N, Makay C, et al. High prevalence of bovine cysticercosis found during evaluation of different post-mortem detection techniques in Belgian slaughterhouses. Vet Parasitol. 2017;244:1–6.

10

Molecular basis of permethrin and DDT resistance in an *Anopheles funestus* population from Benin

Genevieve Tchigossou[1,2*†], Rousseau Djouaka[1†], Romaric Akoton[1,2], Jacob M Riveron[3,5], Helen Irving[3], Seun Atoyebi[4], Kabirou Moutairou[2], Akadiri Yessoufou[2] and Charles S Wondji[3,5]

Abstract

Background: Insecticide resistance in *Anopheles* mosquitoes is threatening the success of malaria control programmes. In order to implement suitable insecticide resistance management strategies, it is necessary to understand the underlying mechanisms involved. To achieve this, the molecular basis of permethrin and DDT resistance in the principal malaria vector, *Anopheles funestus* from inland Benin (Kpome), was investigated.

Results: Here, using a microarray-based genome-wide transcription and qRT-PCR analysis, we showed that metabolic resistance mechanisms through over-expression of cytochrome P450 and glutathione S-transferase genes (GSTs) are a major contributor to DDT and permethrin resistance in *Anopheles funestus* from Kpome. The *GSTe2* gene was the most upregulated detoxification gene in both DDT- [fold-change (FC: 16.0)] and permethrin-resistant (FC: 18.1) mosquitoes suggesting that upregulation of this gene could contribute to DDT resistance and cross-resistance to permethrin. *CYP6P9a* and *CYP6P9b* genes that have been previously associated with pyrethroid resistance were also significantly overexpressed with FC 5.4 and 4.8, respectively, in a permethrin resistant population. Noticeably, the GSTs, *GSTd1-5* and *GSTd3*, were more upregulated in DDT-resistant than in permethrin-resistant *Anopheles funestus* suggesting these genes are more implicated in DDT resistance. The absence of the L1014F or L1014S *kdr* mutations in the voltage-gated sodium channel gene coupled with the lack of directional selection at the gene further supported that knockdown resistance plays little role in this resistance.

Conclusions: The major role played by metabolic resistance to pyrethroids in this *An. funestus* population in Benin suggests that using novel control tools combining the P450 synergist piperonyl butoxide (PBO), such as PBO-based bednets, could help manage the growing pyrethroid resistance in this malaria vector in Benin.

Keywords: *Anopheles funestus*, Insecticide resistance, Permethrin, DDT, Kpome, Resistance mechanisms

Background

There were an estimated 216 million cases of malaria worldwide in 2016 and 445,000 deaths with 80% of all malaria deaths occurring in Africa [1]. Despite extensive control efforts, over half the world's population remains at risk and the disease has a massive impact on health and economic development, particularly in Africa [2]. Four species of *Anopheles*, *An. gambiae* Giles, *An. coluzzii* Coetzee & Wilkerson, *An. arabiensis* Patton and *An. funestus* Giles, are responsible for most of the malaria transmission in this continent. The transmission role of *An. funestus* (*sensu stricto*) is further supported by observations that in many regions of Africa, its infection rate even surpasses that of *An. gambiae* [3]. Long-lasting insecticidal nets (LLINs) and indoor residual spraying (IRS) are the main malaria prevention interventions [4]. However, the success of these control methods is jeopardised by the development of resistance by *Anopheles* species to insecticides such as pyrethroids and DDT as seen in the past with loss of efficacy of dieldrin for IRS in west/central Africa [5, 6]. In Benin, due

* Correspondence: tchigossougenevieve@yahoo.fr
†Genevieve Tchigossou and Rousseau Djouaka contributed equally to this work.
[1]International Institute of Tropical Agriculture, Cotonou 08 BP 0932, Benin
[2]University of Abomey Calavi, BP 526 Cotonou, Benin
Full list of author information is available at the end of the article

to vector resistance to pyrethroids across the country [7–10], two insecticides of two different classes were used in rotation for IRS: bendiocarb (a carbamate) and pirimiphos-methyl (an organophosphate) [11]. However, DDT is still retained for use in IRS, due to the limited number of cost-effective alternatives [12]. Field studies on insecticide susceptibility carried out as baseline surveys for malaria control programs showed *An. funestus* to be resistant to various insecticides at various localities [9, 10, 13]. Metabolic resistance is the main resistance mechanism recorded, and cytochrome P450 genes are playing a major role while target-site resistance like the knockdown resistance (kdr) is absent [9, 14–17]. Target site resistance was investigated in the pyrethroid/DDT-resistant population and the fifth and sixth segments of domain II in the sodium channel sequence and no polymorphism associated with resistance was identified [9, 14, 16, 18–20] although some mutations have been detected in Cameroon [21] and Uganda [22] but with no association yet established with resistance phenotype. A significant increase in mono-oxygenase activities confers resistance to pyrethroids in *An. funestus* in Mozambique and South-Africa (southern Africa) [15, 23–25], Uganda (east Africa) [16, 22, 26], western Kenya (east Africa) [18, 22], Cameroon (central Africa) [21] and in Senegal (west Africa) [19]. Characterisation of the molecular basis of resistance to pyrethroids and DDT in *An. funestus* from the coastal area of Benin [27] revealed a predominant role played by the glutathione S-transferase *GSTe2*. The enzyme encoded by this gene was highly upregulated in association with the presence of an L119F mutation in the substrate binding site conferring a high level of DDT and permethrin resistance [27]. Recently, *An. funestus* from Kpome, an inland region of Benin has also been shown to be resistant to DDT and permethrin with mortality rates of 9.1 ± 2.5% and 13.0 ± 3%, respectively [10]. However, it remains unknown if the resistant mechanism is the same as observed in Pahou, the coastal area of Benin [9] or whether different resistance mechanisms are responsible for the spread of resistance across the country. Such information is essential in designing suitable control interventions nationwide and to improve the implementation of resistance management strategies against *An. funestus*. In this study, using a genome-wide microarray-based transcription analysis, the underlying molecular mechanisms conferring DDT and permethrin resistance in Kpome were characterised revealing that both glutathione S-transferases, notably the *GSTe2*, and cytochrome P450 genes are the main drivers of resistance.

Methods

Area of study and mosquito collection

Blood-fed adult female *An. funestus* mosquitoes resting indoors were collected in houses between 06:00 and 10:00 h from the rural area of Kpome (6°23'N, 2°13'E) a southern inland region of Benin from December 2013 to February 2014. Kpome is a large agricultural setting with the intensive production of tomatoes which mainly serve a commercial purpose and insecticides, mainly pyrethroids (deltamethrin and lambda-cyalothrin), used in public health are also used to protect tomatoes against pest attacks. Mosquito collections and rearing were performed as described previously [10]. Adult female mosquitoes were collected indoor between 06:00 to 10:00 h using electric aspirators. F1 adults were generated from field-collected female mosquitoes using the forced-egg laying method [16] and were randomly mixed in cages for subsequent experiments. All females used for individual oviposition were morphologically and molecularly identified as *An. funestus* (*s.s.*) [10, 28].

Insecticide susceptibility assays

Two to five day-old F1 adult female mosquitoes pooled from different F0 mosquitoes collected from Kpome were used for this test. Twenty to twenty-five mosquitoes per tube with at least four replicates were exposed to DDT (4%) and permethrin (0.75%) for 1 h before transferring into clean holding tube with 10% sugar solution. Final mortality was scored 24 h post-exposure. Survivors and dead mosquitoes were conserved for further analysis. In this study, we used the same mosquitoes from the previously published research results [10] to further describe the molecular basis of the observed resistance in this malaria vector population. Mosquito samples generated from the previous investigation were used for genetic analysis in this work. The susceptible strain used in this study has the same age as the exposed mosquitoes.

Microarrays

A genome-wide transcription profiling was performed to detect the sets of genes differentially expressed in relation to observed resistance phenotypes in *An. funestus* populations from Kpome. The microarray hybridisation for *An. funestus* was carried out using the 8 × 60 k (60 mer) Agilent *An. funestus* chip. This Agilent microarray chip was designed using the eArray program (Agilent, Santa Clara, CA, US) (A-MEXP-2374) by adding the 15,527 expressed sequence tags (ESTs) generated from another transcriptome sequencing of *An. funestus* [29] to the previous 4 × 44 k array (A-MEXP-2245) [24]. Each array was designed using 8540 ESTs generated from *An. funestus* transcriptome 454 sequencing [30], 2850 *An. funestus* cDNAs from GenBank and a set of P450 genes from the *rp1* and *rp2* QTL BAC sequence [31, 32], and the 13,000 transcripts of the complete *An. gambiae* genome. Moreover, *An. gambiae* detoxification genes previously present on the *An. gambiae* detox chip

[33] were added to this. RNA was extracted from three batches of 10 *An. funestus* females (2–5 days-old) from the following sample sets: alive after exposure to 0.75% permethrin (Resistant permethrin: R_{perm}) and 4% DDT (Resistant DDT: R_{DDT}), un-exposed to insecticides (Control: C), and from the fully susceptible laboratory strain FANG (Susceptible: S) [a strain originating from Calueque in southern Angola in 2002 which is completely susceptible to insecticides (Hunt et al. [34]) using the Picopure RNA Isolation Kit (Arcturus, Waltham, MA, USA). The FANG colony was kept in insectary conditions (temperature of 25–28 °C with a relative humidity of 80%) at the Liverpool School of Tropical Medicine where assays were performed. RNA quantity and quality were assessed using a NanoDrop ND1000 spectrophotometer (Thermo Fisher Scientific, Waltham, MA, USA) and Bioanalyzer (Agilent, Santa Clara, CA, USA), respectively. Each RNA sample was used to generate complementary RNA (cRNA) using the Agilent Quick Amp Labeling Kit (two-colour) following the manufacturer's protocol. cRNAs from the resistant samples (R) were labelled with a cy5 dye, and cRNAs from the susceptible strain FANG (S) were labelled with the cy3 dye. cRNA quantity and quality were assessed using the NanoDrop and Bioanalyzer before labelling. Labelled cRNAs were hybridised to the arrays for 17 h at 65 °C according to the manufacturer's protocol. Five hybridisations were performed for each comparison including two dyes swap per comparison. Microarray data were analysed using Genespring GX 13.0 software purchased from Agilent (Agilent). A normalisation of the data was performed with the GeneSpring feature extraction program using the lowess normalisation approach. To identify differentially expressed genes, a cut-off of 2-fold-change (FC) and a statistical significance of $P \leq 0.05$ with Benjamini-Hochberg correction for multiple testing and Storey with bootstrapping (with a cut-off of 1.5-fold--change for the R-C comparison) were applied. A false discovery analysis was also performed using the Benjamini-Hochberg correction test for multiple testing as implemented in GeneSpring.

Quantitative reverse transcriptase PCR

A qRT-PCR was used to validate the microarrays results for seven of some upregulated detoxification genes. These genes include three cytochromes P450s (*CYP6M7, CYP6P9a, CYP9K1*), two glutathione transferases (*GSTd1-5, GSTe2*), and one aldehyde oxidase (*Ald oxi*). Also, the expression level of *CYP6P9b* previously found to be strongly associated with pyrethroid resistance [19, 31, 35] and *GSTd1-3*, a gene shown as possibly associated with pyrethroid resistance by 454 transcriptome profiling [19, 30] were analysed (Table 1). One microgram of the three biological replicates for resistant (permethrin: R_{perm} and DDT: R_{DDT}), control (C), and FANG (S) was used for cDNA synthesis using Superscript III (Invitrogen, Carlsbad, CA, USA) with oligodT20 and RNase H according to the manufacturer's instructions. Standard curves were established for each gene using serial dilution of cDNA. qRT-PCR amplification was performed using the MX 3005P (Agilent) system. The relative expression level and fold change (FC) of each target gene in resistant and control samples relative to susceptible were calculated according to the 2-ΔΔCT method incorporating the PCR efficiency [36] after normalisation with the housekeeping genes *ribosomal protein S7* (*RSP7*; AFUN007153-RA), and *actin* (*Act5C*; AFUN006819).

Investigation of the role of the knockdown resistance mutation in DDT and permethrin resistance

A fragment spanning a portion of the voltage-gated sodium channel gene (*VGSC*), including the 1014 codon (a portion of intron 19 and the entire exon 20, domain II, segment 6 of the *VGSC* gene) associated with resistance in *An. gambiae*, was amplified in eleven field-collected females of *An. funestus* from Kpome using the Exon 19F/KdrFunR2 primers (Exon 19F: 5'-TTT TTA AGC TCG CTA AAT CGT G-3'; KdrFunR2: 5'-CCG AAA TTT GAC AAA AGC AAA-3') [9, 15, 22]. The PCR products were purified using the QIAquick Purification Kit (Qiagen, Hilden, Germany) and directly sequenced. The polymorphic positions were detected through manual analysis of sequence traces using BioEdit. Sequences were aligned using ClustalW [37], and haplotype reconstruction and analysis were done using DnaSP v5.10 [38]. Kpome sequences were also compared to those previously obtained from Pahou in coastal Benin [9] and Gounougou in North Cameroon [21]. After the selection of the best model, a maximum likelihood phylogenetic tree was generated for the VGSC haplotypes in the different populations using Mega 6.06 [39]. The level of *Kst* of pairwise genetic differentiation between the populations was estimated in Dnasp v5.10, and the neighbour-Joining tree was built using Mega 6.06.

Results

Genome-wide microarray-based transcriptional profiling of permethrin resistance

A set of transcripts were differentially expressed (≥ 2-fold change, $P \leq 0.05$) between permethrin resistant (R_{perm}), susceptible (S) and control (C) mosquitoes (Fig. 1) from microarray analysis. Overall, 3669 transcripts were differentially expressed when permethrin resistant mosquitoes were compared to susceptible strains (1460 overexpressed and 2209 underexpressed), 3617 between C-S (1211 overexpressed and 2406 underexpressed) and 210 for R_{perm}-C (91 overexpressed and 119 underexpressed). Overall, a

Table 1 List of primers used for qRT-PCR

Primers	Forward	Reverse	Expected size (bp)
CYP6M7	CCAGATACTGAAAGAGAGCCTTCG	CAAGCACTGTCTTCGTACCG	102
CYP6P9a	CAGCGCGTACACCAGATTGTGTAA	TCACAATTTTTCCACCTTCAAGTAATTACCCGC	92
CYP6P9b	CAGCGCGTACACCAGATTGTGTAA	TTACACCTTTTCTACCTTCAAGTAATTACCCGC	97
GSTe2	GTTTGAAGCAGTTGCCATACTACGAGG	TCAAGCTTTAGCATTTTCCTCCTTTTTGGC	101
GSTd3	CACGGCCAGTCCTCTTTTAG	AAGCTTCTTCGCCACCAGTA	128
GSTd1-5	TGGAGAAATACGGCAAGGAC	CTTGGCGAAGATTTGTGGAT	140
Aldehyde oxidase	GCTCTGAACATTGCACCTCA	TGGTGTCGAACGATTGTGTT	109
CYP9K1	AGGGCTTCTGGATACGGTTC	CGTACGGTTCGGTTTTGATT	103
RSP7	GTGTTCGGTTCCAAGGTGAT	TCCGAGTTCATTTCCAGCTC	98
Actin	TTAAACCCAAAAGCCAATCG	ACCGGATGCATACAGTGACA	111

total of 40 transcripts were differentially expressed in all the three comparisons.

Genes commonly overexpressed in R_{perm}-S, C-S and R_{perm}-C comparisons

Only the transcript, AGAP011496-PA (*Anopheles gambiae* str. PEST) was upregulated in R_{perm}-S, R_{perm}-C and C-S comparisons with FC of 2.7, 1.5 and 2.3, respectively. No detoxification gene was found in the comparison of the three groups of mosquitoes.

Genes commonly overexpressed in R_{perm}-S and C-S comparisons

Several detoxification genes were commonly overexpressed in the R_{perm}-S and C-S. Among these genes, the transcripts for *glycogenin* (Afun000500) and *CYP6M7*, belonging to the cytochrome P450 gene family, were the most commonly overexpressed detoxification gene in R_{perm}-S (FC of 36.2 for Afun000500 and 34.6 for *CYP6M7*) and C-S (FC of 38.1 for Afun000500 and 28.9 for *CYP6M7*). A transcript from *CYP6AA1* was also commonly upregulated in the R_{perm}-S and C-S samples with FC of 5.2 and 3.8, respectively. This gene is the ortholog of *CYP6AA3* in *An. minimus*, which was shown to metabolise pyrethroids [40]. Other upregulated detoxification genes identified in R_{perm}-S and C-S comparisons include *CYP6Y2* located in the genomic region spanning the pyrethroid resistance *rp2* QTL detected in the FUMOZ-R pyrethroid-resistant laboratory strain [32], as well as *CYP6M4, CYP6S1, CYP4K2* and *CYP315A1* that were

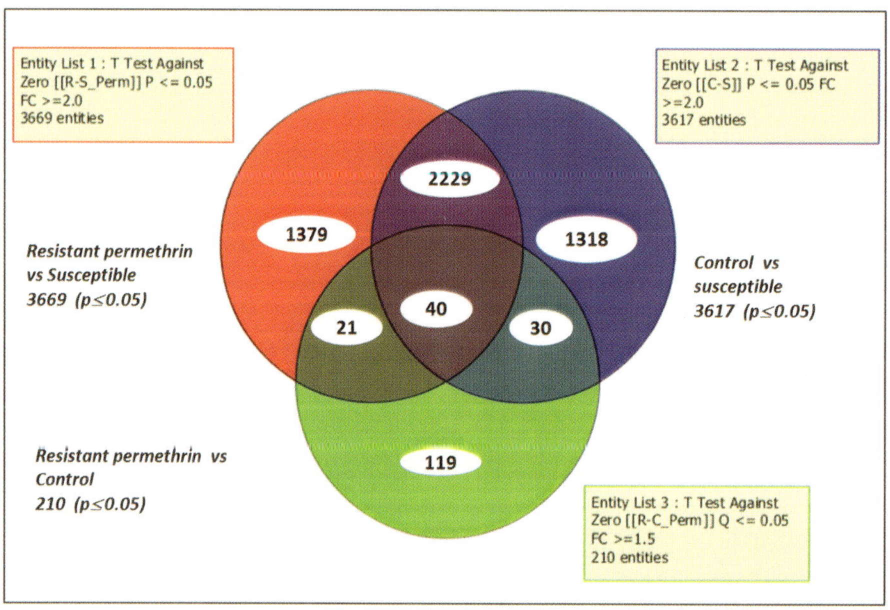

Fig. 1 Summary of transcripts differentially expressed in permethrin resistance. The Venn diagrams show the number of transcripts significantly ($P \leq 0.05$) up- or downregulated (FC ≥ 2) in each comparison as well as the commonly expressed transcripts

Table 2 Top detoxification genes upregulated in Rperm-S, C-S and Rperm-C

Probe name	Systematic name	Rperm-S fold change (FC)	C-S fold change (FC)	Rperm-C fold change (FC)	Ortholog in *An. gambiae*	Description
CUST_5822_PI426302897	Afun005822	2.7	2.31	1.5	AGAP011496-PA	AGAP011496-PA [*Anopheles gambiae* str. PEST]
CUST_500_PI426302897	Afun000500	36.2	38.1		na	Glycogenin
CUST_7663_PI426302897	Afun007663 (CYP6M7)	34.6	28.9		AGAP008213-PA	Cytochrome p450 6a8
CUST_8887_PI426302897	Afun008887	34.0	16.8		AGAP011997-PA	Nucleotide binding protein 2
CUST_9227_PI426302897	Afun009227	23.3	25.6		AGAP008141-PA	Argininosuccinate lyase
CUST_1459_PI406199769	combined_c738	22.0	34.5			Short-chain dehydrogenase
CUST_13921_PI426302897	Afun013921	19.1	21.1		AGAP006709-PA	Chymotrypsin 1
CUST_9492_PI426302897	Afun009492	16.4	3.7		AGAP001722-PA	Carboxylesterase
CUST_1822_PI406199769	combined_c920	11.1	11.4			Glutathione-S-transferase gst
CUST_45_PI426302897	Afun000045 (GSTE2)	10.9	15.2		AGAP009194-PA	Glutathione-S-transferase gst
CUST_4223_PI426302897	Afun004223	10.6	9.4		AGAP008358-PA	Cytochrome p450 4d1
CUST_12461_PI426302897	Afun012461	8.4	10.9		AGAP000288-PA	Alcohol dehydrogenase
CUST_3220_PI426302897	Afun003220	5.7	7.0		AGAP002867-PA	Cytochrome p450
CUST_8615_PI426302897	Afun008615 (CYP6AA1)	5.2	3.8		AGAP002862-PA	Cytochrome p450
CUST_9697_PI426302897	Afun009697	4.8	6.8		AGAP006364-PA	Abc transporter
CUST_9_PI426302915	CYP6M4.seq	4.8	3.5			Cytochrome p450
CUST_13797_PI426302897	Afun013797	4.1	3.0		AGAP000289-PA	Alcohol dehydrogenase
CUST_8445_PI426302897	Afun008445 (GSTE4)	3.9	4.7		AGAP009193-PA	Glutathione-S-transferase gst
CUST_25_PI426302915	CYP6Y2_rvcpl.seq	3.7	3.8			Cytochrome p450
CUST_1392_PI426302897	Afun001392	3.3	3.4		na	Glycine dehydrogenase
CUST_3394_PI426302897	Afun003394 (CYP315A1)	3.1	2.4		AGAP000284-PA	Cytochrome p450
CUST_8909_PI426302897	Afun008909 (CYP4K2)	2.4	2.0		AGAP002416-PA	Cytochrome p450
CUST_20_PI426302915	CYP6S1.seq	2.3	2.2			Cytochrome p450
CUST_7499_PI426302897	Afun007499 (GSTD1)	2.0	2.6		AGAP004164-PA	Glutathione transferase
CUST_11942_PI426302897	Afun011942	6.1			AGAP011509-PA	Carboxylesterase
CUST_4048_PI406199772	CD577343.1	5.3				Cuticle protein
CUST_12343_PI426302897	Afun012343 (CYP4H18)	5.0			AGAP008358-PA	Cytochrome p450 4d1
CUST_10836_PI426302897	Afun010836	4.8			AGAP006228-PA	Esterase b1
CUST_11042_PI426302897	Afun011042	3.9			AGAP003321-PA	Glycine dehydrogenase
CUST_11037_PI426302897	Afun011037	3.7			AGAP003581-PA	Alcohol dehydrogenase
CUST_1_PI426302915	CYP6M1a.seq	2.9				Cytochrome p450
CUST_7501_PI406199798	AGAP007662-RA_2L	2.6			AGAP007662-RA_2L	Short-chain dehydrogenase
CUST_9335_PI426302897	Afun009335 (CYP6AG1)	2.4			AGAP003343-PA	Cytochrome p450
CUST_7769_PI426302897	Afun007769 (CYP9K1)	2.2			AGAP000818-PA	Cytochrome p450 cyp9k1
CUST_11899_PI426302897	Afun011899	2.1			AGAP012514-PA	Short-chain dehydrogenase
CUST_4043_PI406199772	CD577345.1		3.7			Cuticle protein
CUST_7722_PI426302897	Afun007722		3.2		AGAP009850-PA	Abc transporter
CUST_12261_PI426302897	Afun012261		2.8		AGAP005758-PA	Carboxylesterase
CUST_13481_PI426302897	Afun013481 (GSTE1)		2.7		AGAP009195-PA	Glutathione-S-transferase gst
CUST_25_PI406199775	CYP6P9a		2.3			Cytochrome p450
CUST_15331_PI426302897	Afun015331 (CYP307A1)		2.2		AGAP001039-PB	Cytochrome p450 307a1
CUST_493_PI426302897	Afun000493		2.1		AGAP006225-PA	Aldehyde oxidase

Abbreviation: *na* not available

expressed at lower levels (FC < 5) (Table 2). Transcripts from the glutathione S-transferase (GST) family notably from epsilon [*GSTe2* (FC of 10.9 in R_{perm}-S and 15.2 in C-S) and *GSTe4* (FC of 3.9 in R_{perm}-S and 4.7 in C-S)] and delta, *GSTd1-5* (FC 2.0 and 2.6 in R_{perm}-S and C-S, respectively) classes were upregulated. Other genes such as *ABC transporter* (Afun009697), *alcohol dehydrogenases* (Afun012461, Afun013797), *carboxylesterase* (Afun009492), *short chain dehydrogenase* (combined_c738) and *chymotrypsin* (Afun013921) were also overexpressed (Table 2 and Additional file 1: Table S1).

Comparative transcriptional profiling of DDT and permethrin resistance

A comparative analysis of transcriptomes associated with DDT resistance in Kpome showed a total of 2158 transcripts differentially expressed (≥ 2-fold change, FC at $P \leq 0.05$) in R_{DDT}-S with 715 upregulated and 1443 downregulated. The comparison between R_{DDT}-S, R_{perm}-S and C-S revealed 1311 transcripts differentially expressed. A set of 212 transcripts was commonly expressed between R_{DDT}-S and R_{perm}-S, 958 transcripts and 270 transcripts were also expressed when comparing R_{perm}-S and R_{DDT}-S to C-S (Fig. 2).

Genes commonly overexpressed in R_{DDT}-S, Rperm-S and C-S comparisons

Many genes were commonly overexpressed in the three comparisons with *glycogenin* (Afun000500) and *argininosuccinate lyase* (Afun009227) been the most overexpressed and were consistent in all the three comparisons with fold change of (FC 36.2, 38.1 and 41.4) and (FC 22.2, 23.3 and 25.6) in R_{DDT}-S, R_{perm}-S and C-S, respectively. Among the common detoxification gene families identified, the *GSTe2* gene (Afun000045) was the one that remained highly upregulated with FC of 13.3, 10.9 and 15.2 for R_{DDT}-S, R_{perm}-S and C-S, respectively. The *CYP6M7* gene was also overexpressed in all three comparisons; FC was 34.6 in R_{perm}-S and FC 28.9 in C-S but with lower FC of 4 in R_{DDT}-S. Several other genes of the family of P450 such as *CYP6AA1*, *CYP6M4*, *CYP6Y2*, *CYP4K2* and *CYP315A1* were also upregulated. Other transcripts of the GST family were also upregulated such as the *Gste4* (FC 4.3, 3.9 and 4.7 in R_{DDT}-S, R_{perm}-S and C-S, respectively) and the *GSTd1* (FC 2.2, 2.0 and 2.6 in R_{DDT}-S, R_{perm}-S and C-S, respectively (Table 3 and Additional file 1: Table S2).

Overexpressed genes in the comparison between R_{DDT}-S and Rperm-S

A limited number of genes were commonly overexpressed in these two "resistant" comparisons, potentially as a result of induction or greater involvement in resistance than in control samples. The transcript of *alcohol dehydrogenase* (Afun011037) was the most overexpressed in R_{DDT}-S, and R_{perm}-S comparison with FC 6.5 and 3.7, respectively. Other genes of the P450 family including *CYP4H18*, *CYP9K1*, *CYP9J3*, and the *esterase b1* were also overexpressed (Table 3 and Additional file 1: Table S2).

Overexpressed genes in the comparison between R_{DDT}-S and C-S

The transcript (combined_c738) belonging to *the short-chain dehydrogenase* gene was the most commonly

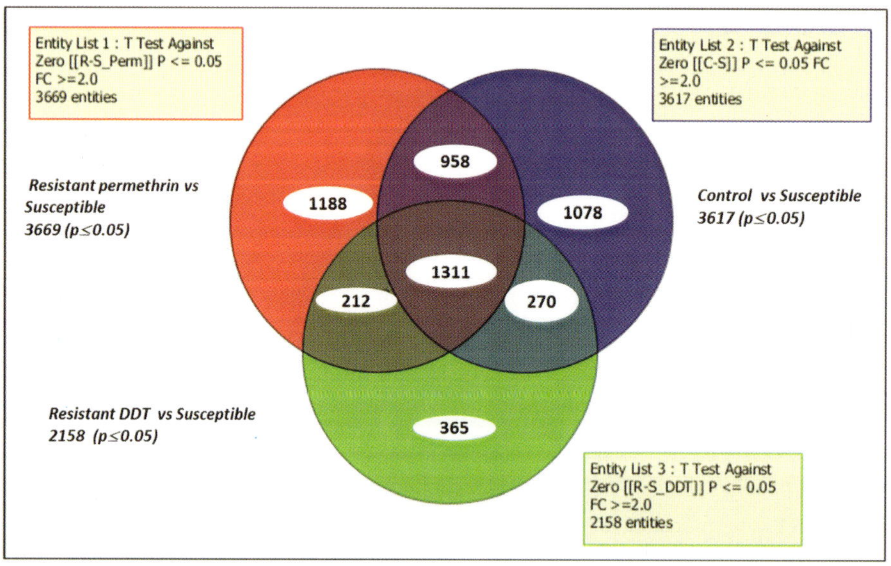

Fig. 2 Summary of transcripts differentially expressed in DDT and permethrin resistance. The Venn diagrams show the number of transcripts significantly ($P \leq 0.05$) up- or downregulated (FC ≥ 2) in each comparison as well as the commonly expressed transcripts permethrin

Table 3 Top detoxification genes upregulated in R_{DDT}-S, Rperm-S and C-S

Probe name	Systematic name	R_{DDT}-S fold change (FC)	Rperm-S fold change (FC)	C-S fold change (FC)	Ortholog in *An. gambiae*	Description
CUST_500_PI426302897	Afun000500	36.2	38.1	41.4	na	Glycogenin
CUST_9227_PI426302897	Afun009227	22.2	23.3	25.6	AGAP008141-PA	Argininosuccinate lyase
CUST_45_PI426302897	Afun000045 (GSTE2)	13.3	10.9	15.2	AGAP009194-PA	Glutathione-S-transferase
CUST_4223_PI426302897	Afun004223	12.8	10.6	9.4	AGAP008358-PA	Cytochrome p450 4d1
CUST_9697_PI426302897	Afun009697	11.6	4.8	6.8	AGAP006364-PA	Abc transporter
CUST_1822_PI406199769	combined_c920	11.5	11.1	11.4		Glutathione-S-transferase
CUST_3220_PI426302897	Afun003220	10.8	5.7	7.0	AGAP002867-PA	Cytochrome p450
CUST_9492_PI426302897	Afun009492	7.9	16.4	3.7	AGAP001722-PA	Carboxylesterase
CUST_8615_PI426302897	Afun008615 (CYP6AA1)	5.1	5.2	3.8	AGAP002862-PA	Cytochrome p450
CUST_9_PI426302915	CYP6M4.seq	4.9	4.8	3.5		Cytochrome p450
CUST_8445_PI426302897	Afun008445 (GSTE4)	4.3	3.9	4.7	AGAP009193-PA	Glutathione-S-transferase
CUST_6930_PI426302897	Afun006930 (CYP6M7)	4.0	34.6	28.9	AGAP008212-PA	Cytochrome p450 6a8
CUST_25_PI426302915	CYP6Y2_rvcpl.seq	3.4	3.7	3.8		Cytochrome p450
CUST_20_PI426302915	CYP6S1.seq	3.0	2.3	2.2		Cytochrome p450
CUST_8909_PI426302897	Afun008909 (CYP4K2)	2.8	2.4	2.0	AGAP002416-PA	Cytochrome p450
CUST_1392_PI426302897	Afun001392	2.5	3.3	3.4	na	Glycine dehydrogenase
CUST_13218_PI426302897	Afun013218 (CYP315A1)	2.3	2.9	2.6	AGAP000284-PA	Cytochrome p450
CUST_7499_PI426302897	Afun007499 (GSTD1)	2.2	2.0	2.6	AGAP004164-PA	Glutathione transferase
CUST_11037_PI426302897	Afun011037	6.5	3.7		AGAP003581-PA	Alcohol dehydrogenase
CUST_12343_PI426302897	Afun012343 (CYP4H18)	5.2	5.0		AGAP008358-PA	Cytochrome p450 4d1
CUST_10836_PI426302897	Afun010836	4.3	4.8		AGAP006228-PA	Esterase b1
CUST_7769_PI426302897	Afun007769 (CYP9K1)	3.0	2.2		AGAP000818-PA	Cytochrome p450 cyp9k1
CUST_7469_PI426302897	Afun007469 (CYP9J3)	2.0	2.1		AGAP012296-PA	Cytochrome p450
CUST_12461_PI426302897	Afun012461		8.4	10.9	AGAP000288-PA	Alcohol dehydrogenase
CUST_3489_PI406199769	combined_c1762		2.2	2.2		Abc transporter
CUST_8026_PI426302897	Afun008026		2.1	2.2	AGAP003578-PA	Aldehyde dehydrogenase
CUST_1458_PI406199769	combined_c738	10.4		15.9		Short-chain dehydrogenase
CUST_4043_PI406199772	CD577345.1	4.4		3.7		Cuticle protein
CUST_15331_PI426302897	Afun015331 (CYP307A1)	3.4		2.2	AGAP001039-PB	Cytochrome p450 307a1
CUST_25_PI406199775	CYP6P9a	2.8		2.3		Cytochrome p450
CUST_13481_PI426302897	Afun013481 (GSTE1)	2.5		2.7	AGAP009195-PA	Glutathione-S-transferase gst
CUST_4048_PI406199772	CD577343.1		5.3			Cuticle protein
CUST_11042_PI426302897	Afun011042		3.9		AGAP003321-PA	Glycine dehydrogenase
CUST_1_PI426302915	CYP6M1a.seq		2.9			Cytochrome p450
CUST_9335_PI426302897	Afun009335 (CYP6AG1)		2.4		AGAP003343-PA	Cytochrome p450
CUST_13475_PI426302897	Afun013475	3.2			AGAP003582-PA	Alcohol dehydrogenase
CUST_5448_PI426302897	Afun005448 (CYP302A1)	2.6			AGAP005992-PA	Cytochrome p450
CUST_4047_PI406199772	CD577343.1	2.4				Cuticle protein
CUST_8823_PI426302897	Afun008823 (CYP4D15)	2.4			AGAP002418-PA	Cytochrome p450
CUST_7301_PI426302897	Afun007301 (CYP4J5)	2.2			AGAP006048-PA	Cytochrome p450
CUST_208_PI406199788	gb-CYP12F3	2.1				Cytochrome p450
CUST_10630_PI426302897	Afun010630	2.1			AGAP002866-PA	Cytochrome p450
CUST_7722_PI426302897	Afun007722			3.2	AGAP009850-PA	Abc transporter

Table 3 Top detoxification genes upregulated in R_{DDT}-S, Rperm-S and C-S *(Continued)*

Probe name	Systematic name	R_{DDT}-S fold change (FC)	Rperm-S fold change (FC)	C-S fold change (FC)	Ortholog in *An. gambiae*	Description
CUST_12261_PI426302897	Afun012261			2.8	AGAP005758-PA	Carboxylesterase
CUST_4088_PI406199772	CD577323.1			2.4		Cuticle protein
CUST_493_PI426302897	Afun000493			2.1	AGAP006225-PA	Aldehyde oxidase

Abbreviation: *na* not available

upregulated in the R_{DDT}-S, and C-S comparison with FC 10.4 and 15.9, respectively. The cytochrome P450 gene *CYP307A1* was also upregulated with FC 3.3 in R_{DDT}-S and FC 2.2 in C-S. The *CYP6P9a* gene, reported to be upregulated in southern Africa mosquitoes, was also upregulated with FC 2.8 and 2.3 in R_{DDT}-S and C-S, respectively. Other genes with a known association with insecticide resistance were also upregulated in Kpome mosquitoes as shown in Table 3 and Additional file 1: Table S2.

Overexpressed genes in the comparison between Rperm-S and C-S

Genes identified from these comparisons include the *alcohol dehydrogenase* gene (Afun012461 ortholog of *AGAP000288* in *An. gambiae*) which is consistently upregulated in R_{perm}-S (FC8.4) and C-S (FC10.9) but not in R_{DDT}-S. Similarly, the *aldehyde dehydrogenase* (Afun0 08026) and the *ABC transporter* (Combined_*c1762*) were also upregulated in R_{perm}-S and C-S exclusively although with lower FC.

Overexpressed genes in the comparison between DDT resistant mosquitoes and a susceptible strain

Some detoxification genes specific for R_{DDT}-S comparison were identified in Kpome. These genes include *alcohol dehydrogenase* Afun013475 (FC 3.2), the most upregulated gene (FC 3.2) as well as *CYP302A1* (FC 2.6), *CYP4D15* (FC 2.4), *CYP4J5* (FC 2.2), *gb-CYP12F3* (FC 2.1) and the cytochrome P450 (Afun010630) (FC 2.1).

Overexpressed genes in the comparison between permethrin resistant mosquitoes and a susceptible strain

For R_{perm}-S comparison, the *ABC transporter* (Afun 007722) was the most upregulated gene with a fold change of 3.2. Also, the *carboxylesterase* (Afun012261) (FC 2.8), the cuticle protein (CD5773231) (FC 2.4) and the *aldehyde oxidase* (Afun00493) (FC 2.4) were upregulated.

Quantitative reverse transcriptase PCR

A qRT-PCR analysis revealed that *GSTe2* is the most overexpressed genes in DDT and permethrin resistant samples (FC 16.0 and 18.1, respectively) analysed in this study. However, the expression level of the detoxification gene, *CYP6M7* recorded with the qRT-PCR analysis was lower (FC 1.4 and 1.7 in permethrin and DDT resistant samples, respectively) compared to expression level from microarray analysis (FC 34.6 and 4.0 in permethrin and DDT resistant samples, respectively). The *GSTd1-5* and the *GSTd3* were significantly upregulated in DDT resistant samples (FC 12.5 and 6.2; $P < 0.01$) compared to permethrin resistant samples (FC 0.72 and 0.86; $P < 0.05$) (Fig. 3a, b).

Role of the knockdown resistance gene in DDT and permethrin resistance profiles recorded in *An. funestus* from Kpome

Amplification and sequencing of a fragment (a portion of intron 19 and the entire exon 20, domain II, segment 6) of the VGSC gene showed that both L1014F (TTA-to-TTT) and L1014S (TTA-to-TCA) kdr mutation commonly found in *An. gambiae* are absent in this mosquito species. However, further analysis with 837 bp of common sequences generated from the eleven mosquitoes analysed revealed 12 polymorphic sites with 12 haplotypes (Table 4, Fig. 4) showing a high genetic diversity of this gene within the *An. funestus* mosquitoes of Kpome. No amino acid change was detected in the Benin population. Furthermore, the Tajima D and Fu and Li D* statistics (Table 4) were not statistically significant. The Neighbour-joining tree showed low genetic differentiation between Benin populations compared to Cameroon samples with respect to geographical distance (Fig. 4).

Discussion

The WHO Global Plan for Insecticide Resistance Management [12] highlights the necessity to detect and monitor the development of insecticide resistance and characterise the underlying resistance mechanisms to maintain the successes in the reduction of malaria cases across Africa. In this study, we elucidated the molecular basis driving DDT and pyrethroids resistance in an inland *An. funestus* population from Benin.

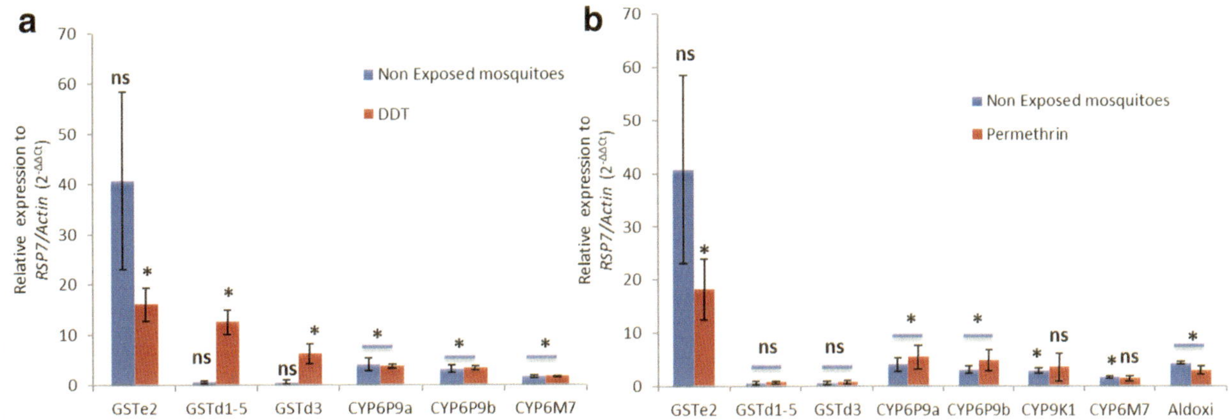

Fig. 3 Quantitative PCR results: differential expression by qRT-PCR of some candidate genes upregulated in microarray assays in *An. funestus* resistant to DDT (**a**) and permethrin (**b**). Error bars represent SD ($n = 3$). The presence of * on top of the two-fold changes for each gene indicates a statistically significant ($P < 0.05$) over-expression in resistant or non-exposed mosquitoes compared to the FANG susceptible strain; "ns" is shown when the difference was not significant

Permethrin and DDT resistance in *An. funestus* from Kpome is driven by metabolic resistance

Transcriptional profiling results and the absence of *kdr* mutation points out to a possible metabolic mechanism driving permethrin and DDT resistance in *An. funestus* from Kpome notably through overexpression of genes involved in insecticide detoxification such as cytochrome P450 genes, GSTs, aldehyde oxidases, and other gene families previously associated with resistance of *An. funestus* to insecticides [41].

The cytochrome P450, *CYP6M7* was the most overexpressed detoxification gene in permethrin exposed mosquitoes compared to the FANG susceptible strain as well as to the unexposed mosquitoes from microarrays analysis. However, this consistent information from microarray analysis was not confirmed by qRT-PCR. This discrepancy could be associated with the high genetic redundancy of some P450 genes and a high level of sequence similarity between different genes. These factors could lead to cross amplification contributing to homogenise the expression between samples. It is more likely that *CYP6M7* could also be a key pyrethroid resistance gene in Benin, but further validation is required. New approaches with RNAseq could help to confirm the expression pattern of this gene. On the other hand, only one gene (*AGAP011496-PA*) was commonly expressed in R_{perm}-S, C-S and R_{perm}-C comparisons. This could be due to the high resistance recorded against permethrin suggesting a less significant difference between the resistant and the control. Such a low number of differentially expressed genes between R-S and C-S comparison is commonly observed in similar studies when the resistance level is high in the population as it is the case here in Kpome [24, 27]. This is because both non-exposed (control; C) and alive mosquitoes after exposure (resistant; R) are all resistant which leads to less difference in the level of gene expression fold change between these two comparisons. The *GSTe2* gene was the most upregulated gene in both DDT and permethrin resistant samples showing that this gene is likely to be involved in both DDT and permethrin resistance as previously shown in coastal Benin [27]. Hence, such genes could confer cross-resistance to both insecticides, and this represents a challenge for the success of the malaria control

Table 4 Summary statistics for polymorphism in the voltage-gated sodium channel gene in F_0 *An. funestus* from Kpome compared to Pahou and Cameroon population

	N	S	π	k	h	hd	Syn	Nonsyn	D (*P*-value)	D* (*P*-value)
Kpome	22	12	0.00351	2.93939	12	0.909	0	0	0.37 (*P* > 0.10)	0.32 (*P* > 0.10)
Pahou	20	10	0.00260	2.17895	12	0.905	0	0	0.79 (*P* > 0.10)	0.96 (*P* > 0.10)
Cameroon	40	37	0.00514	4.30128	29	0.977	2	3	1.81 (*P* > 0.10)	2.75 (*P* > 0.10)

Abbreviations: *N* number of sequences (2n), *S* number of polymorphic sites, *h* number of haplotypes, *hd* haplotype diversity, *π* nucleotide diversity, *k* mean number of nucleotide differences, *D* Tajima's test, *D** Fu and Li's test, *Syn* synonymous mutation, *Nonsyn* non synonymous mutation

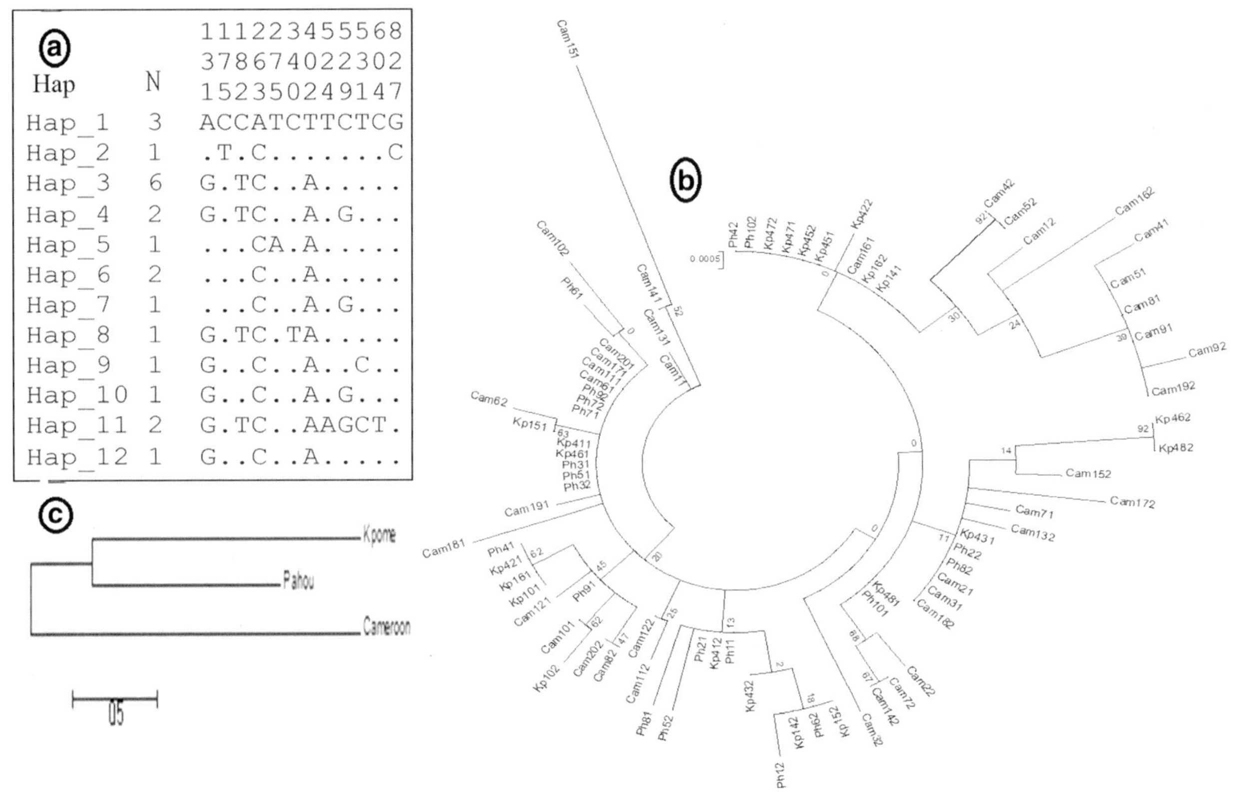

Fig. 4 *kdr* polymorphism in *Anopheles funestus* of Kpome. **a** Schematic representation of haplotypes of Exon20 fragment of the voltage-gated sodium channel gene (*VGSC*) observed in wild type *An. funestus* from Kpome. Only polymorphic sites are shown and these are numbered from the beginning of each aligned sequence. Dots indicate identity with the first sequence. A number has been given to each haplotype. The column (N) indicates the number of individuals sharing the haplotype. **b** Maximum-likelihood tree based on *kdr* data for samples from Kpome, Pahou and Cameroon. **c** Neighbour-joining tree based on the *VGSC* gene data for samples of Kpome, Pahou and Cameroon. *Abbreviations*: Kp, Kpome; Ph, Pahou, Cam: Cameroon

program. The enzyme encoded by this gene was shown to be able to metabolize both DDT and permethrin [27]. QRT-PCR confirmed the expression level of *GSTe2* in permethrin, DDT resistant and unexposed mosquitoes compared to the susceptible FANG. This observation is in line with the common implication of the *GSTe2* gene in permethrin and DDT resistance in the *An. funestus* population from Pahou (Benin) reported by Riveron et al. [27]. Furthermore, the potential role of *GSTe2* in permethrin resistance observed here has been shown in previous reports that suggested that orthologs of *GSTe2* in other insects are associated with pyrethroids resistance. Indeed, the elevated *GSTe2* expression has been associated with pyrethroid resistance by acting as a pyrethroid-binding protein and sequestering the insecticide [42] or by protecting against oxidative stress and lipid peroxidation induced by pyrethroid exposure [43]. In the yellow fever mosquito *Ae. aegypti*, a partial knockdown of the ortholog of *GSTe2* led to increased mortality to pyrethroids (deltamethrin), indicating that *GSTe2* is also associated with deltamethrin resistance in *Ae. aegypti* [44]. Moreover, the over-expression of *GSTe2* was observed with the high frequency of the 119F resistant allele in Kpome (91% of 119F/F homozygote resistant genotype) [10]. The near fixation of 119F-GSTe2 resistant allele in Kpome, which enlarges the substrate binding sites to increase DDT metabolism [27], coupled with the high overexpression of *GSTe2* highlights the key role played by this gene in DDT resistance as previously observed in Pahou. Orthologs of *GSTe2* have also been shown to be associated with DDT resistance in other mosquito species such as *An. gambiae* and *Ae. aegypti* [33, 44, 45]. Overall, *GSTe2* can confer resistance to DDT and permethrin, and this cross-resistance to pyrethroids is of significant concern for malaria control as *GSTe2* could protect mosquitoes against the major insecticides used to impregnate LLINs in public health. However, the overexpression of several genes from other gene families in this study highlights the complexity of resistance mechanisms suggesting the involvement of other genes than just *GSTe2*. In addition, the transcription profile of the duplicated genes *CYP6P9a* and *CYP6P9b* (which can metabolise both types I and II pyrethroids as shown by Riveron et al. [27]) in pyrethroid resistance in Kpome is different to that observed for *An. funestus* population in southern Africa. Indeed these P450 genes were highly upregulated in pyrethroid-resistant laboratory and field population from southern Africa [9, 15, 16, 31, 46, 47] while a lower level of over-expression was recorded in Kpome. The level of expression of *CYP6P9a* and *CYP6P9b* recorded in Kpome *An. funestus* population is similar to what was observed previously in Pahou population (coastal Benin). This result suggests that the two duplicated P450 genes are not strongly associated with permethrin resistance in Benin as observed in Mozambique (southern Africa) [15, 35]. Therefore, the molecular basis of the pyrethroid resistance in Benin is most likely different to that in southern Africa pointing to independent selection events of the pyrethroid resistance across Africa probably under different local selective forces. These different selective pressures could be increased of ITNs coverage across Benin, agricultural use of pesticides [48, 49] and spilt petroleum products [50]. In most African urban areas, insecticides are used for domestic purposes, including the control of mosquitoes in the form of mosquito coils, fumigation bombs or sprays [51]. These insecticides are used in an uncontrolled and heterogeneous manner in term of coverage and doses of insecticides in each household. Such practices may represent an additional selective pressure favouring pyrethroid resistance. The presence of agrochemicals, or industrial pollutants and plant compounds in mosquito breeding sites could also affect insecticide tolerance by modulating mosquito detoxification systems [52]. Concerning DDT resistance, in addition to the *GSTe2* gene, two other detoxification genes of GST family were also upregulated: *GSTd1-5* and *GSTd3*. *GSTd3* was shown to be upregulated in DDT-resistant *An. arabiensis* from an urban site in Burkina Faso [53]. *GSTd1-5* have been previously implicated in coding for enzymes that directly metabolise DDT or have at least been previously associated with the DDT-resistant phenotype [54, 55]. Further validation of the role of these genes in DDT resistance is required. The two duplicated cytochrome P450 genes, *CYP6P9a* (FC = 3.7) and *CYP6P9b* (FC = 3.9), which confer pyrethroid resistance in southern African populations of *An. funestus* [24] were also upregulated in the Benin population. However, because their encoded proteins are unable to metabolise DDT [24], these genes are not likely involved in DDT resistance observed in Kpome mosquitoes. Nevertheless, further investigation is required to validate this hypothesis. Monitoring the insecticide resistance mechanisms that occur within a population should be an essential component to all insecticide-based vector control programs and improving resistance management involves a better understanding of resistance mechanisms. These data contribute to the growing body of knowledge focussed on pyrethroid and DDT resistance in Benin. This situation emphasises the need for natural resistance and vector monitoring so that adjustments to control programmes can be made timeously and accurately.

Analysis of polymorphisms of the VGSC gene supports a limited role of knockdown resistance

Mechanisms of DDT and permethrin resistance are likely not associated with target site resistance as no kdr mutation was detected in analysed mosquitoes from Kpome. L1014F or L1014S change commonly associated with pyrethroid/DDT resistance in *An. gambiae* was not detected in this population of *An. funestus*, as it was also the case for all populations of this species, analysed so far [9, 19–22]. This suggests that the VGSC is probably evolving neutrally in DDT and permethrin resistance in *An. funestus* population.

Furthermore, the neutrality tests with Tajima D and Fu and Li D* statistics revealed no signature of directional selection on the sodium channel gene suggesting the limited role of knockdown resistance in both DDT and pyrethroid resistance in *An. funestus* in Kpome. The neighbour-joining tree revealed that Kpome mosquitoes cluster with Pahou mosquitoes while they are different to Cameroon mosquitoes. This reveals a reduced gene flow between these populations probably through isolation by distance which can also affect the spread of insecticide resistance genes in this species as previously shown for *An. funestus* populations across the continent [56].

Conclusions

Metabolic resistance is likely driving resistance to both pyrethroids (permethrin) and DDT in the major malaria vector *An. funestus* in Benin. The glutathione s-transferase gene, *GSTe2* is playing a key role in DDT resistance and most likely is responsible for the observed cross-resistance to pyrethroids in *An. funestus* populations from Kpome and such cross-resistance should be taken into account for the implementation of future insecticide resistance management strategies. Moreover, this study provides knowledge on the resistance profile and underlying resistance mechanisms to the available insecticides in *An. funestus*, a less studied malaria vector in Benin, in order to develop better insecticide resistance diagnostics. Further investigation should be performed on the expression level of target genes to ascertain the role of metabolic mechanisms in DDT and permethrin resistance in this *An. funestus* population. Resistance mechanisms detected in this studied population appear to be different from those identified in other African regions

showing the need to characterise mosquito populations at country-level for more appropriate and tailored control interventions.

Abbreviations

DDT: Dichlorodiphenyltrichloroethane; LSTM: Liverpool School of Tropical Medicine; qRT-PCR: Quantitative reverse transcriptase polymerase chain reaction; VGSC: Voltage-gated sodium channel; WHO: World Health Organisation

Acknowledgements

We appreciate Kpome community for their cooperation during fieldwork. We thank Innocent Djegbe, Eric Tossou, Gareth Weedall, Claude Gande and Murielle Soglo for their technical assistance and relevant advice.

Funding

The Wellcome Trust supports this work grants Reference 099864/Z/12/Z awarded to RD and a Wellcome Trust Senior Research Fellowship in Biomedical Sciences to CSW (101893/Z/13/Z).

Authors' contributions

RD and CSW designed the study. GT and RA carried out mosquito collection and GT, RA, AM and JR reared mosquitoes and performed WHO bioassays. GT and HI performed microarray, qRT-PCR analyses and sequencing of resistance genes. GT, JMR and CSW analyzed data. AY gave advise on the study design and contributed to the implementation of the study. GT, RD, AY, JMR and CSW wrote the manuscript. All authors read and approved the final manuscript.

Competing interests

The authors declare that they have no competing interests.

Author details

[1]International Institute of Tropical Agriculture, Cotonou 08 BP 0932, Benin. [2]University of Abomey Calavi, BP 526 Cotonou, Benin. [3]Liverpool School of Tropical Medicine, Pembroke Place, Liverpool L3 5QA, UK. [4]Cell Biology and Genetics Unit, Department of Zoology, University of Ibadan, Ibadan, Oyo State, Nigeria. [5]LSTM Research Unit at the Centre for Research in Infectious Diseases (CRID), P.O. Box 13591, Yaoundé, Cameroon.

References

1. WHO. World Malaria Report 2016. Geneva: World Health Organisation; 2016. http://www.who.int/malaria/publications/world-malaria-report-2016.
2. WHO. World Malaria Report 2011. Geneva: World Health Organisation; 2011. http://www.who.int/malaria/world_malaria_report_2011/en/.
3. Fontenille D, Simard F. Unravelling complexities in human malaria transmission dynamics in Africa through a comprehensive knowledge of vector populations. Comp Immunol Microbiol Infect Dis. 2004;27:357–75.
4. WHO. World Malaria Report 2014. Geneva: World Health Organisation; 2014. http://www.who.int/malaria/publications/world_malaria_report_2014/report/en/.
5. Ranson H, Lissenden N. Insecticide resistance in African *Anopheles* mosquitoes: a worsening situation that needs urgent action to maintain malaria control. Trends Parasitol. 2016;32:187–96.
6. Hamon J, Abonnenc E, Noel E. Contribution à l'étude des Culicidés de l'Ouest du Sénégal. Ann Parasitol Hum Comp. 1955;30:278–308.
7. Akogbéto M, Yakoubou S. Resistance of malaria vectors to pyrethrins used for impregnating mosquito nets in Benin, West Africa. Bull Soc Pathol Exot. 1999;92:123–30.
8. Corbel V, N'Guessan R, Brengues C, Chandre F, Djogbenou L, Martin T, et al. Multiple insecticide resistance mechanisms in *Anopheles gambiae* and *Culex quinquefasciatus* from Benin, West Africa. Acta Trop. 2007;101:207–16.
9. Djouaka R, Irving H, Tukur Z, Wondji CS. Exploring mechanisms of multiple insecticide resistance in a population of the malaria vector *Anopheles funestus* in Benin. PLoS One. 2011;6:e27760.
10. Djouaka R, Riveron JM, Yessoufou A, Tchigossou G, Akoton R, Irving H, et al. Multiple insecticide resistance in an infected population of the malaria vector *Anopheles funestus* in Benin. Parasit Vectors. 2016;9:453.
11. Akogbéto MC, Aïkpon RY, Azondékon R, Padonou GG, Ossè RA, Agossa FR, et al. Six years of experience in entomological surveillance of indoor residual spraying against malaria transmission in Benin: lessons learned, challenges and outlooks. Malar J. 2015;14:242.
12. WHO. Global plan for insecticide resistance management in malaria vectors. Geneva: World Health Organization Press; 2012.
13. Djouaka RJ, Atoyebi SM, Tchigossou G, Riveron JM, Irving H, Akoton R, et al. Evidence of a multiple insecticide resistance in the malaria vector *Anopheles funestus* in south-west Nigeria. Malar J. 2016;15:565.
14. Okoye PN, Brooke BD, Koekemoer LL, Hunt RH, Coetzee M. Characterisation of DDT, pyrethroid and carbamate resistance in *Anopheles funestus* from Obuasi, Ghana. Trans R Soc Trop Med Hyg. 2008;102:591–8.
15. Cuamba N, Morgan JC, Irving H, Steven A, Wondji CS. High level of pyrethroid resistance in an *Anopheles funestus* population of the Chokwe District in Mozambique. PLoS One. 2010;5:e11010.
16. Morgan JC, Irving H, Okedi LM, Steven A, Wondji CS. Pyrethroid resistance in an *Anopheles funestus* population from Uganda. PLoS One. 2010;5:e11872.
17. Wondji CS, Dabire RK, Tukur Z, Irving H, Djouaka R, Morgan JC. Identification and distribution of a GABA receptor mutation conferring dieldrin resistance in the malaria vector *Anopheles funestus* in Africa. Insect Biochem Mol Biol. 2011;41:484–91.
18. Kawada H, Dida GO, Ohashi K, Komagata O, Kasai S, Tomita T, et al. Multimodal pyrethroid resistance in malaria vectors, *Anopheles gambiae s.s.*, *Anopheles arabiensis*, and *Anopheles funestus s.s.* in western Kenya. PLoS One. 2011;6:48.
19. Samb B, Konate L, Irving H, Riveron JM, Dia I, Faye O, et al. Investigating molecular basis of lambda-cyhalothrin resistance in an *Anopheles funestus* population from Senegal. Parasit Vectors. 2016;9:449.
20. Irving H, Charles WS. Investigating knockdown resistance (kdr) mechanism against pyrethroids/DDT in the malaria vector *Anopheles funestus* across Africa. BMC Genet. 2017;18:76.
21. Menze BD, Riveron JM, Ibrahim SS, Irving H, Antonio-Nkondjio C, Awono-ambene PH, et al. Multiple insecticide resistance in the malaria vector *Anopheles funestus* from northern Cameroon is mediated by metabolic resistance alongside potential target site insensitivity mutations. PLoS One. 2016;11:e0163261.
22. Mulamba C, Riveron JM, Ibrahim SS, Irving H, Barnes KG, Mukwaya LG, et al. Widespread pyrethroid and DDT resistance in the major malaria vector *Anopheles funestus* in east Africa is driven by metabolic resistance mechanisms. PLoS One. 2014;9:e110058.
23. Brooke BD, Hunt R, Koekemoer L, Temu E, Taylor M, Small G, et al. Bioassay and biochemical analyses of insecticide resistance in southern African *Anopheles funestus* (Diptera: Culicidae). Bull Entomol Res. 2001;91:265–72.

24. Riveron JM, Ndula M, Barnes KG, Ibrahim SS, Paine MJI, Wondji CS. Directionally selected cytochrome P450 alleles are driving the spread of pyrethroid resistance in the major malaria vector *Anopheles funestus*. Proc Natl Acad Sci USA. 2013;110:252–7.
25. Hargreaves K, Koekemoer LL, Brooke BD, Hunt RH, Mthembu J, Coetzee M. *Anopheles funestus* resistant to pyrethroid insecticides in South Africa. Med Vet Entomol. 2000;14:181–9.
26. Mulamba C, Irving H, Riveron JM, Mukwaya LG, Birungi J, Wondji CS. Contrasting *Plasmodium* infection rates and insecticide susceptibility profiles between the sympatric sibling species *Anopheles parensis* and *Anopheles funestus s.s.*: a potential challenge for malaria vector control in Uganda. Parasit Vectors. 2014;7:71.
27. Riveron JM, Yunta C, Ibrahim SS, Djouaka R, Irving H, Menze BD, et al. A single mutation in the *GSTe2* gene allows tracking of metabolically based insecticide resistance in a major malaria vector *Anopheles funestus*. Genome Biol. 2014;15:1–20.
28. Koekemoer LL, Kamau L, Hunt RH, Coetzee M. A cocktail polymerase chain reaction assay to identify members of the *Anopheles funestus* (Diptera: Culicidae) group. Am J Trop Med Hyg. 2002;66:804–11.
29. Crawford J, Guelbeogo W, Sanou A, Traore A, Vernick K, Sagnon N, Lazzaro S. *De novo* transcriptome sequencing in *Anopheles funestus* using Illumina RNA-seq technology. PLoS One. 2010;5:e14202.
30. Gregory R, Darby AC, Irving H, Coulibaly MB, Hughes M, Koekemoer LL, et al. A *de novo* expression profiling of *Anopheles funestus*, malaria vector in Africa, using 454 pyrosequencing. PLoS One. 2011;6:e17418.
31. Wondji CS, Irving H, Morgan J, Lobo NF, Collins FH, Hunt RH, et al. Two duplicated P450 genes are associated with pyrethroid resistance in *Anopheles funestus*, a major malaria vector. Genome Res. 2009;19:452–9.
32. Irving H, Riveron J, Ibrahim S, Lobo N, Wondji C. Positional cloning of rp2 QTL associates the P450 genes *CYP6Z1*, *CYP6Z3* and *CYP6M7* with pyrethroid resistance in the malaria vector *Anopheles funestus*. Heredity. 2012;109:383–92.
33. David J-P, Strode C, Vontas J, Nikou D, Vaughan A, Pignatelli PM, et al. The *Anopheles gambiae* detoxification chip: a highly specific microarray to study metabolic-based insecticide resistance in malaria vectors. Proc Natl Acad Sci USA. 2005;102:4080–4.
34. Hunt RH, Brooke BD, Pillay C, Koekemoer LL, Coetzee M. Laboratory selection for and characteristics of pyrethroid resistance in the malaria vector *Anopheles funestus*. Med Vet Entomol. 2005;19(3):271–5.
35. Riveron JM, Ibrahim SS, Chanda E, Mzilahowa T, Cuamba N, Irving H, et al. The highly polymorphic *CYP6M7* cytochrome P450 gene partners with the directionally selected *CYP6P9a* and *CYP6P9b* genes to expand the pyrethroid resistance front in the malaria vector *Anopheles funestus* in Africa. BMC Genomics. 2014;15:817.
36. Schmittgen D, Livak J. Analyzing real-time PCR data by the comparative CT method. Nat Protoc. 2008;3:1101–8.
37. Thompson JD, Higgins DG, Gibson TJ. CLUSTAL W: Improving the sensitivity of progressive multiple sequence alignment through sequence weighting, position-specific gap penalties and weight matrix choice. Nucleic Acids Res. 1994;22:4673–80.
38. Librado P, Rozas J. DnaSP v5: a software for comprehensive analysis of DNA polymorphism data. Bioinformatics. 2009;25:1451–2.
39. Tamura K, Peterson D, Peterson N, Stecher G, Nei M, Kumar S. MEGA5: Molecular Evolutionary Genetics Analysis using maximum likelihood, evolutionary distance, and maximum parsimony methods. Mol Biol Evol. 2011;28:2731–9.
40. Duangkaew P, Pethuan S, Kaewpa D, Boonsuepsakul S, Sarapusit S, Rongnoparut P. Characterization of mosquito *CYP6P7* and *CYP6AA3*: differences in substrate preference and kinetic properties. Arch Insect Biochem Physiol. 2011;76:236–48.
41. Hemingway J, Hawkes NJ, McCarroll L, Ranson H. The molecular basis of insecticide resistance in mosquitoes. Insect Biochem Mol Biol. 2004;34:653–65.
42. Kostaropoulos I, Papadopoulos AI, Metaxakis A, Boukouvala E, Papadopoulou Mourkidou E. Glutathione S-transferase in the defence against pyrethroids in insects. Insect Biochem Mol Biol. 2001;31:313–9.
43. Vontas JG, Small GJ, Hemingway J. Glutathione S-transferases as antioxidant defence agents confer pyrethroid resistance in Nilaparvata lugens. Biochem J. 2001;357:65–72.
44. Lumjuan N, Rajatileka S, Changsom D, Wicheer J, Leelapat P, Prapanthadara LA, et al. The role of the *Aedes aegypti* Epsilon glutathione transferases in conferring resistance to DDT and pyrethroid insecticides. Insect Biochem Mol Biol. 2011;41:203–9.
45. Strode C, Wondji CS, David JP, Hawkes NJ, Lumjuan N, Nelson DR, et al. Genomic analysis of detoxification genes in the mosquito *Aedes aegypti*. Insect Biochem Mol Biol. 2008;38:113–23.
46. Wondji CS, Morgan J, Coetzee M, Hunt RH, Steen K, Iv WCB, et al. Mapping a Quantitative Trait Locus (QTL) conferring pyrethroid resistance in the African malaria vector *Anopheles funestus*. BMC Genomics. 2007;8:34.
47. Amenya D, Naguran R, Lo T, Ranson H, Spillings B, Wood O, et al. Over expression of a cytochrome P450 (*CYP6P9*) in a major African malaria vector, *Anopheles funestus*, resistant to pyrethroids. Insect Mol Biol. 2008;17:19–25.
48. Akogbeto MC, Djouaka R, Noukpo H. Use of agricultural insecticides in Benin. Bull Soc Pathol Exot. 2005;98:400–5.
49. Yadouleton A, Martin T, Padonou G, Chandre F, Asidi A, Djogbenou L, et al. Cotton pest management practices and the selection of pyrethroid resistance in *Anopheles gambiae* population in northern Benin. Parasit Vectors. 2011;4:60.
50. Djouaka RF, Bakare AA, Bankole HS, Doannio JM, Coulibaly ON, Kossou H, et al. Does the spillage of petroleum products in *Anopheles* breeding sites have an impact on the pyrethroid resistance? Malar J. 2007;6:159.
51. Elissa N, Mouchet J, Riviere F, Meunier JY, Yao K. Resistance of *Anopheles gambiae s.s.* to pyrethroids in Côte d'Ivoire. Ann Soc Belg Med Trop. 1993; 73:291–4.
52. Nkya TE, Akhouayri I, Kisinza W, David J-P. Impact of environment on mosquito response to pyrethroid insecticides: facts, evidences and prospects. Insect Biochem Mol Biol. 2013;43:407–16.
53. Jones CM, Toé HK, Sanou A, Namountougou M, Hughes A, Diabaté A, D R, Simard F, et al. Additional selection for insecticide resistance in urban malaria vectors: DDT resistance in *Anopheles arabiensis* from Bobo-Dioulasso, Burkina Faso. PLoS One. 2012;7:e45995.
54. Tang A, Tu C. Biochemical characterization of *Drosophila* glutathione S-transferases D1 and D21. J Biol Chem. 1994;269:27876–84.
55. Brandt A, Scharf M, Pedra J, Holmes G, Dean A, Kreitman M, et al. Differential expression and induction of two *Drosophila* cytochrome P450 genes near the Rst(2)DDT locus. Insect Mol Biol. 2002;11:337–41.
56. Barnes KG, Weedall GD, Ndula M, Irving H, Mzihalowa T, Hemingway J, et al. Genomic footprints of selective sweeps from metabolic resistance to pyrethroids in African malaria vectors are driven by scale up of insecticide-based vector control. PLoS Genet. 2017;13:e1006539.

11

Studies of *Myxidium giardi* Cépède, 1906 infections in Icelandic eels identifies a genetically diverse clade of myxosporeans that represents the *Paramyxidium* n. g. (Myxosporea: Myxidiidae)

Mark A. Freeman[1*] and Árni Kristmundsson[2]

Abstract

Background: The myxosporean *Myxidium giardi* Cépède, 1906 was described infecting the kidney of the European eel, *Anguilla anguilla* (L.), having spindle-shaped myxospores and terminal sub-spherical polar capsules. Since then, numerous anguillid eels globally have been documented to have similar *Myxidium* infections. Many of these have been identified using the morphological features of myxospores or by the location of infection in the host, and some have been subsequently synonymised with *M. giardi*. Therefore, it is not clear whether *M. giardi* is a widely distributed parasite, infecting numerous species of eels, in multiple organs, or whether some infections represent other, morphologically similar but different species of myxosporeans. The aim of the present study was to assess the status of *M. giardi* infections in Icelandic eels, and related fish hosts in Malaysia and to use spore morphology and molecular techniques to evaluate the diversity of myxosporeans present.

Results: The morphologies of the myxospores from Icelandic eels were very similar but the overall dimensions were significantly different from the various tissue locations. Myxospores from the kidney of the Malaysian tarpon, *Megalops cyprinoides* (Broussonet), were noticeably smaller. However, the *SSU* rDNA sequences from the different tissues locations in eels, were all very distinct, with percentage similarities ranging from 92.93% to as low as 89.8%, with the sequence from Malaysia being even more dissimilar. Molecular phylogenies consistently placed these sequences together in a clade that we refer to as the *Paramyxidium* clade that is strongly associated with the *Myxidium* clade (*sensu stricto*). We erect the genus *Paramyxidium* n. g. (Myxidiidae) to accommodate these histozoic taxa, and transfer *Myxidium giardi* as *Paramyxidium giardi* Cépède, 1906 n. comb. as the type-species.

Conclusions: There is not a single species of *Myxidium* (*M. giardi*) causing systemic infections in eels in Iceland. There are three species, confirmed with a robust phylogeny, one of which represents *Paramyxidium giardi* n. comb. Additional species probably exist that infect different tissues in the eel and the site of infection in the host fish is an important diagnostic feature for this group (*Paramyxidium* n. g. clade). Myxospore morphology is generally conserved in the *Paramyxidium* clade, although actual spore dimensions can vary between some species. *Paramyxidium* spp. are currently only known to infect fishes from the Elopomorpha.

Keywords: *Paramyxidium* n. g., *Paramyxidium giardi* n. comb., Elopomorpha, Protacanthopterygii, Myxosporea, *Chloromyxum*

* Correspondence: mafreeman@rossvet.edu.kn
[1]Ross University School of Veterinary Medicine, Basseterre, Saint Kitts and Nevis
Full list of author information is available at the end of the article

Background

The importance of the shape of myxospores and its relative usefulness in myxosporean taxonomy has been scrutinised in recent years, and it has been unambiguously demonstrated that numerous genera are now polyphyletic in molecular phylogenetic analyses due to the use of spore morphology as the principal taxonomic measure [1–3]. However, myxospores remain the primary diagnostic feature of myxosporean infections in fish and other vertebrates [4] and their morphology, especially when combined with other important information from the host, can sometimes be sufficient to make preliminary identifications or diagnoses without the use of DNA analysis. The polyphyletic nature of some myxosporean genera in molecular analyses has occurred, in part, as our systematic framework for deciding which family and genus to place novel species has become less stringent over time, and gives priority to basic myxospore morphology over other characters [4]. This is combined with the fact that there also seems to be a general reluctance to establish new genera when necessary, with the historical preference being to further loosen the descriptive boundaries of existing genera [4]. This has led to artificially high numbers of species being placed in certain genera, which in some cases are clearly not closely related to each other, and has hence contributed to polyphyly in subsequent molecular phylogenies [2, 4].

Myxidium giardi Cépède, 1906 was originally described from the kidney of the European eel, *Anguilla anguilla* (L.), in France, with myxospores described as spindle-shaped with terminal sub-spherical polar capsules [5], but have since been reported in numerous sizes and described as both wide and slender, some with almost spherical polar capsules [6, 7]. Globally, numerous species of anguillid eels have been reported to have similar *Myxidium* spp. infections, many of which have been distinguished using morphological features such as spore size and number or lack of valvular striations [8, 9] or the site of infection in the eel (skin, gills, kidney, stomach, etc.) [10]. However, many descriptions of *Myxidium* spp. infecting eels have subsequently been synonymized with *M. giardi*, as less emphasis was placed on details such as the site of infection [11] and *M. giardi* was considered to have an almost worldwide distribution [12]. Currently, it is not clear whether *M. giardi* is a widely distributed parasite infecting numerous species of eels, in multiple organs, or whether some infections represent other, morphologically similar, species of myxosporeans. One short rDNA sequence exists for *M. giardi* from the urinary system of *A. anguilla* from Scotland, and phylogenetic analyses place this in the freshwater urinary clade, with numerous other myxosporeans found infecting the urinary systems of fish, but none with a similar spore morphology [13].

Anguillid eels (Order Anguilliformes) are catadromous fish consisting of 17 species in a single genus, *Anguilla* Garsault, distributed in all the world's oceans. Two species inhabit the Atlantic Ocean, the European eel, *A. anguilla*, and the American eel, *Anguilla rostrata* (Lesueur) [14]. A dramatic decline has been experienced in populations of the European eel and diseases/parasites are considered to be one of several factors responsible. Consequently, since 2009, the European eel has been on the red list of the International Union for the Conservation of Nature (IUCN) and hence is listed as a 'critically endangered' species [15]. The Indo-Pacific tarpon, *Megalops cyprinoides* (Broussonet) (Order Elopiformes), inhabits tropical coastal and brackish waters of the Indo-Pacific, migrating between the open sea and inland rivers and mangroves [16]. Elopiformes are related to, but do not resemble anguillid eels, and like eels they spawn at sea producing leptocephalic larvae that later migrate inland [17]. Tarpon (Elopiformes) together with their sister group the eels (Anguilliformes) form the Elopomorpha which are one of the oldest major extant teleost lineages [18].

In the present study, we aimed to examine eels from Iceland and genetically characterise *Myxidium giardi*-like parasites from different infection sites in the hosts. In addition, we aim to compare these with morphologically similar parasites previously observed by one of us (MAF) in tarpon from Malaysia.

Methods

Thirty-one live European eels, *A. anguilla*, (growing yellow eels; total length range 42–68 cm) were collected from Lake Vifilsstadavatn in Iceland during May 2013 using fyke nets. The fish were transported to the laboratory, placed in tanks with freshwater and kept alive until examination. Prior to examination, the fish were euthanized in MS-222. All eels were dissected and examined for myxosporeans in the gills, kidney and stomach wall using dissecting and compound microscopes. Images were taken of twenty spores from each tissue location for size estimations using ImageJ. In addition, fourteen mature Pacific tarpon, *Megalops cyprinoides* total length range 22–34 cm, were caught with gill nets in Kilim mangroves on Langkawi Island, Malaysia. Tarpon were examined for gill and kidney myxosporeans, using dissecting and compound microscopes. In Malaysia, myxospores were photographed in the field using a portable compound microscope and a Dino-Eye eyepiece camera. Infected tissues from eels and tarpon were fixed in 10% buffered formalin and processed for standard histology, 3 μm thick sections prepared, stained with Giemsa and mounted in resin-based medium.

Oligochaetes (n = 100) were taken from sediment samples from the lake Vifilsstadavatn in Iceland, isolated and incubated at 10 °C in filtered (pore size 0.45 μm) lake water in 24-well tissue culture plates. Oligochaetes were examined daily using a dissecting microscope for the presence of actinospore production, typically characterized by a cloudy secretion from the anus of the worms, and confirmed using a compound microscope. Every other day, the water in the wells was exchanged. The oligochaetes that produced actinospores were used for DNA analysis and images of the actinospores taken as detailed above.

Infected tissue (kidney, stomach wall) or spore-filled cysts (gills), equal to approximately 20–40 mg, were placed directly into DNA lysis buffer for molecular analysis. Total DNA was extracted using a GeneMATRIX DNA isolation kit (EURx, Gdansk, Poland) following the tissue protocol and used as templates in subsequent PCR reactions. Parasite small subunit ribosomal DNA (*SSU* rDNA) was amplified using the general myxosporean primers and methodology previously described [2] with a new reverse primer M-790r (5'-ACG ACC AAT TAA GGC TAT GC-3'), paired with 18e, utilising the PCR conditions as in [2]. In addition, the primer pair Mg-50f (5'-ACT AAG CCA TGC ATG TCT ATG T-3') and Mg-1170r (5'-TGA TCA ATC GAA ACG GTC TAG G-3') were designed to assist in further studies of these myxosporeans from anguillid eels and amplified a 1150 bp region of the *SSU* rDNA including the phylogenetically informative variable V1-V5 regions; PCR conditions were the same as in [2], except for using an annealing temperature of 58 °C and extension time of 1 min. PCRs were conducted on parasite DNA, from each tissue, from 4 different fish and amplified in triplicate. PCR products of the expected sizes were recovered using a GeneMATRIX PCR products extraction kit (EURx Poland) and sequencing reactions were performed using BigDyeTM Terminator cycle sequencing chemistry utilising the same oligonucleotide primers that were used for the original PCRs. DNA sequencing was performed in both forward and reverse directions for all PCR products and nucleotide BLAST searches performed for each sequence read to confirm a myxosporean origin [19]. The contiguous sequences were obtained manually using CLUSTAL X and BioEdit [20, 21]. CLUSTAL X was used for the initial *SSU* rDNA sequence alignments of the novel sequences to other related myxosporean sequences identified from the BLAST searches and from relevant literature [1, 13, 22, 23]. Percentage divergence matrices were constructed from selected aligned taxa in CLUSTAL X using the neighbour-joining method based on the Kimura 2-parameter model [24].

Phylogenetic analyses were performed using the maximum likelihood methodology in PhyML [25] with the automatic smart model selection (selection criterion: Akaike Information Criterion), running the general time-reversible substitution model (GTR+G6+I) with 1000 bootstrap repeats. Bayesian inference (BI) analysis was performed using MrBayes v. 3.2 [26]. For the BI analysis, models of nucleotide substitution were first evaluated for the alignment using MrModeltest v. 2.2 [27]. The most parameter-rich evolutionary model based on the AIC was the general time-reversible, GTR+I+G model of evolution. Therefore, the settings used for the analysis were nst = 6, with the gamma-distributed rate variation across sites and a proportion of invariable sites (rates = invgamma). The priors on state frequency were left at the default setting (Prset statefreqpr = dirichlet (1,1,1,1)), and *Chloromyxum leydigi* (AY604199) was set as the outgroup. Posterior probability distributions were generated using the Markov Chain Monte Carlo (MCMC) method with four chains being run simultaneously for 1,000,000 generations. 'Burn-in' was set at 2500 and trees were sampled every 100 generations making a total of 7500 trees used to compile the majority rule consensus trees.

Measurements of myxospores from each organ (kidney, gills and stomach wall) were tested for normality using the Shapiro-Wilk test. To test whether there was a significant difference in analogous measurement between the different myxospores, a Student's t-test was applied. Both tests were performed in RStudio (version 0.98.1062).

Results

All the fish examined in this study appeared in good condition and no gross signs of a disease were present. From the 31 eels examined, small myxosporean cysts were observed on the gills of 25 fish (prevalence of 83%) using a dissection stereoscope, ranging between 2–10 cysts per gill arch. Infections in the kidney and the stomach wall were only detected using a compound microscope. Spores were detected in the kidney of 10 fish (32%) and from stomach scrapings from 6 eels (19%). Infections were light in most cases, being more apparent in the gills. All myxospores detected had a similar morphology that conformed to the currently accepted shape and size range for *Myxidium giardi* (Table 1) [12]. No gill cysts were observed from 14 tarpon, examined in Malaysia, but the kidney of 4 fish (29%) were heavily infected with a myxosporean, observed in fresh tissue preparations. The myxospores from tarpon kidney had a similar morphology to the ones from the eels. However, they were noticeably, and significantly, smaller than all three species observed from the Icelandic eels (Tables 1 and 2).

The overall morphology and dimensions of the myxospores from Icelandic eels appeared similar (Fig. 1). However, taking average dimensions from 20 measured spores, they were significantly different with regard to spore length and/or width (Tables 1 and 2). Most fresh spores were typically observed in the sutural plane and had an oval to bluntly-rounded shape with almost spherical polar capsules opening sub-terminally (Fig. 1a-e). The sutural line, when visible, was sigmoidal and striations were visible on the surface of the spore valves (Fig. 1c, f), although these structures were not always clearly visible. In the valvular view, spores were more lemon-shaped than a true spindle or fusiform shape (Fig. 1e), but clearly resembled the original drawings

Table 1 Measurements of twenty fresh myxospores of *Paramyxidium* spp., including dimensions from the original description of *P. giardi*

Species	Host species	Site of infection	Spore body Range (Mean)		Polar capsules Range (Mean)		Reference
			Length	Width	Length	Width	
P. giardi[a]	*A. anguilla*	Kidney	9.0–10.0 (nd)	5.5–6.0 (nd)	3.0–5.0 (nd)	nd (2.0)	Cépède (1906) [5]
P. giardi	*A. anguilla*	Kidney	9.5–11.4 (10.6)	6.5–7.5 (7.0)	3.5–4.2 (4.0)	2.7–3.9 (3.6)	Present study
P. magi n. sp.	*A. anguilla*	Stomach wall	10.8–12.9 (11.6)	7.0–8.4 (7.6)	3.6–4.6 (4.0)	3.1–4.0 (3.6)	Present study
P. branchialis n. sp.	*A. anguilla*	Gills	10.7–12.3 (11.6)	6.6–7.8 (7.3)	3.9–4.5 (4.2)	3.2–4.2 (3.8)	Present study
P. bulani n. sp.	*M. cyprinoides*	Kidney	6.1–6.9 (6.7)	4.2–5.1 (4.7)	2.1–2.5 (2.3)	1.5–2.0 (1.8)	Present study

[a]Original description
Abbreviation: nd, no data

by Cépède [5], however they did not have terminal capsular foramina. All myxospores in this study were between 62–70% as wide as they were long, which is similar to the original description of *Myxidium giardi* from eels in France (Table 1) [5]. The myxospores from tarpon in Malaysia, had a remarkably similar overall morphology to those from Icelandic eels (Fig. 1g-k), but they were significantly smaller in size (Tables 1 and 2). When myxospores were stained, it was clear that the sporoplasm contained two nuclei, in all cases, as originally described for *M. giardi* [5]. Only one oligochaete, morphologically identified as *Lumbriculus variegatus*, produced actinospores with an Aurantactinomyxon morphology (Fig. 1l, Table 3).

Histological examination

Paramyxidium giardi infecting the kidney of eels forms polysporous plasmodia which vary greatly in size (*c.*55–120 µm in this study). The plasmodia were most commonly found as intratubular, both in the proximal and distal kidney tubules, although they were also, to a lesser extent, observed in the renal interstitium. The associated histopathology was mostly due to mechanical disruption of the tissue as the large plasmodia often caused extensive widening of the kidney tubules followed by atrophy and degeneration of the tubular epithelial cells (Fig. 2a) which is in agreement with the pathology described by Copland [28]. Renal infections described in his study [28] were more extensive than in this study. Consequently, he observed varying degrees of pathology in other parts of the kidney, e.g. the bowman capsule and the kidney interstitium.

Paramyxidium magi n. sp. is histozoic in the stomach wall. It forms polysporous plasmodia of variable sizes (*c.*60–95 µm) in the gastric gland interstitium (Fig. 2b). Large spore masses in the gastric glands cause focal compaction and disruption of the adjacent gastric glands similar to previous reports [28].

Parayxidium branchialis n. sp. is histozoic in the gills. As observed by Copland [28], the great majority of infections were observed in the secondary lamellae. The plasmodia are polysporous and differ significantly in size (*c.*35–142 µm). Infections cause separation of the lamellar epithelial cells from the basement membrane and disruption of pillar cells (Fig. 2c) and in some cases oedema in the basal part of the secondary lamellae.

Table 2 Statistical comparison of spore length (above the diagonal) and width (below the diagonal) of the four species observed in the study

Species	*P. giardi*	*P. magi* n. sp.	*P. branchialis* n. sp.	*P. bulani* n. sp.
P. giardi		$t_{(19)} = -6.53$; $P < 0.0001$ ****	$t_{(19)} = -6.42$; $P < 0.0001$ ****	$t_{(19)} = 30.64$; $P < 0.0001$ ****
P. magi n. sp.	$t_{(19)} = -6.22$; $P < 0.0001$ ****		$t_{(19)} = -0.45$; $P = 0.6544$ ns	$t_{(19)} = 51.94$; $P < 0.0001$ ****
P. branchialis n. sp.	$t_{(19)} = -3.61$; $P = 0.0009$ ***	$t_{(19)} = 3.18$; $P = 0.0029$ **		$t_{(19)} = 44.90$; $P < 0.0001$ ****
P. bulani n. sp.	$t_{(19)} = 29.38$; $P < 0.0001$ ****	$t_{(19)} = 31.12$; $P < 0.0001$ ****	$t_{(19)} = 33.70$; $P < 0.0001$ ****	

Abbreviation: ns, not significant
**$P < 0.01$, ***$P < 0.001$, ****$P < 0.0001$

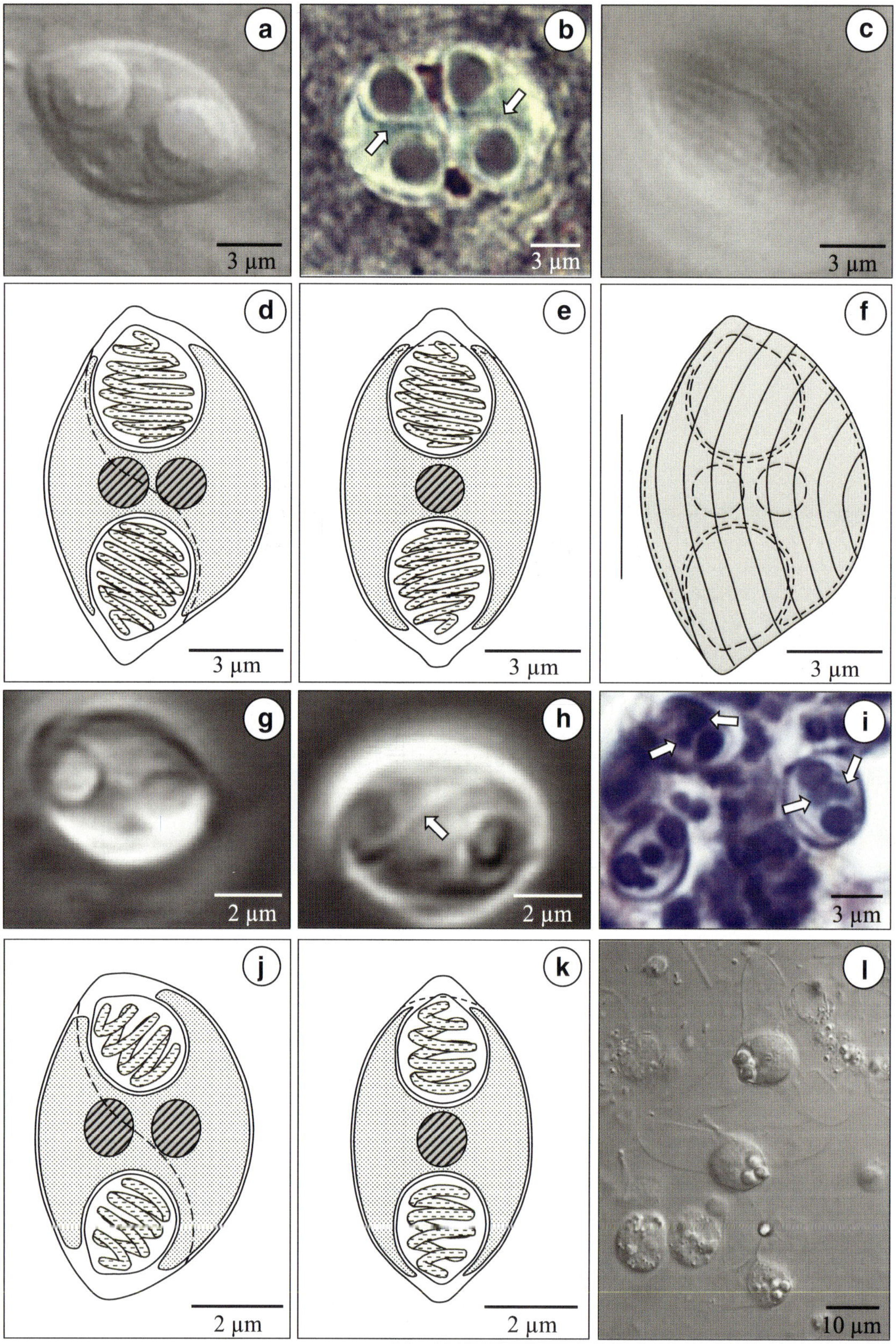

Fig. 1 (See legend on next page.)

(See figure on previous page.)
Fig. 1 a-c *Paramyxidium magi* n. sp. from the stomach wall of *Anguilla anguilla*. Fresh spore in valvular view showing the polar capsules enclosing the polar filaments (**a**), stained imprint of two spores, in the sutural plane, showing a sigmoidal sutural line (arrows) (**b**) and a fresh spore with numerous valvular striations (**c**). **d-f** Line drawings of *P. giardi* from the kidney of an eel; in sutural view (**d**), valvular view (**e**) and one with the valvular striations (**f**). **g-k** *P. bulani* n. sp. from the kidney of *Megalops cyprinoides*. **g, h** Fresh spores in sutural view, showing the polar capsules (**g**) and the sutural line (arrow) (**h**). **i** Histological sections showing the two parallel nuclei (arrows) between the polar capsules. **j, k** Line drawings in sutural (**j**) and valvular (**k**) views. **l** Fresh Aurantiactionmyxon type actinospores from the oligochaete *Lumbriculus variagatus* from Lake Vifilsstadavatn in Iceland

Paramyxidum bulani n. sp. infects the kidney. The plasmodia are polysporous, somewhat elongated (size range: length, 25–75 μm; width, 10–22 μm) and develop as intratubular, both in proximal and distal tubules. They are seen at various stages in development, some of which are fully mature, and commonly attached to the brush border of the proximal kidney tubule epithelium. In the distal kidney tubules, the proportion of mature plasmodia seem higher (Fig 2d). No pathology was associated with infections.

No host response, such as encapsulation by fibroblasts or infiltration of immune cells, was detected in association with any of these four different myxosporeans.

Molecular analyses

SSU rDNA sequences were successfully sequenced for *P. giardi* (2076 bp) and for the three species recognised here as new, i.e. *P. magi* n. sp. (2070 bp), *P. branchialis* n. sp. (2082 bp), *P. bulani* n. sp. (2056 bp) and the Aurantiactinomyxon (865 bp), which have been assigned accession numbers in GenBank: MH414925-MH414929. BLAST searches confirmed a myxosporean origin for all sequences with closest matches in the database being to numerous actinosporean sequences and also *Myxidium lieberkuehni* Bütschli, 1882, the type-species of the genus *Myxidium*. The *SSU* rDNA sequences from infected tissues from eels, were all very distinct, with percentage similarities ranging from 92.93% to as low as 89.8%, over > 2000 bp of sequence data (Table 4). The *SSU* rDNA sequence from *P. bulani* n. sp. was even more dissimilar, being < 84% similar to any of the other myxospore sequences, and only 81.75% similar to the kidney-infecting *P. giardi* from eels (Table 4); only *M. lieberkuehni* was more dissimilar, being < 79% similar to any of the sequences generated from myxospore infections (Table 4). The Aurantiactinomyxon sequence did not match any of the sequences generated from the myxospores in this study and was most similar (96.07%) to *P. magi* n. sp.

Molecular phylogenetic analyses produced trees with very similar topologies irrespective of the methodology used (Fig. 3). All *Paramyxidium* spp. were fully supported in a clade with numerous actinosporean sequences (*Paramyxidium* clade) shown as the lilac box in Fig. 3. *Paramyxidium bulani* n. sp. from a tarpon in Malaysia, represented the basal sequence of the clade. The *Myxidium* clade (*sensu stricto*), that includes the type-species *M. lieberkuehni*, was also fully supported (red box, Fig. 3) and formed a fully supported sister group to the clade containing *Chloromyxum* spp. (green box, Fig. 3). Together these formed a robustly supported sister clade to the *Paramyxidium* clade. The Platysporina (blue box, Fig. 3) formed a fully supported sister clade to this *Paramyxidium* / *Myxidium* (*s.s.*) / *Chloromyxum* grouping. Basal to this is the hepatic biliary clade, a well-supported clade which contains numerous taxa currently assigned to the Myxidiidae, some of which infect vertebrates other than fish [22].

Taxonomy

Class Myxosporea Bütschli, 1881
Suborder Variisporina Lom & Noble, 1984
Family Myxidiidae Thélohan, 1892

Genus *Paramyxidium* n. g.

Diagnosis

Myxospore length width ratio between 1.4–1.6:1 resulting in a lemon-shaped form in valvular aspect and oval to bluntly-rounded form in sutural view. Valvular striations present, with sigmoidal sutural line. Polar capsules two, almost spherical. Two nuclei in the sporoplasm positioned between polar capsules. Capsular foramina open sub-terminally. Histozoic polysporous plasmodia develop in various host tissues with different species infecting different host tissues.

Type-species: *Paramyxidium giardi* (Cépède, 1906) n. comb.

Table 3 Measurements of twenty fresh actinospores observed in this study

Actinospore type	Host species	Diameter of spherical spore body Range (Mean)	Length of caudal process Range (Mean)	Width of caudal process Range (Mean)	Largest span between end of caudal processes Range (Mean)	Reference
Aurantiactinomyxon	*L. variegatus*	9.0–12.5 (10.4)	14.5–16.3 (15.4)	7.5–10 (8.5)	29.9–32.5 (30.8)	Present study

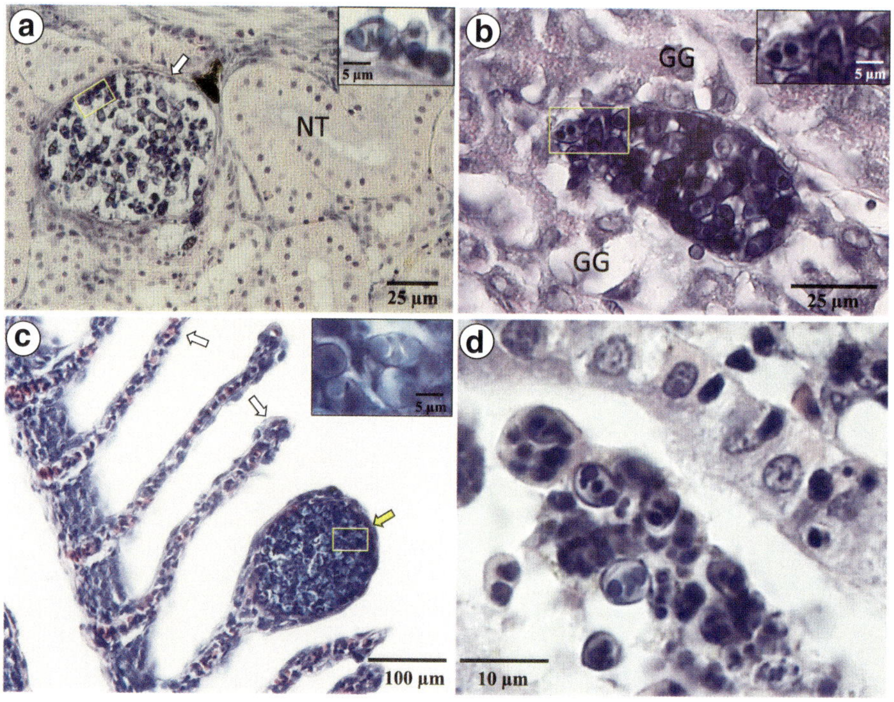

Fig. 2 **a** A polysporous plasmodium of *Paramyxidium giardi* inside a kidney tubule of *Anguilla anguilla*, where is causes extensive widening of the tubules causing atrophy and necrosis of the tubular epithelial cell (arrow); insert shows higher magnification of spores from within the yellow box. **b** A polysporous plasmodium of *P. magi* n. sp. in the gastric gland of stomach wall; insert shows higher magnification of spores from within the yellow box. **c** Normal secondary gill lamellae of *A. anguilla* (white arrow) and one infected with *P. branchialis* n. sp. (yellow arrow). The large plasmodium causes disruption of epithelium and the pillar cells of the secondary lamella; insert shows higher magnification of spores from within the yellow box. **d** *P. bulani* n. sp. infection in the kidney of a Pacific tarpon. The parasite develops inside the kidney tubules, often attached to the brush border of the tubular epithelial cells, without causing any apparent pathology. *Abbreviations*: GG, gastric glands; NT, normal tubule

Other species: *Paramyxidium branchialis* n. sp.; *Paramyxidium bulani* n. sp.; *Paramyxidium magi* n. sp.
Etymology: The new genus is named *Paramyxidium* n. g. as it is placed next to the type-species of the genus *Myxidium* (*s.s.*) in phylogenetic analyses.
ZooBank registration: To comply with the regulations set out in article 8.5 of the amended 2012 version of the *International Code of Zoological Nomenclature* (ICZN) [29], details of the new genus have been submitted to ZooBank. The Life Science Identifier (LSID) of the article is: urn:lsid:zoobank.org:pub:716F81BB-DAFC-4-B33-89ES-A57684065765. The LSID for the new genus name *Paramyxidium* is: urn:lsid:zoobank.org:act:27B9FBC6-345A-4DD9-93D6-A13EACB82A18.

Remarks

Paramyxidium spp. are sufficiently different with respect to either myxospore morphology/ characteristics, tissue location, host type or DNA sequences to necessitate the erection of a novel genus within the family

Table 4 Percentage identities of *SSU* rDNA sequences (above the diagonal) and number of bases compared (below the diagonal) for the new sequences in the *Paramyxidium* clade (bold), related actinospores and the type-species of the genus *Myxidium*, *M. lieberkuehni*

		1	2	3	4	5	6	7	8
1	***Paramyxidium giardi***	–	92.93	89.80	98.29	89.91	94.79	81.75	77.98
2	***Paramyxidium magi*** **n. sp.**	2051	–	91.34	92.50	91.12	96.07	82.61	79.90
3	***Paramyxidium branchialis*** **n. sp.**	2058	2055	–	89.17	95.77	90.35	83.08	78.70
4	*Aurantiactinomyxon* (AF483598)	1931	1933	1930	–	89.58	94.07	81.27	77.60
5	*Synactinomyxon* (AY787784)	1605	1599	1606	1602	–	91.31	82.15	77.53
6	***Aurantiactinomyxon***	864	865	860	860	863	–	83.55	80.05
7	***Paramyxidium bulani*** **n. sp.**	2044	2041	2039	1917	1585	863	–	78.70
8	*Myxidium lieberkuehni* (X76638)	2021	2014	2028	1893	1562	827	2009	–

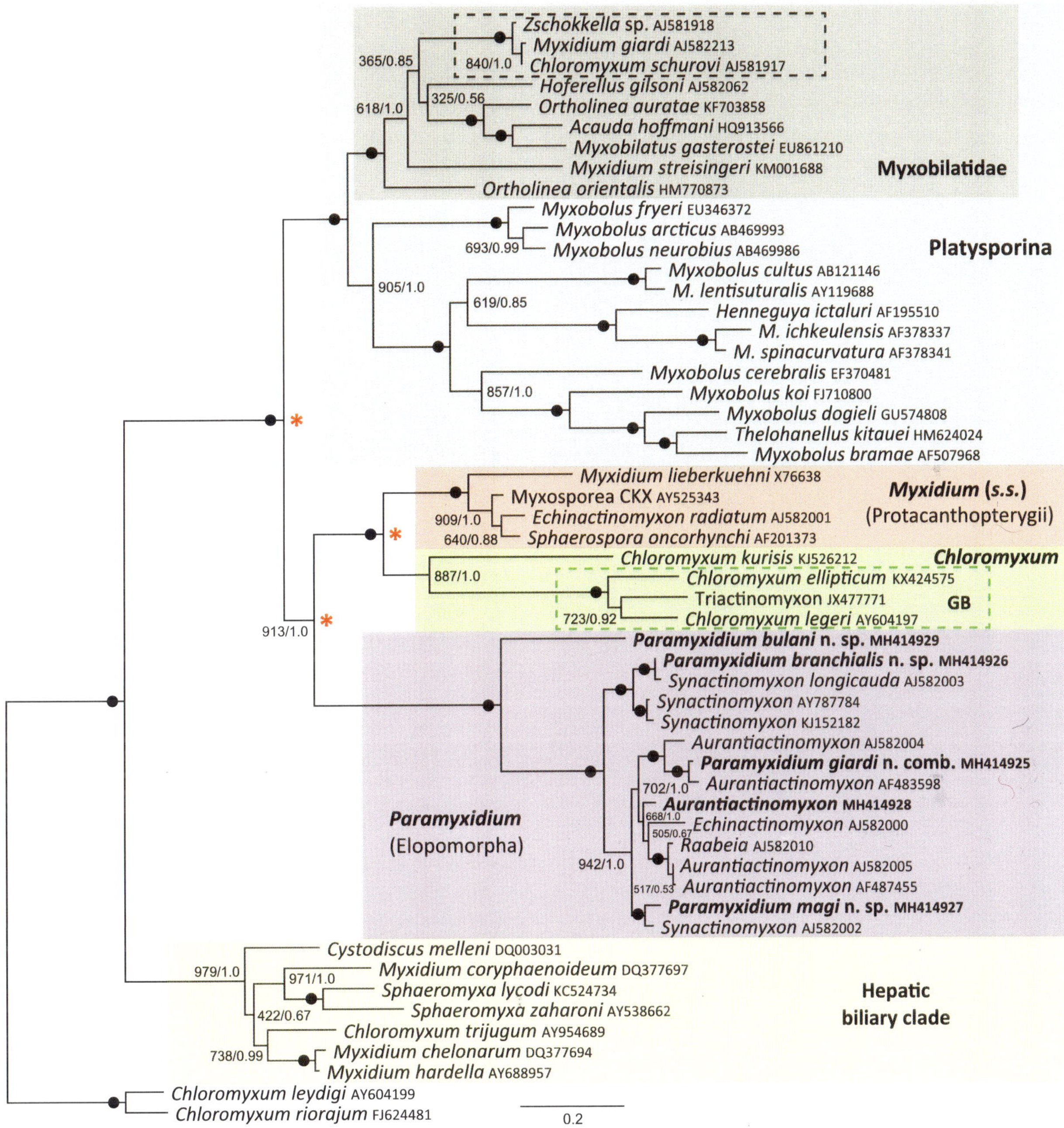

Fig. 3 Maximum likelihood topology of small subunit ribosomal DNA from 54 myxosporeans, rooted to *Chloromyxum leydigi* and *C. riorajum* (infecting cartilaginous fishes). Bootstrap support values and posterior probabilities are shown at the nodes; solid black dots indicate full support for that node. Novel sequences from this study are in bold and contained within the *Paramyxidium* Clade (lilac box). The *Paramyxidium* clade forms a robust sister clade relationship with *Myxidium* clade (*sensu stricto*) (red box) and the *Chloromyxum* clade (green box). The dashed green box within the *Chloromyxum* clade shows species that infect the gall-bladder (GB) of cypriniform fishes. Nodes with a red asterisk indicate that the common ancestor was likely to have been a renal-infecting myxosporean. The Platysporina (blue box) forms a fully supported sister clade to this *Paramyxidium* / *Myxidium* (*s.s.*) / *Chloromyxum* grouping and includes the Myxobilatidae (grey box). Highlighted within the Myxobilatidae, by a dashed black box, is the *Chloromyxum schurovi* sub-clade that contains other renal isolates from eels that have been reported as *Myxidium giardi* and *Zschokkella* sp. Basal to these main clades is the hepatic biliary clade, a well-supported clade which contains numerous taxa, some of which infect vertebrates other than fish

Myxidiidae Thélohan, 1892 to accommodate them. The family Myxidiidae currently contains five genera: *Myxidium* Bütschli, 1882; *Coccomyxa* Léger & Hesse, 1907; *Cystodiscus* Lutz, 1889; *Enteromyxum* Palenzuela, Redondo & Alvarez-Pellitero, 2002; *Soricimyxum* Prunescu, Prunescu, Pucek & Lom, 2007; and

Zschokkella Auerbach, 1910. Species of *Cystodiscus* and *Soricimyxum* are only found in non-fish hosts [22]. *Enteromyxum* spp. have very large and elongated polar capsules, spores that lack valvular striations, and are phylogenetically associated with morphologically similar forms from the gastrointestinal tract of marine fishes [4]. *Coccomyxa* spp. are typically found in the gall-bladder of marine fishes, are more ellipsoidal in morphology, and are phylogenetically distantly placed in the marine gall-bladder (marine *Myxidium*) clade [2]. The genera *Myxidium* and *Zschokkella* are more complicated to decipher for as both are polyphyletic, with many species likely being wrongly attributed to each genus [1, 2, 4]. However, DNA sequence data convincingly placed all *Paramyxidium* taxa in a robust clade which is sister to the *Myxidium* clade (*s.s.*). In addition, host differences and tissue tropism are apparent, with *Paramyxidium* taxa infecting the Elopomorpha in numerous organs and *Myxidium* spp. (*s.s.*) infecting the renal system of members of the Protacanthopterygii.

Therefore, we erect the genus *Paramyxidium* to accommodate these myxosporeans, and transfer *Myxidium giardi* as *Paramyxidium giardi* Cépède, 1906 n. comb. as the type-species. The annelid hosts for *Paramyxidium* spp. are likely to be oligochaetes. Currently known species are restricted to freshwater environments and fish hosts from the Elopomorpha, presumably becoming infected during migratory periods into fresh water.

Paramyxidium magi n. sp.

Type-host: *Anguilla anguilla* (L.) (Anguilliformes: Anguillidae).
Type-locality: Lake Vifilsstadavatn (64°4'47.39"N, 21° 52'26.45"W), Iceland.
Type-specimens: Hapantotypes (histological sections and phototypes) were deposited at the Natural History Museum, London, UK, under the accession number NHMUK 2018.235.
Site in host: Stomach.
Prevalence: 19% (6/31).
Representative DNA sequences: A partial *SSU* rDNA sequence (2070 bp) was deposited in the GenBank database under the accession number MH414927.
ZooBank registration: To comply with the regulations set out in article 8.5 of the amended 2012 version of the *International Code of Zoological Nomenclature* (ICZN) [29], details of the new species have been submitted to ZooBank. The LSID for the new species name *Paramyxidium magi* is: urn:lsid:zoobank.org:act:FEC23203-00E5-4862-8D24-FA5D6D8FFB0C.
Etymology: Specific name derived from Icelandic for stomach 'magi'

Description

Spore. Mature spores lemon-shaped in valvular aspect (Fig. 1a), oval to bluntly-rounded in sutural view with sigmoidal sutural line (Fig. 1b), measuring 10.8–12.9 × 7.0–8.4 (11.6 × 7.6) (L × W) (n = 20). Polar capsules almost spherical, 3.6–4.6 × 3.1–4.0 (4.0 × 3.6) (n = 20), opening sub-terminally (Fig. 1a-b). Fine spore striations visible across both spore valves (Fig. 1c).

Remarks

Histozoic in the stomach wall forming polysporous plasmodia of variable sizes (*c*.60–95 μm) in the gastric gland interstitium (Fig. 2b). Differs from other *Paramyxidium* spp. primarily on the site of infection and genetic distance.

Paramyxidium bulani n. sp.

Type-host: *Megalops cyprinoides* Broussonet (Elopiformes: Megalopidae).
Type-locality: Kilim mangroves, Langkawi Island, Malaysia.
Other localities: Pangkor Island, Malaysia.
Type-specimens: Hapantotypes (histological sections and phototypes) were deposited at the Natural History Museum, London, UK, under the accession number NHMUK 2018.237.
Site in host: Kidney.
Prevalence: 29% (4/14).
Representative DNA sequences: A partial *SSU* rDNA sequence (2059 bp) was deposited in the GenBank database under the accession number MH414929.
ZooBank registration: To comply with the regulations set out in article 8.5 of the amended 2012 version of the *International Code of Zoological Nomenclature* (ICZN) [29], details of the new species have been submitted to ZooBank. The LSID for the new species name *Paramyxidium bulani* is: urn:lsid:zoobank.org:act:DA7B51B0-590F-45A5-88CF-32A015B99593.
Etymology: Specific name refers to the local Malay name for the fish host (ikan bulan).

Description

Spore. Mature spores oval to bluntly-rounded in sutural view, lemon-shaped in valvular aspect, 6.1–6.9 × 4.2–5.1 (6.7 × 4.7) (L × W) (n = 20). Polar capsules almost spherical, 2.1–2.5 × 1.5–2.0 (2.3 × 1.8) (n = 20), opening sub-terminally. Sutural line sigmoidal and inconspicuous (Fig. 1g-k), spore valves with fine striations.

Remarks

Plasmodia are elongated and polysporous (size range: length, 25–75 μm; width, 10–22 μm) and develop as intratubular, in both proximal and distal kidney tubules. Differs from other *Paramyxidium* spp. by having much smaller myxospores and infecting the kidney of Pacific tarpon. Stained spores have a sporoplasm containing two nuclei (Figs. 1i and 2d)

Paramyxidium branchialis n. sp.

Type-host: *Anguilla anguilla* (L.) (Anguilliformes: Anguillidae).
Type-locality: Lake Vifilsstadavatn (64°4'47.39"N, 21° 52'26.45"W), Iceland.
Type-specimens: Hapantotypes (histological sections and phototypes) were deposited at the Natural History Museum, London, UK, under the accession number NHMUK 2018.236.
Site in host: Gills.
Prevalence: 83% (25/31).
Representative DNA sequence: A partial *SSU* rDNA sequence (2082 bp) was deposited in the GenBank database under the accession number MH414926.
ZooBank registration: To comply with the regulations set out in article 8.5 of the amended 2012 version of the *International Code of Zoological Nomenclature* (ICZN) [29], details of the new species have been submitted to ZooBank. The LSID for the new species name *Paramyxidium branchialis* is: urn:lsid:zoobank.org:act:2481F7F4-5B9F-42C8-B2EB-FED264FA7283.
Etymology: Specific name refers to site of infection in the host.

Description

Spore. Mature spores oval to bluntly-rounded in sutural view, lemon-shaped in valvular aspect, 10.7–12.3 × 6.6–7.8 (11.6 × 7.3) (L × W) (n = 20). Polar capsules almost spherical, 3.9-4.5 × 3.2-4.2 (4.2 × 3.8) (n = 20), opening sub-terminally. Sutural line sigmoidal and inconspicuous. Fine spore striations visible across both spore valves.

Remarks

Plasmodia are polysporous, differ significantly in size (*c*.35–142 µm), and develop in the gills (Fig. 2c), whereas other species in the genus develop in different host tissues. Differs from other *Paramyxidium* spp. primarily on the site of infection and genetic distance.

Discussion

Morphological features, such as myxospore size and number of valvular striation, have been used to identify or differentiate between species of *Myxidium* infecting eels in the past [6–10]. However, with such conserved myxospore morphology within the *Paramyxidium* n. g. clade, we do not find this to be a reliable feature to successfully differentiate between species. The location of the parasite within certain specific host tissues would appear to be a far more useful characteristic, with similar tissue tropism being reported for other myxosporean clades in the past [1, 2, 4]. The European eel and its parasites have been extensively studied [5–7, 14] and there have been numerous reports of *Myxidium giardi* infecting the European eel [7, 12, 30]. However, many of these reports of *M. giardi* infections are from tissues other than kidney and it is therefore highly likely that many of these diagnoses are in fact detailing a morphologically similar parasite from the genus *Paramyxidium* but not *M. giardi*. Numerous taxa that fit within the *Paramyxidium* may already be described [8–12], or have been synonymised with other species due to similar spore morphologies [7, 12]. Given the clear differences in *SSU* rDNA data that exist between the known members of this new genus, it is imperative that such data is supplied when validating or describing novel species within this group. The *Paramyxidium* clade currently contains sequences from myxospores that infect various tissues of fish from the superorder Elopomorpha (tarpon/ladyfish and eels). The clade is also comprised of numerous sequences generated from actinospores that probably represent a hidden diversity of unidentified myxosporeans infecting various tissues from anguillid eels; as the sequences have all been generated from European freshwater systems that lack elopiform fish other than eels and *Myxidium*-like infections have been noted in numerous tissues from the European eel [31, 32].

Our phylogenies show that the *Paramyxidium* group is robustly supported as a sister clade to the *Myxidium* clade (*s.s.*) / *Chloromyxum* grouping that form as fully supported subclades (Fig. 3). These three clades all demonstrate levels of fish host association and degrees of tissue tropism. All currently known members of the *Myxidium* clade (*s.s.*) are described from the renal systems of either pike or salmonids (Protacanthopterygii), whilst the adjacent *Chloromyxum* sister group are all described from Cypriniformes, when infecting the gall-bladder (dashed green box, Fig. 3), with the basal species from the clade, *Chloromyxum kurisis* (GenBank: KJ526212), being from the urinary tract of an Atheriniformes fish. This suggests that these two clades have evolved from a common ancestor that infected the renal system of fish potentially having a *Chloromyxum*-like form. The *Paramyxidium*, as a sister to these two groups, have only been described from the Elopomorpha, with the basal species in the clade again coming from a renal infection, further indicating that the common ancestor for the whole grouping was likely to have been a renal myxosporean. A deeper extension of this phenomenon can also be applied to our tree topology. The node from which the Platysporina clade forms as a sister to the *Paramyxidium*/ *Myxidium* (*s.s.*) clade, could also represent a common ancestor that infected the renal system of fish. Recently the Myxobilatidae (all renal-infecting) have been shown to be phylogenetically placed within the platysporinids [33], therefore, a renal myxosporean ancestry for the Platysporina is plausible, which could also be associated with a *Chloromyxum*-form. This outcome is not unexpected, as it has been previously demonstrated that the *Chloromyxum* morphotype is important in phylogenetic studies and appears to represent a basal morphotype for numerous myxosporean clades [22, 23, 34]. Therefore, additional sequence data from this basal morphotype, in particular when infecting more ancient fish lineages (Atheriniformes, Cypriniformes, Elopomorpha and Protacanthopterygii), will assist in future phylogenetic studies of the Myxosporea and help to better resolve the relationships between certain reproducible clades.

Certain anomalies do exist in our phylogenetic tree, which can be explained as follows. The *Myxidium* clade (*s.s.*) currently contains myxosporeans that infect the urinary system of fish from the Protacanthopterygii, a superorder of more basal teleosts, which includes the Salmoniformes (salmonids) and Esociformes (pikes). The sequence in the tree representing *Sphaerospora oncorhynchi* Kent, Whitaker & Margolis, 1993 (GenBank: AF201373) is, therefore, more likely to be from a fish that was co-infected with a *Myxidium*, likely related to the *Myxidium* sp. described as the CKX myxosporean from coho salmon in Canada [35]. Indeed, studies have found both *S. oncorhynchi* and *Myxidium salvelini* Konovalov & Shul'man, 1966, in the renal systems from the same *Oncorhynchus* spp. [36, 37] and other striated *Myxidium* spp. have been reported from the urinary systems of salmonids: *Myxidium minteri* Yasutake & Wood, 1957; *M. salvelini* Konovalov et Shul'man, 1966; *Myxidium noblei* Konovalov, 1966; *Myxidium* sp. of Mavor & Strasser, 1918.

The positioning of the sequences *Zschokkella* sp. (GenBank: AJ581918), *Chloromyxum schurovi* (GenBank: AJ581917) and *Myxidium giardi* (GenBank: AJ582213) (dashed black box, Fig. 3), all generated from the same study [13], within a sub-clade of the Myxobilatidae (Platysporina) remains puzzling, especially the *Myxidium*/*Zschokkella* spore forms that exclusively belong to the Variisporina and should not therefore be present in the Platysporina [33]. This concern is reinforced, as the sequence given for *M. giardi* in eels from Scotland is almost identical to that of *C. schurovi* from salmonids [13]. In his description of the genus *Acauda*, Whipps [38] demonstrated the clustering of the genera *Acauda*, *Myxobilatus* and *Hoferellus* in phylogenetic analyses and noted that the myxospores shared similar morphological features, all having longitudinally striated spore valves and a sutural plane that bisects a pair of polar capsules. This combination of features justified the reuse of the family Myxobilatidae Shul'man, 1953, to accommodate these three genera. In addition, it has been demonstrated that *Ortholinea* should be included in the family Myxobilatidae, as *Ortholinea* spp. share similar morphological features, group within the same clade, and collectively they are all parasitic in the renal system of fish [33]. *Chloromyxum* myxospores also share some synapomorphies with this group, having subspherical or elongated spores that may have caudal appendages, with a straight central suture. *Chloromyxum* is known to be polyphyletic genus and the retention of some features (4 polar capsules) in some derived species could explain why evolved chloromyxid forms are present in some clades, such as the Myxobilatidae clade (*C. schurovi*) and the hepatic biliary clade (*Chloromyxum trijugum*). Indeed, Holzer et. al. [39], reported that *C. schurovi*, whilst being genetically similar to members of the clade it occupied (Myxobilatidae), it shares less than 70% identity to other more basal *Chloromyxum* species and concluded it had evolved further than all other sequenced chloromyxids [39]. Therefore, the inclusion of *C. schurovi* with the Myxobilatidae can potentially be explained in terms of DNA sequence, spore morphology and tissue tropism. However, the presence of *Myxidium giardi* (GenBank: AJ582213) and *Zschokkella* sp. (GenBank: AJ581918) still cannot, as spores with these morphologies share no synapomorphies with any members of the clade or the predicted ancestral morphotypes, which are assumed to be chloromyxids. One possibility is that the sequences generated for *M. giardi* and *Zschokkella* sp. either do not correspond to the myxospores that were observed in the tissue samples, or that they were misidentified. They may represent variants of a sequence for *Zschokkella stettinensis* Wierzbicka, 1987, described from the urinary bladder of the European eel [40]. Indeed, the author of the sequences in question also indicated, in their PhD thesis, that *Z. stettinensis* was a possible identity for this myxosporean [41]. The myxospores of *Z. stettinensis* look superficially like those of *M. giardi* but are also very similar to the *Neomyxobolus* morphotype (known to infect the renal system of freshwater fishes), being described as spores having two delicate streaks running parallel to the suture [40], a feature almost unique to *Neomyxobolus* spp. [42]. Therefore, we suggest that these sequences represent variations of *Z. stettinensis* or genetically related forms, which are better placed in the genus *Neomyxobolus* Chen et Hsieh, 1960. *Myxidium streisingeri* Whipps, Murray & Kent, 2015 also groups in the Myxobilatidae and is another species showing several traits in common with the genus *Neomyxobolus* [33], indicating that it has been mistakenly placed as *Myxidium*. Furthermore, these species also have the tissue location (renal system) and spore characteristics to allow placement in the Myxobilatidae.

In the present study, coinfections with other myxosporeans were not observed in Icelandic eels, only *Paramyxidium* morphologies were observed. However, the Pacific tarpon is known to have other myxosporean parasites [4]. Therefore, it is possible when sampling tissues such as the kidney, that blood-borne stages of non-target myxosporean could be amplified in error. This is considered to be unlikely in this case, as most of the myxosporean taxa from the Pacific tarpon from the type location have been identified [4, 43] (MAF, unpublished data). In addition, the fact that these distantly related parasites form a robust monophyletic clade, support the fact that the sequences were derived from the myxospore forms observed.

Conclusions

Paramyxidium giardi n. comb. (syn. *Myxidium giardi*) does not cause systemic infections in eels. In Iceland there are three species now confirmed, using morphological and molecular data. Additional species probably exist that infect different tissues, such as the skin, and a further member of this clade was identified here from an *Aurantiactinomyxon* sequence. Therefore, the site of infection in the host eels is an important diagnostic feature for this group (*Paramyxidium* clade). Myxospore morphology is highly conserved in the *Paramyxidium* clade, and although some myxospore dimensions are noted as significantly different between isolates, differentiating species based on spore dimension alone is not recommended. Despite very similar myxospore morphologies being present across the group there are relatively low genetic similarities between *SSU* rDNA sequences. The *Paramyxidium* clade is a well-supported sister to the *Myxidium* (*s.s.*) and *Chloromyxum* clades, each demonstrating a degree of fish host group specificity.

Abbreviations

BLAST: Basic Local Alignment Search Tool; LSID: Life Science Identifier; *s.s: sensu stricto*; SEM: Scanning electron microscopy

Acknowledgements

The authors would like to thank the technical services for assistance with histology and SEM.

Funding

Funding for the study was provided by a University of Malaya Research Grant (UMRG) No: RG201-12SUS. Funding for publication costs was provided by the Centre for Conservation Medicine and Ecosystem Health, Ross University School of Veterinary Medicine.

Authors' contributions

MAF and AK sampled the fish and isolated the parasites. AK performed the histology and MAF the PCR and phylogenetics. MAF drafted the manuscript. Both authors read and approved the final manuscript.

Competing interests

The authors declare that they have no competing interests.

Author details

[1]Ross University School of Veterinary Medicine, Basseterre, Saint Kitts and Nevis. [2]Institute for Experimental Pathology, University of Iceland, Reykjavík, Iceland.

References

1. Fiala I. The phylogeny of Myxosporea (Myxozoa) based on small subunit ribosomal RNA gene analysis. Int J Parasitol. 2006;36:1521–34.
2. Freeman MA, Yokoyama H, Ogawa K. Description and phylogeny of *Ceratomyxa anko* sp. n. and *Zschokkella lophii* sp. n. from the Japanese anglerfish, *Lophius litulon* (Jordan). J Fish Dis. 2008;31:921–30.
3. Bartošová P, Freeman MA, Yokoyama H, Caffara M, Fiala I. Phylogenetic position of *Sphaerospora testicularis* and *Latyspora scomberomori* n. gen. n. sp. (Myxozoa) within the marine urinary clade. Parasitology. 2011;138:381–93.
4. Freeman MA, Kristmundsson Á. Histozoic myxosporeans infecting the stomach wall of elopiform fishes represent a novel lineage, the Gastromyxidae. Parasit Vectors. 2015;8:517.
5. Cépède C. *Myxidium giardi* Cépède, et la prétendue immunité des Anguilles a l'ègard des infections myxosporidiennes. Compt Rend Séances Soc Biol Ses Fil. 1906;6:170–3.
6. Treasurer JW, Cox D. The occurrence of *Myxidium giardi* Cépède, in cultured eels, *Anguilla anguilla* L., in West Scotland. Bull Eur Ass. Fish Pathol. 1997;17:171–3.
7. Copland JW. The occurrence and distribution of *Myxidium giardi* Cépède, 1906 in wild and cultured European eels, *Anguilla anguilla* L., in England. J Fish Dis. 1981;4:231–42.
8. Fujita T. Studies on Myxosporidia of Japan. J Fac Agric Hokkaido Imp Univ. 1927;16:229–47.
9. Hine PM. Three new species of *Myxidium* (Protozoa: Myxosporidia) parasitic in *Anguilla australis* Richardson, 1848 and *A. dieffenbachii* Gray, 1842 in New Zealand. J R Soc N Z. 1975;5:153–61.
10. Ishii S. Myxosporidiosis of the Japanese eel. Zool Magazine Tokyo. 1915;27:372–82.
11. Hine PM. Variations in the spores of *Myxidium zealandicum* Hine, 1975 (Protozoa: Myxosporidia). N Z J Mar Freshwater Res. 1978;12:189–95.
12. Hine PM. A review of some species of *Myxidium* Bütschli, 1882 (Myxosporea) from eels (*Anguilla* spp.). J Protozool. 1980;27:260–7.
13. Holzer AS, Sommerville C, Wootten R. Molecular relationships and phylogeny in a community of myxosporeans and actinosporeans based on their 18S rDNA sequences. Int J Parasitol. 2004;34:1099–111.
14. Tesch FW. The Eel. 5th ed. Edited by Thorpe JE. Oxford, UK: Blackwell Publishing; 2003. p. 73–119.
15. Jacoby D, Gollock M. *Anguilla anguilla*. The IUCN Red List of Threatened Species 2014: e.T60344A45833138. https://doi.org/10.2305/IUCN.UK.2014-1.RLTS.T60344A45833138.en.
16. Shen KN, Chang CW, Iizuka Y, Tzeng WN. Facultative habitat selection in Pacific tarpon *Megalops cyprinoides* as revealed by otolith Sr:Ca ratios. Mar Ecol Prog Ser. 2009;387:255–63.
17. Tsukamoto Y, Okiyama M. Growth during the early life-history of the Pacific tarpon *Megalops cyprinoides*. Japan J Ichthyol. 1993;39:379–86.
18. Chen JN, López JA, Lavoué S, Miya M, Chen WJ. Phylogeny of the Elopomorpha (Teleostei): evidence from six nuclear and mitochondrial markers. Mol Phylogenet Evol. 2014;70:152–61.
19. Altschul SF, Gish W, Miller W, Myers EW, Lipman DJ. Basic local alignment search tool. J Mol Biol. 1990;215:403–10.
20. Thompson JD, Gibson TJ, Plewniak F, Jeanmougin F, Higgins DG. The CLUSTAL-X windows interface: flexible strategies for multiple sequence alignment aided by quality analysis tools. Nucl Acids Res. 1997;24:4876–82.
21. Hall TA. BioEdit: a user-friendly biological sequence alignment editor and analysis program for Windows 95/98/ NT. Nucleic Acids Symp Ser. 1999;41:95–8.
22. Kristmundsson A, Freeman MA. Sphaeromyxids form part of a diverse group of myxosporeans infecting the hepatic biliary systems of a wide range of host organisms. Parasit Vectors. 2013;6:13.
23. Sanders JL, Jaramillo AG, Ashford JE, Feist SW, Lafferty KD, Kent ML. Two myxozoans from the urinary tract of topsmelt, *Atherinops affinis*. J Parasitol. 2015;101:577–86.
24. Saitou N, Nei M. The neighbour-joining method: a new method for reconstructing phylogenetic trees. Mol Biol Evol. 1987;4:406–25.
25. Guindon S, Dufayard JF, Lefort V, Anisimov M, Hordijk W, Gascuel O. New algorithms and methods to estimate maximum-likelihood phylogenies: assessing the performance of PhyML 3.0. Syst Biol. 2010;59:307–21.

26. Ronquist F, Huelsenbeck JP. MrBayes 3: Bayesian phylogenetic inference under mixed models. Bioinformatics. 2003;19:1572–4.
27. Nylander JAA, Ronquist F, Huelsenbeck JP, Nieves-Aldrey JL. Bayesian phylogenetic analysis of combined data. Syst Biol. 2004;53:47–67.
28. Copland JW. The pathology of *Myxidium giardi* Cépède, 1906 infections in wild and cultured eels, *Anguilla anguilla* L. J Fish Dis. 1983;6:451–60.
29. ICZN. *International Commission on Zoological Nomenclature*: Amendment of articles 8, 9, 10, 21 and 78 of the International Code of Zoological Nomenclature to expand and refine methods of publication. Bull Zool Nomencl 2012;69:161–9.
30. Jakob E, Walter T, Hanel R. A checklist of the protozoan and metazoan parasites of European eel (*Anguilla anguilla*): checklist of *Anguilla anguilla* parasites. J Appl Ichthyol. 2016;32:757–804.
31. Kristmundsson Á, Helgason S. Parasite communities of eels *Anguilla anguilla* in freshwater and marine habitats in Iceland in comparison with other parasite communities of eels in Europe. Folia Parasitol. 2007;54:141–53.
32. Kristmundsson Á. Sjúkdómar/sníkjudýr í villtum álum, *Anguilla* spp. á Íslandi [Diseases/parasites of wild eels, *Anguilla* spp., in Iceland]. MSc Thesis, University of Iceland, Reykjavík, Iceland; 2003, 1–78 (In Icelandic).
33. Karlsbakk E, Kristmundsson Á, Albano M, Brown P, Freeman MA. Redescription and phylogenetic position of *Myxobolus aeglefini* and *Myxobolus platessae* n. comb. (Myxosporea), parasites in the cartilage of some North Atlantic marine fishes, with notes on the phylogeny and classification of the Platysporina. Parasitol Int. 2017;66:952–9.
34. Fiala I, Bartošová P. History of myxozoan character evolution on the basis of rDNA and EF-2 data. BMC Evol Biol. 2010;10:228.
35. Jones S, Prosperi-Porta G, Dawe S, Blackbourn J, Taylor K, Lowe G, Osborn A. Proliferative renal myxosporidiosis in spawning coho salmon (*Oncorhynchus kisutch*) in British Columbia and Washington. Folia Parasitol. 2004;51:221–7.
36. Kent ML, Khattra J, Hervio DML, Devlin RH. Ribosomal DNA sequence analysis of isolates of the PKX myxosporean and their relationship to members of the genus *Sphaerospora*. J Aquat Anim Health. 1998;10:12–21.
37. Kent ML, Margolis L, Whitaker DJ, Hoskins GE, McDonald TE. Review of Myxosporea of importance in salmonid fisheries and aquaculture in British Columbia. Folia Parasitol. 1994;41:27–37.
38. Whipps CM. Interrenal disease in bluegills (*Lepomis macrochirus*) caused by a new genus and species of myxozoan. J Parasitol. 2011;97:1159–65.
39. Holzer AS, Sommerville C, Wootten R. Molecular identity, phylogeny and life cycle of *Chloromyxum schurovi* Shul'man & Ieshko 2003. Parasitol Res. 2006; 99:90–6.
40. Wierzbicka J. *Zschokkella stettinensis* sp. n. (Myxospora, Bivalvulida) a parasite of eel, *Anguilla anguilla* (L.). Acta Protozool. 1987;26:79–82.
41. Holzer AS. Molecular studies on *Sphaerospora truttae* and other freshwater myxozoans. PhD Thesis, Stirling University, Stirling, UK, 2001. http://hdl.handle.net/1893/21826.
42. Chen CL, Hsieh SR. Studies on sporozoa from the freshwater fishes *Ophiocephalus maculatus* and *O. argus* of China. Acta Hydrobiol. 1960;2:171–96.
43. Fiala I, Hlavničková M, Kodádková A, Freeman MA, Bartošová-Sojková P, Atkinson SD. Evolutionary origin of *Ceratonova shasta* and phylogeny of the marine myxosporean lineage. Mol Phylogenet Evol. 2015;86:75–89.

12

Lymphatic filariasis transmission in Rufiji District, southeastern Tanzania: infection status of the human population and mosquito vectors after twelve rounds of mass drug administration

Clarer Jones[1*], Billy Ngasala[1,2], Yahya A. Derua[3], Donath Tarimo[1], Lisa Reimer[4], Moses Bockarie[5] and Mwelecele N. Malecela[6]

Abstract

Background: Control of lymphatic filariasis (LF) in most of the sub-Saharan African countries is based on annual mass drug administration (MDA) using a combination of ivermectin and albendazole. Monitoring the impact of this intervention is crucial for measuring the success of the LF elimination programmes. This study assessed the status of LF infection in Rufiji district, southeastern Tanzania after twelve rounds of MDA.

Methods: Community members aged between 10 and 79 years were examined for *Wuchereria bancrofti* circulating filarial antigens (CFA) using immunochromatographic test cards (ICTs) and antigen-positive individuals were screened for microfilaraemia. All study participants were examined for clinical manifestation of LF and interviewed for drug uptake during MDA rounds. Filarial mosquito vectors were collected indoor and outdoor and examined for infection with *W. bancrofti* using a microscope and quantitative real-time polymerase chain reaction (qPCR) techniques.

Results: Out of 854 participants tested, nine (1.1%) were positive for CFA and one (0.1%) was found to be microfilaraemic. The prevalence of hydrocele and elephantiasis was 4.8% and 2.9%, respectively. Surveyed drug uptake rates were high, with 70.5% of the respondents reporting having swallowed the drugs in the 2014 MDA round (about seven months before this study). Further, 82.7% of the respondents reported having swallowed the drugs at least once since the inception of MDA programme in 2000. Of the 1054 filarial vectors caught indoors and dissected to detect *W. bancrofti* infection none was found to be infected. Moreover, analysis by qPCR of 1092 pools of gravid *Culex quinquefasciatus* collected outdoors resulted in an estimated infection rate of 0.1%. None of the filarial vectors tested with qPCR were found to be infective.

Conclusion: Analysis of indices of LF infection in the human population and filarial mosquito vectors indicated a substantial decline in the prevalence of LF and other transmission indices, suggesting that local transmission was extremely low if occurring at all in the study areas. We, therefore, recommend a formal transmission assessment survey (TAS) to be conducted in the study areas to make an informed decision on whether Rufiji District satisfied WHO criteria for stopping MDA.

Keywords: Lymphatic filariasis, Mass drug administration, Microfilaremia, Circulating filarial antigens, Hydrocele, Elephantiasis, *Wuchereria bancrofti*, Tanzania

* Correspondence: clarajones2003@yahoo.co.uk
[1]Department of Parasitology and Medical Entomology, Muhimbili University of Health and Allied Sciences, P. O. Box 65011, Dar es Salaam, Tanzania
Full list of author information is available at the end of the article

Background

Lymphatic filariasis (LF) is the second most common vector-borne parasitic disease after malaria and is found in over 83 tropical and subtropical countries [1]. It is estimated that one billion people are at risk of infection and 120 million are affected by LF. Of those at risk of infection, 65% reside in the Southeast Asia, 30% in Africa, and the remainder live in other parts of the tropical world [2, 3]. In sub-Saharan Africa, LF is caused by infection with the parasitic nematode *Wuchereria bancrofti* and transmitted by night-biting mosquitoes of the genera *Anopheles* and *Culex* [4]. The most important filarial vectors in sub-Saharan Africa are *Culex quinquefasciatus* (widespread in urban and semi-urban areas) and members of the *Anopheles gambiae* complex and *An. funestus* group found in rural areas [5].

In 1997, the World Health Assembly passed a resolution calling for the elimination of LF as a public health problem globally [6, 7]. As a result, the Global Programme to Eliminate Lymphatic Filariasis (GPELF) was launched in 2000 by the World Health Organization (WHO). The programme had a principle objective of interrupting the transmission of *W. bancrofti* and *Brugia malayi* through the application of annual mass drug administration (MDA) to the entire at-risk population as well as management and prevention of LF-related disabilities [8]. The fundamental assumption behind the MDA approach is that once the community has been treated long enough, levels of microfilariae will remain below that required to sustain transmission [9]. It has been suggested that after four to six consecutive rounds of MDA, microfilariae load in the endemic population is expected to fall below 1%, and this reduction in microfilaraemia will lead to the reduced acquisition of new infections [10].

LF is endemic in many parts of mainland Tanzania where nearly 70% of the population is at risk, and six million people are estimated to have disabilities due to the disease [11]. LF endemicity varies across the country, with high antigenemia levels of 45–60% along the coast to 2–4% in western Tanzania [11]. Tanzania was one of the first countries in sub-Saharan Africa to adopt the WHO recommended strategy of applying annual MDA to eliminate LF, and the Tanzanian National Lymphatic Filariasis Elimination Programme (NLFEP) was launched on Mafia Island in 2000 [12]. Since then, the programme has expanded to cover a total population of 13 million people treated at least once with ivermectin and albendazole, with a target to extend the coverage to the entire estimated at-risk population of around 34 million people [11].

Monitoring of the transmission dynamics during MDA implementation is essential for measuring the progress and defining MDA endpoints. The main measures used to assess the impact of LF MDA have relied upon detection of parasites, parasite antigens, parasite DNA and/or anti-parasite antibodies in humans [13]. However, detecting these indicators of LF infection in humans are not always definitive of local transmission as they may not account for immigration of infected individuals to areas where transmission has been controlled [13]. On the other hand, detection of filarial parasites in mosquito vectors indicates infection uptake from human hosts while the presence of infective third-stage larvae (L3) indicates a possibility of local transmission [14, 15]. Thus, monitoring *W. bancrofti* infection in humans together with vector infectivity provides a more sensitive measure of local transmission. The present study monitored *W. bancrofti* infection status of the human population and mosquito vectors after twelve annual rounds of MDA with a combination of ivermectin (150–200 mg/kg) and albendazole (400 mg) delivered to individuals aged five years and above in the highly endemic area of southeastern Tanzania.

Methods

Study area

This study was conducted in Rufiji District (7°57'S, 38° 43'E) southeastern Tanzania about 150 km south of Dar es Salaam. Based on 2012 census data, the district had a total population of 217,274 people [16]. The district lies within the floodplain of Rufiji River, *c.*500 m above sea level. The district has two main rain seasons; a long rainy season between February and May and a shorter less intense one from October to December. The annual rainfall ranges between 800–1000 mm. Rufiji District was purposively selected for the study due to its history of high LF prevalence before the start of elimination activities based on ivermectin and albendazole MDA in 2002. Twelve rounds of annual MDA were completed in Rufiji District between 2002 and 2014 (Table 1).

The district has a total of 83 registered villages across 19 administrative wards. Using stratified random sampling, five villages (Bungu, Nyambili, Nyanjati, Mchukwi and Nyamisati) were selected for the study representing three main ecological settings of the district. Nyamisati is located along the coast of the Indian Ocean while both Bungu and Nyanjati are inland villages with high and low population, respectively. Nyambili is a lowland village at the basin of Rufiji River prone to flooding during the rainy season, and Mchukwi is a relatively highland village. Before MDA in 2000, the prevalence of *W. bancrofti* circulating filarial antigens (detected using immunochromatographic test (ICT) cards), microfilaraemia, hydrocele, and elephantiasis were 49, 18, 12 and 4%, respectively (Tanzanian Ministry of Health and Social Welfare (MoHSW) 2000, unpublished). The present study was conducted in April 2015, about seven months after the 12th annual round of MDA based

Table 1 Reported treatment coverage during ivermectin and albendazole MDA intervention in Rufiji District, southeastern Tanzania

MDA No.	Treatment year	Target population	Treated population (% coverage)
1	2002	138,370	75,135 (54.3)
2	2003	141,628	123,216 (87.0)
3	2004	144,962	136,267 (94.0)
	2005[a]	–	–
4	2006	151,868	85,046 (56.0)
5	2007	155,443	116,583 (75.0)
6	2008	159,103	115,350 (72.5)
7	2009	162,848	130,279 (80.0)
8	2010	166,682	113,677 (68.2)
9	2011	170,606	150,133 (88.0)
10	2012	236,614	146,060 (61.7)
11	2013	243,835	149,163 (61.2)
12	2014	217,274	168,930 (77.7)

[a]MDA was not implemented in 2005

on a combination of ivermectin and albendazole delivered in September 2014.

Study population and sampling

Study participants were selected from a list of names of heads of households obtained from the respective village executive officers. Forty heads of households were randomly selected from the list, and all members of the household included for the survey. In 2012, the average household size in Rufiji was reported to be five individuals [16], and thus it was estimated to screen 200 individuals from each village. On the survey date, participants were invited to a central place (dispensary or school premises) for blood testing and interviews. Participants who did not turn up for screening in the central place were followed at their homes.

LF prevalence, burden and MDA compliance

Consented community members aged between 10 and 79 years) in the study villages were examined for *W. bancrofti* CFA using immunochromatographic test (ICT) cards (Binax Now® Filariasis, Inverness Medical Innovations Inc., Massachusetts, USA) following the manufacturer's instructions. Briefly, 100 μl of finger-prick blood was collected from each participant and applied to the test card. Test results were read after precisely 10 min as positive, negative or undetermined. All CFA positive cases detected during the daytime were further examined for microfilaria (MF) by using counting chamber technique [17]. For MF testing, 100 μl of finger-prick blood was collected with sterile heparinised capillary tubes starting from 22:00 to 00:00 h and transferred to sample tubes with 900 μl of 3% acetic acid. In the laboratory, the samples were transferred into the counting chamber and examined for MF under a compound microscope. Moreover, participants were examined in privacy by the study clinicians for clinical manifestation of LF. Using pre-designed forms, demographic information such as sex, age, marital status, occupation, and duration of residence in Rufiji were recorded for all participants. Moreover, participants were interviewed on whether they had swallowed ivermectin and albendazole distributed in the community in September 2014 and also their participation in drug uptake in any of the previous 12 annual MDA campaigns.

Vector and transmission surveys

Filarial mosquito vectors were collected from 10 selected houses from each village using Centre for Disease Control (CDC) light traps (John W. Hock Company, Gainesville, USA). To optimize trap yield, households with thatched roof and open eaves were selected from different parts of each of the trapping village in a non-random approach. Sleeping rooms with a bed and a willing occupant was selected for trapping. CDC light trap was placed beside an occupied bed (with occupant protected with a long-lasting insecticide-treated net) in each household for two consecutive nights. Light traps were switched on between 17:00 and 18:00 h and then turned off between 06:00 and 07:00 h the following morning. Mosquitoes collected from each light trap type were transferred separately into labeled paper cups covered with a netting material and offered cotton pads soaked in a 10% glucose solution and transported to the field laboratory. In the laboratory, they were knocked down with chloroform, sorted, and then identified based on morphological characters. Freshly-killed female filarial mosquito vectors were dissected and examined under a microscope for parity and infection with *W. bancrofti* as described previously [18].

CDC gravid traps were also set outdoors (in the same households used for setting a light trap) to collect gravid mosquitoes for two consecutive nights in each house. The traps were set in peri-domestic areas, and the trappings were conducted as described by Irish et al. [19]. In brief, the traps were switched on between 17:00 and 18:00 h and switched off the next morning between 06:00 and 7:00 h. Collected mosquitoes were treated as described for light trap catch except that the filarial vectors from gravid traps were preserved individually in Eppendorf tubes containing silica gel desiccants for later detection of infection using the quantitative real-time polymerase chain reaction (qPCR) technique.

For qPCR processing, gravid *Cx. quinquefasciatus* were dissected to separate head, thorax, and abdomen. Combined thorax and abdomen segments were processed separately from the heads in pools of five mosquitoes. DNA was extracted from pooled mosquito segments by using the Livak method [20]. In brief, mosquitoes were homogenized in Livak buffer (0.5% sodium dodecyl sulphate (SDS), 0.08M sodium chloride (NaCl), 0.16M sucrose, 0.5M ethylenediaminetetraacetic acid (EDTA) and 0.12M Tris-HCl), proteins and debris separated with 8M potassium acetate, and DNA precipitated with ethanol. The resultant DNA was rinsed in 70% cold ethanol, dried and re-suspended in tris-acetate-EDTA (TAE) buffer. An aliquot of extracted DNA from heads was combined with those from the thorax and abdomen segments and screened in the initial qPCR run to detect infection with *W. bancrofti*. After that, the heads of the positive pools were re-tested in the follow-up qPCR screening to establish whether the positive signal from the initial qPCR run was obtained from the head segment.

The extracted DNA was analysed for the presence of *W. bancrofti* DNA by qPCR using the method of Rao et al. [15]. In brief, the long DNA repeat (LDR) of *W. bancrofti* was targeted with specific forward and reverse primers (LDR1 and LDR2) and *Taq*Man probe for amplification and detection. In the reaction mixture, each 10 µl of PCR consisted of 0.5 µM of each of the two primers (LDR1 and LDR2), 12.5 µl of *Taq*Man probe (Applied Biosystems, Foster City, CA, USA), 1:1 SensiMix™ (Bioline, Meridian Bioscience Asia Pte Ltd, Queenstown, Singapore) and 1 µl of DNA extract. Thermal cycling conditions included 95 °C for 10 min followed by 40 cycles of denaturation at 92 °C for 15 s and annealing at 60 °C for 60 s. Each batch of samples was run with positive and negative controls. Thermal cycling and sample analysis were performed with Agilent MX 3005P qPCR systems, with MXPro software (5301 Stevens Creek Blvd, Santa Clara, CA 95051, USA).

Data analysis

Data were entered in Excel spreadsheets (Microsoft Corp., Redmond, WA, USA) and subsequently analyzed with SPSS version 20.0 (SPSS, Inc., Chicago, IL, USA). Blood test results for CFA and MF, the presence of hydrocele or elephantiasis, demographic characteristics, and MDA compliance were compared by using the Chi-square test and *P*-values ≤ 0.05 were considered statistically significant. The lower and upper limits of the 95% confidence interval for the prevalence of MF and CFA were calculated according to the method described by Newcombe [21]. For pool screening qPCR, the probability that any one mosquito in the pool was infected with *W. bancrofti* was estimated by pool-screen v2.0.2 software providing maximum likelihood estimates for infection rates as previously described [22].

Results

LF prevalence and disease burden

A total of 854 individuals above five years-old in five villages of Rufiji District were examined for CFA, MF, hydrocele and elephantiasis. The overall male to female ratio was 1.3, and the mean age of the participants was 32.3 years (range of 10–79 years). Of 854 individuals screened for LF infection, 9 (1.1%) and 1 (0.1%) had CFA and MF, respectively (Table 2). Males were significantly more infected (CFA) than females (χ^2 = 3.921, *df* = 1, *P* = 0.048). Of the 48 individuals found with the chronic clinical manifestation of LF, 23/481 (4.8%) and 25/854 (2.9%) had hydrocele and elephantiasis, respectively (Table 2). None of the individuals with hydrocele or elephantiasis were found to have MF or CFA.

LF transmission indices

A total of 3334 mosquitoes were caught using CDC light traps of which 69 (2.1%) were identified as species of the *Anopheles gambiae* complex, 1054 (31.6%) were *Culex quinquefasciatus*, and 2211 (66.3 %) were non-filarial vector species. In the laboratory, filarial mosquito vectors were dissected for parity, and 558 parous vectors were examined under microscopy for infection with *W. bancrofti*. None of the mosquitoes examined for infection was found to carry *W. bancrofti* larvae of any stage (Table 3).

A total of 5460 gravid *Cx. quinquefasciatus* were collected outdoors using CDC gravid traps and dissected to separate head, thorax and abdomen. An aliquot of DNA from the head, thorax and abdomen of the 5460 *Cx. quinquefasciatus* was tested in pools of five mosquitoes (a total of 1092 pools) with qPCR. Of 1092 pools of *Cx. quinquefasciatus* tested, five pools were positive for *W. bancrofti* DNA. Further analysis by pool screen (v2.0.2 software) gave an estimate that 0.1% of the tested mosquitoes were infected (Table 3). Further analysis of an aliquot of DNA from head segments of the infected pools revealed the absence of infective mosquitoes (i.e. mosquitoes harboring third-stage larvae of *W. bancrofti*).

MDA compliance concerning LF infection status

Of the 854 individuals interviewed, 82.4% reported having participated in at least one previous MDA round, while 70.6% participated in an MDA that was conducted in September 2014 (about seven months before the present study). Individuals who did not participate in any of the previous rounds of MDA were significantly more infected (CFA) compared with those with a recent history of participating in MDA (χ^2 = 8.723, *df* = 1, *P* = 0.003). The proportion of males with hydrocele was significantly higher in individuals who did not swallow drugs in any MDA round while the prevalence of elephantiasis was not significantly different between these two groups of participants (Table 4).

Discussion

LF elimination activities based on annual MDA with a combination of ivermectin and albendazole have been

Table 2 Prevalence of CFA, microfilariae and clinical manifestation of lymphatic filariasis infection by gender, age and village location in Rufiji District, southeastern Tanzania

Characteristic	No. (%) examined	No. (%) with CFA [95% CI]	No. (%) with MF [95% CI]	No. (%) with hydrocele[a]	No. (%) with elephantiasis
Gender					
Male	481 (56.3)	8 (1.7) [0.8–3.2]	1 (0.2) [0.0–1.2]	23 (4.8)	18 (3.7)
Female	373 (43.7)	1 (0.3) [0.1–1.5]	0 (0.0) [0.0–1.0]	–	7 (1.9)
Total	854	9 (1.1) [0.6–2.0]	1 (0.1) [0.0–0.7]	23 (4.8)	25 (2.9)
Age (years)					
5–14	188 (22.1)	1 (0.5) [0.1–3.0]	0 (0.0) [0.0–2.0]	0 (0.0)	1 (1.0)
15–34	307 (35.9)	4 (1.3) [0.5–3.3]	1 (0.3) [0.1–1.8]	8 (4.7)	13 (7.8)
≥ 35	359 (42.0)	4 (1.1) [0.4–2.8]	0 (0.0) [0.0–1.1]	15 (7.0)	11 (5.2)
Total	854	9 (1.1) [0.6–2.0]	1 (0.1) [0.0–0.7]	23 (4.8)	25 (2.9)
Village					
Nyamisati	213 (24.9)	0 (0.0) [0.0–1.8]	0 (0.0) [0.0–1.8]	7 (4.1)	5 (2.3)
Nyambili	196 (23.0)	6 (3.1) [1.4–6.5]	1 (0.5) [0.1–2.8]	5 (5.0)	10 (5.1)
Nyanjati	189 (22.1)	0 (0.0) [0.0–2.0]	0 (0.0) [0.0–2.0]	3 (3.6)	7 (4.1)
Bungu	172 (20.1)	3 (1.7) [0.6–5.0]	0 (0.0) [0.0–2.2]	4 (5.1)	3 (1.7)
Mchukwi	84 (9.8)	0 (0.0) [0.0–4.4]	0 (0.0) [0.0–4.4]	4 (8.3)	0 (0.0)
Total	854	9 (1.1) [0.6–2.0]	1 (0.1) [0.0–0.7]	23 (4.8)	25 (2.9)

[a]Denominator included only males

ongoing in Tanzania for more than a decade. Thus, regular monitoring is essential to evaluate the progress and make informed decisions on when it is safe to stop MDA intervention. Studies on the impact of MDA on LF transmission and infection in areas implementing diethylcarbamazine (DEC) and albendazole regimes such as American Samoa, India, Egypt and Papua New Guinea, have documented good progress towards elimination [23–25]. In sub-Saharan Africa, many LF-endemic countries are co-endemic with onchocerciasis and thus ivermectin is used to avoid the potential DEC-induced side effects on onchocerciasis patients. Using a combination of ivermectin and albendazole MDA strategy, some West African countries are showing good progress toward elimination of LF [26, 27], and Togo has been declared to have achieved LF elimination target [28, 29]. In northeastern Tanzania, the impact of MDA with this drug combination has shown a remarkable decline in LF infection and transmission [30]. The documented declining trend in LF transmission suggests the need to conduct a WHO-approved transmission assessment survey (TAS) to determine whether MDA can be stopped in endemic areas showing good progress.

The findings of this study have shown that after 12 rounds of ivermectin and albendazole MDA in the Rufiji District there has been a progressive decline in LF prevalence and transmission since the start of MDA intervention in 2002. Before the MDA intervention, the prevalence of CFA, MF, hydrocele and elephantiasis was 49%, 18%, 12% and 4%, respectively (MoH 2000, unpublished). In this study, no children tested positive for CFA in 2015 surveys (after 12 rounds of MDA). This shows a significant decline in CFA rates compared to our previous findings in the same study area in 2012 (after 9 MDA rounds), which showed CFA rate of 14.3% among pupils screened [31]. This decline in CFA suggests a substantial reduction in the acquisition of new infection in children from 2012 to 2014. The prevalence of MF and CFA recorded in the current study (0.1% and 1.1%, respectively) were below the WHO-recommended elimination thresholds of 1% (for MF) and 2% (for CFA) [3]. Our findings on the decline of

Table 3 Filarial mosquito vectors caught and analyzed for infection and or/infectivity with *W. bancrofti* using microscopy and qPCR

Collection method	Vector collected	Parous vectors	Method of analysis	No. analyzed	No. infected (%)	No. infective (%)
Light trap	1123[a]	558[b]	Microscopy	558	0 (0)	0 (0)
Gravid trap	5460	–	qPCR	1092[c]	5 (0.1)[d]	0 (0)

[a]Filarial vector composition: *Anopheles gambiae* complex ($n = 69$) and *Culex quinquefasciatus* ($n = 1054$)
[b]Parous vectors: *An. gambiae* complex ($n = 45$) and *Cx. quinquefasciatus* ($n = 513$)
[c]Pools of 5 *Cx. quinquefasciatus* each
[d]Infection rate (Pool Screen V2.0.2; Likelihood ratio method; 95% CI: 0.03–0.22%)

Table 4 Demographic characteristics of the study population and their reported drug uptake in relation to their LF infection status

Characteristic	No. (%) of total	No. (%) with CFA	χ^2-value (*P*-value)	No (%)[a] with hydrocele	χ^2-value (*P*-value)	No (%) with elephantiasis	χ^2-value (*P*-value)
Gender (*n* = 854)							
Males	481 (56.3)	8 (1.6)	3.921 (0.048)	23 (4.8)	–	18 (3.7)	2.573 (0.109)
Females	373 (43.7)	1 (0.3)				7 (1.9)	
Age groups in years (*n* = 854)							
≤ 29	450 (52.7)	4 (0.9)	0.248 (0.618)	5 (2.0)	8.723 (0.003)	13 (2.9)	0.005 (0.944)
≥ 30	404 (47.3)	5 (1.2)		18 (7.8)		12 (3.0)	
Reported drug uptake in previous MDAs (*n* = 854)							
Yes	704 (82.4)	4 (0.6)	8.723 (0.003)	9 (2.4)	22.743 (0.001)	19 (2.7)	0.737 (0.391)
No	150 (17.6)	5 (3.3)		14 (13.7)		6 (4.0)	
Reported drug uptake in 2014 MDA (*n* = 854)							
Yes	603 (70.6)	6 (1.0)	0.068 (0.794)	8 (2.5)	10.243 (0.001)	16 (2.7)	0.542 (0.462)
No	251 (29.4)	3 (1.2)		15 (9.1)		9 (3.6)	

[a]Denominator included only males: for age group ≤ 29 and ≥ 30 there were 249 and 232 males; drug uptake in any previous MDA, 379 males swallowed the drugs while 102 did not swallow the drugs; drug uptake in 2014 MDA, 316 males swallowed the drugs while 165 did not

LF infection and transmission due to MDA intervention corroborate those reported by Simonsen et al. [30] in northeastern Tanzania.

Detection of *W. bancrofti* infection in mosquito vectors is an essential aspect of monitoring LF transmission as it provides real-time information on the presence of local transmission [14]. CDC light and gravid traps have been considered efficient tools for the collection of filarial vectors in areas where *Anopheles* and *Cx. quinquefasciatus* are the primary vectors [32]. Important filarial mosquito vectors found elsewhere in Tanzania, such as the species of the *An. gambiae* complex, *An. funestus* group and *Cx. quinquefasciatus* have also been reported in Rufiji District [33]. In this study, none of the dissected filarial vectors examined for infection (*Cx. quinquefasciatus* and *An. gambiae* complex) were found to carry *W. bancrofti* larvae of any stage. Using qPCR with high throughput and precision, the probability of finding an infected mosquito in any of the analysed pools of gravid *Cx. quinquefasciatus* was estimated at 0.1%. Importantly in the transmission, none of the mosquitoes tested with qPCR was found to carry an infective stage of *W. bancrofti*. The fact that we did not identify any LF-infective vector by either qPCR or dissection suggests that local transmission is extremely low if occurring at all in the study areas.

The present study showed that the prevalence of hydrocele and elephantiasis was lower than that reported by the MOH before MDA (MoHSW 2000, unpublished), but the survey methods differed and a statistical comparison of prevalence in the two studies could not be made. In contrast, the proportion of individuals with elephantiasis in the present study was similar to that reported by Gasarasi et al. [34] who conducted a study in the same area in 2000. Other studies conducted elsewhere have indicated a moderate to no reduction in the prevalence of lymphoedema after several rounds of MDA [35, 36]. Therefore, the observed low rate of hydrocele in this study might be explained by the ongoing hydrocelectomy intervention in the district.

Treatment coverage and compliance are crucial factors to observe when assessing the impact of MDA on LF transmission. For MDA strategy to be effective, sustained high treatment coverage is critical to reach the elimination target within a reasonable time-frame [37]. Moreover, empirical evidence suggested that endemic areas with high baseline infection levels will require higher treatment coverage and a more sustained MDA intervention [38]. However, it has been documented that attaining optimal drug uptake during MDA is a challenge in LF control programmes in most of the endemic areas [39–41]. In this study, the surveyed drug uptake was 70.6 and 82.4% for the last MDA round (September 2014, seven months before the present study) and participation in any previous MDA rounds, respectively. The surveyed MDA coverage in our study was at the recommended range of 60–70% drug uptake rates required for interruption of transmission [37]. Although drug uptake was found to be significantly lower in respondents with hydrocele, previous studies have reported a low prevalence of microfilaraemia in individuals with hydrocele and elephantiasis [42, 43].

Our study has recorded a progressive and substantial decline in LF prevalence in the study areas when compared to the baseline values before MDA and also to a more recent survey conducted in the same villages in 2012 [31]. In addition to the impact of MDA, the universal distribution of long-lasting insecticide-treated nets which was implemented in 2012 could contribute to the drastic decline in LF disease prevalence. Insecticide-treated nets distributed for malaria control have been shown to reduce LF prevalence in some settings [44–47].

Despite a substantial decline in LF in this study areas, a recommendation to stop MDA could not be made because the current study methods did not follow WHO-approved TAS. The design of the present study was adopted as a result of limited funding and time to implement an elaborated WHO-approved TAS protocol. Moreover, the direct statistical comparison between the baseline study in 2000 and the present study could not be made due to the unavailability of a detailed methodology for the baseline study. With these limitations, it is advisable that a formal TAS is conducted before MDA can be stopped the area.

Conclusions

Analysis of indices of LF infection in the human population and filarial mosquito vectors demonstrated a substantial decline in the prevalence of LF in the study areas when compared with baseline values before the start of elimination activities based on MDA. We recommend a formal TAS to be conducted in the study areas to make an informed decision on whether MDA can be stopped in Rufiji District.

Abbreviations

LF: Lymphatic filariasis; MDA: Mass drug administration; CFA: Circulating filarial antigens; ICT: Immunochromatographic test cards; qPCR: Quantitative real time polymerase chain reaction; TAS: Transmission assessment survey; WHO: World health organization; CDC: Centers for Disease Control and prevention; DNA: Deoxyribonucleic acid; GPELF: Global Programme to Eliminate Lymphatic Filariasis; NLFEP: National Lymphatic Filariasis Elimination Programme

Acknowledgements

The authors extend their gratitude to the residents of the study area for participating in the study. Maembe Mzee Maembe (deceased) and Justine Mkeni are thanked for their technical assistance in mosquito collection, identification and dissections. The authors wish to thank the district authorities for allowing researchers to conduct this study. We are also grateful to the members of the general community for participating in the surveys.

Funding

The study received financial support from the Special Programme for Research and Training in Tropical Diseases (TDR), co-sponsored by UNICEF, UNDP, the World Bank and WHO. The funding bodies had no role in the design, data collection, analysis and interpretation of data and in writing the manuscript.

Authors' contributions

Conceived and designed the study: CJ, BN, YAD, DT and MNM. Performed the field experiments: CJ, BN, LR, YAD and MB. Supervised laboratory work: LR and MB: Wrote the paper: CJ, BN, YAD, LR, MB and MNM. All authors read and approved the final manuscript.

Ethics approval and consent to participate

The study was approved by Muhimbili University of Health and Allied Sciences Research Ethical Review Board as well as the WHO Ethics Review Committee. Before the fieldwork, permission to conduct the study was obtained from the District Executive Director for Rufiji. Members of the community were informed of the purpose of the study during the village meetings in order to obtain their cooperation. Before any examination, a written informed consent was obtained from all adults. For children below 15 years, their parents/guardians signed the informed the consent on their behalf. Before setting the CDC light and gravid traps, written informed consent was obtained from the heads of the households and individuals sleeping in the mosquito collection rooms were provided with long-lasting insecticide-treated nets (LLINs). Study participants who were positive for CFA or MF were treated with ivermectin (150–200 mg/kg) and albendazole (400 mg) as done during MDA.

Competing interests

The authors declare that they have no competing interests.

Author details

[1]Department of Parasitology and Medical Entomology, Muhimbili University of Health and Allied Sciences, P. O. Box 65011, Dar es Salaam, Tanzania. [2]Department of Women's and Children's Health International Maternal and Child Health (IMCH), Uppsala Universitet, Uppsala, Sweden. [3]National Institute for Medical Research, P. O. Box 9653, Dar es Salaam, Tanzania. [4]Liverpool School of Tropical Medicine, Liverpool, UK. [5]European and Development Countries Clinical Trials Partnership, Cape Town, South Africa. [6]WHO Regional Office for Africa, Brazzaville, Republic of the Congo.

References

1. Ottesen EA. The global programme to eliminate lymphatic filariasis. Trop Med Int Health. 2000;5:591–4.
2. WHO. Preparing and implementing a national plan to eliminate lymphatic filariasis. Geneva: World Health Organization; 2000. WHO/CDS/CPE/CEE/2000.16.
3. WHO. Global programme to eliminate lymphatic filariasis: progress report 2000–2009 and strategic plan 2010–2020. Geneva: World Health Organization; 2010. WHO/HTM/NTD/PCT/2010.6.
4. Bockarie MJ, Pedersen EM, White GB, Michael E. Role of vector control in the global program to eliminate lymphatic filariasis. Annu Rev Entomol. 2009;54:469–87.
5. Simonsen PE, Fischer PU, Hoerauf A, Weil GJ. The Filariases. In: Farrar J, Hotez PJ, Junghanss T, Kang G, Lalloo D, White NJ, editors. Manson's Tropical Diseases. 23rd ed. London: Elsevier Saunders; 2014. p. 737–65.
6. Knight R, Molyneux D. Lymphatic filariasis. In: Warrell DA, Cox TM, Firth JD. Oxford Textbook of Medicine. Oxford: Oxford University Press; 2012. doi: https://doi.org/10.1093/med/978099204854.001.1.
7. Gyapong JO, Kumaraswami V, Biswas G, Ottesen EA. Treatment strategies underpinning the global programme to eliminate lymphatic filariasis. Expert Opin Pharmacother. 2005;6:179–200.
8. Molyneux DH. Filaria control and elimination: diagnostic, monitoring and surveillance needs. Trans R Soc Trop Med Hyg. 2009;103:338–41.
9. Michael E, Malecela MN, Zervos M, Kazura JW. Global eradication of lymphatic filariasis: the value of chronic disease control in parasite elimination programmes. PLoS One. 2008;3:e2936.
10. WHO. Global programme to eliminate lymphatic filariasis: annual report on lymphatic filariasis 2001. Geneva: World Health Organization; 2002. WHO/CDS/CPE/CEE/2002.28
11. Malecela MN, Lazarus W, Mwingira U, Mwakitalu E, Makene C, Kabali C, et al. Eliminating LF: a progress report from Tanzania. J Lymphol. 2009;4:10–2.
12. Malecela MN, Kilima P, Mackenzie CD. Implementation and management of lymphatic filariasis control and elimination programmes: the Tanzanian experience.

In: Simonsen PE, Malecela MN, Michael E, Mackenzie CD, editors. Lymphatic Filariasis Research and Control in Eastern and Southern Africa. Copenhagen: DBL - Centre for Health Research and Development; 2008. p. 112–23.
13. Chu BK, Deming M, Biritwum NK, Bougma WR, Dorkenoo AM, El-Setouhy M, et al. Transmission assessment surveys (TAS) to define endpoints for lymphatic filariasis mass drug administration: a multicenter evaluation. PLoS Negl Trop Dis. 2013;7:e2584.
14. Goodman DS, Orelus JN, Roberts JM, Lammie PJ, Streit TG. PCR and mosquito dissection as tools to monitor filarial infection levels following mass treatment. Filaria J. 2003;2:11.
15. Rao RU, Atkinson LJ, Ramzy RM, Helmy H, Farid HA, Bockarie MJ, et al. A real-time PCR-based assay for detection of *Wuchereria bancrofti* DNA in blood and mosquitoes. Am J Trop Med Hyg. 2006;74:826–32.
16. URT. Population and housing census 2012. Dar es Salaam: United Republic of Tanzania; 2013.
17. McMahon JE, Marshall TF, Vaughan JP, Abaru DE. Bancroftian filariasis: a comparison of microfilariae counting techniques using counting chamber, standard slide and membrane (nucleopore) filtration. Ann Trop Med Parasitol. 1979;73:457–64.
18. Rwegoshora RT, Pedersen EM, Mukoko D, Meyrowitsch DW, Masese N, Malecela MN, et al. Bancroftian filariasis: patterns of vector abundance and transmission in two East African communities with different levels of endemicity. Ann Trop Med Parasitol. 2005;99:253–65.
19. Irish SR, Stevens WM, Derua YA, Walker T, Cameron MM. Comparison of methods for xenomonitoring in vectors of lymphatic filariasis in northeastern Tanzania. Am J Trop Med Hyg. 2015;93:983–9.
20. Livak KJ. Organization and mapping of a sequence on the *Drosophila melanogaster* x and y chromosomes that is transcribed during spermatogenesis. Genetics. 1984;107:611–34.
21. Newcombe RG. Two-sided confidence intervals for the single proportion: comparison of seven methods. Stat Med. 1998;17:857–72.
22. Katholi CR, ToeÂ L, Merriweather A, Unnasch TR. Determining the prevalence of *Onchocerca volvulus* infection in vector populations by polymerase chain reaction screening of pools of black flies. J Infect Dis. 1995;172:1414–7.
23. Ramzy RM, El Setouhy M, Helmy H, Ahmed ES, Abd Elaziz KM, Farid H, et al. Effect of yearly mass drug administration with diethylcarbamazine and albendazole on bancroftian filariasis in Egypt: a comprehensive assessment. Lancet. 2006;367:992–9.
24. Weil GJ, Kastens W, Susapu M, Laney SJ, Williams S, King CL, et al. The impact of repeated rounds of mass drug administration with diethylcarbamazine plus albendazole on bancroftian filariasis in Papua New Guinea. PLoS Negl Trop Dis. 2008;2:e344.
25. Liang JL, King JD, Ichimori K, Handzel T, Pa'au M, Lammie PJ. Impact of five annual rounds of mass drug administration with diethylcarbamazine and albendazole on *Wuchereria bancrofti* infection in American Samoa. Am J Trop Med Hyg. 2008;78:924–8.
26. King JD, Eigege A, Umaru J, Jip N, Miri E, Jiya J, et al. Evidence for stopping mass drug administration for lymphatic filariasis in some, but not all local government areas of Plateau and Nasarawa States, Nigeria. Am J Trop Med Hyg. 2012;87:272–80.
27. Richards FO, Eigege A, Miri ES, Kal A, Umaru J, Pam D. Epidemiological and entomological evaluations after six years or more of mass drug administration for lymphatic filariasis elimination in Nigeria. PLoS Negl Trop Dis. 2011;5:e1346.
28. Sodahlon YK, Dorkenoo AM, Morgah K, Nabiliou K, Agbo K, Miller R, et al. A success story: Togo is moving toward becoming the first sub-Saharan African nation to eliminate lymphatic filariasis through mass drug administration and countrywide morbidity alleviation. PLoS Negl Trop Dis. 2013;7:e2080.
29. Budge PJ, Dorkenoo AM, Sodahlon YK, Fasuyi OB, Mathieu E. Ongoing surveillance for lymphatic filariasis in Togo: assessment of alternatives and nationwide reassessment of transmission status. Am J Trop Med Hyg. 2014;90:89–95.
30. Simonsen PE, Derua YA, Magesa SM, Pedersen EM, Stensgaard A, Malecela MN, et al. Lymphatic filariasis control in Tanga Region, Tanzania: status after eight rounds of mass drug administration. Parasit Vectors. 2014;7:507.
31. Jones C, Ngasalla B, Derua YA, Tarimo D, Malecela MN. Lymphatic filariasis elimination efforts in Rufiji, southeastern Tanzania: decline in circulating filarial antigen prevalence in young school children after twelve rounds of mass drug administration and utilization of long-lasting insecticide-treated nets. Int J Infect Dis. 2017;61:38–43.
32. Derua YA, Rumisha SF, Batengana BM, Max DA, Stanley G, Kisinza WN, Mboera LG. Lymphatic filariasis transmission on Mafia Islands, Tanzania: evidence from xenomonitoring in mosquito vectors. PLoS Negl Trop Dis. 2017;11:e0005938.
33. Kigadye ESP, Nkwengulila G, Magesa SM, Abdulla S. Spatial variability in the density, distribution and vectorial capacity of anopheline species in Rufiji District, southeastern Tanzania. Tanzan J Health Res. 2011;13:112–8.
34. Gasarasi DB, Premji ZG, Mujinja PG, Mpembeni R. Acute adenolymphangitis due to bancroftian filariasis in Rufiji District, southeast Tanzania. Acta Trop. 2000;75:19–28.
35. Pani SP, Yuvaraj J, Vanamail P, Dhanda V, Michael E, Grenfell BT, et al. Episodic adenolymphangitis and lymphoedema in patients with bancroftian filariasis. Trans R Soc Trop Med Hyg. 1995;89:72–4.
36. Kazura JW, Bockarie MJ. Lymphatic filariasis in Papua New Guinea: interdisciplinary research on a national health problem. Trends Parasitol. 2003;19:260–3.
37. Michael E, Malecela-Lazaro MN, Simonsen PE, Pedersen EM, Barker G, Kumar A, et al. Mathematical modelling and the control of lymphatic filariasis. Lancet Infect Dis. 2004;4:223–34.
38. Michael E, Malecela-Lazaro MN, Kabali C, Snow LC, Kazura JW. Mathematical models and lymphatic filariasis control: endpoints and optimal interventions. Trends Parasitol. 2006;22:226–33.
39. Kisoka WJ, Simonsen PE, Malecela MN, Tersbøl PB, Mushi DL, Meyrowitsch DW. Factors influencing drug uptake during mass drug administration for control of lymphatic filariasis in rural and urban Tanzania. PLoS One. 2014;9:e109316.
40. Babu BV, Mishra S. Mass drug administration under the programme to eliminate lymphatic filariasis in Orissa, India: a mixed-methods study to identify factors associated with compliance and non-compliance. Trans R Soc Trop Med Hyg. 2008;102:1207–13.
41. Gunawardena S, Ismail M, Bradley M, Karunaweera N. Factors influencing drug compliance in the mass drug administration programme against filariasis in the Western Province of Sri Lanka. Trans R Soc Trop Med Hyg. 2007;101:445–53.
42. Derua YA, Kisinza WN, Simonsen PE. Lymphatic filariasis control in Tanzania: infection, disease perceptions and drug uptake patterns in an endemic community after multiple rounds of mass drug administration. Parasit Vectors. 2018;11:429.
43. Dissanayake S. In *Wuchereria bancrofti* filariasis, asymptomatic microfilaraemia does not progress to amicrofilaraemic lymphatic disease. Int J Epidemiol. 2001;30:394–9.
44. Pedersen EM, Mukoko DA. Impact of insecticide-treated materials on filaria transmission by the various species of vector mosquito in Africa. Ann Trop Med Parasitol. 2002;96(Suppl. 2):S91–5.
45. Odermatt P, Leang R, Bin B, Bunkea T, Socheat D. Prevention of lymphatic filariasis with insecticide-treated bednets in Cambodia. Ann Trop Med Parasitol. 2008;102:135–42.
46. Njenga SM, Mwandawiro CS, Wamae CN, Mukoko DA, Omar AA, Shimada M, et al. Sustained reduction in prevalence of lymphatic filariasis infection despite missed rounds of mass drug administration in an area under mosquito nets for malaria control. Parasit Vectors. 2011;4:90.
47. Ashton RA, Kyabayinze DJ, Opio T, Auma A, Edwards T, Matwale G, et al. The impact of mass drug administration and long-lasting insecticidal net distribution on *Wuchereria bancrofti* infection in humans and mosquitoes: an observational study in northern Uganda. Parasit Vectors. 2011;4:134.

13

Identification of mosquitoes (Diptera: Culicidae): an external quality assessment of medical entomology laboratories in the MediLabSecure Network

Frédéric Jourdain[1], Marie Picard[1], Tatiana Sulesco[2], Nabil Haddad[3], Zoubir Harrat[4], Samer Saleh Sawalha[5], Filiz Günay[6], Khalil Kanani[7], Taher Shaibi[8], Denys Akhramenko[9], M'hammed Sarih[10], Enkelejda Velo[11], Lusine Paronyan[12], Igor Pajovic[13], Chafika Faraj[14], Irakli Sikharulidze[15], David Putkaradze[15], Jelena Maric[16], Golubinka Bosevska[17], Elizabeta Janceska[17], Ali Bouattour[18], Afrim Hamidi[19], Kurtesh Sherifi[19], Bülent Alten[20], Dušan Petrić[21] and Vincent Robert[22]*

Abstract

Background: Identification of vectors is of prime importance in the field of medical entomology for both operational and research purposes. An external quality assessment of mosquito identification capacities was carried out within the MediLabSecure Network, which is composed of laboratories located in 19 countries close to the European Union around the Mediterranean and Black seas.

Methods: A set of blind samples consisting of 7 or 8 adult mosquitoes and 4 larvae was given to each participant laboratory. In all, 138 adult mosquitoes and 76 larvae of different species were distributed for genus and species identification.

Results: All identifications were exclusively morphology based. Overall, 81% of identifications were correct at the genus level, 64% at the species level. The results were highly varied among the 19 participating laboratories. The levels of correct identifications were: 100% (three laboratories), 90–95% (four laboratories), 50–75% (six laboratories) and < 50% (six laboratories).

Conclusions: This evaluation showed the need to maintain efforts in capacity building and quality control in the field of medical entomology and, more specifically, in the morphological identification of the Culicidae.

Keywords: EQA medical entomology, Mediterranean Sea, Mosquito species, Capacity building, Quality control, International network

Background

The MediLabSecure project aims to develop capacities of preparedness and response to viral emergencies by establishing an integrated network covering the fields of human virology, animal virology, medical entomology and public health in 19 non-European Union countries in the Mediterranean and Black Sea regions (Fig. 1). One medical entomology laboratory in each country (two in one of the countries) were selected for inclusion in the network.

In the broad sense, vectors encompass any organism involved in the transmission of an infectious agent. More specifically, in medical and veterinary entomology, vectors designate any haematophagous arthropod which actively transmits an infectious pathogen from an infected host to a new host [1]. In a given zoological group, vector species are ordinarily outnumbered by other non-vector species. For instance, among the 540 species of mosquito in the subfamily Anophelinae, about 60

* Correspondence: vincent.robert@ird.fr
[22]French National Research Institute for Sustainable Development, Research Unit MiVEGEC, IRD-CNRS-Montpellier University, Montpellier, France
Full list of author information is available at the end of the article

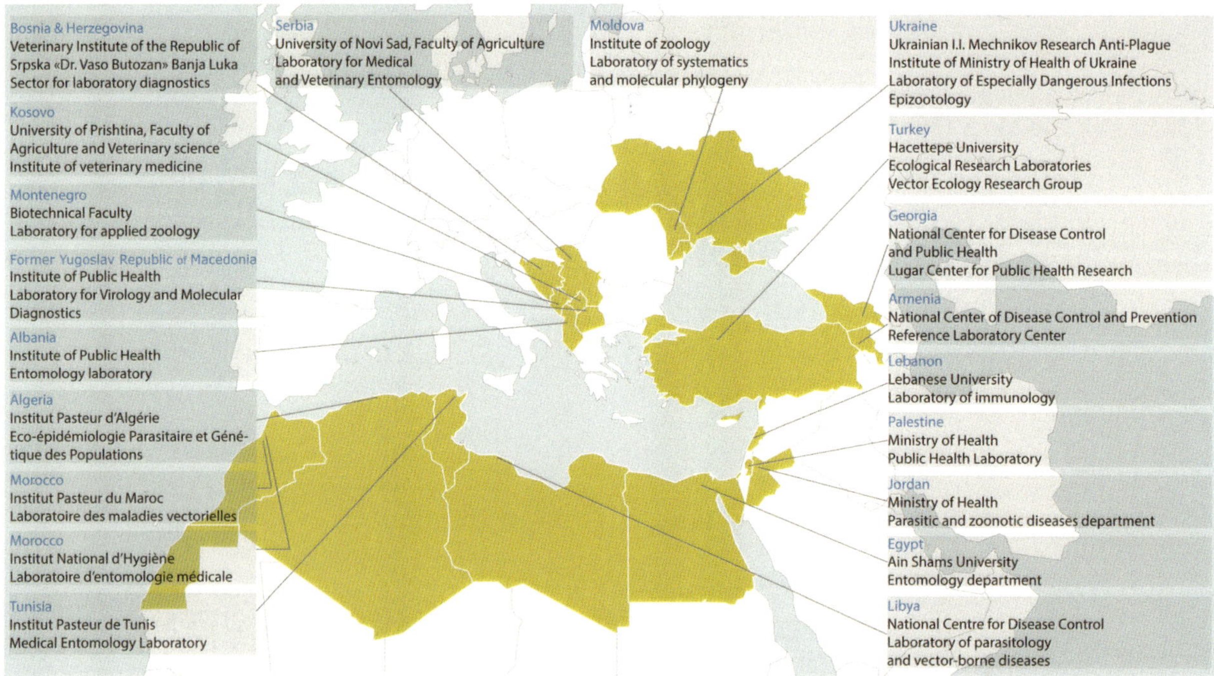

Fig. 1 Map of the member countries of MediLabSecure and the locations of the laboratories constituting the medical entomology network

species are recognised vectors of *Plasmodium*, the agent of malaria [2]. Identification of arthropod species, both vectors and non-vectors, is a core capacity in the field of medical and veterinary entomology. Accurate identification of a species involved in transmitting a pathogen is essential for a proper understanding of the mechanisms that govern any biological system. Knowing which arthropod species transmit vector-borne diseases is also vital to providing species-specific focused control programmes and to correctly identifying disease risk and exposure [3].

Determining the quality of taxonomic data is a matter of recent concern. Where data of unknown quality are used, they naturally lead to conclusions of unknown quality. It is, therefore, crucial that uncertainty associated with taxonomic identification is documented and reported. This issue is central to any monitoring programme in biology [4–6] as well as in ecology [7].

Different approaches to mosquito identification are available: morphological, molecular (PCR and nucleic acids sequencing), proteomics tools, isozyme analysis, etc. [8, 9]. However, for historical and technical reasons, morphological identification is still the reference method for both research purposes and operational surveillance as it requires little technical equipment, is easy to implement in the field and is inexpensive even when large numbers of individuals need to be identified. The method has three principal limitations, the first being that it relies on expert entomologists performing the identification, especially when many species are present in the collection area. The second limitation resides in the level of preservation of the morphological characters used in the sample handling process. The third concerns species complexes and a few morphologically similar species where identification should be based on more than one developmental stage, which is not always accessible.

Most traditional morphological identification keys are organised in a series of alternative statements, which may be dichotomous (every choice has two alternatives) or polytomous (two or more options at each choice). In practice, most of them are a mixture of dichotomous and polytomous sequential choices. Importantly, they are structured as single-access keys because they trace a unique path in the decision tree. An alternative to this type of fixed sequence of choice is the multi-access key (or matrix key), where the sequence choices are largely up to the user [10]. Dichotomous keys are printable and multi-access keys are the most suitable tools for computer-aided identification. Dichotomous keys tend to be used linearly; identification choices must be made stepwise and missing out a step or choice can result in a sample being misidentified. Multi-access keys have the advantage of allowing steps to be missed out, so it may still be possible to identify a damaged sample or to look for other morphological characters when one cannot be clearly determined. Within these two types of key, the dichotomous keys by Becker et al. [11] and the computer-aided MosKeyTool [12] are among the most commonly used for identifying mosquitoes in the Euro-Mediterranean Sea region.

External quality assessments (EQA) have for decades been regularly implemented in medical laboratories to appraise a wide range of analyses [13]. They are essential for quantifying the quality of routine laboratory work and ensuring the quality of biological test results, which are often the basis for clinical decision making. A quick search in PubMed using the phrase "External Quality Assessment" OR "External Quality Assurance" OR "External Quality Control" found 2883 occurrences (accessed 15 May 2018). However, we found no published EQAs on insects as nuisances or vectors, with the exception of Chaki et al. [14], who dealt with operational field quality control issues rather than vector determination. A self-assessment of the quality of mosquito identification was therefore performed within the medical entomology activities of MediLabSecure. While EQAs are often carried out in quality control in medical laboratories, we present here what is, to the best of our knowledge, the first EQA in the field of identifying arthropods of medical interest.

Methods

The EQA was designed and coordinated by Medical Entomology Work Package leaders of the MediLabSecure Network, none of whom belonged to any of laboratories that took part in the EQA. A full list of the 19 participating laboratories is given in Additional file 1: Table S1.

A set of blind samples consisting of seven or eight adult specimens plus four stage IV larvae in alcohol was given to each participant laboratory. The adults were double-mounted on micro-pins while fresh, then preserved in insect boxes for a period not exceeding 2 years. A senior entomologist double-checked the previously identified samples before they were taken to the participating laboratories. An identification code was attributed to each specimen. Overall, 138 adult mosquitoes and 76 larvae (total = 214) were distributed to the laboratories. The precise composition of the different biological sets is given in Additional file 2: Table S2.

Although particular care was taken in handling the biological material, some specimens, especially adults, may have been damaged during transportation, a possibility not uncommon in the identification of vector specimens. Where this occurred, participants were invited to perform the identification as best they could.

Specimen sets were distributed by hand during regional meetings, which provided an opportunity to meet representatives of the target laboratories and reduced the risk of damage during transportation. The following instructions were given: (i) morphological identification should be performed on behalf of the laboratory, meaning that several persons could take part in the process; (ii) all available resources could be used to support identification (dichotomous keys, interactive keys for mosquito species, monographies and publications, molecular methods, etc.) and the choice was left to the participants' discretion; (iii) results of the identification had to be returned within a maximum of two months *via* an online form specifying the specimen's genus and species name.

Identification responses were classified into three categories: Correct, False and Not Responding. Responses limited to identification of the sex of adult specimens were considered False. Each head of laboratory was confidentially informed of the results of the identifications delivered by his/her laboratory. The data were anonymised prior to analysis because the aim of this study was only to evaluate the accuracy of the identifications; we did not intend to applaud, stigmatise or rank the laboratories.

Results

All laboratories performed morphology-based identification using interactive identification keys / dichotomous keys / reference literature, either alone or in combination. None of them used molecular methods (PCR diagnostics, nucleic acid sequencing, MALDI-TOF, etc.). Analysis by identification tool showed that interactive keys were the most commonly used (16/19 laboratories, i.e. 84%), followed by dichotomous keys (12 laboratories; 63%), and lastly reference literature (3 laboratories; 16%). Analysis by laboratory shows that 8 laboratories (42%) relied on both interactive and dichotomous keys for identification, 6 (32%) used only interactive keys, 2 (11%) used only dichotomous keys, 1 (5%) used interactive keys and reference literature, 1 (5%) used dichotomous keys and reference literature, and 1 (5%) based its identifications on the three tools together (Fig. 2). One laboratory mentioned also using their own expertise (especially for mosquito species regularly recorded in their region) and another used web-based images to complete identification.

Eight adult specimens out of 138 (6%) were considered by the identifiers as being too damaged to allow identification, even at the genus level. This was probably due to transportation in a suitcase in the hold of an aircraft. Identification was not performed on these specimens, which were classified as Not Responding and were not included in the subsequent analysis.

Table 1 presents the percentages of correct identifications from all the respondents. Overall, 81% of identifications were correct at the genus level, while the percentage was lower (64%) at the species level. Accuracy of identification was similar for the larval and adult stages and for males and females.

The results from the different laboratories varied considerably, with accuracy of identification ranging from

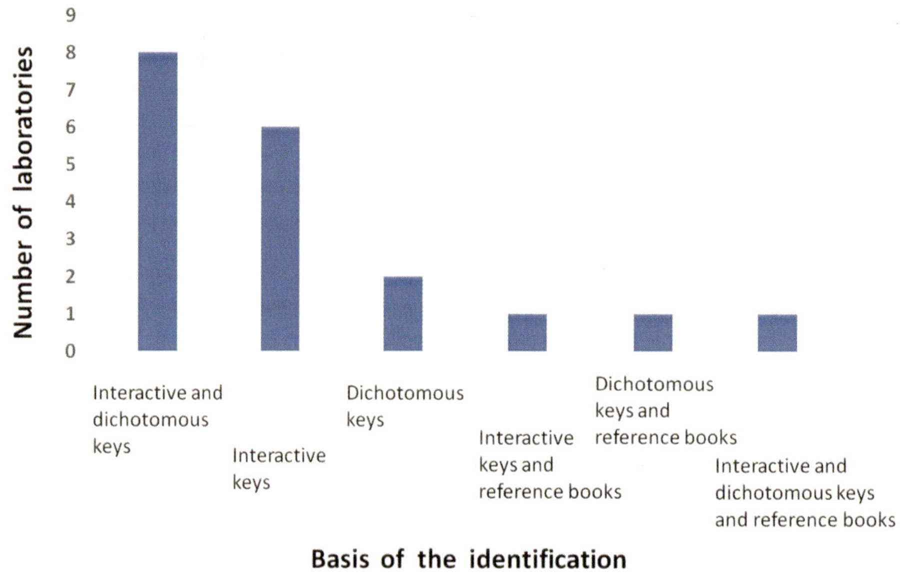

Fig. 2 The various methodologies used to identify mosquito species according to the number of laboratories using them (19 laboratories in total)

100% to 8%. Three laboratories correctly identified 100% of specimens (adults and larvae) at the species level, four laboratories between 90–95%, six between and 50–75%, and six less than 50%. Details are given in Fig. 3.

Table 2 presents the results by mosquito species. The results for larvae ranged from 84% to 37% correct identifications. More than 50% of *Aedes* spp. were incorrectly identified.

Regarding adults, *Aedes albopictus*, a species of some importance, was correctly identified at 95%, but another important species, *Culex pipiens* (*s.l.*), was correctly identified at 50%. As it is useful for all new mosquito taxonomists to be aware of common pitfalls, the following recurrent errors deserve to be highlighted: three Culicinae males were misidentified as Anophelinae (both have long maxillary palps); *Orthopodomyia pulcripalpis* adults were misidentified five times as *Ae. aegypti* (both have more or less similar scutum patterns); larvae of *Ae. vittatus* were identified three times as *Ae. aegypti* (both have siphon without acus or with indistinct acus); larvae of *Ae. detritus* were confused with *Ae. vexans* three times.

Discussion

This EQA aimed to evaluate objectively the quality of mosquito identification within the MediLabSecure Network and offers useful perspectives in terms of capacity building to strengthening skills, competencies and abilities in the field of morphological identification of mosquitoes.

Taxonomy and systematics are endangered disciplines but are nonetheless a core capacity of medical entomology [15]. Reliable identification is crucial in order to support capacities for responding to vector-borne disease threats, as effective management measures can only be implemented when species are correctly identified. Misidentifications can have significant costs and consequences when decisions are needed for public health purposes. Morphological descriptions and identification keys (dichotomous or interactive) are still needed, as biological molecular tools and other "emerging" means

Table 1 Identifications of mosquito genera and species, according to development stage and sex

	Percentage of correct genus identification	Fisher's exact test (*P*-value)	Percentage of correct species identification	Fisher's exact test (*P*-value)
All mosquitoes (*n* = 206)	81.1	–	63.6	–
All larvae (*n* = 76)	88.2	ns (0.064)	60.5	ns (0.5489)
All adults (*n* = 130)	76.9	–	65.4	–
Adult females (*n* = 96)	81.3	ns (0.060)	68.8	ns (0.2098)
Adult males (*n* = 34)	64.7	–	55.9	–

Abbreviations: ns, not significant

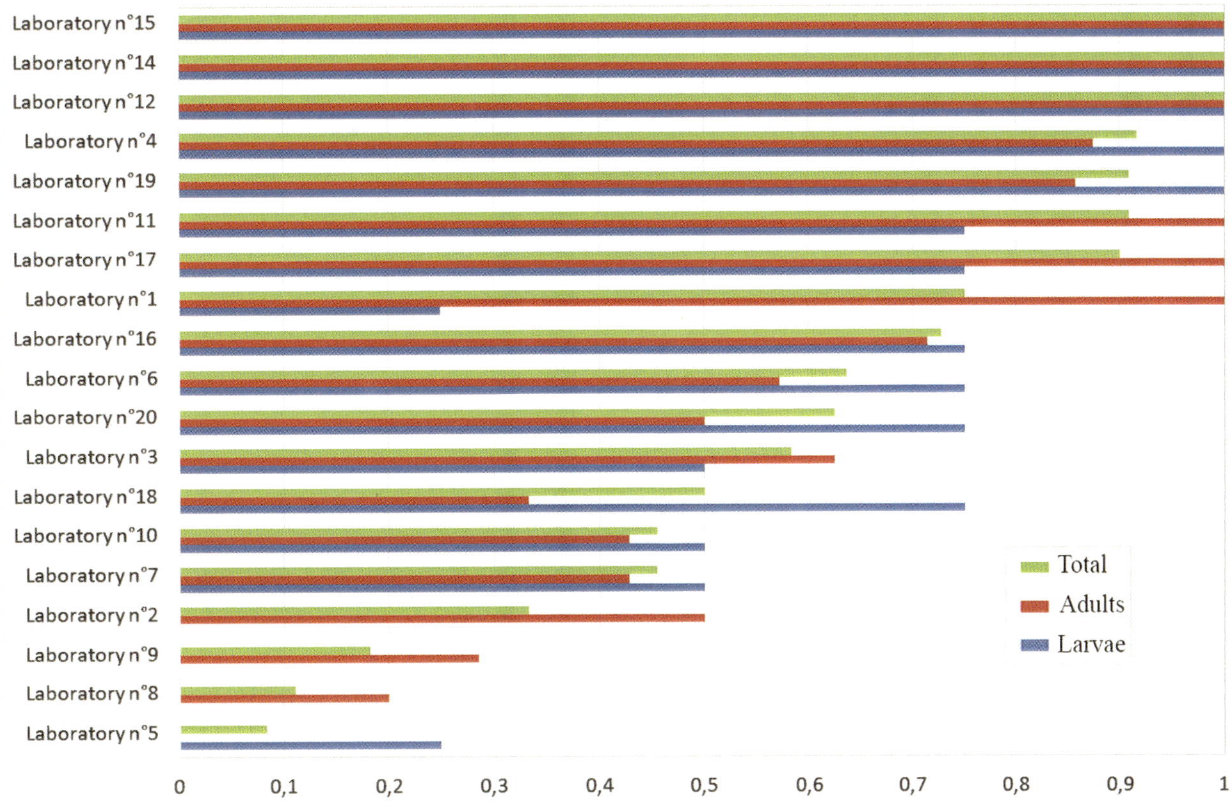

Fig. 3 Percentages of correct identifications at the species level by country for all samples (adults and larvae), and for adults and larvae separately

of identification (such as MALDI-TOF mass spectrometry profiling, geometric morphometrics using landmarks on the wings, and optically-refracted wing interference patterns) are not viable alternatives [16]. However, there have been calls for decades to fill the gap in expertise in insect systematics [17], including vectors [18].

It is worth noting that, although there were no restrictions on using molecular methods, all the laboratories in our study used morphological identification alone. This may be related to the dedicated training, known as 'MosPictoQuizz', routinely carried out every two months within the MediLabSecure Network, in which a series of pictures of an unknown mosquito are presented for identification [19]. It may also have to do with the fact that only half the participant laboratories are properly equipped for molecular identification.

The results of this EQA highlight the great need for improving the quality and reliability of mosquito identification. Finding solutions that may help to improve the situation is a huge task because many factors interfere with the accuracy of identification, including the suitability of the key used for the mosquito (with regard to

Table 2 Identifications of mosquito species ordered by decreasing rightness of identification of adult specimens. Only species where six or more adults were correctly identified were retained for analysis

	Percentage of correct species identification (adults)	Percentage of correct species identification (larvae)
Aedes albopictus	95 (*n* = 19)	– (*n* = 0)
Culiseta longiareolata	71 (*n* = 17)	74 (*n* = 19)
Aedes vittatus	68 (*n* = 19)	37 (*n* = 19)
Orthopodomyia pulcripalpis	63 (*n* = 19)	84 (*n* = 19)
Aedes vexans	60 (*n* = 15)	– (*n* = 0)
Culex hortensis	55 (*n* = 11)	– (*n* = 0)
Anopheles maculipennis (*s.l.*)	50 (*n* = 6)	– (*n* = 0)
Culex pipiens (*s.l.*)	50 (*n* = 18)	– (*n* = 0)
Aedes detritus (*s.l.*)	– (*n* = 0)	47 (*n* = 19)

the geographical area, the development stage or the sex of the specimen), the light source, and the microscope and its adjustment to the observer and focussing, etc. The keys themselves and how they are written may also be a factor in incorrect identifications. Simple questions may check the reasonableness of identification: is it a first record in the area? If yes, is there a senior entomologist around that may confirm the identification? Is the species known to be abundant in the area and in the season of sampling? Clearly, there is a need for standards of accuracy of identification in all entomology laboratories (not just those in this network) that report mosquito vector species information.

The results of this EQA also highlight the need to pursue efforts and obtain funding for capacity building in medical entomology to improve preparedness and response to vector-borne diseases. Here, we may want to ask what the best strategy is to improve the overall situation around the Mediterranean. In our opinion, there are two key options. The first consists in increasing the training sessions in those laboratories identified as reference centres in the various countries. However, training is only a step in the process of skill acquisition, which is gradually built through personal experience and regular practice. This means that in designating reference laboratories there must be a political, or at least institutional, solution to include taxonomy as a fundamental competence wherever arthropods of medical and public health importance are dealt with. The second option would be to identify a regional reference laboratory with the capacity to deal with numerous samples and to provide expertise to the different countries in the zone. However, expertise in taxonomy requires significant investment and there is currently a global lack of such expertise. Furthermore, control would be conceded to one country in the zone, on which the others would be dependent for this type of activity with consequent loss of sovereignty.

As with any technical activity delivering results, quality control is useful to check the performance of laboratories. This type of external assessment should be repeated and extended to other methods such as molecular assays, and to other activities and processes, such as sample collection or receipt, in order to maintain standards.

Conclusions

Identification of vectors is a core capacity in the field of medical and veterinary entomology and is needed to support response capacities to vector-borne disease threats. The results of this EQA highlight the need to maintain efforts in capacity building and quality control in the field of medical entomology and, more specifically, in the morphological identification of Culicidae.

Abbreviations

EQA: External quality assessment

Acknowledgements

The authors thank the Euro-Mediterranean project MediLabSecure.

Funding

The MediLabSecure project is supported by the European Commission (DEVCO: IFS/21010/23/_194), http://www.medilabsecure.com.

Authors' contributions

MP and VR conceived the EQA. FJ, MP, FG and VR analyzed the results and wrote the first draft. TS, NH, ZH, SSS, KK, TS, DA, MS, EV, LP, IP, CF, IS, DP, JM, GB, EJ, AB, AH, KS, BA and DP responded to the EQA. All authors read and approved final manuscript.

Competing interests

The authors declare that they have no competing interests.

Author details

[1]Research Unit MiVEGEC, French National Research Institute for Sustainable Development, IRD-CNRS-Montpellier University, Montpellier, France. [2]Institute of Zoology, Ministry of Education, Culture and Research, Chisinau, Moldova. [3]Laboratory of Immunology and Vector Borne Diseases, Lebanese University, Fanar, Lebanon. [4]Laboratoire Éco-épidémiologie Parasitaire et Génétique des Populations, Institut Pasteur d'Algérie, Algiers, Algeria. [5]Ministry of Health, Public Health General Directorate, Environmental Health Department, Vector Control Unit, Ramallah, Palestine. [6]Faculty of Science, Biology Department, Ecology Section, Vector Ecology Research Group Laboratories, Hacettepe University, Ankara, Turkey. [7]Parasitic and Zoonotic Diseases Department, Vector-Borne Diseases Programmes Manager, MOH, Amman, Jordan. [8]Reference Laboratory of Parasites & Vector Borne Diseases, NCDC Libya, and Zoology Department, Faculty of Science, University of Tripoli, Tripoli, Libya. [9]State Body I.I. Mechnikov Ukrainian Anti-Plague Research Institute of Ministry of Health, Odessa, Ukraine. [10]Laboratoire des Maladies Vectorielles, Institut Pasteur du Maroc, Casablanca, Morocco. [11]Control of Infectious Diseases Department, Institute of Public Health, Tirana, Albania. [12]Vector-borne and Parasitic Diseases Epidemiology Department, NCDC, Ministry of Health, Yerevan, Armenia. [13]Biotechnical Faculty, University of Montenegro, Podgorica, Montenegro. [14]Laboratoire d'Entomologie Médicale, Institut National d'Hygiéne, Rabat, Morocco. [15]Zooentomology Laboratory, National Center for Disease Control and Public Heath, Tbilisi, Georgia. [16]P.I. Veterinary Institute of the Republic of Srpska "Dr. Vaso Butozan", Banja Luka, Bosnia and Herzegovina. [17]Laboratory for virology and molecular diagnostics, Institute of Public Health of R. Macedonia, Skopje, Former Yugoslav Republic of Macedonia. [18]Université de Tunis El Manar, Institut Pasteur de Tunis, LR11IPT03 Service d'Entomologie Médicale, Tunis, Tunisia. [19]Faculty of Agriculture and Veterinary Sciences, University of Prishtina, Pristina, Republic of Kosovo. [20]Faculty of Science, Biology Department, Ecology Section, Vector Ecology Research Group Laboratories, Hacettepe University, Ankara, Turkey. [21]Faculty of Agriculture, Laboratory for Medical and Veterinary Entomology, University of Novi Sad, Novi Sad, Serbia. [22]French National Research Institute for Sustainable Development, Research Unit MiVEGEC, IRD-CNRS-Montpellier University, Montpellier, France.

References

1. Duvallet G, Boulanger N, Robert V. Arthropods: definition and medical importance. In: Boulanger N, editor. Skin and Arthropod Vectors. London: Academic Press; 2018. p. 29–54.
2. Cohuet A, Harris C, Robert V, Fontenille D. Evolutionary forces on *Anopheles*: what makes a malaria vector? Trends Parasitol. 2010;26:130–6.
3. Failloux AB, Bouattour A, Faraj C, Gunay F, Haddad N, Harrat Z, et al. Surveillance of arthropod-borne viruses and their vectors in the Mediterranean and Black Sea regions within the MediLabSecure network. Curr Trop Med Rep. 2017;4:27–39.
4. Stribling JB, Moulton SR II, Lester GT. Determining the quality of taxonomic data. J N Am Benthol Soc. 2003;22:621–31.
5. Stribling JB, Pavlik KL, Holdsworth SM, Leppo EW. Data quality, performance, and uncertainty in taxonomic identification for biological assessments. J N Am Benthol Soc. 2008;27:906–19.
6. Stribling JB. Partitioning error sources for quality control and comparability analysis in biological monitoring and assessment. In: Eldin AB, editor. Modern Approaches to Quality Control. Rijeka, Croatia: InTech; 2011. p. 59–84.
7. Bortolus A. Error cascades in the biological sciences: the unwanted consequences of using bad taxonomy. AMBIO. 2008;37:114–8.
8. Fontenille D, Almeras L, Garros C. Concepts et méthodes d'identification des espèces d'arthropodes. In: Duvalet G, Fontenille D, Robert V, editors. Entomologie Médicale et Vétérinaire. Marseille: IRD Editions & Quae Editions; 2017. p. 61–78.
9. Nayduch D. Molecular tools used in medical and veterinary entomology. In: Mullen GR, Durden LA, editors. Medical and Veterinary Entomology. 2nd ed. London: Academic Press; 2009. p. 543–55.
10. Hagedorn G, Rambold G, Martellos S. Types of identification keys. In: Nimis PL, Vignes-Lebbe R, editors. Tools for Identifying Biodiversity: Progress and Problems. Trieste: Edizioni Universitàdi Trieste; 2010. p. 59–64.
11. Becker N, Petrić D, Zgomba M, Boase C, Madon M, Dahl S, et al. Mosquitoes and Their Control. 2nd ed. Heidelberg: Springer; 2010.
12. Gunay F, Picard M, Robert V. MosKeyTool, an interactive identification key for mosquitoes of Euro-Mediterranean. Version 2.1. 2018. http://medilabsecure.com/moskeytool. Accessed 03 Aug 2018.
13. Ceriotti F. The role of External Quality Assessment Schemes in monitoring and improving the standardization process. Clin Chim Acta. 2014;432:77–81.
14. Chaki PP, Mlacha Y, Msellemu D, Muhili A, Malishee AD, Mtema ZJ, et al. An affordable, quality-assured community-based system for high-resolution entomological surveillance of vector mosquitoes that reflects human malaria infection risk patterns. Malar J. 2012;11:172.
15. Almeida APG, Fouque F, Launois P, Sousa CA, Silveira H. From the laboratory to the field: updating capacity building in medical entomology. Trends Parasitol. 2017;33:664–8.
16. Erlank E, Koekemoer LL, Coetzee M. The importance of morphological identification of African anopheline mosquitoes (Diptera: Culicidae) for malaria control programmes. Malar J. 2018;17:43.
17. Daly H. Endangered species: doctoral students in systematic entomology. Am Entomol. 1995;41:55–9.
18. Cuisance D, Rioux JA. Current status of medical and veterinary entomology in France: endangered discipline or promising science? Comp Immun Microbiol Infect Dis. 2004;27:377–92.
19. MediLabSecure Project. Mosquito Fact Sheet repository. 2014. http://www.medilabsecure.com/resources_factsheets.html. Accessed 03 Aug 2018.

14

Eugenol-hyperactivated nymphs of *Triatoma infestans* become intoxicated faster than non-hyperactivated nymphs when exposed to a permethrin-treated surface

Mercedes María Noel Reynoso, Alejandro Lucia, Eduardo Nicolás Zerba and Raúl Adolfo Alzogaray*

Abstract

Background: Eugenol is a botanical monoterpene that hyperactivates the blood-sucking bug *Triatoma infestans*, and permethrin is a pyrethroid with a strong triatomicide effect. In the present work, we tested the hypothesis that eugenol-hyperactivated nymphs of *T. infestans* pick up more insecticide, and then become intoxicated faster, than non-hyperactivated nymphs when exposed to a permethrin-treated surface.

Results: Values of knockdown time 50% (KT50) for third-instar *T. infestans* exposed to a paper impregnated with permethrin were obtained under the following situations: (a.i.) immediately after topical application of eugenol (KT50: 66.75 min for acetone pre-treated controls, and 46.27 min for eugenol pre-treated nymphs); (a.ii.) 30 min after topical application of eugenol (KT50: 66.79 min for controls, and 66.79 min for eugenol pre-treated nymphs); (b) simultaneously with exposure to eugenol vapors (KT50: 51.90 min for controls, and 39.5 min for nymphs exposed to an eugenol-treated filter paper); and (c) immediately after an injection of eugenol (on average, controls were knocked down after 63.00 min, whereas nymphs injected with eugenol were knocked down after 65.30 min). In other experimental series, the distance traveled (DT) by nymphs exposed to eugenol was quantified in the same situations previously described, but without exposure to permethrin. In (a.i.), the DT in interval 0–30 min after topical application of eugenol was 487.00 (control) and 1127.50 (eugenol) cm; in (a.ii.), the DT in the interval 31–60 min after topical application was 336.75 (control) and 256.75 (eugenol) cm; in (b), DT was 939.08 (control) and 1048.53 (eugenol) cm; and in (c), it was 589.20 (control) and 700.00 (eugenol) cm. The KT50 values for permethrin decreased significantly in situations (a.i.) and (b), and eugenol only produced a significant hyperactivity in the same situations. Finally, the amount of permethrin picked up by non-hyperactivated and hyperactivated nymphs exposed to a film of permethrin was quantified by gas chromatography. Non-hyperactivated nymphs picked up 0.34 μg/insect of permethrin, while hyperactivated nymphs picked up 0.65 μg/insect.

Conclusion: Results support the hypothesis that eugenol-hyperactivated nymphs of *T. infestans* pick up more insecticide, and then become intoxicated faster, than non-hyperactivated nymphs when exposed to a permethrin-treated surface.

Keywords: *Triatoma infestans*, Triatominae, Eugenol, Permethrin, Hyperactivity, Increased intoxication, Insecticide pick up, Chagas disease

* Correspondence: ralzogaray@hotmail.com
UNIDEF-CITEDEF-CONICET- CIPEIN, Juan B. de La Salle 4397, (1603) Villa Martelli, Buenos Aires, Argentina

Background

Eugenol is a botanical monoterpene present in the essential oils of clove, cinnamon, nutmeg, basil and other plants [1]. Its very low toxicity in mammals allows it to be used in odontology (for surgical dressings, temporary fillings, pulp capping agents and cavity liners), as a food flavoring and in perfumes [2]. It also shows insecticidal and repellent activities in several insect species [3–7]. An almost unexplored sublethal effect of monoterpenes consists in the modification of insect locomotor activity [8, 9]. For example, eugenol hyperactivates nymphs of the blood-sucking bug *Triatoma infestans*, vector of *Trypanosoma cruzi*, the causal agent of Chagas disease in Latin America [8]. The primary sites of action of the vast majority of insecticidal monoterpenes are unknown, but there is evidence suggesting that eugenol is a ligand of the octopamine receptor of the insects' nervous system [10].

When an organism is exposed to a mixture of two or more substances, their biological activity can be modified by the presence of the other compound. As a consequence of their interaction, the effect of the resulting combination can be higher or lower than the addition of the effects of each substance alone (synergism and antagonism, respectively) [11]. Both types of interactions have been observed in binary combinations of monoterpenes [12–15].

The classical concept of toxicological interactions considers the processes of absorption, distribution, metabolism, reaching sites of action and excretion of the components of the mixtures [16]. Some of these processes have been suggested as responsible for the toxicological interactions observed between monoterpenes [17–19]. In the cabbage looper, *Trichoplusia ni*, topical application of a mixture of *p*-cymene and thymol has a synergic effect since the first substance increases cuticle penetration, increasing the toxicity of the second substance [14, 20].

Other interactions involve changes in insect behavior. Incorporation of volatile host-plants increased the attraction of the boll weevil, *Anthonomus grandis*, and the palm weevil, *Rhynchophorus ferrugineus*, to their respective aggregation pheromones [21, 22]. In these cases, the behavioral response of insects exposed to a mixture of volatile substances was greater than the response to the components applied individually. This type of interaction has been named "behavioral synergism" [23].

The behavior of an insect can modify its exposure to a surface treated with insecticide. For example, hyperactive larvae of the tobacco budworm, *Heliothis virescens* picked up more permethrin from a treated surface than less active larvae of the same species [24].

Considering the information summarized above, the aim of this work was to test the hypothesis that eugenol-hyperactivated nymphs of *T. infestans* become intoxicated faster than non-hyperactivated nymphs when exposed to a permethrin-treated surface.

Methods

Biological material

We used third-instar nymphs of *T. infestans*, 1–14 days-old and starved after molt, from a colony at the Centro de Investigaciones de Plagas e Insecticidas (UNIDEF-CITEDEF-CONICET-CIPEIN, Buenos Aires, Argentina). This colony was established from a sample of insects donated by the Instituto Nacional de Parasitología "Dr. Mario Fatala Chaben" (Buenos Aires, Argentina). Insects were reared at a temperature of 25 ± 2 °C, 60–90% relative humidity and under a 12:12 h (L:D) photoperiod. Insects were fed on pigeon blood once per week according to a protocol approved by the Institutional Animal Care and Use Committee of CIPEIN (IACUC/CICUAL 1531/13).

Chemicals

Permethrin (94.5%) was provided by Chemotecnica S.A. (C. Spegazzini, Buenos Aires, Argentina), eugenol (99%) was purchased from Sigma-Aldrich (Buenos Aires, Argentina), acetone (technical grade) from Merck (Darmstadt, Germany) and silicone oil (556 cosmetic grade fluid) from Daltosur S.R.L. (Buenos Aires, Argentina).

We used eugenol due to its reported effect on the locomotor activity of *T. infestans* nymphs [8]. On the other hand, we chose permethrin because, in addition to its proved lethal effect on *T. infestans* [25], we found that the concentrations needed for our toxicity assays did not modify the locomotor activity of the nymphs. This was a key requirement, as in order to test our hypothesis we needed only eugenol to produce hyperactivity.

Bioassays of toxicity

Topical application of eugenol followed by exposure to a permethrin-treated surface

A disc of filter paper 11 cm in diameter (102 FAST, Hangzhou Xinxing Paper Industry & Co. Ltd., Funyang, China) was impregnated with 0.5 ml permethrin dissolved in an acetone:silicone (1:1) solution (1840 mg/m^2). The solvent was left to evaporate for an hour and then a glass ring (4 cm high and 10 cm in diameter) was placed over the paper disc.

Using a microsyringe (Hamilton, Reno, NE), 1 µl of eugenol dissolved in acetone was dropped onto the dorsal side of the abdomen of ten nymphs (0.1 µg/insect). They were then placed on the disc of filter paper impregnated with permethrin (a.i) immediately or (a.ii) 30 min after the topical application of eugenol. As controls, ten nymphs were treated with acetone alone in each case. The number of knockdown individuals was registered every 5 min. A nymph was considered knocked down if it remained in the same place for 30 s after being gently touched with a soft pair of tweezers (controls walked away immediately after being touched). Three independent replicates were carried out and each included a group of ten nymphs exposed to a filter paper impregnated only with the solvent. Knockdown time 50% (KT50) values were calculated with the results.

Simultaneous exposure to eugenol vapors and a permethrin-treated surface

The source of vapors was a piece of rectangular filter paper impregnated with eugenol (3.0 × 29.1 cm) (Fig. 1). One of the longer sides of the rectangle had six square lapels (0.5 × 0.5 cm) separated by 4.3 cm, that were turned up at a 90° angle. The surface of the rectangle was treated with 0.5 ml of eugenol dissolved in acetone (33 μg/cm^2). Once the solvent had evaporated, the inner side of the glass ring was lined with the paper rectangle, leaving the lapels to hang over the upper side of the ring. Thus, when the glass ring was placed over the circle of filter paper impregnated with permethrin, the bottom side of the paper rectangle hung 1 cm above the filter paper and was out of reach from the ten nymphs that were subsequently placed inside the ring. Finally, the upper side of the ring was covered with a glass square (10 × 10 cm) to create a micro-atmosphere with eugenol. Four independent replicates were carried out and each included a group of ten nymphs exposed to a piece of rectangular filter paper treated with acetone alone.

Injection of eugenol followed by exposure to a permethrin-treated surface

The upper side of a slide was covered by double-sided adhesive tape and a nymph was placed in a supine position and attached dorsally. Using a microsyringe and a binocular Nikon SMZ-10 10× magnifying glass (Tokyo, Japan), 0.2 μl of eugenol dissolved in acetone was injected into the nymph (2 ng/insect). The injection was performed in the left pleura of the first abdominal segment using a microsyringe (Hamilton, Reno, NE, USA). The nymph was then gently unstuck from the adhesive tape and placed in the center of a permethrin-impregnated filter paper disc. A nymph injected with acetone alone was used as control. As the immobilization and injection of the nymphs took longer than a topical application, in this series of experiments nymphs were individually exposed to a permethrin-treated filter paper. The time until each nymph was knocked down was registered. Each treatment was independently repeated ten times.

Bioassays of locomotor activity

Experiments were carried out inside a wooden box coated with melamine (1.0 × 0.5 × 0.5 m). The experimental arena was a filter paper disc (11 cm in diameter) (102 FAST; Hangzhou Xinxing Paper Industry & Co. Ltd.) placed on the floor of the box. A glass ring (4 cm high and 10 cm in diameter) was placed over the paper disc. A video camera was located 20 cm above the

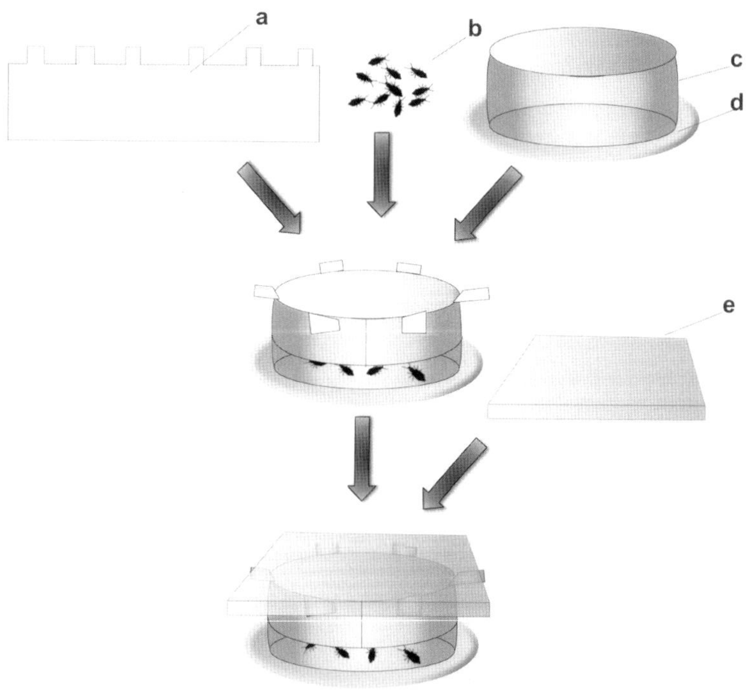

Fig. 1 Experimental arena used for simultaneous exposure of *T. infestans* nymphs to eugenol (vapors) and permethrin (contact): eugenol-impregnated piece of rectangular filter paper with six square lapels (**a**), *T. infestans* nymphs (**b**), glass ring (**c**), filter paper impregnated with permethrin (**d**), and glass square (**e**)

experimental arena (HD Webcam C525, Logitech, Lausanne, Switzerland) and connected to a personal computer. The camera had a resolution of 640 × 480 pixels with an acquisition and image processing speed of 30 frames/second. Lighting was provided by a cold light bulb (22 watts; Luxa, Shanghai, China) placed in the center of the top of the box.

A nymph was placed on the center of the filter paper and its movement was registered for 60 min. This experimental time allowed determining the duration of the effect of eugenol on locomotor activity and observing the way nymphs behaved once the hyperactive effect disappeared.

The video was analyzed using EthoVision XT 10.0 software [26]. This program quantifies the distance an insect moves expressed in cm.

The four experimental series described below (a'-d') were carried out using the same doses and concentrations of eugenol and permethrin as used in the toxicity bioassays. After testing that there were no variations in nymph locomotor activity between 11 am and 15 pm, trials were always performed within that time frame.

(a') Topical application of eugenol. Three independent replicates were performed, each including a nymph treated with acetone alone and another one treated with 0.1 μg eugenol/insect;
(b') Exposure to eugenol vapors. Six independent replicates were carried out, each including a nymph exposed to a piece of rectangular filter paper treated with acetone alone and another one exposed to a piece of rectangular filter paper impregnated with a solution of eugenol in acetone (33 μg/cm^2);
(c') Eugenol injection. One nymph was injected with acetone alone and another with 2 ng eugenol/insect. Each treatment was independently repeated ten times;
(d') Exposure to a paper filter disc impregnated with permethrin. Three independent replicates were carried out, each including a nymph exposed to a disc of filter paper treated with solvent alone and another one exposed to a disc of filter paper treated with permethrin (1840 mg/m^2).

Each of these four experimental series included one or two untreated control groups as follows: in series (a'), nymphs with no topical application; in (b'), nymphs exposed to an untreated piece of rectangular filter paper; in (c'), a group of nymphs pricked with the microsyringe needle but not injected with any substance, and a group of non-pricked nymphs; and in (d'), nymphs exposed to an untreated filter paper disc.

Extraction of the permethrin picked up by the nymphs

The procedure published by Pennell et al. [27] was adopted in this study with major modifications. Five hundred microliters of permethrin in acetone (0.035 g/ml) were applied on a circle of filter paper to obtain a concentration of 1840 mg/m^2. After solvent evaporation, the filter paper was placed on a horizontal surface and a glass ring was placed over it. Then, a group of ten nymphs topically pre-treated with 0.1 μg/insect of eugenol in acetone was placed on the permethrin-treated filter paper. After 10 min, the insects were transferred to a glass vial (2 ml) and fully immersed in 0.5 ml of acetone. The glass vial was gently shaken for 2 min after which the insects were discarded. Finally, an additional volume of acetone was added to the vial to complete 1 ml.

GC-MS analysis for determining the quantity of permethrin picked up

The analysis of permethrin was performed using a GC-2010 instrument coupled with a QP2010 mass spectrometer detector (Shimadzu, Kyoto, Japan) in the electron impact mode (70 eV). Samples were analyzed following the methodology used by Pinheiro et al. [28]. An apolar GC capillary column DB-5 (30 m × 0.25 mm i.d. and 0.25 μm coating thickness; J&W Scientific, Folsom, CA, USA) was used. The GC column temperature was maintained at 60 °C for 1 min, then programmed to increase from 60 to 150 °C at a rate of 20 °C/min, held for 4 min and then increased to 290 °C at a rate of 15 °C/min. This final temperature was held for 5.17 min. The injector was held at 280 °C. Helium (99.99%) was used as the carrier gas at a 1.2 ml/min caudal. The detector temperature was 250 °C and all injections were performed in the splitless mode (sampling time: 2 min). The volume of sample injected was 1 μl. The mass spectrometer scanned mass range m/z 40 and 400 was used for quantitative determinations of permethrin. For quantitative determination using selective ion monitoring (SIM), permethrin was identified by an ion of mass 183 (retention time: 20.15 min). The quantification was performed by calculating the absolute peak areas and a calibration curve was constructed by plotting the peak area of technical permethrin (purity 95.4%; cis: 52.4) *versus* permethrin concentration using a linear regression model (R^2: 0.99). With this calibration curve, the amount of permethrin in 1 ml (volume used for the extraction of 10 individuals) was obtained. These values were divided by 10 to obtain the amount of permethrin recovered per nymph (permethrin recovered expressed as μg per insect) of the insects previously treated by topical application of eugenol (treatment) or acetone alone (control).

In summary, the experiment for determining the amount of permethrin picked up by the nymphs consisted of two parts: (a) extraction of the permethrin picked up by the nymphs, and (b) GC-MS analysis for determining the permethrin picked up. This experiment (a + b) was performed five times. Thus, the values of the amount of permethrin picked up are representative of five independent experiments. Additionally, as the error was greater than in a routine analysis (by total scan mode), each sample was injected three times and the resulting values were used to calculate the total amount of permethrin. The average variation coefficient obtained for 30 injections by GC-MS was 18.76%.

Statistical analyses

Values of knockdown time 50% (KT50) and their corresponding 95% confidence intervals (95% CI) were calculated with the software for correlated data developed by Throne et al. [29]. Differences among KT50 values were consider significant if their 95% CI did not overlap. The results of the locomotor activity bioassays were analyzed using ANOVA, and those from the permethrin pick up quantification using Student's t-test.

Results

The toxicity of permethrin applied as a film on filter paper (1840 mg/m^2) was quantified in nymphs previously treated topically with eugenol (0.1 μg/insect) (Table 1). When nymphs were exposed to permethrin immediately after the pre-treatment with eugenol, their KT50 (46.27 min) was significantly lower compared to the control group (66.75 min) ($P < 0.05$). However, when the nymphs were exposed to permethrin 30 min after the pre-treatment, no significant differences were observed between the KT50 values of the group treated with eugenol (66.79 min) and the control group (66.79 min).

The second experiment assessed the effect of eugenol and permethrin on nymphs locomotor activity (Fig. 2). The same doses used in the previous experiment were evaluated. Topical application of eugenol significantly hyperactivated the nymphs but only for 30 min (for time interval 0–10 min, $F_{(2, 6)} = 169.8$, $P < 0.001$; 11–20 min, $F_{(2, 6)} = 15.7$, $P = 0.001$; 21–30 min, $F_{(2, 6)} = 6.22$, $P = 0.02$) (Fig. 2a). Exposure to filter paper impregnated with permethrin did not initially affect the locomotor activity of nymphs, but during the last minutes of the assay the activity decreased significantly (for the time interval 0–10 min: $F_{(2, 6)} = 4.2$, $P = 0.052$; 11–20 min: $F_{(2, 6)} = 1.4$, $P = 0.29$; 21–30 min: $F_{(2, 6)} = 0.37$, $P = 0.70$; 31–40 min: $F_{(2, 6)} = 9.95$, $P = 0.005$; 41–50 min: $F_{(2, 6)} = 27.3$, $P < 0.001$; 51–60 min: $F_{(2, 6)} = 8.83$, $P = 0.008$) (Fig. 2b). This decrease in locomotor activity coincided with the appearance of spasms, convulsions, and paralysis of the third pair of legs. These are the first symptoms of intoxication with pyrethroids, which manifest before knockdown.

Next, we assessed the toxicity of permethrin (1840 mg/m^2) on nymphs simultaneously exposed to eugenol vapors released by an impregnated paper (33 μg/cm^2) (Table 2). The KT50 values of nymphs exposed to both substances (39.50 min) was significantly lower than the values for the control group (51.90 min) ($P < 0.05$). Additionally, exposure to eugenol vapors in the absence of permethrin only produced a significant increase in locomotor activity during the first 10 min ($F_{(2, 9)} = 10.86$, $P = 0.001$) (Fig. 3).

We then determined the mean KT50 values of nymphs injected with eugenol (2 ng/insect) and immediately exposed to a paper disc impregnated with permethrin. On average, the KT50 value of nymphs injected with eugenol was 65.30 ± 4.80 min while the KT50 of nymphs injected with acetone alone was 63.0 ± 2.63 min. The difference between these values was not significant ($P > 0.05$), indicating that eugenol injection did not significantly modify the locomotor activity of nymphs compared to the control group (for the time interval 0–10 min: $F_{(3, 36)} = 1.94$, $P = 0.14$; 11–20 min: $F_{(3, 36)} = 0.04$, $P = 0.99$; 21–30 min: $F_{(3, 36)} = 0.45$, $P = 0.72$; 31–40 min: $F_{(3, 36)} = 0.43$, $P = 0.73$; 41–50 min: $F_{(3, 36)} = 1.32$, $P = 0.28$; 51–60 min: $F_{(3, 36)} = 0.90$, $P = 0.45$) (Fig. 4).

Finally, we assessed the amount of permethrin picked up by nymphs treated topically with eugenol and immediately exposed to permethrin impregnated filter papers for 10 min (Fig. 5). Nymphs pre-treated with eugenol picked up significantly higher quantities of permethrin than individuals pre-treated with acetone alone ($t_{(8)} = 8.17$, $P = 0.001$).

Discussion

In the present study, we report that nymphs of *T. infestans* hyperactivated by eugenol pick up more insecticide

Table 1 Knockdown time 50% (KT50) for permethrin in *T. infestans* nymphs topically pre-treated with eugenol

Pre-treatment (topical application)	Time before exposure to a permethrin-treated filter paper (min)	KT50 for permethrin (min)	95% CI	Slope ± SE
Acetone	0	66.75^a	60.43–74.43	8.99 ± 1.51
Eugenol (0.1 μg/insect)	0	46.27^b	40.90–52.29	7.40 ± 1.15
Acetone	30	66.79^a	62.16–71.94	12.68 ± 2.07
Eugenol (0.1 μg/insect)	30	66.79^a	61.87–72.32	11.90 ± 1.98

Abbreviations: *KT50*, knockdown time 50%; *95% CI*, 95% confidence interval; *SE*, standard error

Notes: Permethrin was applied as a film on filter paper (1840 mg/m^2). KT50 values followed by different letters are significantly different (based on their respective 95% CI not overlapping; $P < 0.05$)

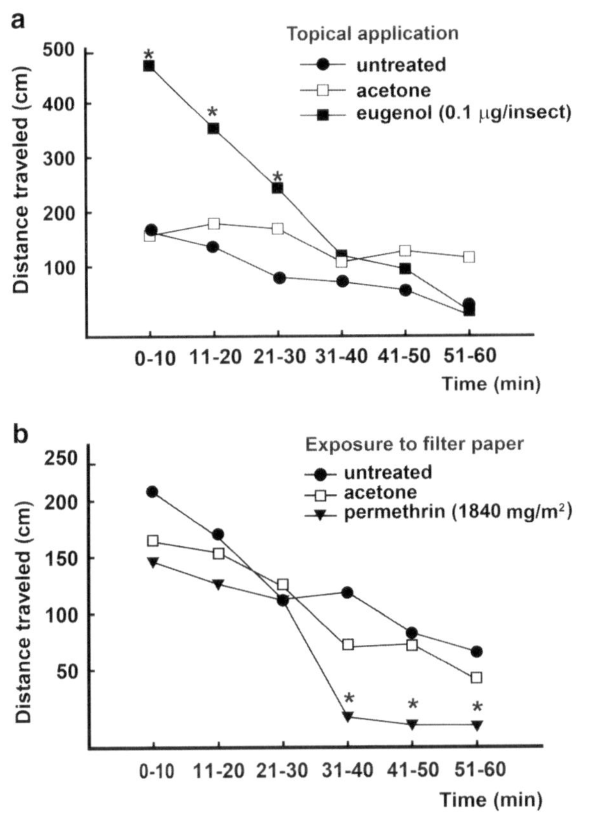

Fig. 2 Locomotor activity of *T. infestans* nymphs topically treated with eugenol or exposed to permethrin. **a** Nymphs were topically treated with acetone alone (control, empty squares) or a solution of eugenol in acetone (filled squares). **b** Nymphs were exposed to a filter paper impregnated with acetone alone (empty squares) or a solution of permethrin in acetone (filled triangles). Each symbol represents the mean of four independent replicates. Means in each time interval were analyzed using ANOVA. Symbols marked with an asterisk are significantly different from both untreated and acetone controls ($P < 0.05$)

from a permethrin-treated surface, thus becoming intoxicated faster than non-hyperactivated nymphs.

We quantified knockdown values produced by permethrin in four different situations: (a.i) immediately after a topical application of eugenol; (a.ii) 30 min after a topical application of eugenol; (b) simultaneously with the exposure to eugenol vapors; and (c) immediately after eugenol injection. The KT50 values of permethrin

Table 2 Knockdown time 50% (KT50) for permethrin in *T. infestans* nymphs exposed simultaneously to eugenol vapor

Simultaneous exposure to:	KT50 (min)	95% CI	Slope ± SE
Acetone	51.90^{a}	46.9–56.7	8.70 ± 1.39
Eugenol (33 μg/cm^2)	39.50^{b}	34.9–44.8	6.30 ± 0.89

Abbreviations: *KT50*, knockdown time 50%; *95% CI*, 95% confidence interval
Notes: Permethrin was applied as a film on filter paper (1840 mg/m^2). KT50 values followed by different letters are significantly different (based on their respective 95% CI not overlapping; $P < 0.05$)

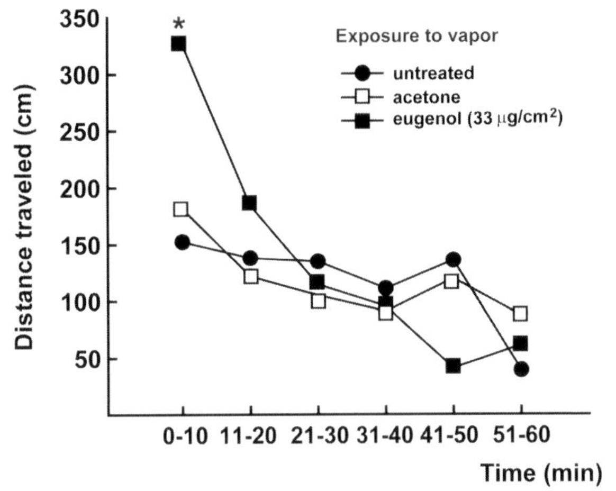

Fig. 3 Locomotor activity of *T. infestans* nymphs exposed to vapors of eugenol. Nymphs were exposed to a filter paper impregnated with acetone (control, empty squares) or a solution of eugenol in acetone (filled squares). Each symbol represents the mean of four independent replicates. Means in each time interval were analyzed using ANOVA. Symbols marked with an asterisk are significantly different from both untreated and acetone controls ($P < 0.05$)

were significantly lower than the controls in situations (a.i) and (b). Moreover, when eugenol was applied in the absence of permethrin, it only produced hyperactivity in those same two situations.

Locomotor activity is a complex characteristic that is directly or indirectly involved in almost all the activities of an insect and is regulated by a neurophysiological mechanism [30]. It has a very important role in survival and depends on both internal (age, hormonal state) and

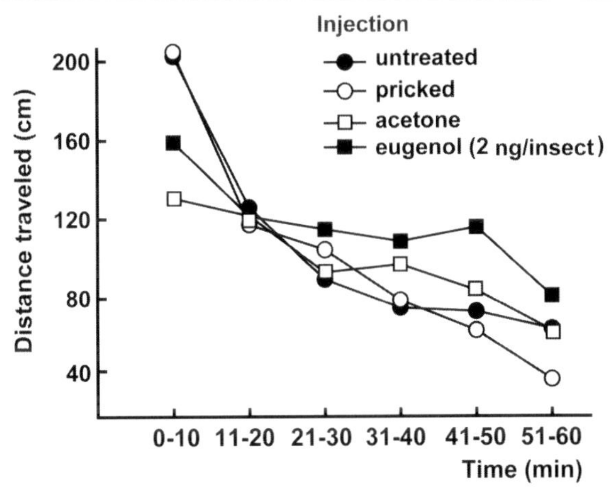

Fig. 4 Locomotor activity of *T. infestans* nymphs injected with eugenol. Nymphs were injected with acetone alone (control, empty squares) or a solution of eugenol in acetone (filled squares). Each symbol represents the mean of ten independent repetitions. Means in each time interval were analyzed using ANOVA. No significant differences were detected in any case ($P > 0.05$)

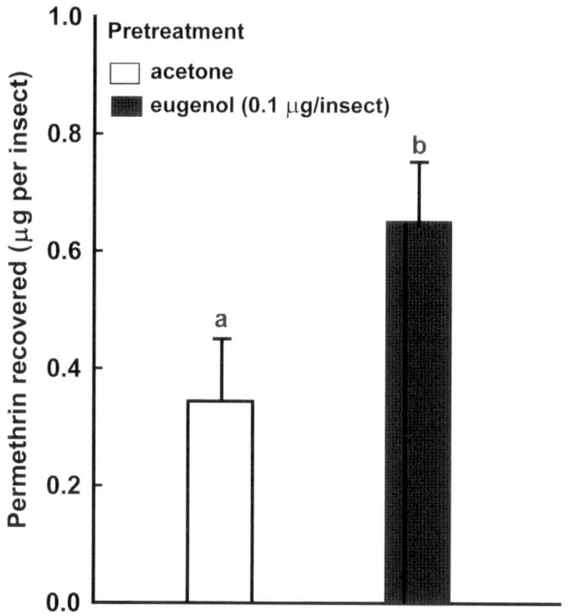

Fig. 5 Permethrin picked-up by hyperactivated *T. infestans* from an impregnated filter paper. Nymphs were topically pre-treated with acetone alone (empty bar) or a solution of eugenol in acetone (filled bar), then exposed to a filter paper treated with permethrin (1840 mg/m^2). Each bar represents the mean of five independent replicates. Vertical lines represent the SE. Bars marked with different letters are significantly different (Student's t-test, $P < 0.05$)

external (presence or absence of predators and conspecifics) factors [31–34]. Of particular interest is the recent discovery that infection with *T. cruzi* increases the locomotor activity of *R. prolixus*, whereas infection with *T. rangeli* causes a decrease [35].

Exposure to DDT and other insecticides increases the locomotor activity of insects [36–38]. Nymphs of *T. infestans* resistant to deltamethrin showed a reduced sensitivity to the hyperactivity produced by this insecticide when compared to deltamethrin-susceptible individuals [39]. Hyperactivity was also observed in insects exposed to components of essential oils [10], but it was only quite recently that this effect was quantified exposing *T. infestans* and *R. prolixus* to alcoholic monoterpenes [8, 9].

In the present study, the effect of eugenol on the locomotor activity of the nymphs varied considerably according to the form of administration. Topical application produced the highest effect, followed by exposure to vapors, whereas eugenol injection caused no modification in nymph locomotor activity.

The amount of compound that reaches an insect depends strongly on the type of exposure [40]. For example, insects exposed to an insecticidal film mainly pick up the compound by their legs, whereas topical application generates a more extensive distribution on the body cuticle [41].

In the present study, nymphs treated topically received a larger amount of eugenol than those exposed to vapors. Therefore, the difference observed in the effect on locomotor activity could be due to the fact that a higher dose produces a greater effect.

Why did eugenol fail to produce hyperactivity when injected? The dose applied (2 ng of eugenol/insect) might have been too low to modify the nymphs' locomotor activity. In fact, hyperactivity by eugenol and other monoterpenes is dose-dependent in *T. infestans* and *R. prolixus* [8, 9]. We were unable to test higher doses because they rapidly produced symptoms of intoxication (lateral walking, proboscis extension, leg tremors). Applying a substance that hyperactivates the nymphs at a dose that is much lower than the threshold producing intoxication symptoms could help solve this issue.

On the other hand, the effect of eugenol on hyperactivity could be induced *via* the neurons of sensory structures on the cuticle that react to different environmental stimuli. If this is true, stimulation would not occur when the monoterpene is injected into the hemolymph. The very rapid manifestation of hyperactivity when nymphs were exposed to eugenol vapors (Fig. 4) provides evidence that supports this explanation.

The mode of action of most monoterpenes remains unknown. Eugenol is one of the few exceptions, as evidence suggests that its primary site of action is the octopaminergic receptor [10]. The octopaminergic system is widely distributed throughout the central and peripheral nervous systems of invertebrates, where it participates in many physiological and behavioral aspects [42]. Within the context of the present study, it is important to note that the octopaminergic system is involved in the initiation and maintenance of rhythmic behaviors such as walking [43–45]. Based upon this knowledge, an interaction between eugenol and octopaminergic receptors could explain the hyperactivity observed in our experiments.

After demonstrating that hyperactivated nymphs become intoxicated more rapidly than the non-hyperactivated ones when exposed to a permethrin-treated surface, we quantified the amount of insecticide permethrin picked up in both situations. For this we adapted two protocols, one used for extracting dieldrin picked up by mosquitoes exposed to a surface treated with this insecticide [27], and another used to quantify permethrin and other insecticides in water samples [28]. This way, we managed to detect minute quantities of permethrin picked up by the nymphs exposed to treated filter papers. Our results showed that the nymphs hyperactivated by eugenol picked up more permethrin than the non-hyperactivated ones.

As mentioned in Background, a similar result was observed by other authors working with two strains of *H. virescens*, one susceptible and the other resistant to permethrin [24]. When exposed to a permethrin-treated surface, larvae from the resistant strain were less active and picked up less insecticide, than larvae from the susceptible strain. This behavioral response was considered partially responsible for the resistance to permethrin.

In summary, here we have gathered a significant amount of evidence that support our hypothesis: eugenol-hyperactivated nymphs of *T. infestans* pick up more insecticide, and then become intoxicated faster, than non-hyperactivated nymphs when exposed to a permethrin-treated surface.

Future studies should investigate the effects of other monoterpenes as possible enhancers of the toxicity of different insecticides on triatomines. Mixtures of monoterpenes should also be evaluated, to establish whether synergistic interactions occur. The application of mixtures of monoterpenes and conventional insecticides under field conditions is a possibility that is worth exploring, since hyperactivity could increase the exposure to recently applied insecticides, increasing the efficacy of control. Another issue to be investigated is the effect of eugenol on the locomotor activity of both trypanosomes-infected and resistant to pyrethroids *T. infestans*. These studies could elucidate for the physiological basis of the hyperactivity induced by insecticides in insects.

Conclusion

Results from toxicological, behavioral and analytical assays performed in this work support the hypothesis that eugenol-hyperactivated nymphs of *T. infestans* pick up more insecticide, and then become intoxicated faster, than non-hyperactivated nymphs when exposed to a permethrin-treated surface.

Abbreviations

95% CI: 95% confidence interval; DT: Distance traveled; GC-MS: Gas chomatography - mass spectrometry; KT50: Knockdown time 50%

Acknowledgements

AL and RAA are members of the Carrera del Investigador Científico del Consejo Nacional de Investigaciones Científicas y Técnicas of Argentina (CONICET). MMNR is a fellowship holder of the CONICET for her doctoral studies at Universidad de San Martín. We thank Catriona Kirkwood for translating the manuscript into English.

Funding

This work was funded by the Agencia Nacional de Promoción Científica y Tecnológica, Argentina (PICT 2012/1471 to ENZ).

Authors' contributions

MMNR conceived, designed and performed the experiments, analyzed the data, prepared figures and tables, and wrote and reviewed drafts of the paper. AL conceived, designed and performed the experiments, and wrote and reviewed drafts of the paper. ENZ and RAA conceived and designed the experiments, and wrote and reviewed drafts of the paper. All authors read and approved the final manuscript.

Competing interests

The authors declare that they have no competing interests.

References

1. Kamatou GP, Vermaak I, Viljoen AM. Eugenol - from the remote Maluku islands to the international market place: a review of a remarkable and versatile molecule. Molecules. 2012;17:6953–81.
2. Barceloux DG. Medical toxicology of natural substances: Foods, fungi, medicinal herbs, plants, and venomous animals. Hoboken: John Wiley & Sons; 2008.
3. Obeng-Ofori D, Reichmuth C. Bioactivity of eugenol, a major component of essential oil of *Ocimum suave* (Wild.) against four species of stored-product Coleoptera. Int J Pest Manage. 1997;43:89–94.
4. Huang H, Ho SH, Lee HC, Yap IL. Insecticidal properties of eugenol, isoeugenol and methyleugenol and their effects on nutrition of *Sitophilus zeamais* Motsch. (Coleoptera: Curculionidae) and *Tribolium castaneum* (Herbst) (Coleoptera: Tenebrionidae). J Stored Prod Res. 2002;38:403–12.
5. Waliwitiya R, Kennedy CJ, Lowenberger CA. Larvicidal and oviposition-altering activity of monoterpenoids, trans-anithole and rosemary oil to the yellow fever mosquito *Aedes aegypti* (Diptera: Culicidae). Pest Manag Sci. 2009;65:241–8.
6. Tabanca N, Bernier UR, Ali A, Wang M, Demirci B, Blythe EK, et al. Bioassay-guided investigation of two Monarda essential oils as repellents of yellow fever mosquito *Aedes aegypti*. J Agr Food Chem. 2013;61:8573–80.
7. Ali A, Cantrell CL, Khan KA. New *in vitro* bioassay system for the discovery and quantitative evaluation of mosquito repellents. J Med Entomol. 2017;54: 1328–36.
8. Moretti A, Zerba EN, Alzogaray RA. Behavioral and toxicological responses of *Rhodnius prolixus* and *Triatoma infestans* (Hemiptera: Reduviidae) to ten monoterpene alcohols. J Med Entomol. 2013;50:1046–54.
9. Moretti AN, Seccacini EA, Zerba EN, Canale D, Alzogaray RA. The botanical monoterpenes linalool and eugenol flush-out nymphs of *Triatoma infestans*. J Med Entomol. 2017;54:1293–8.
10. Enan EE. Insecticidal activity of essential oils: octopaminergic sites of action. Comp Biochem Phys C. 2001;130:325–37.
11. Wilkinson CF. Insecticide Interaction: Insecticide Biochemistry and Physiology. New York: Plenum Press; 1976.
12. Savelev S, Okello E, Perry NSL, Wilkins RM, Perry EK. Synergistic and antagonistic interactions of anticholinesterase terpenoids in *Salvia lavandula efolia* essential oil. Pharmacol Biochem Behav. 2003;75:661–8.
13. Ntalli NG, Ferrari F, Giannakou I, Menkissoglu-Spiroudi U. Synergistic and antagonistic interactions of terpenes against *Meloidogyne incognita* and the nematicidal activity of essential oils from seven plants indigenous to Greece. Pest Manag Sci. 2011;67:341–51.
14. Tak JH, Jovel E, Isman MB. Comparative and synergistic activity of *Rosmarinus officinalis* L. essential oil constituents against the larvae and anovarian cell line of the cabbage looper, *Trichoplusia ni* (Lepidoptera: Noctuidae). Pest Manag Sci. 2016;72:474–80.
15. Pavela R. Acute, synergistic and antagonistic effects of some aromatic compounds on the *Spodoptera littoralis* Boisd. (Lep., Noctuidae) larvae. Ind Crop Prod. 2014;60:247–58.
16. Cedergreen N. Quantifying synergy: a systematic review of mixture toxicity studies within environmental toxicology. PLoS One. 2014;9:e96580.
17. Passreiter CM, Wilson Andersen JR, Isman MB. Metabolism of thymol and trans-anethole in larvae of *Spodoptera litura* and *Trichoplusia ni* (Lepidoptera: Noctuidae). J Agr Food Chem. 2004;52:2549–51.
18. Taylor WG, Fields PG, Sutherland DH. Insecticidal components from field pea extracts: soyasaponins and lysolecithins. J Agric Food Chem. 2004;52:7484–90.
19. Fields PG, Woods S, Taylor WG. Triterpenoid saponins synergize insecticidal pea peptides: effect on feeding and survival of *Sitophilus oryzae* (Coleoptera: Curculionidae). Can Entomol. 2010;142:501–12.
20. Tak JK, Isman MB. Enhanced cuticular penetration as the mechanism of synergy for the major constituents of thyme essential oil in the cabbage looper, *Trichoplusia ni*. Ind Crop Prod. 2017;101:29–35.

21. Dickens J. Green leaf volatiles enhance aggregation pheromone of boll weevil, *Anthonomus grandis*. Entomol Exp Appl. 1989;52:191–203.
22. Hallett RH, Oehlschlager AC, Borden JH. Pheromone trapping protocols for the Asian palm weevil, *Rhynchophorus ferrugineus* (Coleoptera: Curculionidae). Int J Pest Manage. 1999;45:231–7.
23. Reinecke A, Hilker M. Plant semiochemicals - Perception and behavioural responses by insects. Annu Rev Plant Biol. 2014;47:115–54.
24. Sparks TC, Lockwood JA, Byford RL, Graves JB, Leonard BR. The role of behavior in insecticide resistance. Pestic Sci. 1989;26:383–99.
25. Casabé N, Melgar F, Wood EJ, Zerba EN. Insecticidal activity of pyrethroids against *Triatoma infestans*. Int J Trop Insect Sci. 1988;9:233–6.
26. Noldus. Software Ethovision XT 10.0. Leesburg: Noldus Information Technology Inc; 2013.
27. Pennell JT, Miskus R, Craig R. The use of gas chromatography for the quantitative determination of micro-amounts of insecticide picked up by mosquitos. Bull World Health Organ. 1964;30:91–5.
28. Pinheiro AS, Rocha GO, Andrade JB. A SDME/GC-MS methodology for determination of organophosphate and pyrethroid pesticides in water. Microchem J. 2001;99:303–8.
29. Throne JE, Weaver DK, Chew V, Baker JE. Probit analysis of correlated data: multiple observations over time at one concentration. J Econ Entomol. 1995;88:1510–2.
30. Klowden MJ. Physiological Systems in Insects. Idaho: Academic Press; 2007.
31. Hoffmann AA. The influence of age and experience with conspecifics on territorial behavior in *Drosophila melanogaster*. J Insect Behav. 1990;3:1–12.
32. Rakshit K, Wambua R, Giebultowicz TM, Giebultowicz JM. Effects of exercise on circadian rhythms and mobility in aging *Drosophila melanogaster*. Exp Gerontol. 2013;48:1260–5.
33. Van Der Bijl W, Thyselius M, Kotrschal A, Kolm N. Brain size affects the behavioural response to predators in female guppies (*Poecilia reticulata*). P Roy Soc B-Bio Sci. 2015;282:20151132.
34. Pflüger HJ, Duch C. Dynamic neural control of insect muscle metabolism related to motor behavior. Physiol. 2011;26:293–303.
35. Marliere NP, Latorre-Estivalis JM, Lorenzo MG, Carrasco D, Alves-Silva J, de Oliveira RJ, et al. Trypanosomes modify the behavior of their insect hosts: effects on locomotion and on the expression of a related gene. PLoS Negl Trop Dis. 2015;9:e0003973.
36. Gammon DW. Neural effects of allethrin on the free walking cockroach *Periplaneta americana*: an investigation using defined doses at 15 and 32 °C. Pestic Sci. 1978;9:79–81.
37. Toth SJ, Sparks TC. Effect of temperature on toxicity and knockdown activity of cis-permethrin, esfenvalerate, and lambda-cyhalothrin in the cabbage looper (Lepidoptera: Noctuidae). J Econ Entomol. 1990;83:342–6.
38. Alzogaray RA, Fontán A, Zerba EN. Evaluation of hyperactivity produced by pyrethroid treatment on third instar nymphs of *Triatoma infestans* (Hemiptera: Reduviidae). Arch Insect Biochem. 1997;35:323–33.
39. Sfara V, Zerba EN, Alzogaray RA. Toxicity of pyrethroids and repellency of diethyltoluamide in two deltamethrin resistant colonies of *Triatoma infestans* Klug, 1834 (Hemiptera: Reduviidae). Mem Inst Oswaldo Cruz. 2006; 101:89–94.
40. Matsumura F. Toxicology of Insecticides. 2nd ed. Berlin: Springer Science & Business Media; 2012.
41. Miller TP, Gold RE, Ball HJ. Tissue analysis and hemolymph translocation of [^{14}C] chlorpyrifos sorbed from treated surfaces by American cockroaches. Pestic Biochem Phys. 1983;20:19–24.
42. Farooqui T. Review of octopamine in insect nervous systems. Insect Physiol. 2012;4:1–17.
43. Yang NW, Li AL, Wan Liu FH, Johnson D. Effects of plant essential oils on immature and adult sweetpotato whitefly, *Bemisia tabaci* biotype B. Crop Prot. 2010;29:1200–7.
44. Saraswati S, Fox LE, Soll DR, Wu CF. Tyramine and octopamine have opposite effects on the locomotion of *Drosophila* larvae. J Neurobiol. 2004; 58:425–41.
45. Yellman C, Tao H, Biao H, Jay H. Conserved and sexually dimorphic behavioral responses to biogenic amines in decapitated *Drosophila*. Proc Natl Acad Sci USA. 1997;94:4131–6.

15

Functional analysis of a novel parasitic nematode-specific protein of *Setaria digitata* larvae in *Culex quinquefasciatus* by siRNA mediated RNA interference

Magalla Bastian Chalitha Lakmal Somarathne[1], Yasanthi Illika Nilmini Silva Gunawardene[2], Naduvilath Vishvanath Chandrasekharan[1], Arjuna Nisantha Bandara Ellepola[3] and Ranil Samantha Dassanayake[1*]

Abstract

Background: Functional analysis of animal parasitic nematode genes is often quite challenging due to the unavailability of standardised *in vitro* culture conditions and lack of adequate tools to manipulate these genes. Therefore, this study was undertaken to investigate the suitability of *Culex quinquefasciatus*, as an *in vivo* culture platform for *Setaria digitata* larvae and RNA interference (RNAi), as a post-transcriptional gene silencing tool to study the roles of a vital gene that encodes a novel parasitic nematode-specific protein (*SDNP*).

Results: The red colour fluorescence detected following RNAi injection to the thorax of *C. quinquefasciatus* indicated the uptake of dsRNA by *S. digitata* larvae. The reduction of *SDNP* transcripts in siRNA treated larvae compared to non-treated larvae, as determined by qPCR, indicated that the siRNA pathway is operational in *S. digitata* larvae. The observation of motility reductions and deformities during the development indicated the association of *SDNP* in larvae locomotion and development processes, respectively. The irregularities in the migration of larvae in mosquitoes and elevated survival rates of mosquitoes compared to their untreated counterparts indicated reduced parasitism of *S. digitata* larvae in mosquitoes upon targeted downregulation of *SDNP* by siRNA treatment.

Conclusion: SDNP plays vital roles in muscle contraction, locomotion, development processes, larval development and parasitism of *S. digitata*. Its ubiquitous presence in parasitic nematodes and its absence in their hosts provide a tantalising prospect of the possibility of targeting SDNP for future development of anthelmintic drugs. The susceptibility of the larval stages of *S. digitata* for RNAi in *Culex quinquefasciatus* was also demonstrated for the first time in this study.

Keywords: *Setaria digitata*, *SDNP*, RNAi, *Culex quinquefasciatus*, Gene knockdown

Background

Nematodes are the most abundant metazoans, capable of inhabiting both terrestrial and aquatic habitats. This facilitates their ability to cause both human and animal health problems, as well as to impair crop production worldwide. Gastrointestinal nematodes infect 3.5 billion humans annually worldwide, and cause around 125,000 deaths per year, whereas filarial nematodes infect 120 million people in the globe annually, disabling around 40 million of them [1–3]. Additionally, plant-parasitic nematodes destroy approximately 12.3% of the annual crop yield, and animal parasitic nematodes kill millions of livestock animals. This contributes to a loss of billions of US dollars annually and necessitates the allocation of additional billions of US dollars for anthelminthic drugs for livestock [4, 5]. Strategies for controlling this problem have mainly focused on chemical treatments [5]. However, due to the limited efficiency and high toxicity of the available drugs, adverse effects on the environment, and emergence of drug resistance in parasites, these chemical treatment methods have become somewhat ineffective [6–8]. Hence, global interest has recently arisen in

* Correspondence: rsdassanayake@chem.cmb.ac.lk
[1]Department of Chemistry, Faculty of Science, University of Colombo, Colombo 03 00300, Sri Lanka
Full list of author information is available at the end of the article

developing more effective controlling strategies for parasitic nematodes. In this context, screening of the nematode genome will enable us to gain a comprehensive knowledge of the molecular mechanisms associated with the development of the nematode, which may facilitate the control of parasitic nematodes [9, 10].

RNA mediated gene silencing has become a promising and unbiased tool in genetic screening [11]. RNA interference (RNAi) is a double-stranded RNA (dsRNA) induced post-transcriptional, homology-dependent gene silencing mechanism, naturally occurring in organisms, assumed to be involved in defence against virus attacks, heterochromatinisation and retrotransposon silencing [11–13]. RNAi was initially utilised in the genetic screening of *Caenorhabditis elegans*, and after that, this technique was expanded to other invertebrates (nematodes, insects, molluscs), vertebrates (fish, mice, humans), plants, fungi and algae [14–17]. RNAi allows the temporary shut-down of gene expression more specifically and rapidly and gives an insight into gene function [18, 19].

Setaria digitata is a parasitic nematode that naturally resides in the peritoneum and mesentery of cattle, zebu and water buffalo. Under normal circumstances, the nematode does not show any pathogenicity towards the natural hosts. The microfilariae produced by the adult female worm travel into the bloodstream of the cattle and are transmitted into new hosts *via* mosquito bites. However, when the larvae are transfected into non-permissive hosts such as goats, sheep and horses, they invade the brain, spinal cord, and eyes, causing cerebrospinal setariosis, conjunctivitis, and filariasis oculi, respectively [20]. Intriguingly, studies on *S. digitata* have revealed that it has a high resemblance to the human parasitic nematode *Wuchereria bancrofti* with regard to its morphology, antigenicity and histology [21, 22]. Hence *S. digitata* has been recommended as a model organism for studying *W. bancrofti* and *Brugia malayi* [23].

Unveiling the biology of the parasitic nematodes genes, which are specific and functionally crucial for their survival, is crucial in identifying targets to control the nematode population [16]. *SDNP* is such a gene found in *S. digitata*. Intriguingly, this gene has demonstrated high sequence similarities with putative proteins of *W. bancrofti* (79%), *Brugia malayi* (77%) and *Loa loa* (81%). Moreover, bioinformatics studies of *SDNP* revealed that this protein contains a nuclear localisation signal, an RNAP_Rpb7_N_like domain, and an inter-domain linker of muscle-specific twitchin kinase similar to that of *C. elegans* [24]. Considering the background, our study focused on the functional characterisation of *SDNP*.

Commonly, RNAi protocols are practised by isolation of the nematodes from their natural hosts and maintaining them in artificial liquid cultures (*in vitro*). These *in vitro* protocols reduce the efficiency of RNAi due to several shortcomings such as difficulty in maintaining the worms' viability in the culture, poor RNAi trigger delivery, and compatibility issues of the culture medium with different life stages of the worm [25]. To overcome these drawbacks of *in vitro* protocols, in our study an *in vivo* approach was developed, where *S. digitata* larval stages were cultured in its intermediate host, *Culex quinquefasciatus*, and the RNAi trigger (siRNA) was directly injected into the mosquito [19], and the possibility of using the mosquito as a better siRNA delivery platform examined. Furthermore, we focused on developing an effective RNAi protocol to specifically shut down the gene of interest to study its function and explore the gene's potential as a likely drug target.

Methods

Mosquito colony establishment

Culex quinquefasciatus were collected from a cattle trap and maintained at 27 °C with 80% relative humidity, with cycles of 16 h of light and 8 h of darkness, in 12 × 12 × 12-inch cages [26]. The eggs obtained from these mosquitoes were hatched in cups containing pre-boiled water, and the larvae which emerged from the eggs were fed with a larval diet (brewer yeast, bovine liver powder, tuna meal) until pupae appeared. The pupae were then separated from the larvae and placed in containers with fresh water in separate cages for 36 h until adult mosquitoes emerged. These were then fed with 10% sucrose solution [27]. They were used as an *in vivo* culturing medium for *S. digitata* microfilariae.

Mosquito infection with *S. digitata*

Adult female worms obtained from a cattle slaughterhouse in Welisara, Ragama, Sri Lanka were cut into small pieces after washing three times with mosquito physiological saline (MPS) [28] to release microfilariae (MF) into a tube containing 300 μl MPS. This was vortexed and centrifuged at 1500× *rpm* for 30 s, and the supernatant recovered was then re-centrifuged at 1500× *rpm* for 3 min to obtain a pellet containing MF, which was then re-suspended in MPS to achieve a microfilariae (MF) concentration of 40 MF/μl.

The thorax of anaesthetized adult mosquitoes (aged 3 days) on ice [29] was injected with a volume of 0.5 μl of microfilariae suspension using a pre-pulled borosilicate glass capillary attached to a manual injector [29–31]. The injected mosquitoes were kept in paper cups covered with a net while providing them with cotton pads soaked with the sucrose solution.

siRNA synthesis, Cy3 labelling and RNAi treatment

The entire coding sequence of *SDNP* was divided into four overlapping regions, and each of them was amplified by separate PCR reactions using four separate primer sets containing T7 promoter sequence at 5' ends (Table 1) to enrich the total yield of the template and PCR products of overlapping regions were used to synthesize siRNA. The PCR conditions used for the amplification were initial denaturation at 94 °C for 2 min, followed by 40 cycles of denaturation at 94 °C for 30 s, annealing at 55 °C for the primer sets SDNP-1-F/R, SDNP-2-F/R and SDNP-3-F/R and 45 °C for the primer set SDNP-4-F/R, and extension at 72 °C for 30 s with a final extension of 10 min at 72 °C (Table 1).

The resulting PCR fragments were transcribed separately *in vitro* by T7 RNA polymerase (New England Biolabs, Hitchin, UK) using slightly modified manufacturer's protocols, to yield a high amount of dsRNA. Briefly, the *in vitro* transcription reaction was carried out overnight at 37 °C in a 120 µl reaction mix containing 81.5 µl of nuclease-free H_2O, 12.0 µl of 10× T7 buffer, 3.0 µl of DTT (100 mM), 10 µl (2 µg) of PCR product, 12 µl of rNTP mix (80 mM), 1.5 µl of T7 RNA polymerase (18 U/µl). The RNA products of *in vitro* transcribed DNA were first treated with DNase 1 (New England BioLabs) to remove DNA templates and then incubated at 75 °C for 5 min before cooling them down to room temperature for the complementary strands of synthesized RNA to anneal to make dsRNA. The dsRNA (assessed by gel electrophoresis) was digested with RNase III (New England Biolabs) according to the manufacturer's protocol to produce 21–23 mer siRNA. They were analyzed by polyacrylamide gel electrophoresis before labelling with Cy3 fluorescent dye using a Silencer® siRNA Labeling Kit - Cy™3 dye (Ambion, Life Technologies, California, USA) according to the manufacturer's instructions [32].

The ds-RNA synthesized from the gene encoding for the green fluorescent protein (GFP) of *Aequorea victoria* was also used as the non-specific siRNA control as this gene neither has any homologous sequences in *S. digitata* nor mosquito. pCRII TOPO vector (pCRII TOPO-*GFP*) containing *GFP* was used in the synthesis of GFP dsRNA. The vector was digested with *Kpn* I [7.5 µl nuclease free H_2O, 2.0 µl 10× buffer, 0.5 µl *Kpn* I (15 U/µl), 10 µl DNA (200 ng/µl); incubated 1 h at 37 °C] and *Xho* I [10 µl nuclease free H_2O, 3.0 µl 10× buffer, 0.3 µl BSA, 0.5 µl *Xho* I (20 U/µl), 16.2 µl DNA (200 ng/µl); incubated 3 h at 37 ° C] separately. The *Kpn* I digested vector was *in vitro* transcribed by T7 RNA polymerase using the same protocol indicated above. The *Xho* I digested vector was *in-vitro* transcribed by Sp6 RNA polymerase using the following reaction; 60 µl of nuclease-free H_2O, 8.0 µl of 10x Sp6 buffer, 2 µg (10 µl) of pCR II-TOPO vector, 8 µl of rNTP mix (80 mM), 2 µl of Sp6 RNA polymerase (20 U/µl), incubated at 40°C for 4 h. The separately *in vitro* transcribed RNA was mixed and incubated at 75 °C for 5 min and cooled down to room temperature for the complementary strands of synthesised RNA to anneal to make dsRNA.

The *S. digitata* infected mosquitoes were initially injected with 150 ng of Cy3 labelled *SDNP* siRNA mix into their thorax at 12 h post infection (hpi) to monitor the uptake of siRNA by larvae. To target the L2 to L3 larvae transformation, non-labelled siRNA mix was injected at eight days post infection (dpi). The *GFP* siRNA (150 ng) was injected as a negative control.

Mosquito dissection

The mosquitoes infected with *S. digitata* and injected with *SDNP* siRNA, non-injected, *GFP* siRNA-injected and buffer-injected were dissected at different time intervals (24 hpi, 8–14 dpi) under a dissection microscope. In this process, the bodies of cold anaesthetized mosquitoes were separated into the thorax, midgut, and head, and each of these body parts was further dissected to release the larvae on to glass slides. The MF obtained from the smeared content on the slides at 24 hpi were visualized under the fluorescent microscope using Cy3 filter set (excitation: 550 nm, emission: 570 nm) to detect the uptake of siRNA. The transformation of L2 larvae to L3 was recorded from the mosquitoes dissected at 8 to 14 dpi, and the following data were recorded only from the mosquitoes dissected at 14 dpi: (i) larvae length and

Table 1 Primer sets used for the synthesis of dsRNA. The positions of the primers with respect to *SDNP* sequence (GenBank: GU222920), sequence corresponding to T7 promoter region of primers (underlined), the size of the PCR products, and the optimized annealing temperatures of primer sets are given

Primer	Position	Sequence (5'-3')	Product size (bp)	Annealing T (°C)
SDNP-1-F	1	TAATACGACTCACTATAGGGCGACGAGGGTTCCATTGAGTGA	154	55
SDNP-1-R	134	TAATACGACTCACTATAGGGGCTTCCTGACAAGCCAAACAT		
SDNP-2-F	155	TAATACGACTCACTATAGGGCGACGAGGGTTCCATTGAGTGA	150	55
SDNP-2-R	282	TAATACGACTCACTATAGGGTTGGAATATAAACATGCGGTATA		
SDNP-3-F	305	TAATACGACTCACTATAGGGCTACCGGTATCAGAACTCAGAA	157	55
SDNP-3-R	462	TAATACGACTCACTATAGGGTAGCGCTGGACCGAATTCTTTT		
SDNP-4-F	463	TAATACGACTCACTATAGGGGGAAATGGAACTTGTGAAATAA	155	45
SDNP-4-R	618	TAATACGACTCACTATAGGGTCAGTAATTAATCAAATT		

Abbreviation: *T* temperature

Table 2 Primers used for qPCR. The primer sequences of the target (SDNP) and internal control (Actin) are given

Primer	Sequence (5'-3')	Position	Product size (bp)	Annealing T (°C)
SDNP amplification				
SDNP-RTPCR-FP	AAGACTTGCAACTCCATCTCGAT	219	170	60
SDNP-RTPCR-RP	ATTTTCTCGCTGACCACCACAACT	366		
S. digitata actin amplification (reference gene)				
SDACT-RTPCR-FP	CGCTCGAGAAATCTTACGAATTGC	707	147	55
SDACT-RTPCR-RP	TCCTTTCTGATATCGATATCACATT	854		

Abbreviation: *T* temperature

width (Image J software was utilized in obtaining the measurements); (ii) larvae location in the mosquito (larvae in the head, thorax and abdomen of the mosquito; (iii) larvae motility (motility of the RNAi treated and control worms were compared according to a previously used pre-fashioned 5-point scheme based on Song et al. [19]). The scoring scheme was as follows: 1, immobile, dead; 2, compromised motility; 3, partial movement of the body; 4, slightly reduced motion in the body; and 5, all parts of the body are vigorously twisting. Values in

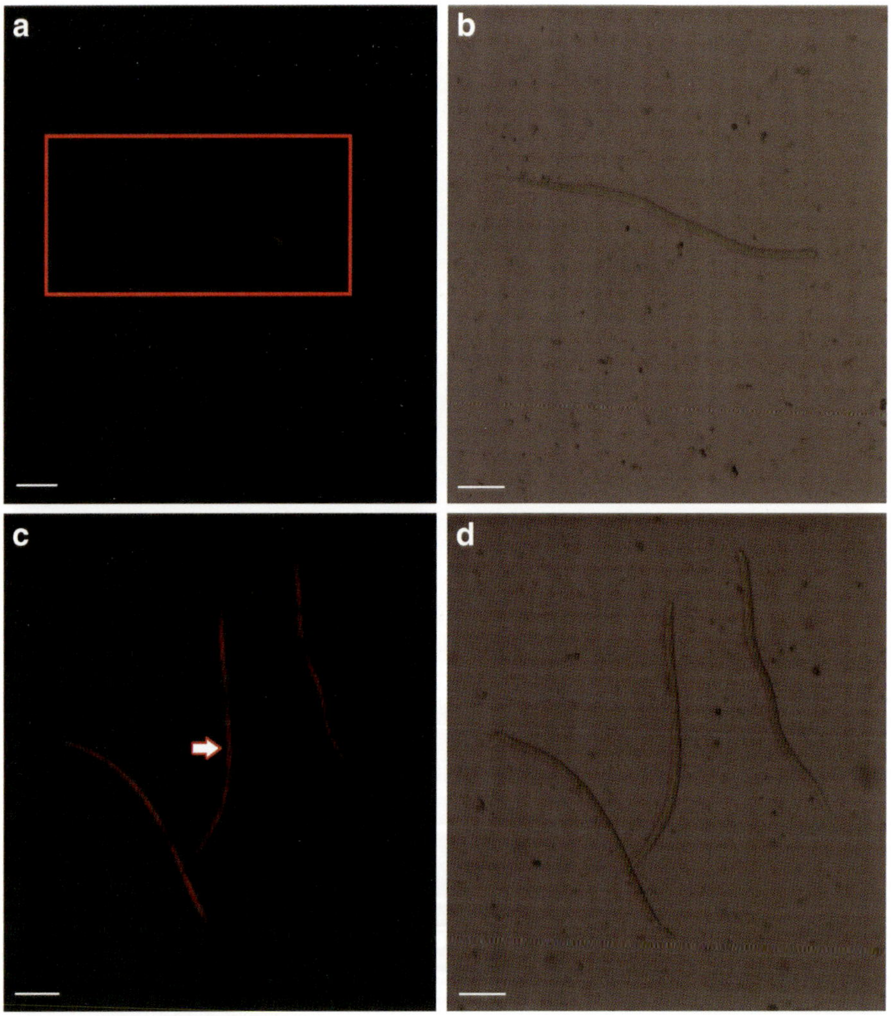

Fig. 1 Uptake and distribution of Cy3 labelled *SDNP* siRNA by microfilariae at 24 hpi. **a** Fluorescent image of microfilariae from siRNA non-injected mosquitoes (position indicated by a red square). **b** Bright field image of microfilariae from siRNA non-injected mosquitoes. **c** Fluorescent image of microfilariae from Cy3 labelled *SDNP* siRNA-injected mosquitoes (arrow indicates the dispersion of Cy3 labelled siRNA). **d** Bright field image of microfilariae from Cy3 labelled *SDNP* siRNA-injected mosquitoes. Fluorescence was visualised using Olympus BX53 using Cy3 filter. Magnification 400×. *Scale-bars*: **a-d**, 20 μm

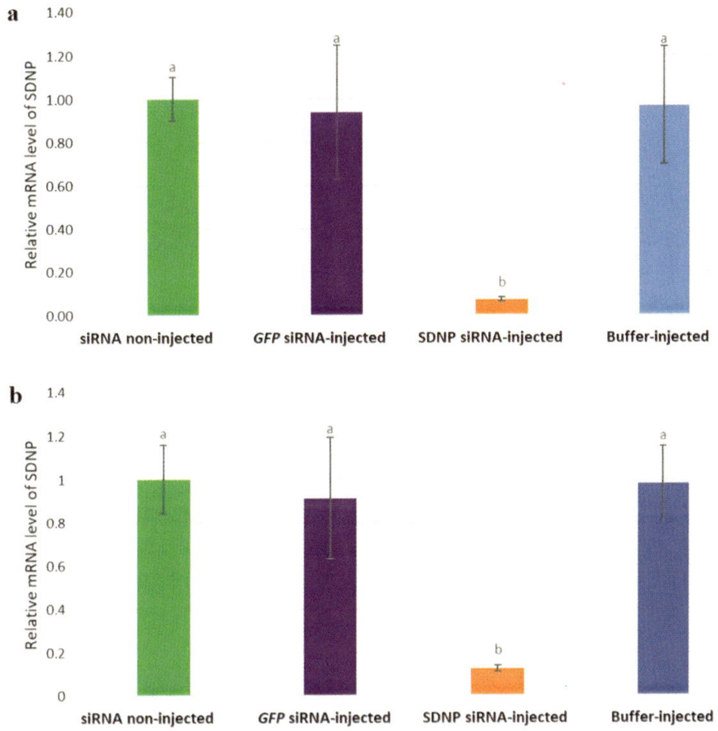

Fig. 2 Relative mRNA expression changes owing to the RNAi. **a** Relative mRNA levels of *SDNP* at two dpi. **b** Relative mRNA levels of *SDNP* at 14 dpi. Changes of *SDNP* specific transcript levels were analysed by qPCR, and the $2^{\Delta\Delta CT}$ method was used in evaluating the results. For the reference gene, *S. digitata* actin gene was used. *GFP* was used as the non-specific control. *SDNP* transcript level was presented as relative to that of non-treated worms. Each experiment was performed in triplicate. Bars display mean ± SD. Statistical analysis was performed using Student's t-test ($P < 0.05$). Significant differences are represented by different lowercase letters

between 5 and 1 in the scale were assigned according to the decreasing motility blindly by an independent evaluator; (iv) at 14 dpi, mosquito survival rate was also measured by counting the live mosquitoes.

Relative quantification of SDNP mRNA level

Total RNA was extracted at two dpi and 14 dpi from non-injected, *GFP* siRNA injected, *SDNP* siRNA-injected and buffer-injected mosquitoes infected with S. *digitata* using a GenoSpin R^{TM} Total RNA Extraction Kit (CEYGEN Biotech, Colombo, Sri Lanka) according to the manufacturer's instructions. Five mosquitoes were used from each batch. DNA contamination in extracted RNA was removed by treating with DNase I and heat inactivating the DNase I at 75 °C for 5 min. cDNA synthesis was carried out using RNA (2 μg) purified using an RNeasy Plus Mini Kit (Qiagen, California, USA) in a 20 μl reaction mix containing 5.0 μl of M-MLV transcription buffer, 1.0 μl of oligo dT primers (5 nM), 1.25 μl of dNTP mix (10 nM), 1.0 μl RNase inhibitor (20 U), 1.0 μl M-MLV reverse transcriptase (200 U, Promega, California, USA), RNA (2 μg), and RNase free water according to the vendor's protocol.

Relative quantification of *SDNP* mRNA levels was carried out by quantitative real-time PCR [CFX96 RealTime PCR System (Bio-Rad)] using SYBR green as the DNA binding dye. qPCR conditions were initial denaturation at 95 °C for 2 min, followed by 40 cycles of denaturation at 95 °C for 30 s annealing at 60 °C for SDNP primers and 55 °C for actin primers for 45 s (Table 2), and with an extension at 72 °C for 30 s. In qPCR, the actin gene (GenBank: AF079359.1) was used as the internal amplification control in a separate tube for each qPCR reaction. In calculating the relative mRNA expression level, the $2^{-\Delta\Delta CT}$ method was used as mentioned in qPCR Application Guide (BioRad). The data obtained were presented as the mean ± standard deviation (SD). A P value < 0.05 was considered statistically significant.

Results and discussion

siRNA uptake by *S. digitata* microfilariae in the mosquito host

A previous study demonstrated the possibility of *in vivo* suppression of the cathepsin L-like cysteine protease gene of *B. malayi* using RNAi in *Aedes aegypti* [19]. Therefore, in this study, the possibility of using *C. quinquefasciatus* as an *in vivo* siRNA delivery platform for developing *S. digitata* larvae was tested, where the transformation of MF to L3 larvae of the latter organism has been observed. Since the previously stated study revealed

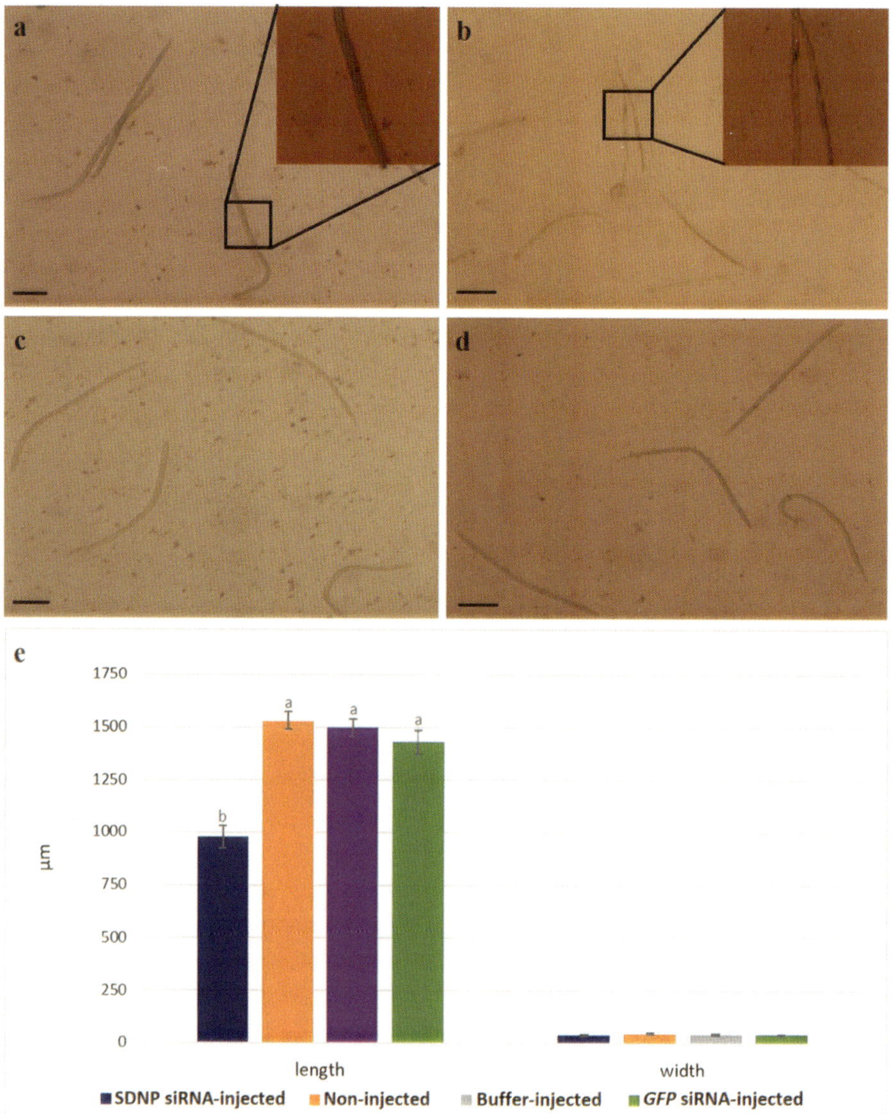

Fig. 3 Larvae development in *C. quinquefasciatus* mosquitoes at 14 dpi. **a** Larvae in siRNA non-injected mosquito. **b** Larvae in *SDNP* siRNA-injected mosquito. **c** Larvae in *GFP* siRNA-injected mosquito. **d** Larvae in buffer-injected mosquito (magnification 400×). **e** Mean length and width of larvae form *SDNP* siRNA-injected, non-injected, buffer-injected and *GFP* siRNA-injected mosquitoes. To target L2 to L3, siRNA injections were made at 8 dpi. Triplicates were performed for each experiment. Bars represent mean ± SD. Significant differences at $P < 0.05$ are represented by different lowercase letters. *Scale-bars*: **a**-**d**, 400 µm

the dissemination of siRNA to the MF of *B. malayi* through the mosquito, in the current study the uptake of the Cy3 labeled RNAi trigger by MF was investigated by, comparing the internal fluorescence of the MF with the mosquito physiological saline (MPS) injected control under a fluorescent microscope (Fig. 1a). A dispersion of the fluorescent signal was observed throughout the body of the tested MF at 24 hpi (Fig. 1c) indicating that uptake of Cy3 labelled siRNA by MF is occurring in the mosquitoes. Although the mechanism of siRNA uptake is unclear at this point, it is possible that this would occur *via* feeding or through the cuticle of MF. Therefore, here, it was possible to recreate the *in vitro* siRNA soaking conditions for *S. digitata* larvae *in vivo*, and the possibility of utilizing the mosquito as a siRNA delivering platform for parasitic nematodes hosted by the mosquito was affirmed.

The effect of siRNA on SDNP mRNA level of MF

Several recent studies involving RNAi on nematodes showed that genes could be specifically suppressed by soaking the nematode in *in vitro* culture media consisting of RNAi triggers [25, 32–35]. In this study, instead

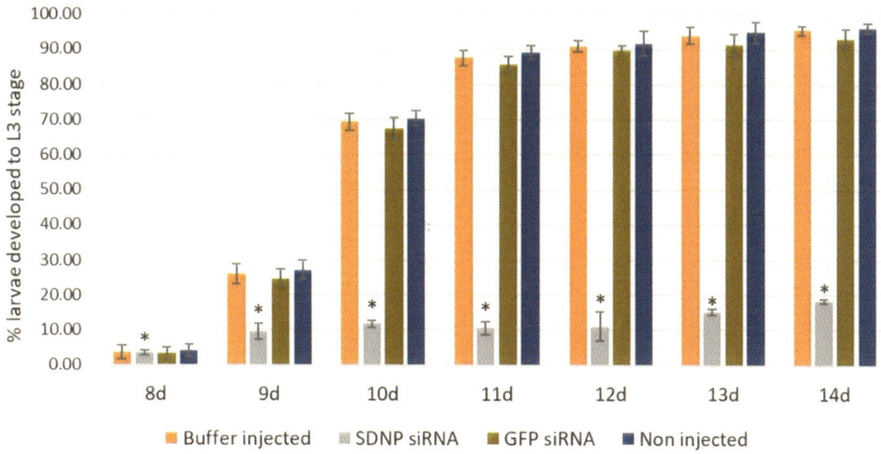

Fig. 4 Percentage of larval development to L3 stage out of total larvae inside the mosquito. *S. digitata* larvae from non-injected, *SDNP* siRNA-injected, *GFP* siRNA-injected and buffer-injected *C. quinquefasciatus* are represented by four different patterns in the graph. To target L2 to L3, siRNA injections were made at 8 dpi. Triplicates were performed for each experiment. Bars represent mean ± SD. Significant differences at $P < 0.05$ are indicated by *

of using the *in vitro* culture conditions, we recreated the soaking conditions *in vivo* by injecting the mosquitoes harbouring nematode larvae with siRNA. The RNAi effect on *SDNP* transcript level was assessed two dpi, and 14 dpi of siRNA using qPCR and the knockdown of the gene was determined by comparing the transcript levels of the worms derived from non-injected, buffer-injected and *GFP* siRNA-injected mosquitoes. A significant suppression of the target gene expression was observed in this study, and the transcript abundance of the *SDNP* was reduced by 93% (unpaired two-tailed t-test, $t_{44} = 15.8716$, $P = 0.05$) and 87.4 % (unpaired two-tailed t-test, $t_{44} = 15.2220$, $P = 0.05$) in the worms from *SDNP* siRNA-injected mosquitoes, compared to the non-injected at 2 dpi and 14 dpi, respectively, compared to worms from non-injected mosquitoes (Fig. 2a, b). Worms from the buffer-injected, and *GFP* siRNA-injected mosquitoes displayed no significant changes in the *SDNP* transcript levels (Fig. 2a, b). The qPCR results obtained proved the worms' susceptibility to specific RNAi while showing the effectiveness of the new siRNA delivery platform developed in this study and the capability of siRNA to knockdown the targeted gene specifically in this parasitic nematode.

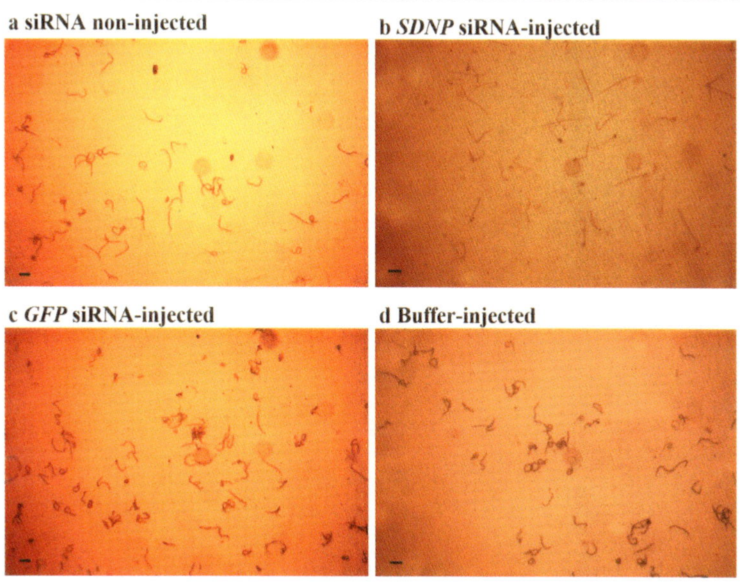

Fig. 5 Motility comparison of larvae at 14 dpi in, **a** non-injected, **b** *SDNP* siRNA-injected, **c** *GFP* siRNA-injected, **d** buffer-injected mosquitoes (Magnification 40×) *Scale-bars*: **a**-**d**, 400 μm

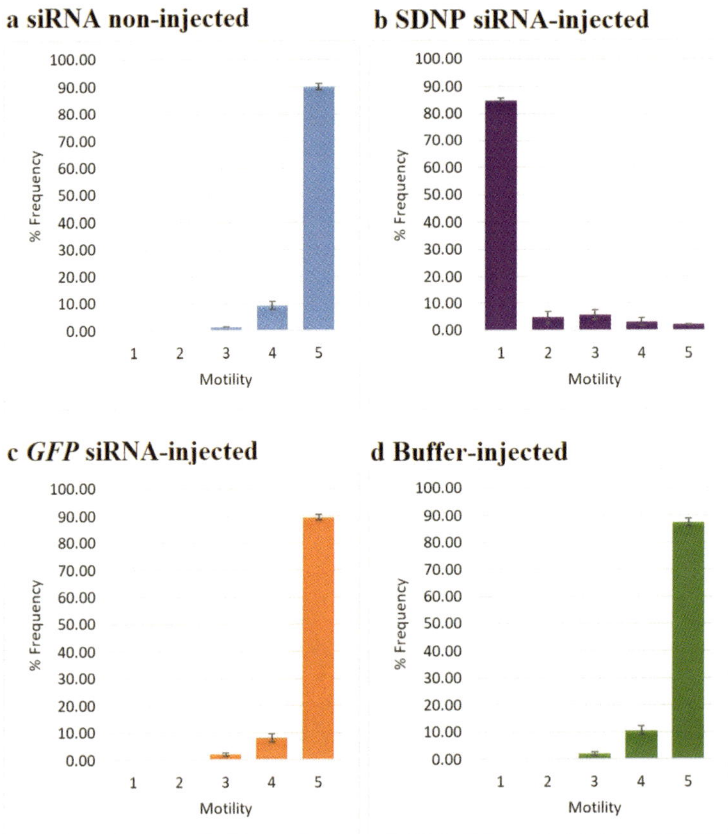

Fig. 6 Frequency distribution for motility of *S. digitata* larvae at 14 dpi in, **a** siRNA non-injected, **b** *SDNP* siRNA-injected, **c** *GFP* siRNA-injected and **d** buffer-injected mosquitoes. The scoring scheme was: 1, immobile or dead; 2, compromised motility; 3, partial movement of the body; 4, slightly reduced motion in the body; 5, all parts of the body are vigorously twisting. Values in between 5 and 1 in the scale were assigned according to the decreasing motility blindly by an independent evaluator. Five replicates were performed for each experiment. Bars represent mean ± SD

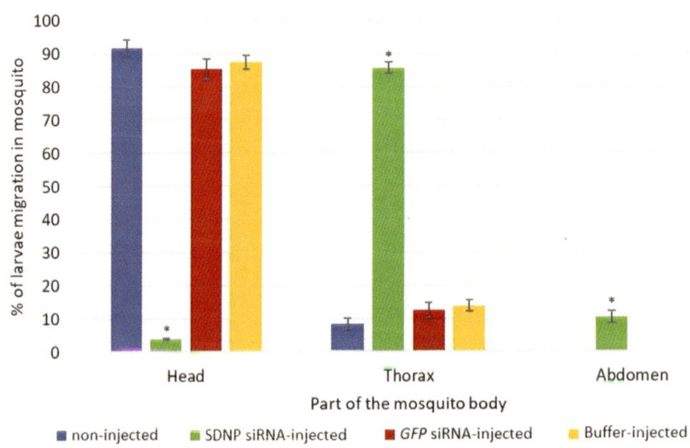

Fig. 7 Frequency distribution of *S. digitata* larvae in *C. quinquefasciatus* head, thorax, or abdomen. Migration of the larvae was monitored at 14 dpi in non-injected, *SDNP* siRNA-injected, *GFP* siRNA-injected and buffer-injected mosquitoes. Mosquitoes were dissected into head, thorax and abdomen and larvae in each part was counted. Five replicates were performed for each experiment. Bars represent mean ± SD. Statistical analysis was performed using Student's t-test ($P < 0.05$). Significant differences at $P < 0.05$ are indicated by *

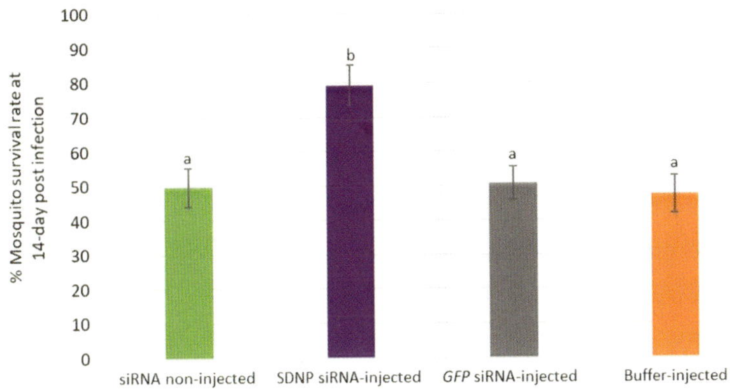

Fig. 8 Mosquito survival rate. Survivability of the non-injected, *SDNP* siRNA-injected, *GFP* siRNA-injected and buffer-injected mosquitoes at 14 dpi was measured. Five replicates were performed for each experiment. Bars represent mean ± SD. Significant differences at $P < 0.05$ are indicated with different lowercase letters

Changes in developmental phenotypes and motility of larvae because of RNAi

To study the phenotypic changes, if any, associated with the transformation of L2 to L3 in the *SDNP* siRNA-injected group in comparison to the control mosquito groups, the infected mosquitoes were dissected to recover the larval stages at eight dpi to 14 dpi following the RNAi trigger. A significant reduction in body length and width together with deformities in the body structure was observed in the larvae from *SDNP* siRNA-injected mosquitoes at 14 dpi (Fig. 3b, e) compared to the non- injected, buffer-injected and *GFP* siRNA-injected counterparts (Fig. 3a, c-e). In addition, aberrations, with larval lethality was also observed in *SDNP* siRNA treated larvae compared to its control groups, and with ~96% of L2 to L3 transformation in non-treated, ~95% in buffer-treated and ~93% in *GFP* siRNA treated compared to ~18% of such transformation in treated at 14 dpi (Fig. 4). The L2 and L3 larvae were differentiated based on their length of the body. No significant developmental changes were observed in the worms from *GFP* siRNA-injected mosquitoes suggesting the phenotypic changes are specific to *SDNP* siRNA and not due to the injection of non-specific siRNA. Therefore, it is reasonable to assume these phenotypic changes are most likely due to the downregulation of *SDNP* transcripts, which in turn affects the larval development. The previous finding reported by us, i.e., the ubiquitous expression of *SDNP* in all life stages of *S. digitata* and also its predominant expression in longitudinal muscle, reproductive systems, and developing embryos [24, 36], together with the findings of the present study, i.e. association of *SDNP* downregulation with irregularities in the larvae development, transformation arrest, changes in phenotypes, etc. in larvae can be used to further strengthen our previous suggestion regarding the involvement of *SDNP* in growth and development of nematodes.

In the motility changes monitored at 14 dpi of the control worms and worms from *SDNP* siRNA-injected mosquitoes, the former displayed a vigorously convoluting body movement (Fig. 5a, c, d) of 4 and 5 in the motility scale (Fig. 6a, c, d) while the *SDNP* siRNA-treated showed a significantly depressed body movement, feeble body twitching, and total body paralysis (Figs. 5b, 6b). Also, the worms from *SDNP* siRNA-injected worms and monitored at 14 dpi displayed irregular migration patterns in the mosquitoes compared to the controls (Fig. 7). Worms from the control mosquitoes were predominantly found in the head (non-injected: ~91%; GFP siRNA-injected: ~85%; buffer-injected: ~87%) of the mosquito, while *SDNP*-suppressed worms were mainly found either in the thorax (~85%) or abdomen (~10%) indicating that motility irregularities of larvae are associated with the migration within the mosquito. It has been previously revealed that *SDNP* had homology with the inter-domain linkers of the muscle-specific twitchin kinase of *C. elegans* and was expressed in the longitudinal muscles of the adult worm [24]. Hence, the downregulation of the *SDNP* could affect the muscle movement of the developing worm, which in turn reduces the migration of the parasite in the mosquito. The increased mosquito survival rate was seen in the *SDNP* siRNA-injected mosquito group compared to the control groups (Fig. 8). This observation suggests that the compromised motility and development of the larvae induced by the *SDNP* siRNA treatment could reduce the parasitic burden on the mosquito, thereby increasing its survival.

Conclusions

In this study, we demonstrated the successful usage of the RNAi approach to turn off the expression of *SDNP* in the larval stages of *S. digitata* in their natural milieu,

C. quinquefasciatus, and the possibility of using this host as an *in vivo* culture platform in the absence of proper culture conditions to study the biological functions of the genes that the *S. digitata* genome encodes. Further, we showed that the specific silencing of *SDNP* is associated with developmental deformities and motility changes in the developing larvae of *S. digitata*, in addition to the reduction of migration of the larvae to the head of the mosquito. Therefore, by taking the outcomes of present and our previous studies into consideration, it can be concluded that *SDNP* plays a vital role in the movement and development of larvae. Hence, it can be suggested that the *SDNP* may be utilised as a candidate anthelminthic drug target.

Abbreviations

RNAi: RNA interference; SDNP: Setaria digitata novel protein; qPCR: Quantitative real-time polymerase chain reaction; siRNA: Small interfering RNA; dsRNA: Double stranded RNA; MPS: Mosquito physiological saline; MF: Microfilariae; hpi: Hour post infection; dpi: Days post-infection; GFP: Green fluorescent protein.

Acknowledgement

The corresponding author wishes to acknowledge Professor Mark Taylor and his team for providing him training in RNA interference at his laboratories in Liverpool School of Tropical Medicine, Liverpool under the Commonwealth Fellowship Programme in 2012.

Funding

The research was funded by a grant (AP/3/2011/CG/03) awarded to Professor R.S. Dassanayake by the University of Colombo, Sri Lanka, to promote collaborative research. The funders had no role in study design, data collection and analysis, decision to publish, or preparation of the manuscript.

Authors' contributions

MBCLS carried out research work, collected samples, analysed data, and wrote the manuscript. YINSG supervised research work, analysed research data and wrote the manuscript. NVC supervised research work data and corrected the manuscript. ANBE analysed research data and corrected the manuscript. RSD designed and supervised the study and corrected the manuscript. All authors read and approved the final manuscript.

Competing interests

The authors declare that they have no competing interests.

Author details

[1]Department of Chemistry, Faculty of Science, University of Colombo, Colombo 03 00300, Sri Lanka. [2]Molecular Medicine Unit, Faculty of Medicine, University of Kelaniya, Ragama 11010, Sri Lanka. [3]Department of Bioclinical Sciences, Faculty of Dentistry, Health Sciences Center, University of Kuwait, Kuwait City, Kuwait.

References

1. Bhadury P, Austen MC, Bilton DT, Lambshead PJD, Rogers AD, Smerdon GR. Development and evaluation of a DNA-barcoding approach for the rapid identification of nematodes. Mar Ecol Prog Ser. 2006;320:1–9.
2. Stepek G, Buttle DJ, Duce IR, Behnke JM. Human gastrointestinal nematode infections: are new control methods required? Int J Exp Pathol. 2006;87:325–41.
3. Global Programme to Eliminate Lymphatic Filariasis. Progress report on mass drug administration 2010. Switzerland: World Health Organization; 2011.
4. Singh S, Singh B, Singh AP. Nematodes: a threat to sustainability of agriculture. Procedia Environ Sci. 2015;29:215–6.
5. Roeber F, Jex AR, Gasser RB. Impact of gastrointestinal parasitic nematodes of sheep, and the role of advanced molecular tools for exploring epidemiology and drug resistance - an Australian perspective. Parasit Vectors. 2013;6:153.
6. Gilleard JS. Understanding anthelmintic resistance: the need for genomics and genetics. Int J Parasitol. 2006;36:1227–39.
7. Kaplan RM. Drug resistance in nematodes of veterinary importance: a status report. Trends Parasitol. 2004;20:477–81.
8. Richard-Lenoble D, Chandenier J, Gaxotte P. Ivermectin and filariasis. Fundam Clin Pharmacol. 2003;17:199–203.
9. Berriman M, Lustigman S, McCarter JP. Genomics and emerging drug discovery technologies. Expert Opin Drug Discov. 2007;2:S83–9.
10. Foster JM, Zhang Y, Kumar S, Carlow CKS. Mining nematode genome data for novel drug targets. Trends Parasitol. 2005;21:101–4.
11. Kuwabara PE, Coulson A. RNAi - prospects for a general technique for determining gene function. Parasitol Today. 2000;16:347–9.
12. Allshire R. Retraction. Hairpin RNAs and retrotransposon LTRs effect RNAi and chromatin-based gene silencing. Science. 2005;310:49.
13. Hall IM, Shankaranarayana GD, Noma K-I, Ayoub N, Cohen A, Grewal SIS. Establishment and maintenance of a heterochromatin domain. Science. 2002;297:2232–7.
14. Behm CA, Bendig MM, McCarter JP, Sluder AE. RNAi-based discovery and validation of new drug targets in filarial nematodes. Trends Parasitol. 2005; 21:97–100.
15. Fire A, Albertson D, Harrison SW, Moerman DG. Production of antisense RNA leads to effective and specific inhibition of gene expression in *C. elegans* muscle. Development. 1991;113:503–14.
16. Grant WN, Behm CA. Target identification and validation for anthelmintic discovery. Expert Opin Drug Discov. 2007;2:S91–8.
17. Pfarr K, Heider U, Hoerauf A. RNAi mediated silencing of actin expression in adult *Litomosoides sigmodontis* is specific, persistent and results in a phenotype. Int J Parasitol. 2006;36:661–9.
18. Kamath RS, Ahringer J. Genome-wide RNAi screening in *Caenorhabditis elegans*. Methods. 2003;30:313–21.
19. Song C, Gallup JM, Day TA, Bartholomay LC, Kimber MJ. Development of an *in vivo* RNAi protocol to investigate gene function in the filarial nematode, *Brugia malayi*. PLoS Pathog. 2010;6:e1001239.
20. Jinkichi F, Soichi I, Toshio I, Tetsuo N, Ken T, Tadashi T, et al. Heterotopic parasitism of *Setaria digitata* (Linstow, 1906) in the heart of a cattle. Japanese J Vet Sci. 1985;47:999–1002.
21. Bal M, Das MK. Antigenicity of a filarial protease from *Setaria digitata* in *Wuchereria bancrofti* infection. Ann Trop Med Parasitol. 1999;93:279–88.
22. Decruse SW, Raj RK. Histological studies on female *Setaria digitata* (von Linstow 1906), a filaria of bovine, *Bos indicus*. Proc Anim Sci. 1990;99:103–12.
23. Hawking F & World Health Organization. Diethylcarbamazine: a review of the literature with special reference to its pharmacodynamics, toxicity, and use in the therapy of onchocerciasis and other filarial infections. Geneva: World Health Organization; 1978. http://www.who.int/iris/handle/10665/70735
24. Rodrigo WWP, Dassanayake RS, Voronin D. Novel parasitic nematode-specific protein of *Setaria digitata* largely localized in longitudinal muscles, reproductive systems and developing embryos. Exp Parasitol. 2014;141:12–20.
25. Lendner M, Doligalska M, Lucius R, Hartmann S. Attempts to establish RNA interference in the parasitic nematode *Heligmosomoides polygyrus*. Mol Biochem Parasitol. 2008;161:21–31.
26. Tung KC, Cheng FP, Lai CH, Wang KS, Wang JS, Lee WM. Demonstration of vector competence of *Culex quinquefasciatus* (Diptera: Culicidae) for *Setaria digitata*. Vet Parasitol. 2004;123:279–84.
27. Gerberg EJ. Manual for mosquito rearing and experimental techniques. Bull Am Mosq Control Assoc. 1970;5:1–109.

28. Hayes RO. Determination of a physiological saline solution for *Aedes aegypti* (L.). J Econ Entomol. 1953;46:624–7.
29. Benedict M, Howell P. 3.8 Mosquito Anesthesia. In: Methods in *Anopheles* Research. 2nd ed. Atlanta: bei RESOURCES; 2010. p. 1–4.
30. Garver L, Dimopoulos G. Protocol for RNAi assays in adult mosquitoes (*A. gambiae*). J Vis Exp. 2007;5:230.
31. Luna BM, Juhn J, James AA. Injection of dsRNA into female *A. aegypti* mosquitoes. J Vis Exp. 2007;215:224.
32. Ford L, Zhang J, Liu J, Hashmi S, Fuhrman JA, Oksov Y, et al. Functional analysis of the cathepsin-like cysteine protease genes in adult *Brugia malayi* using RNA interference. PLoS Negl Trop Dis. 2009;3:e377.
33. Ma HB, Lu Q, Liang J, Zhang XY. Functional analysis of the cellulase gene of the pine wood nematode, *Bursaphelenchus xylophilus*, using RNA interference. Genet Mol Res. 2011;10:1931–41.
34. Aboobaker AA, Blaxter ML. Use of RNA interference to investigate gene function in the human filarial nematode parasite *Brugia malayi*. Mol Biochem Parasitol. 2003;129:41–51.
35. Lustigman S, Zhang J, Liu J, Oksov Y, Hashmi S. RNA interference targeting cathepsin L and Z-like cysteine proteases of *Onchocerca volvulus* confirmed their essential function during L3 molting. Mol Biochem Parasitol. 2004;138:165–70.
36. Dassanayake RS, Rodrigo WWP, Karunanayake EH, Weerasena OVDSJ, Chandrasekharan NV. A putative nuclear growth factor-like globular nematode-specific protein. Bioinformation. 2009;3:370–4.

Spatial distribution and populations at risk of *A. lumbricoides* and *T. trichiura* co-infections and infection intensity classes

Kei Owada[1,2*], Colleen L Lau[2,3], Lydia Leonardo[4], Archie C A Clements[3], Laith Yakob[5], Mark Nielsen[6,7], Hélène Carabin[8] and Ricardo J Soares Magalhães[2,9]

Abstract

Background: Soil-transmitted helminth (STH) infections are highly prevalent in the Philippines. Mapping the prevalence and high-intensity of STH co-infections can help guide targeted intervention programmes to reduce morbidity, especially among vulnerable school-aged children. In this study, we aimed to predict the spatial distribution of the prevalence of *Ascaris lumbricoides* and *Trichuris trichiura* co-infection and infection intensity classes in the Philippines to identify populations most in need of interventions.

Methods: Data on STH infections from 29,919 individuals during the nationwide parasitological survey in 2005 to 2007 were included in the analysis. To geographically predict the prevalence of *A. lumbricoides* and *T. trichiura* co-infections and infection intensity classes, Bayesian multinomial geostatistical models were built including age, sex, environmental variables and a geostatistical random effect. The number of individuals co-infected and belonging to each of the infection intensity classes in 2017 was forecast by combining our predictive prevalence maps with population density maps.

Results: Our models showed that school-aged children (5–19 years) are most at risk of *A. lumbricoides* and *T. trichiura* co-infections and of moderate/high infection intensity compared to other age groups. We identified target provinces where the likelihood of STH-associated morbidity was highest: Luzon (Bulacan, Benguet, Cavite, Sorsogon, Metropolitan Manila, Pampanga and Rizal), the Visayas (Cebu, Iloilo, Leyte and Negros Occidental), and in Mindanao (Agusan Del Norte, Davao Del Sur, Davao Oriental, Lanao Del Sur, Maguindanao, Misamis Oriental, Sulu and Zamboanga Del Sur). Luzon had the highest estimated number of school-aged children with *A. lumbricoides* and *T. trichiura* co-infections (estimated total 89,400), followed by the Visayas (38,300) and Mindanao (20,200).

Conclusions: Our study provided epidemiological evidence to highlight national priority areas for controlling co-infections and high intensity infections in the Philippines. Our maps could assist more geographically targeted interventions to reduce the risk of STH-associated morbidity in the Philippines.

Keywords: Soil-transmitted helminths, *Ascaris lumbricoides*, *Trichuris trichiura*, Co-infection, Infection intensity, Spatial epidemiology, Bayesian geostatistics, The Philippines

* Correspondence: kei.owada@uqconnect.edu.au
[1]School of Medicine, The University of Queensland, QLD, South Brisbane, Australia
[2]Children's Health and Environment Program, Child Health Research Centre, The University of Queensland, QLD, South Brisbane, Australia
Full list of author information is available at the end of the article

Background

Soil-transmitted helminth (STH) infections with *Ascaris lumbricoides*, *Trichuris trichiura* and hookworm species including *Ancylostoma duodenale*, *Ancylostoma ceylanicum* and *Necator americanus* are among the most common infections in school-aged children. These infections are particularly common in impoverished communities where the provision of water, sanitation and hygiene education are limited [1]. Exposure to STH infections is also driven by environmental factors such as vegetation, land cover, elevation, temperature and water availability [2]. Additionally, sex and age have been shown to influence exposure and susceptibility to STH [3–5]. Morbidity caused by STH infections is estimated to incur 4.98 million years lived with disability (YLDs) for an estimated loss of 5.18 million disability-adjusted life years (DALYs) [1]. STH-related morbidity includes anaemia of inflammation and iron-deficiency, chronic nutritional imbalances, stunting, impaired cognitive function and delayed development of fine and gross motor functions [1, 6]. The highest burden for *A. lumbricoides* is observed in South and Southeast Asia and West Africa, and the highest relative burden for *T. trichiura* and hookworm is found in southern Africa [1]. Previous studies have demonstrated that STH-associated morbidity is exacerbated by co-infections and high intensity infections [2, 6–9].

To control STH morbidity, the World Health Organization (WHO) advocates the administration of regular chemotherapy with anthelminthic medicines such as albendazole and mebendazole to at-risk populations [6]. Importantly, the WHO proposes the global target of eliminating morbidity attributable to STH in school-aged children by 2020 by regularly treating at least 75% of school-aged children in STH endemic areas [10]. Treatment is given once a year where the prevalence of STH infections in the community is over 20%, and twice a year where the prevalence exceeds 50% [10] at the commencement of a programme.

The Philippine Department of Health has been implementing an integrated helminth control programme since 2006, using chemotherapy with albendazole or mebendazole, targeting all children aged 12 months to 12 years, pregnant women, adolescents, farmers and indigenous populations [11–13]. The integrated helminth control programme also includes health education approaches and installation of water and sanitation facilities [14]. However, even after one decade of integrated helminth control programme implementation, the WHO target of < 20% prevalence of STH infections and elimination of moderate and high intensity infections in school-aged children has not been reached in the Philippines [15–18]. According to the most recent WHO report, it is estimated that 19.6 million school-aged children live in STH endemic areas of the Philippines and require preventive chemotherapy [10].

The spatial distribution of STH infection prevalence shows significant variation across the Philippines [13, 19]. While mapping the prevalence of STH infections is important to define areas that need regular treatment with albendazole or mebendazole [17], the prevalence of infection alone is not necessarily a good indicator of population-level morbidity. Indicators based on co-infections and intensity of infection, which are linked to morbidity, might be more useful for estimating disease burden [4, 20]. Indeed, modelling the spatial distribution of STH infection intensity classes and co-infections has relevance for identifying communities where the likelihood of morbidity and parasite transmission is at its highest [4, 21]. Targeting treatment, prevention and control activities to communities with high-intensity STH infections, or co-infections, could lead to a more efficient reduction in transmission and severe STH-related morbidity compared to targeting treatment based only on prevalence of single infections [21–23]. Despite intervention schemes being implemented to reduce morbidity attributable to STH infections in the Philippines [11, 17], persistently high prevalence rates among school-aged children continue to be recorded across the country [15, 18, 24, 25]. Available evidence suggests that indicators based on co-infections and infection intensities, which are linked to higher degrees of morbidity, are useful for estimating disease burden. Furthermore, prediction maps based on co-infection and intensity models have made spatially targeted helminth control interventions possible [4, 26]. Studies of this kind have not been conducted in the Philippines. Therefore, in this study we attempt to apply this methodology to provide previously unavailable evidence such as predictive prevalence maps of STH co-infections and infection intensity classes to identify and quantify populations most at risk of STH associated morbidity in the Philippines and thus assist the local governments to focus their resource allocation on these areas.

Methods

Data for analysis

STH infection data

Information on study design, sample size and sampling procedures are detailed elsewhere [13]. In brief, we used STH infection data collected during the National Schistosomiasis Survey in the Philippines in 2005 to 2007 [3, 19]. Our previous study [1] used data collected from the National Schistosomiasis survey and from Western Samar [2]; however, the current study does not include the infection data from Samar due to the lack of reliability of the intensity of infection data. Therefore, to maintain data consistency across all models we only used the data collected by the National Schistosomiasis Survey. This brought the total number of individuals included in this study, after removing those without plausible intensity of infection information, to 2701 for Luzon, 7575 for the Visayas and 19,643 for Mindanao. In the national survey, STH infections were diagnosed by the detection of parasite eggs in two stool samples collected on two separate days from each individual, using a Kato-Katz thick smear examination; however, the submission of the second stool sample was reported to be inconsistent thus only the results from the first examination were taken [3, 19]. Infection intensity was expressed as eggs per gram of faeces (epg) [13]. Each individual was categorized into infected or not infected based on the presence of at least one egg. We only considered data for *A. lumbricoides* and *T. trichiura* because co-infections with these parasites were most prevalent (Additional file 1: Table S1).

We analysed infection intensity data only from Mindanao because the majority of STH infections for Luzon and the Visayas were of light infection intensity. We excluded hookworm from our infection intensity models because the majority of hookworm infections in Mindanao were of light infection intensity (1–1999 epg). Data on infection intensity were categorized according to the WHO classes, i.e. 0; 1–4999; 5000–49,999; and ≥ 50,000 epg for *A. lumbricoides*, and 0; 1–999; 1000–9999; and ≥ 10,000 epg for *T. trichiura* for light, moderate and high infection intensity, respectively [20]. We combined moderate and high infection intensity classes due to low prevalence of high infection intensity classes for all species of STH in our analyses (Table 1).

Data from the regions of Luzon and the Visayas were combined due to the size of the separate datasets, the frequent movement of people between islands of both regions and the similar spatial dependence patterns in these two regions as demonstrated in our spatial analyses. The presence of infection was measured for a total of 10,276 participants for Luzon and the Visayas, and 19,643 for Mindanao, from 187 survey locations (i.e. 79 locations in Luzon and the Visayas; 108 locations in Mindanao), with complete information regarding STH infection status, barangay geolocation and demography (i.e. age and sex). For the purpose of this study, age was stratified as categorical variables (children under 5 years-old, school-aged children defined as 5–19 years-old, and individuals aged 20 years and older).

Environmental data

Environment data for land surface temperature (LST), rainfall and distance to perennial water bodies (DPWB) were obtained from WorldClim (https://www.worldclim.org). Normalized difference vegetation index (NDVI) data, which serves as a proxy measure of rainfall for a 1 × 1 km grid cell resolution, were obtained from the National Oceanographic and Atmospheric Administrations' (NOAA) Advanced Very High Radiometer [27]. Values of these environmental covariates were extracted in ArcGIS version 10.4.0.5524 [28] for each barangay.

Spatial analysis

Geo-referencing of data

The unit of analysis was the barangay (the smallest administrative unit in the Philippines), which has an average diameter of approximately 11 km. Barangay centroids were estimated using the geographical information system (GIS) software Quantum GIS version 1.7.3 (QGIS Development Team, 2011) based on a shapefile of the barangays of the Philippines, obtained from the geographical data warehouse DIVA GIS (https://www.diva-gis.org/Data) and PhilGIS (https://www.philgis.org). Infection data and environmental data were linked to the barangay centroid.

Variable selection

In all models, initial variable selection included sex and age, and environmental variables (rainfall, DPWB, LST and NDVI). LST were considered in the analysis because *A. lumbricoides* and *T. trichiura* have thermal thresholds outside of which the survival of the infective stages in the soil declines [4, 29]. Rainfall, NDVI and DPWB were also considered because these affect the moisture of the soil where the helminth infective stages are found, and therefore their survival. Correlations between environmental covariates were investigated using Pearson's correlation coefficients.

Frequentist fixed-effects multinomial regression models of *A. lumbricoides* and *T. trichiura* co-infections were developed. We used multinomial models for the prevalence of STH infection intensity classes rather than infection intensity data on a continuous scale. This was done to facilitate estimation of the number of population with a particular infection intensity class. The interaction between age and sex was checked in all models using the "*mfpigen*" command in Stata version 13.1 [30]. It was found that an interaction term between age and sex improved the STH co-infection model for Mindanao only. Previous studies indicated that the non-linear relationship between infection and environmental covariates could be addressed parametrically [4, 26]. In all models, non-linearity between STH infection outcomes and environmental data was investigated [4]. Quadratic terms for DPWB and rain were found to improve model fit of non-spatial multinomial models for the prevalence of *A. lumbricoides* infection intensity classes, as per the Akaike's Information Criterion (AIC) [31]. Covariates were included in the final model based on backwards-stepwise regression analysis (with Wald's $P > 0.2$ as the exclusion criterion, and $P < 0.05$ as the entry criterion).

Table 1 Number of individuals with STH infections, and the distribution of intensity among those infected in Mindanao

STH species	Total number of individuals	Age group (in years)		
		Under 5	5–19	20 and older
A. lumbricoides[a]				
With infection, *n*	2447	294	1249	904
Mean infection intensity (95% CI)	8450.8 (7574.1–9327.5)	15,163.9 (11,142.9–19,184.9)	9118.8 (7874.2–10,363.3)	5344.6 (4405.6–6283.7)
Light intensity, *n* (%)	1704 (69.6)	170 (57.8)	830 (66.5)	704 (77.9)
Moderate intensity, *n* (%)	651 (26.6)	99 (33.7)	365 (29.2)	187 (20.7)
High intensity, *n* (%)	92 (3.8)	25 (8.5)	54 (4.3)	12 (1.4)
T. trichiura[b]				
With infection, *n*	2122	164	1064	894
Mean infection intensity (95% CI)	506.7 (384.9–628.5)	525.1 (332.5–717.6)	540.1 (380.2–699.9)	465.5 (250.2–680.8)
Light intensity, *n* (%)	1935 (91.2)	143 (87.2)	955 (89.7)	837 (93.6)
Moderate intensity, *n* (%)	176 (8.3)	21 (12.8)	104 (9.8)	51 (5.7)
High intensity, *n* (%)	11 (0.5)	0	5 (0.5)	6 (0.7)
Hookworm[c]				
With infection, *n*	1503	124	418	961
Mean infection intensity (95% CI)	275.0 (227.3–322.8)	368.4 (162.8–574.1)	243.5 (135.3–351.6)	276.7 (224.8–328.6)
Light intensity, *n* (%)	1473 (98.0)	121 (97.6)	412 (98.6)	940 (97.8)
Moderate intensity, *n* (%)	29 (1.3)	1 (0.8)	2 (0.5)	17 (1.8)
High intensity, *n* (%)	10 (0.7)	2 (1.6)	4 (0.9)	4 (0.4)

[a]Light infection intensity: 1–4999 epg; moderate: 5000–49,999 epg; high: ≥ 50,000 epg [20]
[b]Light infection intensity: 1–999 epg; moderate: 1000–9999 epg; high: ≥ 10,000 epg [20]
[c]Light infection intensity: 1–1999 epg; moderate: 2000–3999 epg; high: ≥ 4000 epg [20]

Analysis of residual spatial dependence

Residuals for non-spatial models with the final set of covariates were extracted and examined for spatial autocorrelation by generating semivariograms using the *geoR* package of R software version 3.1.1 (The R foundation for statistical computing, Vienna, Austria, https://www.r-project.org). Further detailed information regarding analysis and results of residual spatial dependence are provided in detail in Additional file 1: Text S1. The semivariograms for Luzon and the Visayas (Additional file 1: Figure S1) demonstrated similar spatial dependence, justifying the combining of data from these two regions into a single region for subsequent modelling.

Spatial models

Multinomial models with geostatistical random effects were built using OpenBUGS (MRC Biostatistics Unit, Cambridge, and Imperial College London, UK) for Luzon/the Visayas and Mindanao.

In our co-infection models, survey data were aggregated into groups according to age, sex, and location using four infection outcomes (i.e. no infection; *A. lumbricoides* monoinfection; *T. trichiura* monoinfection; and *A. lumbricoides* and *T. trichiura* co-infection). For the Mindanao STH infection intensity class models, we used three infection intensity outcomes for *A. lumbricoides* and *T. trichiura* infections (i.e. no infection; light intensity; and moderate/high intensity). All models included an intercept, individual-level variables such as age (categorized into three age groups: aged < 5 years; 5–19 years; and ≥ 20 years) and sex, the selected environmental variables, and a geostatistical random effect. Due to computational demands, our spatial models for Mindanao did not include quadratic terms for rainfall and DPWB variables (in the infection intensity model for *A. lumbricoides*) or interaction terms between age and sex (in the *A. lumbricoides* and *T. trichiura* infection intensity models and co-infection model). For all models, the reference category was "No infection".

Formal model presentation

For co-infection models and infection intensity class models, we assumed:

$$Y_{ijk} \sim Multinomial(p_{ijk}, n_{ijk}), and\ p_{ijk} = \frac{\phi_{ijk}}{\sum_k \phi_{ijk}}$$

where Y_{ijk} is the observed number of children at location i in age-sex group j and outcome group k. For co-infection models, i = 1,..,187, j = 1,...,6, and k =

1,...,4. The 187 locations come from 79 locations in Luzon and the Visayas, and 108 locations in Mindanao. The six sex-age groups were made of male/female and ages < 5 years, 5–19 years, and ≥ 20 years. The four outcome groups were: No infection (reference group); *A. lumbricoides* monoinfection; *T. trichiura* monoinfection; and *A. lumbricoides* and *T. trichiura* co-infection. In contrast to co-infection models, for infection intensity class models, $i = 1,..,108$, $j = 1,...,6$, and $k = 1,...,3$. The 108 locations come from the survey locations in Mindanao alone. The six sex-age groups were the same as for co-infection models. The three outcome groups were: No infection (reference group); light infection intensity; and moderate/high infection intensity. n_{ijk} is the number tested and p_{ijk} is the probability of infection. Here Φ_{ijk} can be thought of as the overall odds of being in a specific outcome group relative to not being infected. To give a reference value, Φ_{ij1} (for the no infection group) was constrained to equal 1. The nominal regression models were fitted for the other outcome groups for both co-infection models and infection intensity class models as:

$$\log\left(\phi_{ijk}\right) = \alpha_k + \sum_{z=1}^{T} \beta_{zk} \times X_{zij} + \theta_{ik}$$

where α_k is the outcome group-specific intercept, β is a matrix of T coefficients and X is a matrix of T covariates. The θ_{ik} are coefficients representing location-level (i.e. barangay) spatial effects for the prevalence of each mono- and co-infection and of each infection intensity class. They have a multivariate normal distribution $\theta_{ik} \sim MVN(0, \Sigma_{ik})$ and are defined by isotropic powered exponential spatial correlation functions:

$$\sum\nolimits_{ik} = f(d_{ab}, \phi) = \sigma^2 \exp[-(\phi d_{ab})]$$

where d_{ab} are the distances between pairs of survey locations a and b, the parameter phi (Φ) is the rate of decay of spatial correlation per unit of distance, and indicates the size of clusters, and σ^2 is a variance parameter. For the Mindanao model, non-informative priors were used for the intercept alpha (α), and the effect sizes of covariates beta (β) (normal distribution prior with mean zero and precision 0.001). For the Luzon and Visayas model, the prior for the intercept and the effect size of covariates had mean zero and precision 0.01. The geostatistical random effects were assumed to follow a normal distribution, with a mean of zero and a variance of $1/ui$, where the precision of ui was given a non-informative gamma prior distribution with shape and scale parameters = 2, 0.05. The prior distribution of Φ was also given a non-informative gamma prior distribution with shape and scale parameters = 2, 0.05 [26]. The radius of a cluster measured in decimal degrees corresponds to $3/\Phi$. One decimal degree is equivalent to approximately 111 km at the equator (the radii of cluster = $3/\Phi \times 111$ km - the further away from the equator the multiplier increases).

Prediction maps

Model predictions were used to generate representative risk maps of the prevalence of *A. lumbricoides* and *T. trichiura* monoinfections and co-infections across the Philippines, and the prevalence of infection intensity classes across Mindanao region, for females aged 5–19 years, the subgroup with the highest prevalence of monoinfection, co-infections and infection intensity classes (note: all other age and sex groups would have a different overall mean infection prevalence, but the same spatial patterns of infection risk). Predictions were made at the nodes of a 0.05 × 0.05 decimal degree grid (approximately 5 km^2). The mean and standard deviation were extracted from the posterior distributions of predicted risk and plotted in ArcGIS version 10.4.0.5524 [28]. Further detailed information regarding model specification is provided in Additional file 1: Text S2.

Model validation

The WHO recommends that in order to mitigate STH morbidity, an area must attain prevalence less than 20% as well as eliminate moderate/high infection intensities entirely [32]. The models were validated in terms of their ability to predict prevalence of higher or lower than 20% as per WHO guidelines.

The area under the curve (AUC) of the receiver operating characteristic (ROC) was used to determine discriminatory performance of the model predictions relative to observed co-infections prevalence thresholds of 20% at validation locations. Validation was indeed based on holding a random 25% subset of the data and performing AUC ROC to assess the discriminatory ability of the model on the 20% WHO threshold of prevalence. AUC ROC is a valid model validation procedure routinely used in similar studies [13]. For our models of prevalence of STH infection intensity classes, we used the mean prevalence of infection intensity classes of *A. lumbricoides* and *T. trichiura* as our cut-off value to determine discriminatory performance of the model predictions (20% and 15%, respectively). An AUC of 0.50–0.69 was taken to indicate poor discriminative ability; 0.70–0.89 reasonable discriminative ability; and ≥ 0.90 good discriminatory ability [33].

Estimation of the number of infections in population most at risk of STH-associated morbidity in the Philippines in 2017

School-aged children (5–19 years old) were identified as being most at risk of STH-associated morbidity in our analysis. In order to estimate the number of school-aged children aged 5–19 years at risk, we multiplied a raster map of the estimated total number of school-aged children in 2017 by the predicted prevalence of *A. lumbricoides* and *T. trichiura* monoinfection and co-infections, and the prevalence of infection intensity classes. To derive the 2017 population raster map, we multiplied the 2015 population raster map from the AsiaPop project [34] by the reported UNDP annual population growth rate for 2015–2020, which was retrieved from the World Population Prospects 2015 Revision Population Database [35]. To generate a raster map of the estimated total number of school-aged children in 2017 in the Philippines, the 2017 population raster map was multiplied by the proportion of the Filipino population aged 5–19 years to derive a map of the number of school-aged children/km^2, and then summed by region. All estimates were conducted in the ArcGIS Map algebra raster calculator [28].

Results

Descriptive findings

For the purpose of spatial modelling, 10,276 individuals in the combined region (i.e. Luzon and the Visayas) and 19,643 individuals in Mindanao with complete information were included in the analysis (Additional file 1: Table S2). The observed prevalence of infection was higher in females than males in all regions. Among children aged under 5 years and school-aged children (5–19 years), the prevalence of *A. lumbricoides* and *T. trichiura* co-infections was highest in Luzon and the Visayas, whereas the prevalence of *A. lumbricoides* monoinfection was highest in Mindanao. *Trichuris trichiura* monoinfection was highest in individuals aged 20 and older in Luzon and the Visayas. *Ascaris lumbricoides* monoinfection was highest among this age group in Mindanao. In the case of the infection intensity (Mindanao only), among those infected, the majority of *A. lumbricoides* and *T. trichiura* infection intensity classes were of light infection intensity; 30% were of moderate/high infection intensity classes of *A. lumbricoides* and, approximately 9% were of moderate/high intensity of *T. trichiura* infections.

Spatial risk prediction

In Luzon, the Visayas, and Mindanao, females had significantly higher risk of *A. lumbricoides* monoinfection and *A. lumbricoides* and *T. trichiura* co-infections compared to males (Tables 2, 3). Similar results were found in each infection intensity class for both *A. lumbricoides* and *T. trichiura* infections (Table 4).

Similarly, school-aged children (ages 5–19 years) had a significantly higher risk of *A. lumbricoides* monoinfection, *T. trichiura* monoinfection and *A. lumbricoides* and *T. trichiura* co-infections compared to children aged under 5 years in Luzon, the Visayas, and Mindanao (Tables 2, 3). This was also evident in each infection intensity class for both *A. lumbricoides* and *T. trichiura* infections (Table 4). NDVI was significantly and negatively associated with the prevalence of *A. lumbricoides* and *T. trichiura* co-infections in Mindanao (Table 3). DPWB was significantly and negatively associated with the prevalence of the light infection intensity class for *A. lumbricoides* infection in Mindanao (Table 4).

Semivariograms of model residuals for *A. lumbricoides* monoinfection, *T. trichiura* monoinfection, and co-infections demonstrated spatial autocorrelation in Luzon, the Visayas, and Mindanao (Additional file 1: Figure S1). By contrast, semivariograms of the model residuals demonstrated spatial autocorrelation in Mindanao for all infection intensity classes, except for the prevalence of *T. trichiura* light infection intensity, which indicated no residual spatial autocorrelation (Additional file 1: Figure S2). A detailed summary of parameters of semivariograms for prevalence of mono- and co-infections, and infection intensity classes is provided in Additional file 1: Text S1, Table S3, and Table S4.

Spatial prediction maps

Predicted prevalence of *A. lumbricoides* monoinfection was mostly 10–20% across all regions of the Philippines, with the highest predicted prevalence observed in the north-eastern part of Luzon (> 40%; Fig. 1a). The predicted prevalence of *T. trichiura* monoinfection was mostly 20–30% across Luzon and the Visayas and south-eastern part of Mindanao, with the highest predicted prevalence observed in north-west Visayas (> 40%; Fig. 1b). Predicted prevalence of *A. lumbricoides* and *T. trichiura* co-infections showed a wide distribution across the Philippines, with the highest predicted prevalence observed in the south-eastern tip of Luzon; and eastern division of the Visayas; and the northern and south-eastern divisions of Mindanao, the northeast island province (Sulu) and the southernmost island province (Tawi-Tawi) located in the Autonomous Region in Muslim Mindanao (> 50%; Fig. 1c).

In Mindanao, predicted prevalence of light infection intensity classes for *A. lumbricoides* and *T. trichiura* were predominantly 10–20%, with the highest predicted prevalence of *A. lumbricoides* moderate/high infection intensity observed in the south-eastern part of Mindanao - Davao Oriental and Compostela Valley provinces (> 30%; Fig. 2).

Similarly, the highest predicted prevalence of *T. trichiura* moderate/high infection was observed in Davao Oriental and Compostela Valley provinces (> 20%; Fig. 3).

Predicted prevalence corresponded well with the observed values (Additional file 1: Figures S3-S7).

Table 2 Spatial effects for the prevalence of mono- and co-infections in Luzon and the Visayas

Coefficient	*A. lumbricoides* mono mean (95% BCI)[a]	*T. trichiura* mono mean (95% BCI)[a]	Co-infection mean (95% BCI)[a]
Female *vs* male	0.38 (0.23–0.52)	0.07 (-0.05–0.19)	0.18 (0.05–0.30)
Age 5–19 *vs* < 5 years-old	0.54 (0.34–0.75)	1.21 (1.01–1.42)	1.18 (0.98–1.37)
Age ≥ 20 *vs* < 5 years-old	-0.10 (-0.30–0.11)	0.79 (0.58–0.99)	0.07 (-0.13–0.27)
Normalised difference vegetation index[b]	0.10 (-0.15–0.36)	0.046 (-0.30–0.43)	0.24 (-0.26–0.76)
Temperature[b]	-0.16 (-0.39–0.08)	-0.19 (-0.51–0.15)	-0.16 (-0.53–0.22)
Intercept	-1.93 (-2.23– -1.65)	-1.98 (-2.46– -1.55)	-1.97 (-2.54– -1.48)
Phi[c]	47.96 (4.66–97.51)	10.69 (2.53–59.88)	10.04 (2.40–60.54)
Tau, precision	1.11 (0.70–1.65)	0.60 (0.36–0.90)	0.35 (0.21–0.51)

[a] *BCI* Bayesian Credible Interval (The posterior distributions are summarized by the posterior mean and 95% BCI. A variable was considered as influencing the outcome if it excluded 0)

[b] Variables were standardized to have mean of zero, and standard deviation of 1

[c] Rate of decay of spatial autocorrelation, measured in decimal degrees; 3/phi determines the cluster size; one decimal degree is approximately 111 km at the Equator (the size of the radii of the clusters)

Predicted standard deviation (SD) of prevalence of *A. lumbricoides* monoinfections, *T. trichiura* monoinfections, co-infections and infection intensity classes are available in Additional file 1: Figures S8-S10.

Model validation

The *A. lumbricoides* and *T. trichiura* co-infection model for Mindanao performed satisfactorily (reasonable discriminative ability) for two of the following infection outcomes: *A. lumbricoides* monoinfection (AUC = 0.78 for Mindanao), *T. trichiura* monoinfection (AUC = 0.70 for Mindanao). Discriminatory ability of the co-infection model for *A. lumbricoides* and *T. trichiura* co-infections was just below the threshold (0.69 for Mindanao and 0.68 for Luzon); however, the 95% confidence interval included values of reasonable to good discriminatory ability. Discriminatory ability of *A. lumbricoides* monoinfection, and *T. trichiura* monoinfection for Luzon and the Visayas performed poorly with AUC values below 0.70 (Additional file 1: Table S5). Discriminatory ability of the infection intensity class models for *A. lumbricoides* and *T. trichiura* in Mindanao were poor to reasonable (AUC range 0.52–0.75) (Additional file 1: Table S5).

Predicted total number of school-aged children with monoinfections, co-infections and infection intensity classes

Areas within and around the capital Manila in Luzon had the highest number of school-aged children with *A. lumbricoides* monoinfection (Additional file 1: Figure S11), with some areas exceeding 45 persons/km^2. In the Visayas and Mindanao the geographical distribution of the predicted number of school-aged children with *A. lumbricoides* monoinfection was more localised compared to Luzon with some areas exceeding 15 persons/km^2. Similarly, the number of school-aged children predicted with *T. trichiura* monoinfection (Additional file 1: Figure S12) was distributed widely in the capital Manila in Luzon (some areas with more than 26 persons/km^2), while the Visayas and Mindanao had small localized areas with more than 23 persons/km^2 predicted infected. In addition, while in Mindanao the number of school-aged children with *A. lumbricoides* and *T. trichiura* co-infections

Table 3 Spatial effects for the prevalence of mono- and co-infections in Mindanao

Coefficient	*A. lumbricoides* mono mean (95% BCI)[a]	*T. trichiura* mono mean (95% BCI)[a]	Co-infection mean (95% BCI)[a]
Female *vs* male	0.11 (0.02–0.19)	0.12 (0.01–0.23)	0.19 (0.07–0.32)
Age 5–19 *vs* < 5 years-old	0.24 (0.11–0.38)	1.39 (1.16–1.63)	1.39 (1.20–1.59)
Age ≥ 20 *vs* < 5 years-old	-0.43 (-0.57– -0.29)	0.92 (0.70–1.16)	0.30 (0.10–0.51)
Normalised difference vegetation index[b]	-0.01 (-0.21–0.19)	-0.23 (-0.53–0.06)	0.52 (0.86 0.15)
Intercept	-1.87 (-2.08– -1.65)	-4.88 (-5.27– -4.38)	-3.57 (-3.97– -3.19)
Phi[c]	65.9 (23.67–98.44)	0.10 (0.10–0.12)	50.6 (13.35–96.77)
Tau, precision	1.23 (0.88–1.65)	0.01 (0.01–0.02)	0.39 (0.27–0.53)

[a] *BCI* Bayesian Credible Interval (The posterior distributions are summarized by the posterior mean and 95% BCI. A variable was considered as influencing the outcome if it excluded 0)

[b] Variables were standardized to have mean of zero, and standard deviation of 1

[c] Rate of decay of spatial autocorrelation, measured in decimal degrees; 3/phi determines the cluster size; one decimal degree is approximately 111 km at the Equator (the size of the radii of the clusters)

Table 4 Spatial effects for the prevalence of infection intensity classes in Mindanao

Coefficient	*A. lumbricoides* light intensity (95% BCI)[a]	*A. lumbricoides* moderate/high intensity (95% BCI)[a]	*T. trichiura* light intensity (95% BCI)[a]	*T. trichiura* moderate/high intensity (95% BCI)[a]
Female *vs* male	0.16 (0.05–0.27)	0.38 (0.20–0.57)	0.12 (0.02–0.22)	0.49 (0.15–0.86)
Age 5–19 *vs* < 5 years-old	0.72 (0.51–0.91)	1.11 (0.85–1.37)	1.26 (1.05–1.47)	3.17 (2.43–3.93)
Age ≥ 20 *vs* < 5 years-old	0.18 (-0.02–0.37)	0.06 (-0.22–0.35)	0.77 (0.57–0.99)	2.16 (1.34–2.98)
Distance to perennial water bodies[b]	-0.71 (-1.19– -0.03)	0.43 (-0.37–1.4)	ni	ni
Rain[b]	0.42 (-0.45–1.05)	0.15 (-0.69–1.05)	ni	ni
Normalised difference vegetation index[b]	ni	ni	0.18 (-0.18–0.57)	-0.36 (-0.87–0.16)
Intercept	-5.38 (-6.12– -4.33)	-6.36 (-6.92– -5.71)	-4.19 (-4.53– -3.76)	-6.98 (-7.75– -6.02)
Phi[c]	4.80 (1.89–10.55)	4.52 (1.56–9.63)	4.52 (1.69–8.88)	20.38 (1.14–86.09)
Tau, precision	0.10 (0.05–0.17)	0.13 (0.05–0.23)	0.23 (0.11–0.38)	0.72 (0.21–1.61)

[a]*BCI* Bayesian Credible Interval (The posterior distributions are summarized by the posterior mean and 95% BCI. A variable was considered as influencing the outcome if it excluded 0)
[b]Variables were standardized to have mean of zero, and standard deviation of 1
[c]Rate of decay of spatial autocorrelation, measured in decimal degrees; 3/phi determines the cluster size; one decimal degree is approximately 111 km at the Equator (the size of the radii of the clusters)
Abbreviation: *ni* not included

(Additional file 1: Figure S13) was predicted to be higher (exceeding 80 persons/km^2 over a much more localized area around the southernmost tip of Mindanao including Sarangani Province and northern Mindanao including Lanao Del Sur and Misamis Oriental provinces) than in Luzon and the Visayas (27 persons/km^{2}and 35 persons/km^2, respectively), the geographical distribution was more localised in Mindanao compared to Luzon and the Visayas.

In Mindanao, our results showed school-aged children with light or moderate/high infection intensity classes for *A. lumbricoides* were predominantly localised in areas around the southern and northern provinces including Surigao Del Norte and Zamboanga Del Norte (some areas with more than 25 persons/km^2) (Additional file 1: Figures S14 and S15). School-aged children infected with light or moderate/high infection intensity classes for *T. trichiura* were predicted to be in areas around southern Mindanao

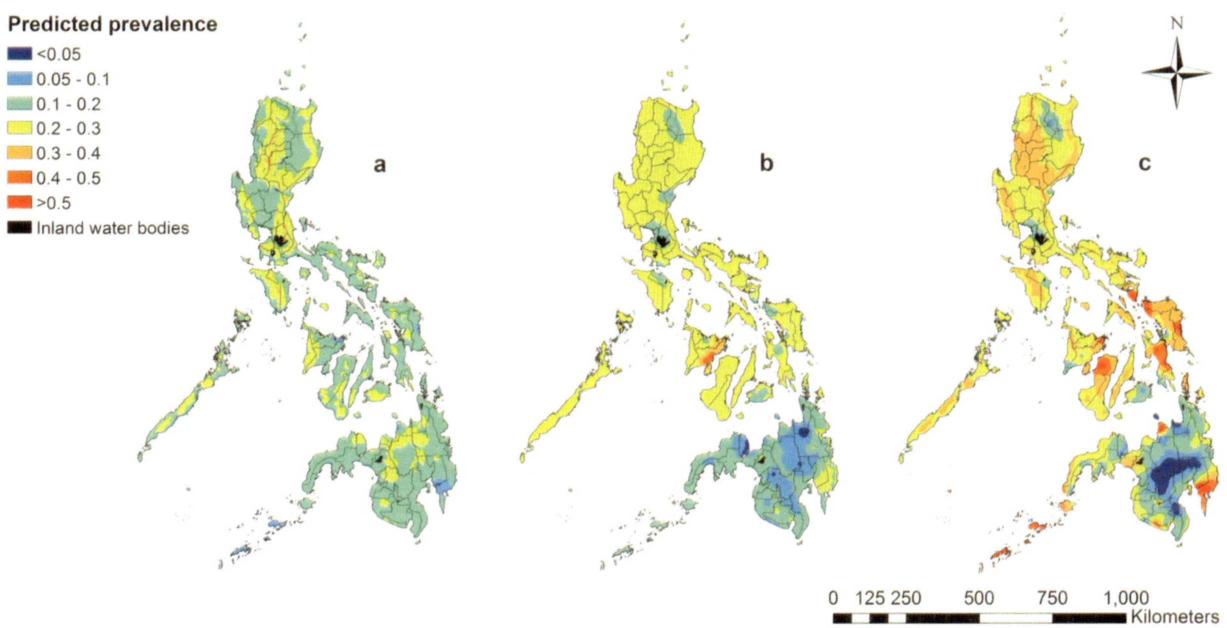

Fig. 1 Predicted prevalence of *A. lumbricoides* mono- (**a**), *T. trichiura* mono- (**b**), and co-infections (**c**) in school-aged children in the Philippines. Note: the overall mean predicted prevalences are specific to the age and sex group (choice of a different age-sex group would result in a different spatial mean), with spatial variation around the mean being influenced by the environmental variables and the spatial correlation component of the model

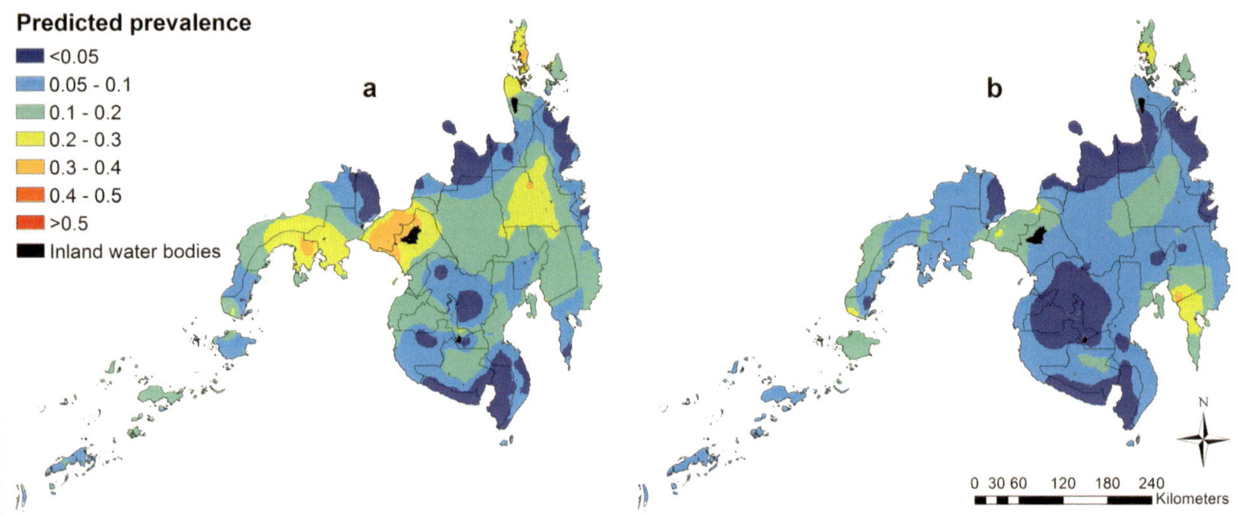

Fig. 2 Predicted prevalence of light infection intensity class (**a**) and moderate/high infection intensity classes (**b**) of *A. lumbricoides* in school-aged children in the Philippines

and around Lake Buluan near South Cotabato and Davao Del Sur, Maguindanao, Sultan Kudarat (some areas with more than 24 persons/km^2) (Additional file 1: Figures S16 and S17).

Based on our school-aged children density maps, using the 1 km^2 grid cells across the Philippines (Additional file 1: Figures S11-S17), our maps of the co-infections identified target provinces where the likelihood of STH-associated morbidity is at its highest, and that spatially targeted integrated helminth control interventions are most needed in Luzon (Bulacan, Benguet, Cavite, Sorsogon, Metropolitan Manila, Pampanga and Rizal) and the central and western islands of the Visayas (Cebu, Iloilo, Leyte and Negros Occidental). Our maps of co-infections and maps of the number of school-aged children with moderate/high infection intensity classes identified target provinces in Mindanao including Agusan Del Norte, Davao Del Sur, Davao Oriental, Lanao Del Sur, Maguindanao, Misamis Occidental, Misamis Oriental, Sulu, Surigao Del Norte, Zamboanga Del Norte, Zamboanga Del Sur and around Lake Buluan.

For 2017, it was estimated that in the Philippines approximately 114,900, 125,200 and 147,900 school-aged children are monoinfected with *A. lumbricoides* and *T. trichiura*, and co-infected with *A. lumbricoides* and *T. trichiura*, respectively. By region, Luzon had the highest estimated number of school-aged children with *A. lumbricoides* and *T. trichiura* co-infections (estimated total

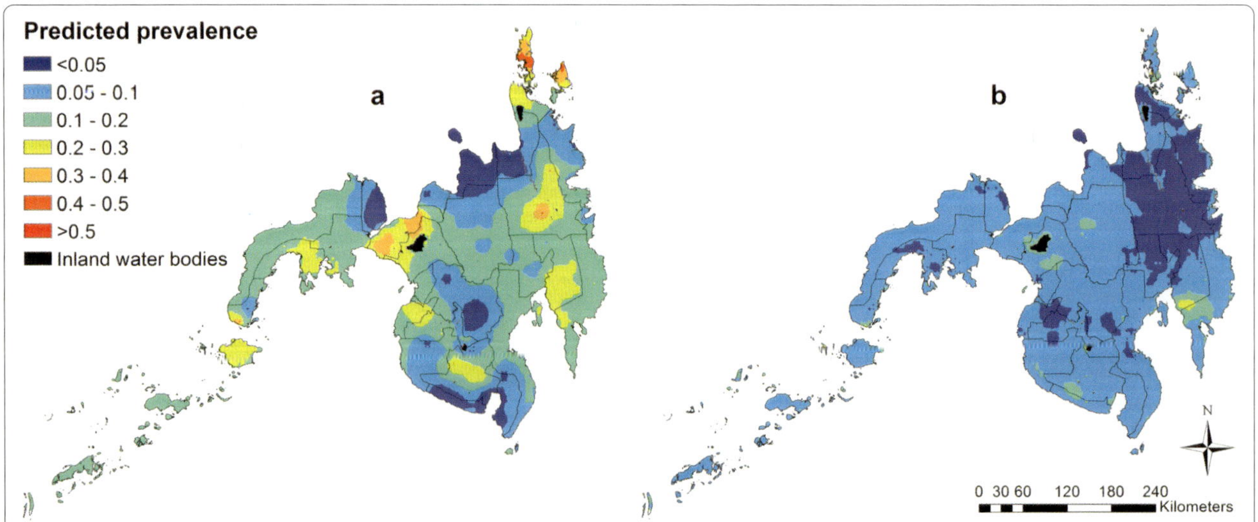

Fig. 3 Predicted prevalence of light infection intensity class (**a**) and moderate/high infection intensity classes (**b**) of *T. trichiura* in school-aged children in the Philippines

Table 5 Predicted number of school-aged children with mono- and co-infection in the Philippines, 2017

Total population for 2015 (millions)[a]	Annual population growth rate for 2015–2020 (%)[b]	Total population for 2017 (millions)[c]	% of individuals aged 5–19 yrs[b]	Region	Number of school-aged children with infection (thousands)[d]						
					Mono- and co-infections			Infection intensity classes			
					Mono-*Asc*	Mono-*Tric*	Co-infection	Light-*Asc*	Moderate/high-*Asc*	Light-*Tric*	Moderate/high-*Tric*
100.7	1.48	103.7	30.2	National	114.9	125.2	147.9	–	–	–	–
				Luzon	68.5	75.7	89.4	–	–	–	–
				The Visayas	22.4	32.7	38.3	–	–	–	–
				Mindanao	24.0	16.8	20.2	15.4	8.3	18.5	6.6

[a]Source: Alpha version 2015 estimates of numbers of people/km^2, with national totals adjusted to match UN population division estimates (https://esa.un.org/wpp/) and remaining unadjusted; Spatial resolution: 0.000833333 decimal degrees (approx. 100 m at the equator); Projection: Geographic, WGS84; Date of production: November 2013 [34, 42]
[b]Source: The World Population Prospects 2015 Revision Population Database [35, 43]
[c]Estimated value based on the ArcGIS Map algebra raster calculator; 2015 population raster map (the AsiaPop Project) was multiplied by the annual population growth rate for 2015 to 2020
[d]Estimated value based on the ArcGIS Map algebra raster calculator; 2017 population raster map was multiplied by the proportion of the Filipino population aged 5–19 years to derive a map of the number of school-aged children aged 5–19 years in 2017 in each grid cell. We then multiplied the map of the total population aged between 5–19 years by our prediction maps of the prevalence of *A. lumbricoides* monoinfection, *T. trichiura* monoinfection, and *A. lumbricoides* and *T. trichiura* co-infection, and the predicted prevalence of infection intensity classes in ArcGIS software (ESRI 2013. ArcGIS Desktop: Release 10. Redlands, CA: Environmental Systems Research Institute
Abbreviations: *Asc A. lumbricoides*; *Tric T. trichiura*

89,400), followed by the Visayas (estimated total 38,300) and Mindanao (estimated total 20,200) (Table 5). In Mindanao, approximately 8300 and 6600 school-aged children were estimated to be infected with moderate/high infection intensity of *A. lumbricoides* and *T. trichiura* infections, respectively, in 2017.

Discussion

Our modelling approach analysed policy-relevant indicators of STH morbidity and allowed the estimation of the number of school-aged children infected with STH infections in greatest need of benzimidazole treatment in the Philippines. In that regard, our study extends previous spatial epidemiological investigations in the Philippines [13] by predicting the spatial variation in the prevalence of STH co-infections and infection intensity classes in order to identify locations in the Philippines where STH-associated morbidity is at its highest.

Individual-level determinants of prevalence of STH monoinfection and co-infections, and infection intensity classes

In a recent study, the prevalence of *A. lumbricoides* and *T. trichiura* in the Philippines was estimated to be significantly higher in males compared to females [13]. However, our results showed the reverse relationship for co-infections suggesting that females are more at risk of co-infections in Luzon, the Visayas and Mindanao. Similarly, this was also the case in each infection intensity class for *A. lumbricoides* and *T. trichiura* infections. Evidence indicates that the pattern of infections in females is different from that of males due to a number of interacting factors including immunity to infection, response to treatment, and differing levels of exposure related to behaviour and occupational differences [36]. For example, higher prevalence of helminth infections observed in female farmers was reported to be associated with household activities that involved access to open latrines and the manipulation of untreated human faeces in agricultural fields [37]. Further research on the different transmission patterns between males and females is required to encourage the development of gender-sensitive helminth control intervention programmes.

Moreover, consistent with available evidence [9, 20], our results show that school-aged children are at increased risk of *T. trichiura* monoinfection and co-infections compared to children under 5 years in Luzon, the Visayas, and Mindanao. This relationship between age and increased risk of infection was also evident in each infection intensity class for *A. lumbricoides* and *T. trichiura* infections. Our finding on school-aged children being at increased risk of *T. trichiura* monoinfection has implications for future studies to evaluate the type of treatment administered for school-aged children with *T. trichiura* infection. A recent study demonstrated that the most widely used cost-effective preventive chemotherapy with the two benzimidazoles (albendazole and mebendazole) has low to moderate efficacy against *T. trichiura* in high STH endemic countries [38]. Nevertheless, our finding reaffirms the importance of implementing targeted helminth-associated morbidity control for the school-age group.

The role of environment in the prevalence of monoinfection and co-infections, and STH infection intensity classes

The environmental variables (rainfall, DPWB, LST and NDVI) used in the spatial modelling were found to not adequately explain the spatial variation of *A. lumbricoides* and *T. trichiura* mono- and co-infections based on 95% BCI. While the relative focality of co-infections may be explained by exposure opportunities to contaminated environments [6], the results of this study suggest that small scale factors such as socioeconomic status, occupational exposure, behaviour and access to safe drinking water and to adequate sanitation facilities may be more important than natural environmental variables at explaining the spatial variation in the prevalence of STH co-infections in Luzon and the Visayas [15].

In contrast, in the southernmost region of the Philippines (Mindanao), we found a strong signal in the environmental variables explaining the spatial variation in the prevalence of *A. lumbricoides* and *T. trichiura* co-infections and *A. lumbricoides* light infection intensity class. Our study found that the prevalence of *A. lumbricoides* and *T. trichiura* co-infections was significantly higher in areas of lower greenness (dry areas), which is consistent with the findings of our previous study [13]. This could be due to a number of reasons. For example, in the past couple of decades Mindanao has experienced severe drought [39], which has led to water shortages limiting the access and utilisation of adequate sanitation facilities, contributing to open defecation and inadequate disposal of human waste [40, 41], which in turn is likely to result in a higher prevalence of STH infections [16]. However, NDVI alone cannot fully explain the role of such environmental conditions in the prevalence of *A. lumbricoides* and *T. trichiura* co-infections. Other environmental variables such as type of soil, slope, and normalised difference water index (NDWI) could be added to the spatial modelling to better understand the role of the environment in the prevalence of *A. lumbricoides* and *T. trichiura* mono- and co-infections and infection intensity.

Populations most in need of interventions to reduce the risk of STH-associated morbidity

Our estimates indicated that for 2017, Luzon had the highest estimated number of school-aged children with *A. lumbricoides* and *T. trichiura* co-infections (estimated total of 89,400 people) followed by the Visayas, (estimated total of 38,300 people) and Mindanao (estimated total of 20,200 people). However, when these estimates were adjusted by population density maps (people/km^2) we found that areas in Mindanao had the highest density of school-aged children with *A. lumbricoides* and *T. trichiura* co-infections (82 people/km^2, compared to 27 people/km^2 in Luzon and 35 people/km^2 in the Visayas). This suggests that spatially targeted integrated helminth control interventions in Mindanao may be effective in order to reduce STH-related morbidity. Maps of infection intensity classes for Mindanao indicated that the number of school-aged children predicted to be infected with light or moderate/high infection intensity classes for *A. lumbricoides* and *T. trichiura* were highest in areas around the northern provinces and southern Mindanao (some areas with more than 24 persons/km^2). Together with the predicted number of co-infections these results suggest that areas of priority in Mindanao would include Agusan Del Norte, Davao Del Sur, Davao Oriental, Lanao Del Sur, Maguindanao, Misamis Occidental, Misamis Oriental, Sulu, Surigao Del Norte, Zamboanga Del Norte, Zamboanga Del Sur and around Lake Buluan.

In addition, spatial variability of the prevalence of co-infection across the Philippines is suggestive of differing impacts of anthropogenic and natural environmental factors. For instance, many suburbs around the capital city of Manila in Luzon are densely populated areas (except the Sorsogon Province which is known for fisheries), which means urbanization (including establishment of slums), overcrowding and sanitation could be influencing the prevalence of STH infections among school-aged children in this region [29]. However, provinces in the Visayas and Mindanao are mostly rural areas known for agriculture and fisheries, which means that school-aged children in these areas may have more contact with the natural environment and agricultural work compared to those living in Luzon.

Limitations of the study

The results of the study should be interpreted in the light of some limitations. First, our study used secondary data collected in 2005–2007 and may not fully reflect the current situation. However, these data constitute the most up to date information on the prevalence of STH infections in the Philippines. The most recent studies only cover the prevalence of STH infections on a regional level [15, 18, 24, 25], but provide sufficient evidence to suggest that the national level of prevalence is still similar to that of the 2005–2007 survey. Therefore, we anticipate our survey data is still relevant. Secondly, parasite egg counts were based on a single sample which limits the Kato-Katz test performance for detecting light infection intensities [4, 18]. Therefore, the results reported in our study may have underestimated the prevalence of STH infections. The accuracy of estimates of the association between covariates and STH infection could be improved by adjusting for potential measurement error in eggs per gram of faeces (epg) counts. Thirdly, while this study was able to produce prediction maps of *A. lumbricoides* and *T. trichiura* co-infections for all three regions, we did not have enough information on infection intensity classes for the Visayas and Luzon. Further studies or surveys are suggested especially targeting the areas predicted to have the high prevalence of co-infections in the Visayas and Luzon. This approach would allow estimation of the number of school-aged children with co-infections and high infection intensity who are at increased risk of severe morbidity, and are most in need of interventions. Fourthly, while the 95% confidence interval of validation statistics (AUC) included values of acceptable discriminatory ability for all models, the discriminatory outcomes of co-infections for Luzon and the Visayas, and Mindanao moderate/high infection intensity classes' models were below the threshold. This may be due to our data on these infections being sparse for these regions and thus additional surveys would be required to improve the accuracy of our prediction models. Fifthly, small scale factors such as socioeconomic status, occupational exposure, behaviour, household or water sanitation factors are also known to be important determinants of the prevalence of STH infections. Unfortunately, data on these factors were not available. This was however was captured by residuals, thus we are accounting for that by including spatial random effects in our models.

Conclusions

Overall, our study generated an important epidemiological resource, highlighting national priority areas for STH morbidity control in the Philippines. Our findings can guide policy makers in the Philippines to design geographically targeted intervention programmes to reduce STH-associated morbidity. This is particularly important in order for the Philippines to achieve the target of less than 20% prevalence of STH infections, and zero prevalence of moderate and high intensity STH infections recommended by the WHO to achieve morbidity control.

Additional file

Additional file 1: Text S1. Analysis of residual spatial dependence. **Text S2.** Model specification. **Table S1.** Number of individuals with two or more STH infections. **Table S2.** Number of individuals with mono- and co-infections. **Table S3.** Summary of parameters of semivariograms for prevalence of mono- and co-infections. **Table S4.** Summary of parameters of semivariograms for prevalence of infection intensity classes. **Table S5.** Summary of validation statistics for models used in study. **Figure S1.** Semivariograms of prevalence of co-infection models. **Figure S2.** Semivariograms of prevalence of infection intensity classes model. **Figure S3.** Map of observed prevalence of mono- and co-infections in Luzon. **Figure S4.** Map of observed prevalence of mono- and co-infections in the Visayas. **Figure S5.** Map of observed prevalence of mono- and co-infections in Mindanao. **Figure S6.** Map of observed infection intensity classes of *A. lumbricoides* in Mindanao. **Figure S7.** Map of observed infection intensity classes of *T. trichiura* in Mindanao. **Figure S8.** Maps of standard deviation of predicted prevalence of *A. lumbricoides* mono-, *T. trichiura* mono-, and co-infection. **Figure S9.** Maps of standard deviation of predicted prevalence of infection intensity classes of *A. lumbricoides*. **Figure S10.** Maps of standard deviation of predicted prevalence of infection intensity classes of *T. trichiura*. **Figure S11.** Maps showing number of individuals with *A. lumbricoides* monoinfection. **Figure S12.** Maps showing number of individuals with *T. trichiura* monoinfection. **Figure S13.** Maps showing number of individuals with co-infections. **Figure S14.** Map showing number of individuals with light intensity class of *A. lumbricoides*. **Figure S15.** Map showing number of individuals with moderate/high intensity classes of *A. lumbricoides*. **Figure S16.** Map showing number of individuals with light intensity class of *T. trichiura*. **Figure S17.** Map showing number of individuals with moderate/high intensity classes of *T. trichiura*. (DOCX 4419 kb)

Abbreviations

AIC: Akaike's information criterion; AUC: Area under the curve; BCI: Bayesian credible interval; DALYs: Disability-adjusted life years; DPWB: Distance to perennial water bodies; EPG: Eggs per gram of faeces; GIS: Geographical Information System; LST: Land surface temperature; MDA: Mass drug administration; NOAA: National Oceanographic and Atmospheric Administrations; NDVI: Normalized difference vegetation index; SD: Standard deviation; STH: Soil-transmitted helminths; UNDP: United Nations Development Programme; WHO: World Health Organization; YLDs: Years lived with disability

Acknowledgements

We would like to acknowledge the National Schistosomiasis Control Programme in the Philippines which provided the dataset. The authors would like to thank the regional coordinators, provincial health teams, municipal health officers and barangay health workers for completing all the phases of the national prevalence survey. KO is a PhD candidate supported by an Australian Government Research Training Programme Scholarship from the University of Queensland; MN is funded by an Australian Research Council Discovery Project Grant (DP140101410); CLL is funded by an Australian National Health and Medical Research Council (NHMRC) Early Career Fellowship (1109035); ACAC is supported by a NHMRC Senior Research Fellowship; LY is funded by the Medical Research Council UK, the Newton Fund, the Wellcome Trust and the European Union.

Authors' contributions

KO performed statistical analyses and drafted the first draft of the manuscript. RJSM supervised the analysis of the study. KO, RJSM, MN, CLL, LY, HC, LL and ACAC assisted in interpretation and revision of the report. All authors read and approved the final manuscript.

Competing interests

The authors declare that they have no competing interests.

Author details

[1]School of Medicine, The University of Queensland, QLD, South Brisbane, Australia. [2]Children's Health and Environment Program, Child Health Research Centre, The University of Queensland, QLD, South Brisbane, Australia. [3]Research School of Population Health, Australian National University, ACT, Canberra, Australia. [4]Department of Parasitology, College of Public Health, University of the Philippines Manila, Manila, Philippines. [5]Department of Disease Control, London School of Hygiene and Tropical Medicine, London, UK. [6]School of Psychology, The University of Queensland, QLD, St Lucia, Australia. [7]Faculty of Humanities, University of Johannesburg, Auckland Park, South Africa. [8]Department of Biostatistics and Epidemiology, College of Public Health, University of Oklahoma Health Sciences Center, Oklahoma, USA. [9]Spatial Epidemiology Laboratory, School of Veterinary Science, The University of Queensland, QLD, Gatton, Australia.

References

1. Pullan RL, Smith JL, Jasrasaria R, Brooker SJ. Global numbers of infection and disease burden of soil-transmitted helminth infections in 2010. Parasit Vectors. 2014;7:37.
2. Soares Magalhaes RJ, Clements AC. Mapping the risk of anaemia in preschool-age children: the contribution of malnutrition, malaria, and helminth infections in West Africa. PLoS Med. 2011;8:e1000438.
3. Leonardo L, Rivera P, Saniel O, Villacorte E, Lebanan MA, Crisostomo B, et al. A national baseline prevalence survey of schistosomiasis in the Philippines using stratified two-step systematic cluster sampling design. J Trop Med. 2012:2012, 936128.
4. Soares Magalhaes RJ, Biritwum NK, Gyapong JO, Brooker S, Zhang Y, Blair L, et al. Mapping helminth co-infection and co-intensity: geostatistical prediction in Ghana. PLoS Negl Trop Dis. 2011;5:e1200.
5. Belizario VY, Totanes FI, de Leon WU, Lumampao YF, Ciro RN. Soil-transmitted helminth and other intestinal parasitic infections among school children in indigenous people communities in Davao del Norte, Philippines. Acta Trop. 2011;120(Suppl. 1):S12–8.
6. World Health Organization. Eliminating STH as a public health problem in children. Geneva: World Health Organization; 2012.
7. Yakob L, Williams GM, Gray DJ, Halton K, Solon JA, Clements AC. Slaving and release in co-infection control. Parasit Vectors. 2013;6:157.
8. Pullan R, Brooker S. The health impact of polyparasitism in humans: are we under-estimating the burden of parasitic diseases? Parasitology. 2008;135:783–94.
9. Brooker S, Clements AC, Bundy DA. Global epidemiology, ecology and control of soil-transmitted helminth infections. Adv Parasitol. 2006;62:221–61.
10. World Health Organization. PCT databank: Soil-transmitted helminthiases. 2016. http://www.who.int/neglected_diseases/preventive_chemotherapy/sth/en. Accessed 8 Dec 2016.
11. Duque IIIFT. Strategic and operational framework for establishing integrated helminth control program (IHCP). In: Administrative Order No. Manila: Republic of the Philippines Department of Health; 2006. p. 2006–0028.
12. Jex AR, Lim YA, Bethony JM, Hotez PJ, Young ND, Gasser RB. Soil-transmitted helminths of humans in Southeast Asia - towards integrated control. Adv Parasitol. 2011;74:231–65.
13. Soares Magalhaes RJ, Salamat MS, Leonardo L, Gray DJ, Carabin H, Halton K, et al. Mapping the risk of soil-transmitted helminthic infections in the Philippines. PLoS Negl Trop Dis. 2015:9, e0003915.
14. Monse B, Benzian H, Naliponguit E, Belizario VY, Schratz A, van Palenstein Helderman W. The Fit for School Health Outcome Study - a longitudinal survey to assess health impacts of an integrated school health programme in the Philippines. BMC Public Health. 2013;13:256.
15. Belizario V, Ng J, Amarillo M, Trinos J, Reyes M, Fudalan O. High burden of soil-transmitted helminthiases in preschool-age children in Masbate: a decade of implementation of the integrated helminth control program in the Philippines. Southeast Asian J Trop Med Public Health. 2016;47:667–79.
16. Belizario VY, Liwanag HJ, Naig JR, Chua PL, Madamba MI, Dahildahil RO. Parasitological and nutritional status of school-age and preschool-age children in four villages in Southern Leyte, Philippines: lessons for monitoring the outcome of Community-Led Total Sanitation. Acta Trop. 2015;141:16–24.
17. World Health Organization. Helminth control in school age children: a guide for managers of control programmes. 2nd ed. Geneva: World Health Organization; 2011.
18. Mationg MLS, Gordon CA, Tallo VL, Olveda RM, Alday PP, Renosa MDC, et al. Status of soil-transmitted helminth infections in schoolchildren in Laguna Province, the Philippines, determined by parasitological and molecular diagnostic techniques. PLoS Negl Trop Dis. 2017;11:e0006022.
19. Leonardo LR, Rivera P, Saniel O, Villacorte E, Crisostomo B, Hernandez L, et al. Prevalence survey of schistosomiasis in Mindanao and the Visayas, The Philippines. Parasitol Int. 2008;57:246–51.
20. World Health Organization. Prevention and control of schistosomiasis and soil-transmitted helminthiasis. In: World Health Organization Technical Report Series 912. Geneva: World Health Organization; 2002.
21. Clements AC, Moyeed R, Brooker S. Bayesian geostatistical prediction of the intensity of infection with *Schistosoma mansoni* in East Africa. Parasitology. 2006;133:711–9.
22. Brooker S, Clements AC. Spatial heterogeneity of parasite co-infection: determinants and geostatistical prediction at regional scales. Int J Parasitol. 2009;39:591–7.
23. Howard SC, Donnelly CA, Kabatereine NB, Ratard RC, Brooker S. Spatial and intensity-dependent variations in associations between multiple species helminth infections. Acta Trop. 2002;83:141–9.
24. Belizario VY, Chua PL, Liwanag HJ, Naig JR, Erfe JM. Soil-transmitted helminthiases in secondary school students in selected sites in two provinces in the Philippines: policy implications. J Trop Pediatr. 2014;60:303–7.
25. Sanza M, Totanes FI, Chua PL, Belizario VY. Monitoring the impact of a mebendazole mass drug administration initiative for soil-transmitted helminthiasis (STH) control in the Western Visayas Region of the Philippines from 2007 through 2011. Acta Trop. 2013;127:112–7.
26. Soares Magalhaes RJ, Clements AC, Patil AP, Gething PW, Brooker S. The applications of model-based geostatistics in helminth epidemiology and control. Adv Parasitol. 2011;74:267–96.
27. Hay SI, Tatem AJ, Graham AJ, Goetz SJ, Rogers DJ. Global environmental data for mapping infectious disease distribution. Adv Parasitol. 2006;62:37–77.
28. ESRI. ArcGIS 10.4 for Desktop. https://www.esri.com. In: ESRI 2015. ArcGIS Desktop: Release 10. Redlands, CA: Environmental Systems Research Institute. p. 2015.
29. Brooker S, Alexander N, Geiger S, Moyeed RA, Stander J, Fleming F, et al. Contrasting patterns in the small-scale heterogeneity of human helminth infections in urban and rural environments in Brazil. Int J Parasitol. 2006;36:1143–51.
30. StataCorp. Stata Statistical Software: Release 13. College Station, TX: StataCorp LP; 2013.
31. Assmann SF, Hosmer DW, Lemeshow S, Mundt KA. Confidence intervals for measures of interaction. Epidemiology. 1996;7:286–90.
32. World Health Organization. Preventive checmotherapy in human helminthiasis in coordinated use of anthelminthic drugs in control interventions: a manual for health professionals and programme managers. Geneva: World Health Organization; 2006.
33. Brooker S, Hay SI, Bundy DA. Tools from ecology: useful for evaluating infection risk models? Trends Parasitol. 2002;18:70–4.
34. Gaughan AE, Stevens FR, Linard C, Jia P, Tatem AJ. High resolution population distribution maps for Southeast Asia in 2010 and 2015. PLoS One. 2013;8:e55882.
35. Population Division of the Department of Economic. Social Affairs of the United Nations Secretariat. In: World Population Prospects 2015 Revision Population Database; 2015. https://esa.un.org/unpd/wpp/. Accessed 26 Nov 2015.
36. Brabin L, Brabin BJ. Parasitic infections in women and their consequences. Adv Parasitol. 1992;31:1–81.
37. Nguyen PH, Nguyen KC, Nguyen TD, Le MB, Bern C, Flores R, et al. Intestinal helminth infections among reproductive age women in Vietnam: prevalence, co-infection and risk factors. Southeast Asian J Trop Med Public Health. 2006;37:865–74.
38. Moser W, Ali SM, Ame SM, Speich B, Puchkov M, Huwyler J, et al. Efficacy and safety of oxantel pamoate in school-aged children infected with *Trichuris trichiura* on Pemba Island, Tanzania: a parallel, randomised, controlled, dose-ranging study. Lancet Infect Dis. 2016;16:53–60.
39. Chandra A, McNamara EK, Dargusch P, Caspe MA, Dalabajan D. Gendered vulnerabilities of smallholder farmers to climate change in conflict-prone areas: a case study from Mindanao, Philippines. J Rural Stud. 2017;50:45–59.
40. Food and Agriculture Organization. The elimination of food insecurity in the Horn of Africa. Rome: Food and Agriculture Organization of the United Nations; 2000.
41. Bhagwan JN, Still D, Buckley C, Foxon K. Challenges with up-scaling dry sanitation technologies. Water Sci Technol. 2008;58:21–7.
42. Stevens FR, Gaughan AE, Linard C, Tatem AJ. Disaggregating census data for population mapping using random forests with remotely-sensed and ancillary data. PLoS One. 2015;10:e0107042.
43. Centre for International Earth Science Information Network (CIESIN). International Food Policy Research Institute (IFPRI), World Resources Institute (WRI). Gridded Population of the World (GPW). Version. 2009:3 http://sedac.ciesin.columbia.edu/theme/population. Accessed 1 Oct 2014.

17

Characterization of tick organic anion transporting polypeptides (OATPs) upon bacterial and viral infections

Vikas Taank[1], Wenshuo Zhou[1], Xuran Zhuang[2], John F. Anderson[3], Utpal Pal[2], Hameeda Sultana[1,4] and Girish Neelakanta[1,4*]

Abstract

Background: *Ixodes scapularis* organic anion transporting polypeptides (OATPs) play important roles in tick-rickettsial pathogen interactions. In this report, we characterized the role of these conserved molecules in ticks infected with either Lyme disease agent *Borrelia burgdorferi* or tick-borne Langat virus (LGTV), a pathogen closely related to tick-borne encephalitis virus (TBEV).

Results: Quantitative real-time polymerase chain reaction analysis revealed no significant changes in *oatps* gene expression upon infection with *B. burgdorferi* in unfed ticks. Synchronous infection of unfed nymphal ticks with LGTV *in vitro* revealed no significant changes in *oatps* gene expression. However, expression of specific *oatps* was significantly downregulated upon LGTV infection of tick cells *in vitro*. Treatment of tick cells with OATP inhibitor significantly reduced LGTV loads, kynurenine amino transferase (*kat*), a gene involved in the production of tryptophan metabolite xanthurenic acid (XA), levels and expression of several *oatps* in tick cells. Furthermore, bioinformatics characterization of OATPs from some of the medically important vectors including ticks, mosquitoes and lice revealed the presence of several glycosylation, phosphorylation and myristoylation sites.

Conclusions: This study provides additional evidence on the role of arthropod OATPs in vector-intracellular pathogen interactions.

Keywords: Organic anion transporting polypeptide, Kynurenine aminotransferase, *Borrelia burgdorferi*, Langat virus, *Ixodes scapularis*, *Anaplasma phagocytophilum*, Xanthurenic acid, Anti-vector vaccine

Background

Blood-feeding arthropods such as ticks, mosquitoes and lice are important vectors for several human pathogens [1]. Based on the disability adjusted life year (DALY) estimates, one sixth of the human population worldwide are prone to infections caused by pathogens transmitted by arthropods, including ticks, mosquitoes and lice [1]. These arthropods have evolved different blood-feeding behaviors [2–4]. The control strategies for these arthropods are limiting, as use of several acaricides have shown to be ineffective in many instances [5]. Recent progress in new methods such as the development of transmission-blocking vaccines targeting conserved proteins across various arthropod species has provided a significant promise for the treatment or control of the diseases transmitted by these arthropods [6–9].

The presence of the multigene family of organic anion transporting polypeptides (OATPs) across various arthropods and vertebrates suggests that it has an important role in various aspects of the physiology of these organisms [10–12]. OATPs in humans are now recognized as determinants of the transmembrane passage of drugs that are important for pharmacokinetics [13]. Human OATPs localize to barrier epithelial cells that facilitate the uptake of several substances including toxins, hormones, metabolites and those involved in cell signaling [10, 11, 13, 14]. The N-terminus and C-terminus parts of vertebrate OATPs are noted to be intracellular

* Correspondence: gneelaka@odu.edu
[1]Department of Biological Sciences, Old Dominion University, Norfolk, VA, USA
[4]Center for Molecular Medicine, College of Sciences, Old Dominion University, Norfolk, VA, USA
Full list of author information is available at the end of the article

[10, 11, 13–15]. However, the remaining part of OATPs is organized into several transmembrane domains linked by short intracellular loops and extracellular loops that face outside the membrane [10, 11, 13–15].

The black-legged *Ixodes scapularis* tick is a medically important vector for various human pathogens including *Borrelia burgdorferi*, *Anaplasma phagocytophilum*, *Babesia microti*, *Ehrlichia muris*-like agent (EMLA), Powassan virus (POWV) and *Borrelia miyamotoi* [16–19]. Other *Ixodes* species transmit tick-borne encephalitis virus (TBEV) [20]. Langat virus (LGTV), a close member of TBEV, is considered as a model biosafety level 2 pathogen to study infection dynamics of TBEV [20, 21]. LGTV readily infects *I. scapularis* ticks and the ISE6 tick cell line derived from these ticks [21, 22]. A recent study reported the presence of nine OATPs in *I. scapularis* ticks [23]. Phylogenetic analysis of *I. scapularis* and other tick OATPs revealed that these OATPs are clustered with various other orthologs from medically important blood-feeding arthropods such as lice and mosquitoes [23].

We recently reported the importance of specific OATPs in *I. scapularis* tick-rickettsial pathogen interactions [12]. We have shown that *A. phagocytophilum* specifically modulates tick OATP, *isoatp4056*, and kynurenine amino transferase (*kat*), a gene involved in the production of tryptophan metabolite xanthurenic acid (XA), for its survival in ticks. RNAi mediated analysis revealed that knockdown of *isoatp4056* and/or *kat*, affected *A. phagocytophilum* survival in ticks. Our results noted interesting cross-talk between tick OATP and XA in the survival of this rickettsial pathogen in its vector host. Arthropod XA mediates malarial parasite gametogenesis in mosquitoes [24, 25]. Collectively, these studies suggest that in addition to their role in physiological processes in various organisms, OATPs also participate in vector-pathogen interactions. The role of OATPs in the interactions of ticks with other pathogens remains to be explored.

In view of the development of anti-vector vaccines as an effective means to target various arthropods, understanding the role of conserved protein families such as OATPs in vector biology and interactions with different pathogens remains important. In this study, we performed molecular analysis of OATPs in the interactions of ticks with an extracellular bacterial pathogen and an intracellular tick-borne virus.

Methods

Bacterial/viral isolates, ticks and tick cell line

Borrelia burgdorferi strain B31-A3 or Langat virus (LGTV) strain (LGT-TP21) was used throughout this study. These strains will be herein referred to as *B. burgdorferi* and LGTV, respectively. *Borrelia burgdorferi*-infected ticks were generated as described [26] and RNA extractions from ticks were performed in the laboratory of Dr Utpal Pal at the University of Maryland, USA. Uninfected nymphs used in generating LGTV-infected ticks were obtained from a tick colony at the Connecticut Agricultural Experiment Station, New Haven, CT, USA. The ISE6 tick cell line was provided by Dr Ulrike Munderloh at the University of Minnesota (St Paul, MN, USA) and maintained as described [12]. Both uninfected and LGTV-infected ticks used in this study were maintained in an environmental chamber (Parameter Generation and Control, Black Mountain, NC, USA) set at a temperature of 23 ± 1 °C, 95% humidity and a 14/10 h light/dark photoperiod regiment.

In vitro generation of LGTV-infected ticks

Synchronous LGTV infection in uninfected ticks was performed as described [21]. Briefly, about 25 nymphal ticks were immersed in 0.5 ml of complete Dulbecco's modified Eagle's medium (DMEM) containing 1×10^7 pfu/ml of LGTV viral stock and incubated at 34 °C for 1 h. Vials containing ticks in the medium were vortexed every 10 min to redistribute the medium over ticks. After incubation, ticks were thoroughly washed five times with 1× phosphate-buffered saline (PBS) and incubated for 17 days in an environmental chamber. RNA from these ticks were extracted and tested for the presence of both positive and negative sense RNA strands of LGTV as described [21, 27].

RNA extraction and quantitative real-time PCR (QRT-PCR) analysis

Total RNA from uninfected or LGTV-infected nymphs and tick cells was generated using an Aurum Total RNA mini kit (Bio-Rad, Hercules, USA) following the manufacturer's instructions. The cDNA was later synthesized using an iScript cDNA synthesis kit (Bio-Rad) and used for QRT-PCR reactions [12, 27]. The amount of tick *beta-actin* transcripts was used to normalize the amount of template in each reaction. QRT-PCR assays were performed using iQ-SYBR Green Supermix (Bio-Rad) and a Bio-Rad CFX96 QPCR machine. *Borrelia burgdorferi flaB* gene transcripts or LGTV positive or negative RNA strands were quantified in the cDNA samples. Serial dilutions (10-fold) ranging from 1 to 0.00001 ng of respective fragments were used to generate a standard curve. QRT-PCR oligonucleotides for *oatps*, actin, *kat*, *B. burgdorferi flaB* and for the detection of LGTV are published in our previous studies [12, 27, 28].

LGTV infection of tick cells

LGTV infection of tick cells was performed as described [27]. All infection experiments in tick cells were performed with 1 MOI of LGTV. 1×10^5 tick cells were seeded in L-15B300 medium onto 12-well plates and incubated for 24 h followed by infection with 1 MOI of LGTV and collection of cells at 24 and 72 h post-infection (pi). RNA from these collected cells was extracted and processed for cDNA synthesis and QRT-PCR analysis.

Tick cell line experiments with OATP inhibitor

Inhibitor treatment was performed as described [12]. 1×10^5 tick cells were plated in 12-well cell culture plates and incubated for 20 h. After incubation, 100 μM of ±-sulfinpyrazone (SPZ, purchased from Santa Cruz Biotechnology Inc., Dallas, USA) was added and cells were incubated for an additional 4 h followed by LGTV infection. 0.5 N NaOH was used to prepare 10 mM SPZ stocks. For experiments, a one-tenth diluted (with 1× PBS) solution (final concentration 1mM SPZ) was used. A mock solution was prepared in a similar way but without SPZ. An equal volume of mock solution (corresponding to 100 μM volume of SPZ) was added to control cell culture wells. After 24 h pi, cells were processed for RNA extractions followed by cDNA synthesis and QRT-PCR analysis to measure *oatp* or *kat* transcripts and LGTV loads.

Bioinformatic analysis

The amino acid sequences that contained OATP signature sequence WxGxWWxG were downloaded from GenBank and individually analyzed at PROSITE (http://prosite.expasy.org/) as described [29–31]. Biology WorkBench (San Diego Supercomputer Center) at http://workbench.sdsc.edu/ and the National Center for Biotechnology Information conserved domain search (NCBI-CD) at http://www.ncbi.nlm.nih.gov/Structure/cdd/wrpsb.cgi were used for the prediction of glycosylation, myristoylation, protein kinase C phosphorylation, casein kinase II phosphorylation, tyrosine phosphorylation, cAMP-dependent protein kinase phosphorylation and identification of Kazal domain sites. For data analysis, the post-translational modification sites that are present either outside or inside regions of OATPs but not on the transmembrane regions were considered. TMHMM http://www.cbs.dtu.dk/services/TMHMM/ server v.2.0 (prediction of transmembrane helices in proteins) was used to predict transmembrane and outside or inside regions of OATP. For Kazal site prediction, full-length OATP sequences were considered.

GenBank accession numbers

The GenBank accession numbers for the OATP sequences used in the study are as follows: *D. melanogaster* (AAF46824-AAF46826, AAF49332, NP_609055, NP_001260417), *Aedes aegypti* (XP_001658583, XP_001659726, XP_001660406, XP_001660407, XP_001661188), *Anopheles gambiae* (XP_314819, XP_316669, XP_319187, XP_557860, XP_001237849), *Culex quinquefasciatus* (EDS26845, EDS34303, EDS45569, EDS45572), *Pediculus humanus corporis* (EEB11548, EEB18131, EEB20444, EEB20468), *Rhipicephalus pulchellus* (JAA58190, JAA59396, JAA59849, JAA64227), *Amblyomma americanum* (ACH98103) and *Ixodes scapularis* (DAA34891, XP_002400770, XP_002412161, XP_002414101, XP_002434179, XP_002404592, XP_002404594, XP_002415171, XP_002435666).

Statistics

A non-paired two-tailed Student's t-test and nonparametric Mann-Whitney tests from GraphPad Prism6 software and Microsoft Excel 2016 were used to calculate statistical significance. Graphs were generated using GraphPad Prism6 software. Horizontal lines in the graphs represent the mean values. $P < 0.05$ was considered significant and shown at relevant places.

Results

Borrelia burgdorferi has no impact on the expression of any of the *I. scapularis oatps* in unfed ticks

Previous studies have reported expression of nine *oatps* in unfed *I. scapularis* ticks [12, 23]. Our recent study reported upregulation of specific *oatps* and *kat* upon *A. phagocytophilum* infection in unfed ticks [12]. To test whether similar observation was evident upon infection with an extracellular pathogen, we used *B. burgdorferi*-infected unfed ticks. We found no significant ($P > 0.05$) differences (Additional file 1: Table S1) in the expression levels of *isoatp-0726* (Fig. 1a), *-2114* (Fig. 1b), *-2116* (Fig. 1c), *-4056* (Fig. 1d), *-4134* (Fig. 1e), *-4548* (Fig. 1f), *-4550* (Fig. 1g), *-5126* (Fig. 1h) and *-5621* (Fig. 1i) between unfed uninfected and *B. burgdorferi*-infected ticks. In addition, no significant ($P > 0.05$) difference (Additional file 1: Table S1) in *kat* gene expression was noted between unfed uninfected and *B. burgdorferi*-infected ticks (Fig. 1j). As expected, QRT-PCR analysis revealed presence of *flaB* transcripts only in *B. burgdorferi*-infected ticks but not in uninfected ticks (Fig. 1k). These results show that unlike the intracellular pathogen *A. phagocytophilum* (as reported in our previous study [12]), the extracellular pathogen *B. burgdorferi* has no impact on the expression of any arthropod *oatps* and *kat* gene in unfed ticks.

Synchronous infection of LGTV does not impact OATP expression in unfed ticks

LGTV readily infects *I. scapularis* ticks [21]. We generated synchronously infected LGTV ticks *in vitro* (as described in Methods) to test whether tick-borne viruses have any impact on *oatp* expression. We found no significant ($P > 0.05$) differences (Additional file 1: Table S1) in the expression levels of *isoatp-0726* (Fig. 2a), *-2114* (Fig. 2b), *-2116* (Fig. 2c), *-4056* (Fig. 2d), *-4134* (Fig. 2e), *-4548* (Fig. 2f), *-4550* (Fig. 2g), *-5126* (Fig. 2h) and *-5621* (Fig. 2i) between unfed uninfected ticks or LGTV-infected ticks. In addition, no significant ($P > 0.05$) difference (Additional file 1: Table S1) in *kat* gene expression was

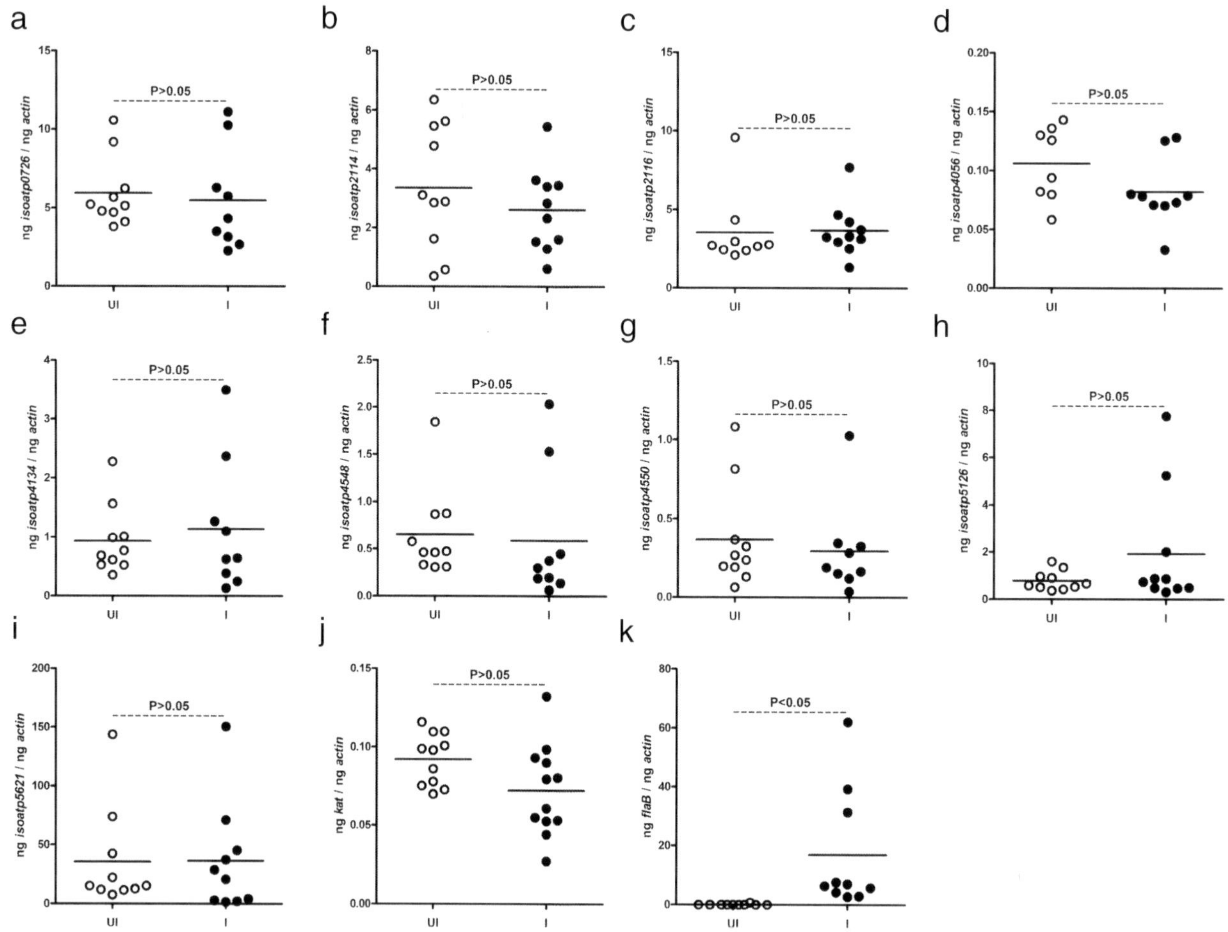

Fig. 1 *B. burgdorferi* has no impact on the expression of nine *I. scapularis oatps* in unfed nymphal ticks. Results from QRT-PCR assays are shown in all panels. **a-i** Expression of nine *I. scapularis* OATPs: *isoatp-0726* (**a**), *-2114* (**b**), *-2116* (**c**), *-4056* (**d**), *-4134* (**e**), *-4548* (**f**), *-4550* (**g**), *-5126* (**h**) and *-5621* (**i**) in unfed uninfected or *B. burgdorferi*-infected ticks. Levels of tick *kat* (**j**) or spirochete *flaB* (**k**) mRNA in *B. burgdorferi*-infected unfed nymphal ticks are also shown. Uninfected ticks were used as controls in all panels. In all panels, open circles represent data from uninfected (UI) and closed circles represent data from infected (I) ticks. Each circle represents data from one tick. The amount of mRNA levels of *flaB* or *oatps* or *kat* was normalized to the amount of tick beta-actin mRNA levels. The *P*-values indicate the results from statistical analyses

noted between unfed uninfected or LGTV-infected ticks (Fig. 2j). QRT-PCR analysis revealed presence of both positive (Fig. 2k) and negative (Fig. 2l) strands of virus in LGTV-infected ticks. As expected, no LGTV RNA was detected in uninfected controls (Fig. 2k, l). These results show that LGTV does not impact *oatp* and *kat* expression in unfed ticks.

Expression of specific *I. scapularis oatp* transcripts was downregulated upon LGTV infection of tick cells

We next tested whether LGTV infection has any impact on the *oatp* mRNA levels in tick cells. We selected 24 and 72 h pi as early and late infection stages, respectively, and expression of all nine *oatp* genes were analyzed (Fig. 3). No significant ($P > 0.05$) differences (Additional file 1: Table S1) in the expression levels of *isoatp-0726* (Fig. 3a), *-2116* (Fig. 3c), *-4056* (Fig. 3d), *-4134* (Fig. 3e) and *-5621* (Fig. 3i) between uninfected and LGTV-infected tick cells at 24 h pi were noted. However, significant downregulation of *isoatps-2114* (Fig. 3b), *-4548* (Fig. 3f), *-4550* (Fig. 3g) and *-5126* (Fig. 3h) was evident in LGTV-infected tick cells in comparison to uninfected control at 24 h pi. No significant ($P > 0.05$) differences (Additional file 1: Table S1) in the expression of all nine *oatps* were noted between LGTV-infected tick cells and uninfected controls at 72 h pi. In addition, no significant ($P > 0.05$) difference (Additional file 1: Table S1) in *kat* gene expression was noted between unfed uninfected and LGTV-infected tick cells (Fig. 3j). LGTV readily infected tick cells with increased viral loads at 72 h pi in comparison to 24 h pi (Fig. 3k). No morphological difference was evident between uninfected or LGTV-infected tick cells at both time points (Additional file 1: Figure S1). These results suggest that specific *oatp* genes are modulated

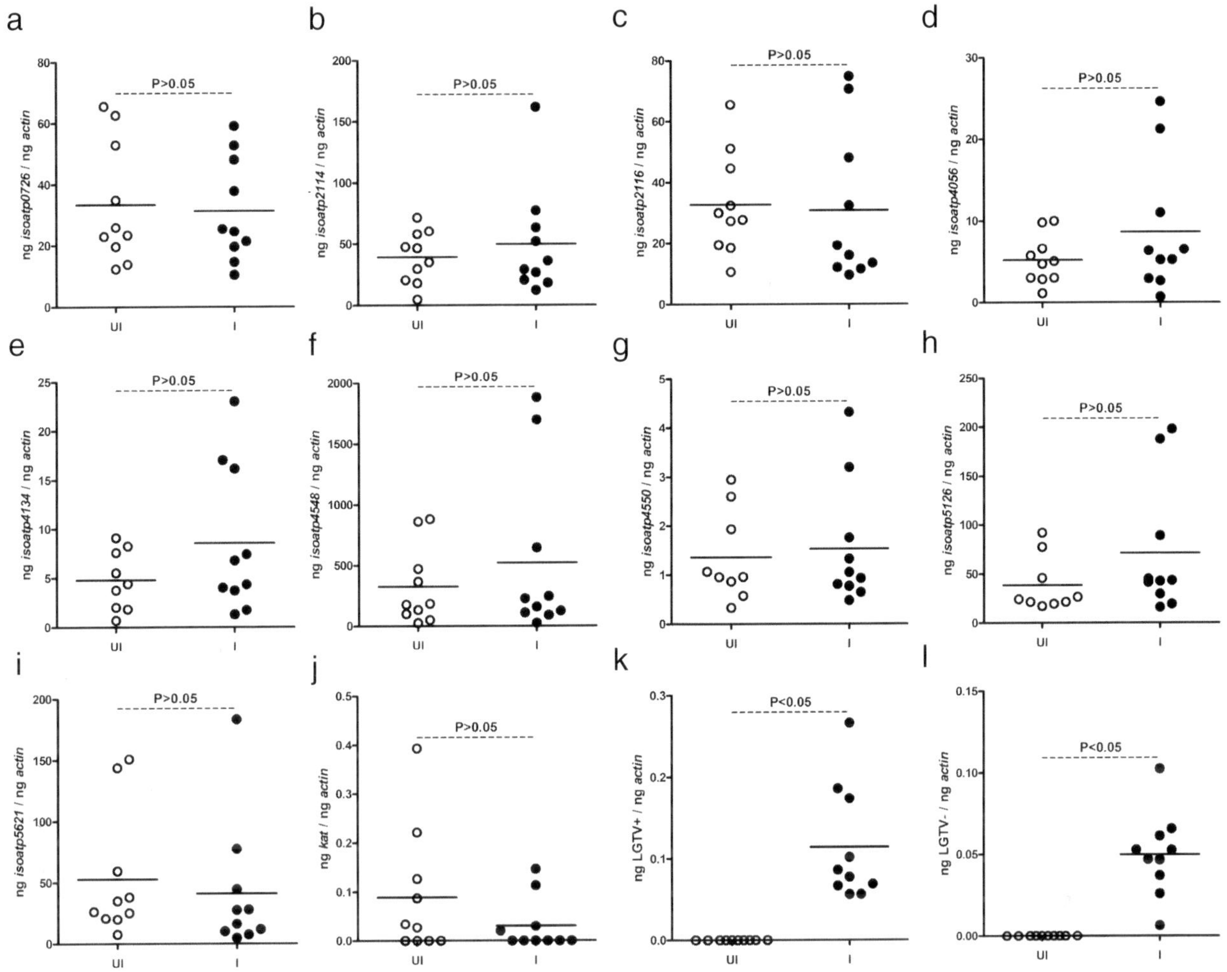

Fig. 2 LGTV has no impact on the expression of nine *I. scapularis oatps* in synchronously-infected unfed nymphal ticks. Data from QRT-PCR assays are shown in all panels. **a-i** Expression of nine *I. scapularis* OATPs: *isoatp-0726* (**a**), *-2114* (**b**), *-2116* (**c**), *-4056* (**d**), *-4134* (**e**), *-4548* (**f**), *-4550* (**g**), *-5126* (**h**) and *-5621* (**i**) in unfed uninfected or LGTV-synchronously-infected ticks is shown. **j** Levels of tick *kat* mRNA in unfed uninfected or LGTV-synchronously-infected ticks. Levels of viral positive-sense strand (**k**) or negative sense strand (**l**) in LGTV-synchronously-infected ticks are shown. Uninfected ticks were used as controls in all panels. In all panels, open circles represent data from uninfected (UI) and closed circles represent data from LGTV synchronously-infected (I) ticks. Each circle represents data from one tick. The amount of mRNA levels of LGTV positive- or negative-sense strands or *oatps* or *kat* was normalized to the amount of tick beta-actin mRNA levels. The *P*-values indicate the results from statistical analyses

at early but not at later stages of LGTV infection of tick cells.

Inhibition of OATP affects LGTV burden in tick cells

The downregulation of specific *oatps* suggests an important role for these molecules in early tick-LGTV interactions. We tested whether treatment of tick cells with SPZ, a general inhibitor of OATP, has any impact on LGTV infection at early stages. Tick cells were treated with 100 μM of SPZ as described [12], followed by LGTV infection for 24 h. Microscopic observations revealed no morphological differences in tick cells that were either mock-treated or SPZ-treated at 4 h post-treatment followed by LGTV-infection for 24 h (Fig. 4a). In addition, no cytotoxicity was observed upon treatment of uninfected tick cells with 100 μM of SPZ at 4, 24, 48 and 72 h post--treatment (Additional file 1: Figure S2). However, significantly ($P < 0.05$) reduced viral loads were evident in SPZ-treated LGTV-infected tick cells in comparison to mock-treated control at 24 h pi (Fig. 4b, Additional file 1: Table S1). These results suggest that OATPs play important roles in the survival of LGTV in tick cells.

Treatment of LGTV-infected tick cells with OATP inhibitor affects expression of several *oatps* and *kat* gene expression

We then assessed whether treatment of tick cells with OATP inhibitor has any effect on the *oatps* mRNA levels (Fig. 5, Additional file 1: Table S1). QRT-PCR analysis

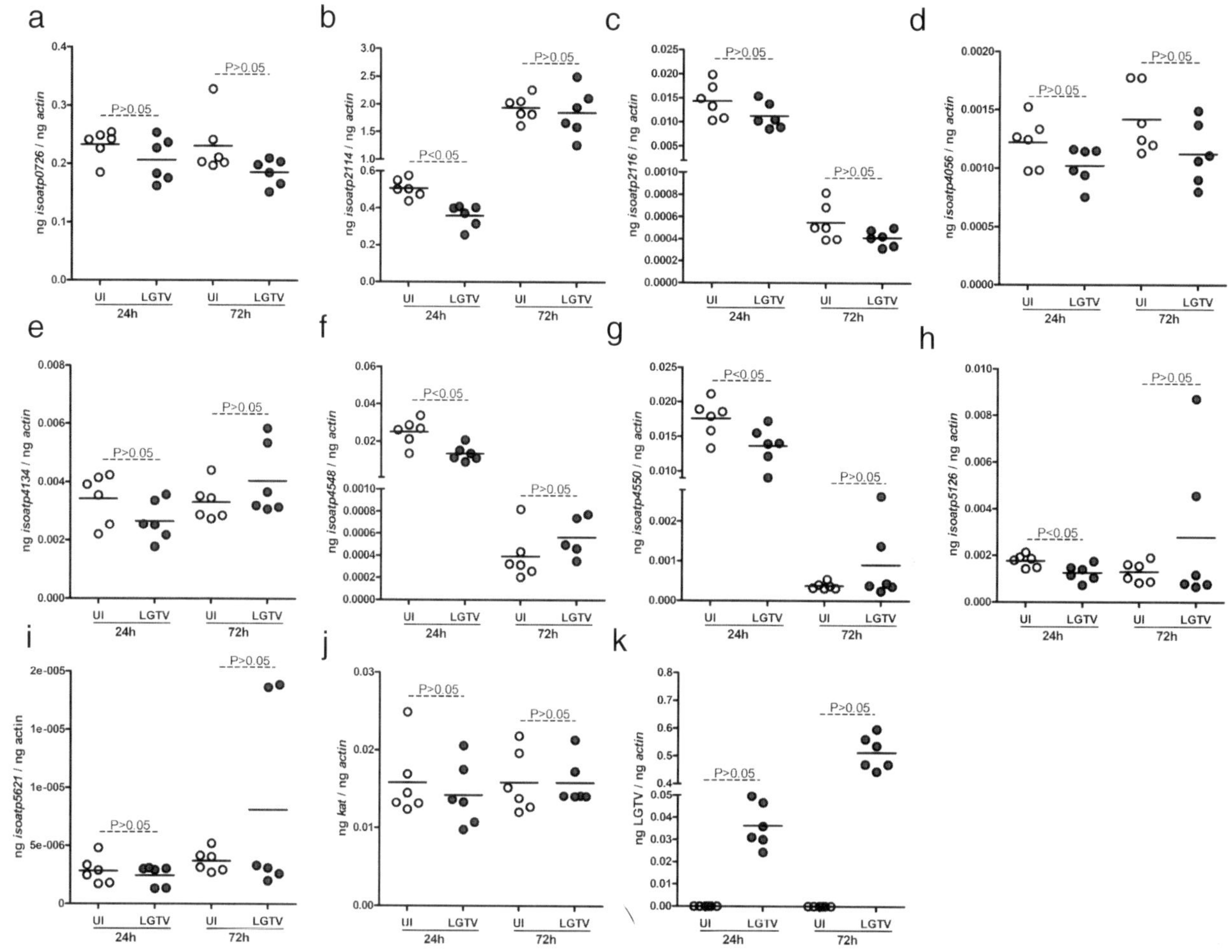

Fig. 3 LGTV infection of tick cells *in vitro* affects expression of *isoatp2114*, *isoatp4548*, *isoatp4550* and *isoatp5126*. Data from QRT-PCR assays are shown in all panels. **a-i** Expression of nine *I. scapularis* OATPs: *isoatp-0726* (**a**), *-2114* (**b**), *-2116* (**c**), *-4056* (**d**), *-4134* (**e**), *-4548* (**f**), *-4550* (**g**), *-5126* (**h**), *-5621* (**i**) and *kat* mRNA (**j**) in unfed uninfected ticks and LGTV-infected tick cells at 24 and 72 h pi. **k** Levels of viral RNA in LGTV-infected ISE6 tick cell line (LGTV) at 24 and 72 h pi. is shown. Uninfected (UI) cells were used as controls in all panels. In all panels, open circles represent data from uninfected (UI) and closed circles represent data from LGTV-infected (LGTV) tick cells. Each circle represents data from one cell culture well. LGTV loads or *oatps* or *kat* mRNA levels was normalized to the amount of tick beta-actin mRNA levels. The *P*-values indicate the results from statistical analyses

revealed significant ($P < 0.05$) downregulation of *isoatps-0726* (Fig. 5a), *-4056* (Fig. 5d), *-4134* (Fig. 5e) and *-5621* (Fig. 5i) in SPZ-treated LGTV-infected tick cells in comparison to mock-treated control at 24 h pi. In addition, we noted a significant ($P < 0.05$) upregulation of *isoatp4550* in SPZ-treated LGTV-infected tick cells in comparison to mock-treated control at 24 h pi (Fig. 5g). No significant ($P > 0.05$) differences in the expression levels of *isoatps 2114* (Fig. 5b), *-2116* (Fig. 5c), *-4548* (Fig. 5f), *-5126* (Fig. 5h) was noted between SPZ-treated LGTV-infected tick cells in comparison to the mock-treated control at 24 h pi. Our previous study suggests KAT as an upstream molecular player that impacts *isoatp4056* expression [12]. QRT-PCR analysis revealed a significant ($P < 0.05$) reduction in *kat* transcripts (Additional file 1: Table S1) in SPZ-treated LGTV-infected tick cells in comparison to the mock-treated control at 24 h pi (Fig. 5j). These results clearly suggest an interplay among OATPs in the early stages of tick-LGTV interactions.

Bioinformatic analysis of OATPs from ticks, mosquitoes and lice

Post-translational modification is a key strategy that pathogens use to modulate functions of host factors that play central roles in cell signaling [32]. Our previous findings on the role of the OATP-KAT pathway in rickettsial pathogen-tick interactions [12] and the present findings on their roles in LGTV-tick interactions suggest that these conserved molecules play central roles in vector-pathogen interactions. Post-translational modifications are critical for OATPs to function efficiently [33–35]. Therefore, understanding putative post-translational modification sites

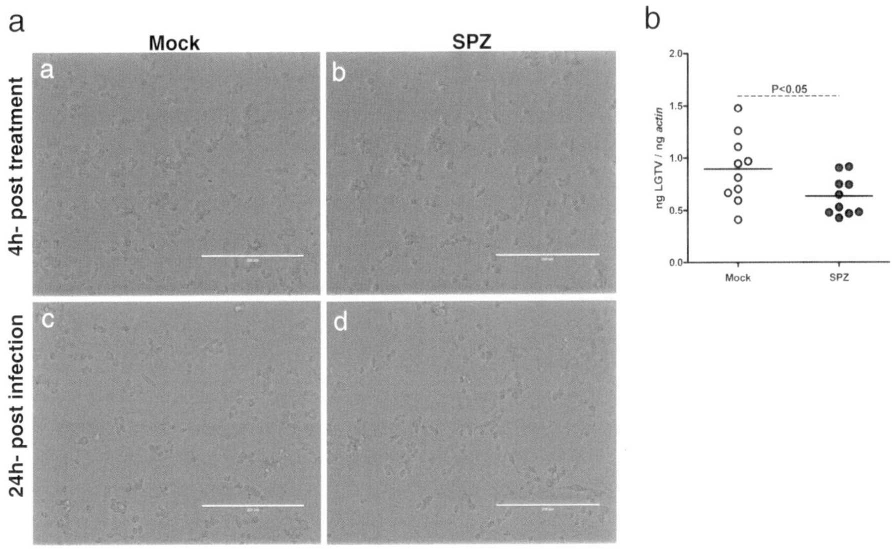

Fig. 4 Inhibition of OATPs affect LGTV loads in tick cells. **a** Representative phase-contrast images of LGTV-infected mock-treated or SPZ-treated tick cells (4 h post-treatment, before infection) followed by 24 h post-LGTV-infection. **b** QRT-PCR analysis showing levels of viral RNA in LGTV-infected mock- or SPZ-treated tick cells at 24 h pi. Open circles represent data from LGTV-infected mock-treated and closed circles represent data from SPZ-treated tick cells at 24 h pi. Each circle represents data from one cell culture well. LGTV loads were normalized to the amount of tick beta-actin levels. In **b**, the *P*-value indicates the result from statistical analysis. *Scale-bars*: 200 μm

on OATPs is highly required. As OATPs are shown to be present in many arthropod species [23, 36–38], we performed a comparative analysis of *I. scapularis* OATPs with orthologs from other medically important vectors and the fruit fly *Drosophila melanogaster*. A previous study reported the phylogenetic analysis of OATPs from different species that revealed *I. scapularis* OATPs are segregated with other tick OATPs [23]. In this study, the primary amino acid sequences (that contained OATP signature sequence, WxGxWWxG) of eight *I. scapularis* OATPs, five *Aedes aegypti* OATPs, five *Anopheles gambiae* OATPs, four *Culex quinquefasciatus* OATPs, four *Pediculus humanus corporis* OATPs, four *Rhipicephalus pulchellus* OATPs, one *Amblyomma americanum* OATP and six *D. melanogaster* OATPs were downloaded from the National Center for Biotechnology Information (NCBI) database. Variable length of amino acid sequences among different tick OATPs was noticed (Additional file 1: Tables S2 and S3). Each OATP amino acid sequence was first individually analyzed at TMHMM server v.2.0 (prediction of transmembrane helices in proteins) followed by selection of regions that are exposed outside the plasma membrane and regions that are inside the plasma membrane (Additional file 1: Tables S2 and S3). The transmembrane regions within each OATP sequence were excluded from the analysis. The regions that are outside and inside the plasma membrane were considered to predict conserved and/or unique post-translational modifications in the sequences. Based on the analysis, all but two OATP sequences were predicted to carry at least two N-glycosylation sites (Fig. 6a and Additional file 1: Table S2). OATP from *Ae. aegypti* (GenBank: XP_001660407) was predicted to carry the highest number (14 sites), while, *I. scapularis* (GenBank: XP_002435666), *A. americanum* (GenBank: ACH98103), *R. pulchellus* (GenBank: JAA59396) and *Cx. quinquefasciatus* (GenBank: EDS26845) were predicted to carry the lowest (2 sites) number of N-glycosylation sites (Fig. 6a and Additional file 1: Table S2). All of the OATPs were predicted to carry at least 2 myristoylation sites (Fig. 6b and Additional file 1: Table S2), where OATP from *An. gambiae* (XP_557860) was predicted to carry the highest number (24 sites) and *I. scapularis* OATPs (DAA34891, XP_002400770, XP_002404592, XP_002415171) were predicted to carry the lowest (3 sites) number of myristoylation sites.

All 37 OATPs analyzed in this study were predicted to carry varying numbers of PKC phosphorylation sites (Fig. 7a and Additional file 1: Table S3). The *D. melanogaster* OATPs (AAF46824, AAF46826) were predicted to carry the highest number (12 sites) and *I. scapularis* OATP (XP_002400770) was predicted to carry the lowest number (1 site) of PKC phosphorylation sites (Fig. 7a and Additional file 1: Table S3). In addition, out of the 37 OATPs analyzed, all were predicted to carry at least one CK2 phosphorylation site (Fig. 7b and Additional file 1: Table S3). *P. humanus corporis* OATP (EEB20444) was predicted to carry the highest number (19 sites) and *I. scapularis* OATP (XP_002404594) was predicted to carry the lowest number (1 site) of CK2 phosphorylation sites

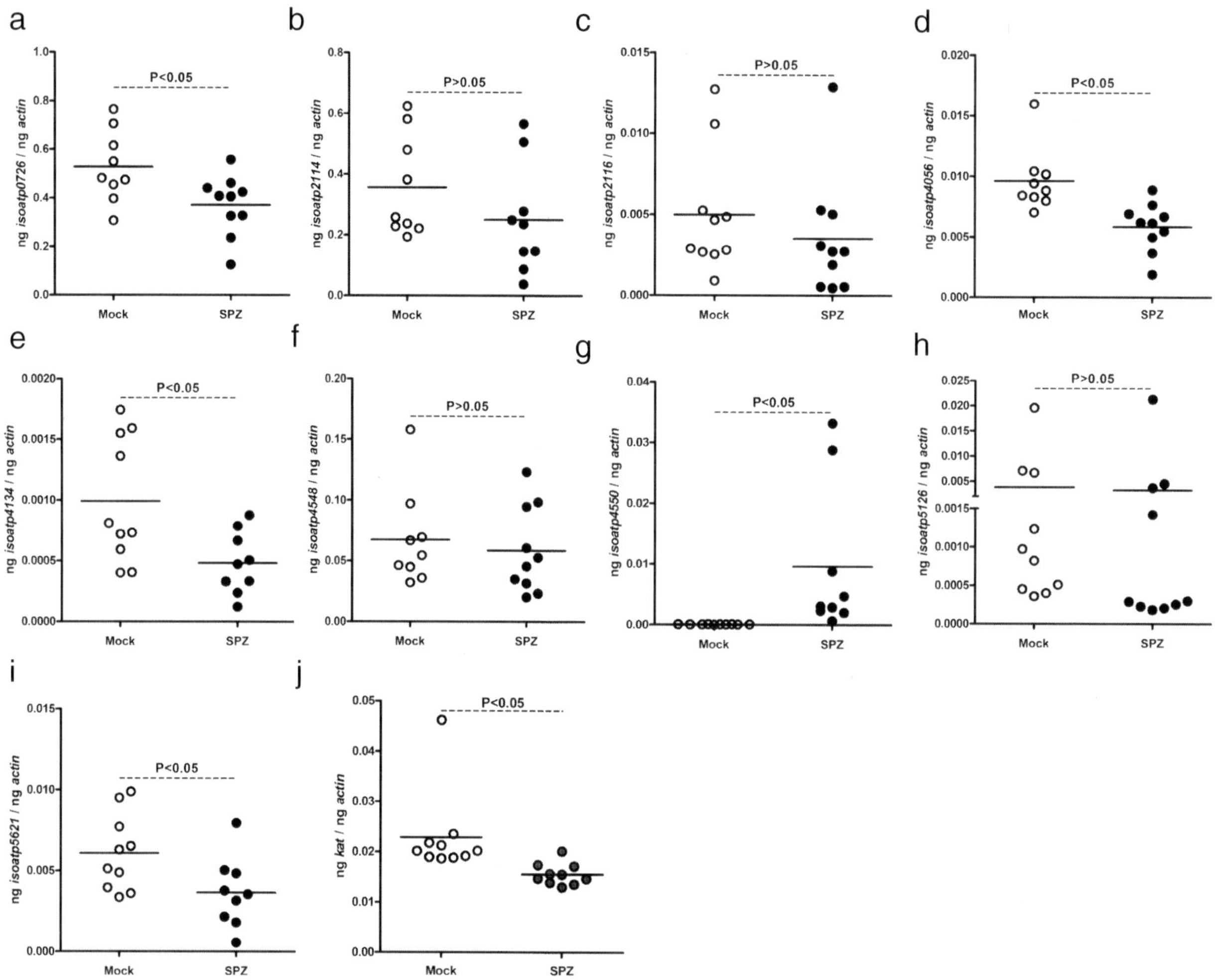

Fig. 5 Treatment of tick cells with OATP inhibitor affects *oatps* and *kat* gene expression. Data from QRT-PCR assays are shown in all panels. Expression of nine *I. scapularis* OATPs: *isoatps-0726* (**a**), *-2114* (**b**), *-2116* (**c**), *-4056* (**d**), *-4134* (**e**), *-4548* (**f**), *-4550* (**g**), *-5126* (**h**), *-5621* (**i**) and *kat* (**j**) mRNA levels in LGTV-infected mock- or OATP-inhibitor (SPZ)-treated tick cells at 24 h pi. In all panels, open circles or closed circles represent data from LGTV-infected mock- or SPZ-treated tick cells at 24 h pi, respectively. Each circle represents data from one cell culture well. The *oatps* and *kat* mRNA levels were normalized to the tick beta-actin mRNA levels. The *P*-values indicate the results from statistical analyses

(Fig. 7b and Additional file 1: Table S3). Tyrosine phosphorylation sites were also evident in 20 out of the 37 OATPs that were analyzed (Fig. 7c and Additional file 1: Table S3). All four sequences from *P. humanus corporis* OATPs, four out of six *D. melanogaster* sequences, three out of four *Cx. quinquefasciatus* sequences and three out of five *An. gambiae* sequences contained at least one tyrosine phosphorylation site (Fig. 7c). Interestingly, out of 13 OATP sequences from ticks, only three sequences from *I. scapularis* (XP_002412161, XP_002414101, XP_002435666) were predicted to carry tyrosine phosphorylation sites (Fig. 7c). Among all OATPs, *Ae. aegypti* OATP (XP_001660407), *P. humanus corporis* OATPs (EEB18131, EEB20468) and *D. melanogaster* OATPs (AAF46824, AAF49332) were predicted to carry the highest number (2 sites) of tyrosine phosphorylation sites (Fig. 7c and Additional file 1: Table S3). Out of 37 OATPs, 27 were predicted to carry at least one cAMP-dependent protein kinase phosphorylation site (Fig. 7d and Additional file 1: Table S3). The *Ae. aegypti* OATP (XP_001660407) and *An. gambiae* OATP (XP_557860) were predicted to carry the highest number (4 sites) of cAMP-dependent protein kinase phosphorylation sites (Fig. 7d and Additional file 1: Table S3). In addition, with the exception of three *I. scapularis* OATPs (XP_002400770, XP_002404594, XP_002415171) and one *D. melanogaster* OATP (AAF46825), all 33 other OATPs were predicted to carry one Kazal domain in their sequences (Additional file 1: Figure S3).

Discussion

The development of a broad-spectrum anti-vector vaccine to control or treat diseases transmitted by ticks, mosquitoes and lice largely depends on the characterization of conserved proteins present in them. Our previous study

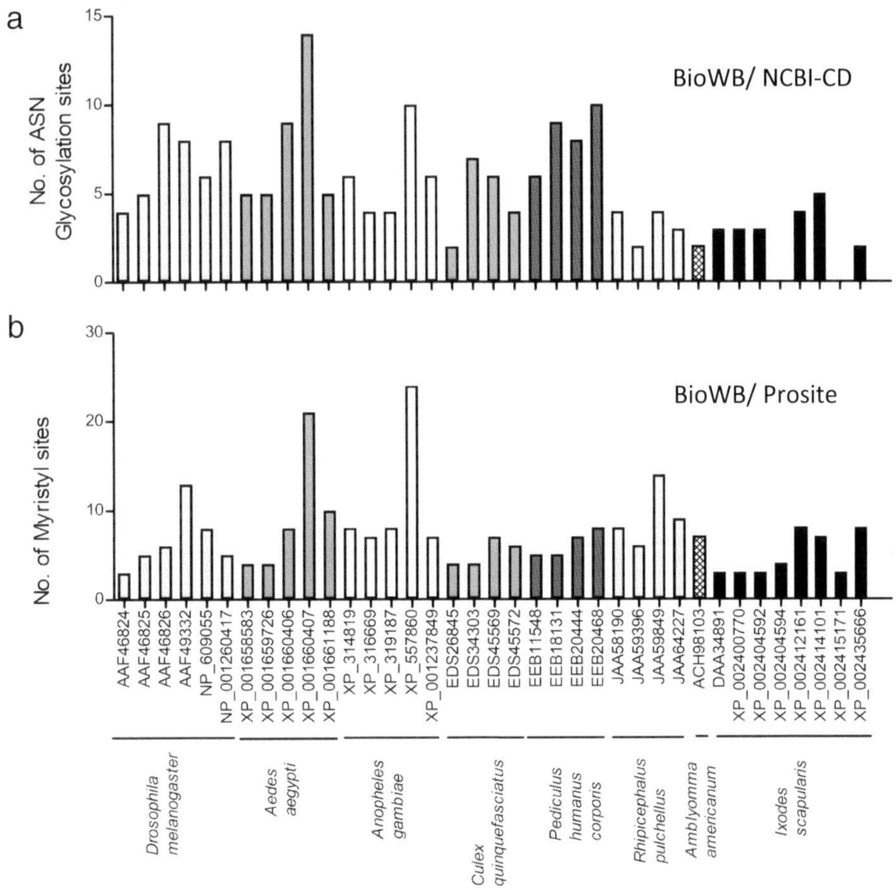

Fig. 6 Analysis of glycosylation and myristoylation sites in OATPs from medically important vectors. Amino acid sequences of several OATPs were individually analyzed at Biology WorkBench (**a**, **b**), NCBI conserved domain search (**a**) and PROSITE (**b**) databases for glycosylation (**a**) and myristoylation (**b**) sites. Histograms represent the number of post-translational modification sites on each OATP. The post-translational modifications in the transmembrane regions within each OATP were not considered for histogram plots. GenBank accession numbers and organism names are shown at the bottom of the figure

provided evidence on the role of OATP family proteins in the survival of rickettsial pathogen in ticks [12]. In this study, we provide evidence on the role of OATP family proteins in the survival of intracellular tick-borne viruses. This study, in conjunction with our previous findings, clearly recognizes arthropod OATPs as molecular players targeted by vector-borne pathogens and in particular by intracellular pathogens for their survival in the vector host.

The observation of no difference in OATP gene expression between *B. burgdorferi* and LGTV-infected ticks in comparison to their uninfected controls in unfed tick developmental stage cannot rule out the possibility that these pathogens may impact *oatp* expression during initial phases of their infection in ticks. We used the ISE6 *in vitro* tick cell line and LGTV-infection model to address whether intracellular pathogens have any impact on *oatp* expression in the early part of their infection of tick cells. We considered 24 and 72 h, as early and late time points of infection, respectively. The significant increase in LGTV burden at 72 h pi in comparison to 24 h pi, and observation of significant downregulation of *oatps* at 24 h pi but not at 72 h pi, clearly suggests an initial vector-host response to control viral replication at an early infection phase. Our data suggest that OATPs may be critical for initial replication of LGTV and that the host is downregulating these arthropod molecules to control viral replication. The observation of a significant reduction in viral loads upon treatment of tick cells with OATP inhibitor supports this hypothesis.

The inhibitor SPZ is a general OATP inhibitor that could block the function of tick OATPs. In addition, SPZ is proposed to be a nonselective uridine 5'-diphospho-glucuronosyltransferase (UGT) inhibitor and a substrate for ATP-binding cassette (ABC) transporters such as multi-drug resistance proteins MRP2 [39, 40]. The observation of differential modulation (up/downregulation) of OATP transcripts upon treatment of LGTV-infected tick cells

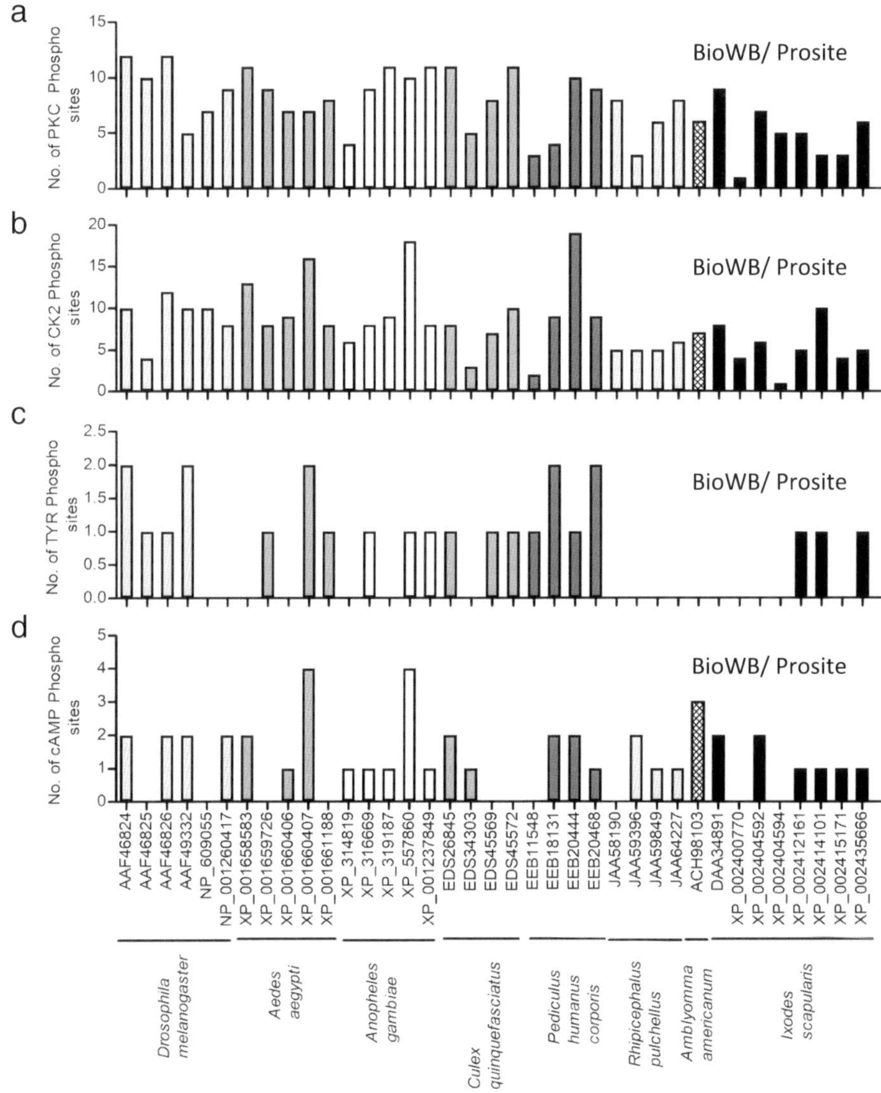

Fig. 7 Analysis of phosphorylation sites in OATPs from medically important vectors. Amino acid sequences of several OATPs were individually analyzed at Biology WorkBench or PROSITE databases for PKC phosphorylation (**a**), CK2 phosphorylation (**b**), tyrosine phosphorylation (**c**) and cAMP-dependent phosphorylation sites (**d**). Histograms represent the number of post-translational modification sites for each OATP. The post-translational modifications in the transmembrane regions within each OATP were not considered for histogram plots. GenBank accession numbers and organism names are shown at the bottom of the figure

with SPZ suggests that the transcriptional regulation of OATPs could be interdependent to each other. The blocking of one OATP may have an effect on the transcription of other OATPs. As SPZ is related to ABC-transporters or affect glucuronosyltransferases, the roles for these molecules in the regulation of OATPs or in LGTV-tick interactions cannot be excluded. In our previous study, we observed that knockdown of *kat* gene expression affected *isoatp4056* expression [12]. We proposed that xanthurenic acid (XA), a metabolite from tryptophan pathway and a product of KAT enzyme, is important in the regulation of *isoatp4056* expression. Consistent with our previous *A. phagocytophilum*-infection model [12], we noticed a low expression of *isoatp4056* and reduced levels of *kat* transcripts upon SPZ-treatment of LGTV-infected tick cells. Collectively, these observations suggest a highly interdependent pathway among OATPs with KAT.

In this study, putative post-translational modifications on various arthropod OATPs were predicted and analyzed. Glycosylation is an important post-translational modification that is commonly observed in membrane proteins [41]. A study has shown that glycosylation could impact membrane targeting and/or maintenance of protein stability [42]. Based on the presence of glycosylation sites on several OATPs analyzed in this study, post-translational modification might be essential for

OATPs function at the host cell membrane during early phase of interactions with intracellular pathogens. As evidenced in our comparative analysis, *Ae. aegypti* OATP (XP_001660407) contains the highest number of glycosylation sites in comparison to the other OATPs from various arthropods. This study opens up an interesting question: does the level of glycosylation have any impact on the membrane targeting and/or maintenance of OATP protein stability during vector-pathogen interactions?

We previously demonstrated that a rickettsial pathogen modulates phosphorylation of actin in its vector host [43]. The observation of a higher number of CK2, PKC and cAMP phosphorylation sites in comparison to tyrosine phosphorylation sites suggests serine/threonine kinases are the important mediators of signaling in the medically important vectors. It was interesting to note that all but four of the OATPs carry one Kazal domain in their primary amino acid sequence (Additional file 1: Figure S3). Kazal domain containing serine proteases plays crucial roles in various physiological mechanisms in several organisms including arthropod blood-feeding [37, 44]. A study by Mulenga et al. [37] has shown that *A. americanum* ticks treated with OATP-dsRNA had lower engorgement weights in comparison to the control group, suggesting the importance of OATP in blood-feeding. The presence of the Kazal domain in most of the OATPs suggests that this domain could be an ideal target for the development of a broad-spectrum anti-vector vaccine against various arthropods.

Conclusions

In conclusion, this study provides additional important evidence on the role of OATP in the interactions of vector with bacteria and viruses, in particular with intracellular pathogens. Studies such as this in understanding the roles of OATPs in vector-pathogen interactions might provide novel universal strategies to combat several tick-borne bacterial and/or viral diseases.

Additional file

Additional file 1: Figure S1. LGTV infection has no impact on tick cell morphology. Representative phase contrast images of uninfected or LGTV-infected tick cells at 24 and 72 h pi. UI indicates uninfected and LGTV indicates LGTV-infected tick cells. *Scale-bars*: 200 μm. **Figure S2.** SPZ treatment has no cytotoxic effects on tick cells. Representative phase contrast images of untreated or mock- or 100 μM of SPZ uninfected tick cells at 4, 24, 48 and 72 h post-treatment (pt). *Scale-bars*: 200 μm. **Figure S3.** Analysis of Kazal domain sites in OATPs from medically important vectors. Amino acid sequences of OATPs were individually analyzed at NCBI conserved domain search and PROSITE databases for prediction of Kazal domain sites in several OATPs. Histograms represent number of KAZAL sites for each OATP. Full-length OATP sequences were considered to determine KAZAL sites. GenBank accession numbers and organism names are shown at the bottom of the figure. **Table S1.** Summarizing statistical test outcomes for the data in this paper. **Table S2.** The numbers of ASN glycosylation and myristoylation sites predicted from either outside (external) or inside (internal) regions of OATPs but not in the transmembrane regions are shown. Aa indicates total number of amino acids and TM indicates number of transmembrane regions. **Table S3.** Summarizing number of phosphorylation sites in different OATPs. The numbers of cAMP, PKC, CK2 and tyrosine phosphorylation sites (predicted either outside or inside regions of OATPs but not in the transmembrane regions) are shown. Aa indicates total number of amino acids, TM indicates number of transmembrane regions, Int. indicates number of sites in the inside region and Ext. indicates number of sites on the outside regions of OATPs. (PDF 12295 kb)

Abbreviations

ASN: Asparagine N-glycosylation; CK2: Casein kinase II; KAT: Kynurenine aminotransferase; LGTV: Langat virus; OATPs: Organic anion transporting polypeptides; pi: Post-infection; PKC: Protein kinase C; QRT-PCR: Quantitative real-time polymerase chain reaction; SPZ: ±-sulfinpyrazone; TBEV: Tick-borne encephalitis virus; XA: Xanthurenic acid

Acknowledgements

We thank Dr Ulrike Munderloh for the supply of tick cell line ISE6.

Funding

This work was supported by independent start-up funds from Old Dominion University to GN and HS and in part by NIAID/NIH R01AI130116.

Authors' contributions

VT, WZ, XZ and HS performed the experiments. VT, HS and GN analyzed the data. HS and GN designed the study. UP and JFA provided ticks and/or reagents. GN conceived the study, wrote the paper and supervised overall investigations. All authors read and approved the final manuscript.

Competing interests

The authors declare that they have no competing interests.

Author details

[1]Department of Biological Sciences, Old Dominion University, Norfolk, VA, USA. [2]Department of Veterinary Medicine, Virginia-Maryland Regional College of Veterinary Medicine, University of Maryland, College Park, MD, USA. [3]Department of Entomology, Connecticut Agricultural Experiment Station, New Haven, CT, USA. [4]Center for Molecular Medicine, College of Sciences, Old Dominion University, Norfolk, VA, USA.

References

1. Hill CA, Kafatos FC, Stansfield SK, Collins FH. Arthropod-borne diseases: vector control in the genomics era. Nat Rev Microbiol. 2005;3:262–8.
2. Scott TW, Takken W. Feeding strategies of anthropophilic mosquitoes result in increased risk of pathogen transmission. Trends Parasitol. 2012;28:114–21.
3. Sonenshine DE, Roe R. Biology of ticks, second edition. Oxford: Oxford University Press; 2014.

4. Veracx A, Raoult D. Biology and genetics of human head and body lice. Trends Parasitol. 2012;28:563–71.
5. George JE, Pound JM, Davey RB. Acaricides for controlling ticks on cattle and the problem of acaricide resistance. In: Bowman AS, Nuttall P, editors. Ticks: Biology, Disease and Control. Cambridge: Cambridge University Press; 2008. p. 408–23.
6. Neelakanta G, Sultana H. Transmission-blocking vaccines: focus on anti-vector vaccines against tick-borne diseases. Arch Immunol Ther Ex. 2015;63: 169–79.
7. Billingsley PF, Foy B, Rasgon JL. Mosquitocidal vaccines: a neglected addition to malaria and dengue control strategies. Trends Parasitol. 2008;24: 396–400.
8. de la Fuente J, Merino O. Vaccinomics, the new road to tick vaccines. Vaccine. 2013;31:5923–9.
9. McNair CM. Ectoparasites of medical and veterinary importance: drug resistance and the need for alternative control methods. J Pharm Pharmacol. 2015;67:351–63.
10. Stieger B, Hagenbuch B. Organic anion-transporting polypeptides. Curr Top Membr. 2014;73:205–32.
11. Hagenbuch B, Meier PJ. Organic anion transporting polypeptides of the OATP/ SLC21 family: phylogenetic classification as OATP/ SLCO superfamily, new nomenclature and molecular/functional properties. Pflug Arch Eur J Phy. 2004;447:653–65.
12. Taank V, Dutta S, Dasgupta A, Steeves TK, Fish D, Anderson JF, et al. Human rickettsial pathogen modulates arthropod organic anion transporting polypeptide and tryptophan pathway for its survival in ticks. Sci Rep. 2017;7: 13256.
13. Kalliokoski A, Niemi M. Impact of OATP transporters on pharmacokinetics. Brit J Pharmacol. 2009;158:693–705.
14. Nigam SK, Bush KT, Martovetsky G, Ahn SY, Liu HC, Richard E, et al. The organic anion transporter (OAT) family: a systems biology perspective. Physiol Rev. 2015;95:83–123.
15. Roth M, Obaidat A, Hagenbuch B. OATPs, OATs and OCTs: the organic anion and cation transporters of the SLCO and SLC22A gene superfamilies. Brit J Pharmacol. 2012;165:1260–87.
16. Anderson JF, Armstrong PM. Prevalence and genetic characterization of Powassan virus strains infecting *Ixodes scapularis* in Connecticut. Am J Trop Med Hyg. 2012;87:754–9.
17. Anderson JF, Magnarelli LA. Biology of ticks. Infect Dis Clin North Am. 2008; 22:195–215.
18. Krause PJ, Narasimhan S, Wormser GP, Barbour AG, Platonov AE, Brancato J, et al. *Borrelia miyamotoi sensu lato* seroreactivity and seroprevalence in the northeastern United States. Emerg Infect Dis. 2014;20:1183–90.
19. Pritt BS, Sloan LM, Johnson DK, Munderloh UG, Paskewitz SM, McElroy KM, et al. Emergence of a new pathogenic *Ehrlichia* species, Wisconsin and Minnesota, 2009. New Engl J Med. 2011;365:422–9.
20. Nuttall PA, Labuda M. Dynamics of infection in tick vectors and at the tick-host interface. Adv Virus Res. 2003;60:233–72.
21. Mitzel DN, Wolfinbarger JB, Long RD, Masnick M, Best SM, Bloom ME. Tick-borne flavivirus infection in *Ixodes scapularis* larvae: development of a novel method for synchronous viral infection of ticks. Virology. 2007;365:410–8.
22. Mlera L, Melik W, Offerdahl DK, Dahlstrom E, Porcella SF, Bloom ME: Analysis of the Langat Virus Genome in Persistent Infection of an Ixodes scapularis Cell Line. Viruses. 2016;8(9):252.
23. Radulovic Z, Porter LM, Kim TK, Mulenga A. Comparative bioinformatics, temporal and spatial expression analyses of *Ixodes scapularis* organic anion transporting polypeptides. Ticks Tick Borne Dis. 2014;5:287–98.
24. Arai M, Billker O, Morris HR, Panico M, Delcroix M, Dixon D, et al. Both mosquito-derived xanthurenic acid and a host blood-derived factor regulate gametogenesis of *Plasmodium* in the midgut of the mosquito. Mol Biochem Parsitol. 2001;116:17–24.
25. Bhattacharyya MK, Kumar N. Effect of xanthurenic acid on infectivity of *Plasmodium falciparum* to *Anopheles stephensi*. Int J Parasitol. 2001;31:1129–33.
26. Nogueira SV, Smith AA, Qin JH, Pal U. A surface enolase participates in *Borrelia burgdorferi*-plasminogen interaction and contributes to pathogen survival within feeding ticks. Infect Immun. 2012;80:82–90.
27. Zhou W, Woodson M, Neupane B, Bai F, Sherman MB, Choi KH, et al. Exosomes serve as novel modes of tick-borne flavivirus transmission from arthropod to human cells and facilitates dissemination of viral RNA and proteins to the vertebrate neuronal cells. PLoS Pathog. 2018;14:e1006764.
28. Neelakanta G, Li X, Pal U, Liu X, Beck DS, DePonte K, et al. Outer surface protein B is critical for *Borrelia burgdorferi* adherence and survival within *Ixodes* ticks. PLoS Pathog. 2007;3:312–22.
29. Sultana H, Patel U, Toliver M, Maggi RG, Neelakanta G. Molecular identification and bioinformatics analysis of a potential anti-vector vaccine candidate, 15-kDa salivary gland protein (Salp15), from *Ixodes affinis* ticks. Ticks Tick Borne Dis. 2016;7:46–53.
30. Sultana H, Patel U, Sonenshine DE, Neelakanta G. Identification and comparative analysis of subolesin/akirin ortholog from *Ornithodoros turicata* ticks. Parasit Vectors. 2015;8:132.
31. Neelakanta G, Sultana H, Sonenshine DE, Andersen JF. Identification and characterization of a histamine-binding lipocalin-like molecule from the relapsing fever tick *Ornithodoros turicata*. Insect Mol Biol. 2018;27:177–87.
32. Ribet D, Cossart P. Pathogen-mediated posttranslational modifications: a re-emerging field. Cell. 2010;143:694–702.
33. Yao J, Hong W, Huang J, Zhan K, Huang H, Hong M. N-Glycosylation dictates proper processing of organic anion transporting polypeptide 1B1. PLoS One. 2012;7:e52563.
34. Powell J, Farasyn T, Kock K, Meng X, Pahwa S, Brouwer KL, Yue W. Novel mechanism of impaired function of organic anion-transporting polypeptide 1B3 in human hepatocytes: post-translational regulation of OATP1B3 by protein kinase C activation. Drug Metab Dispos. 2014;42:1964–70.
35. Alam K, Crowe A, Wang X, Zhang P, Ding K, Li L, Yue W. Regulation of organic anion transporting polypeptides (OATP) 1B1- and OATP1B3-mediated transport: an updated review in the context of OATP-mediated drug-drug interactions. Int J Mol Sci. 2018;19:855.
36. Nene V, Wortman JR, Lawson D, Haas B, Kodira C, Tu ZJ, et al. Genome sequence of *Aedes aegypti*, a major arbovirus vector. Science. 2007;316: 1718–23.
37. Mulenga A, Khumthong R, Chalaire KC, Strey O, Teel P. Molecular and biological characterization of the *Amblyomma americanum* organic anion transporter polypeptide. J Exp Biol. 2008;211:3401–8.
38. Mongin E, Louis C, Holt RA, Birney E, Collins FH. The *Anopheles gambiae* genome: an update. Trends Parasitol. 2004;20:49–52.
39. Evers R, de Haas M, Sparidans R, Beijnen J, Wielinga PR, Lankelma J, Borst P. Vinblastine and sulfinpyrazone export by the multidrug resistance protein MRP2 is associated with glutathione export. Brit J Cancer. 2000;83:375–83.
40. Uchaipichat V, Mackenzie PI, Elliot DJ, Miners JO. Selectivity of substrate (trifluoperazine) and inhibitor (amitriptyline, androsterone, canrenoic acid, hecogenin, phenylbutazone, quinidine, quinine, and sulfinpyrazone) "probes" for human udp-glucuronosyltransferases. Drug Metab Dispos. 2006; 34:449–56.
41. Spiro RG. Protein glycosylation: nature, distribution, enzymatic formation, and disease implications of glycopeptide bonds. Glycobiology. 2002;12:43R–56R.
42. Zhou F, Xu W, Hong M, Pan Z, Sinko PJ, Ma J, You G. The role of N-linked glycosylation in protein folding, membrane targeting, and substrate binding of human organic anion transporter hOAT4. Mol Pharmacol. 2005;67(3):868–76.
43. Sultana H, Neelakanta G, Kantor FS, Malawista SE, Fish D, Montgomery RR, Fikrig E. *Anaplasma phagocytophilum* induces actin phosphorylation to selectively regulate gene transcription in *Ixodes scapularis* ticks. J Exp Med. 2010;207:1727–43.
44. Laskowski MJ, Kato I. Protein inhibitors of proteinases. Ann Rev Biochem. 1980;49:593–626.

Prevalence and genetic diversity of *Enterocytozoon bieneusi* in sheep in China

Heng Yang[1†], Rongsheng Mi[1†], Long Cheng[1], Yan Huang[1], Rui An[2], Yehua Zhang[1], Haiyan Jia[1], Xiaoli Zhang[1], Xu Wang[1], Xiangan Han[1] and Zhaoguo Chen[1*]

Abstract

Background: *Enterocytozoon bieneusi* is a common species of microsporidia that not only influences human health but also threatens animal productive performance and value. However, there have been no systematic studies of the prevalence of *E. bieneusi* in sheep in China.

Results: A total of 953 fecal specimens were collected from sheep from 11 provinces across five regions of China and analyzed for *E. bieneusi* by nested PCR targeting the ribosomal internal transcribed spacer (ITS). *Enterocytozoon bieneusi* infections were detected in four regions, with an overall infection rate of 20.4% (194/953). The highest infection rate was detected in pre-weaned lambs (25.0%), followed by post-weaned lambs (22.2%) and adult sheep (14.6%). *Enterocytozoon bieneusi* was found in nine of the 11 tested provinces, with infection rates between 2.9–51. 7%. Eleven genotypes were identified based on ITS analysis, including seven known genotypes (BEB6, CHG1, CHG3, CHS7, CHS8, COS-I and NESH5) and four novel genotypes (CHHLJS1, CHHLJS2, CHNXS1 and CHXJS1). All 11 genotypes were clustered into group 2, and the zoonotic genotype BEB6 was the dominant genotype (n = 129, 66.5%) in sheep.

Conclusion: The prevalence of *E. bieneusi* was studied in five regions representing most areas where sheep are bred in China. This is the first report of *E. bieneusi* infection in sheep for seven Chinese provinces. Geographical differences were detected in the distribution of *E. bieneusi* genotypes, but no differences were found among sheep in different age groups. The zoonotic genotype BEB6 was the dominant genotype, indicating that sheep are a potential source of zoonotic microsporidiosis in China. These results improve our knowledge of the epidemiology of *E. bieneusi* in sheep in China.

Keywords: *Enterocytozoon bieneusi*, Sheep, Prevalence, Genotyping, China

Background

Microsporidia are obligate intracellular eukaryotic parasites with a wide range of hosts that includes arthropods, birds, mammals and humans [1, 2]. To date, more than 1300 microsporidian species belonging to 150 genera have been reported [3], including at least 14 microsporidian species belonging to eight families that have been reported to infect humans. The most common species, *Enterocytozoon bieneusi* [4, 5], can cause severe diarrhea in immunocompromised humans and animals, and zoonotic genotypes from domestic animals may be a threat to public health [1, 6, 7].

Enterocytozoon bieneusi has frequently been reported in domestic animals and wildlife all over the world [7]. Because it is difficult to distinguish *E. bieneusi* spores using microscopy, and no sophisticated culture approaches have been developed *in vitro*, molecular methods have been widely used for *E. bieneusi* detection [8]. To date, polymorphisms in the ribosomal internal transcribed spacer (ITS) of the rRNA gene have been widely used for *E. bieneusi* genotyping, and more than 200 *E. bieneusi* genotypes have been reported in humans and animals [8, 9]. When analyzed in combination with phylogeny, these genotypes can be grouped into several genetically isolated clusters [10].

* Correspondence: zhaoguochen@shvri.ac.cn
†Heng Yang and Rongsheng Mi contributed equally to this work.
[1]Key Laboratory of Animal Parasitology of Ministry of Agriculture, Laboratory of Quality and Safety Risk Assessment for Animal Products on Biohazards (Shanghai) of Ministry of Agriculture, Shanghai Veterinary Research Institute, Chinese Academy of Agricultural Sciences, Shanghai 200241, China
Full list of author information is available at the end of the article

Group 1 includes zoonotic genotypes that have been reported in humans and animals [11]. Groups 2 to 9 have mainly been reported in animals and wastewater [11, 12], and few genotypes have been detected in humans [8].

In addition to humans, *E. bieneusi* also infects a variety of animals, such as birds, cats, cattle, deer, dogs, donkeys, horses, pigs and wild mammals [5, 7, 13–20]. However, the epidemiology of *E. bieneusi* has rarely been reported in sheep. To date, a few studies have reported *E. bieneusi* infection in sheep in Brazil [21], China [19, 22–26], Iran [27] and Sweden [28] (Table 1). Several genotypes were identified in these studies, including genotypes D, BEB6, BEB7, EbpC, O, I, Peru6, NESH1-NESH 6, CS-4, CM7, COS-I-COS-VII and CHS1-CHS12 [7, 22, 23, 25]. Among these, genotypes BEB6, D, EbpC, O, I and Peru6 have been reported in humans [8, 21]. BEB6 is the most prevalent genotype detected in sheep in Brazil and China [21, 23–25].

In China, *E. bieneusi* infections have been reported in sheep in five provinces, including Heilongjiang, Henan, Inner Mongolia, Liaoning and Qinghai Province, with infection rates ranging between 4.4–69.3% [19, 22–26] (Table 1). At the end of 2016, China had the largest number of sheep in the world (http://www.fao.org/faostat/en/#data/QA), with most being bred in northern areas. However, there have been no systematic studies of *E. bieneusi* infection in sheep in China. Therefore, in order to determine the epidemiology and genetic diversity of *E. bieneusi* in sheep in China, 11 provinces across five regions that represent most areas where sheep are farmed in China were selected for *E. bieneusi* testing. These results lay a foundation for a better understanding of the epidemiology and genotypic features of *E. bieneusi* in China.

Methods

Fecal specimen collection

Between June 2013 and September 2015, a total of 953 fecal samples were collected from sheep in the following 11 provinces in China: Henan Province in central China; Anhui Province, Shandong Province and Shanghai City in eastern China; Beijing City and Inner Mongolia Autonomous Region in northern China, Heilongjiang Province and Jilin Province in northeast China; and Ningxia Hui Autonomous Region, Qinghai Province and Xinjiang Uyghur Autonomous Region in northwest China (Fig. 1). One fecal specimen was collected from each sheep. The three age groups selected for this study were pre-weaned (< 3 months) and post-weaned (3–12 months) lambs, and adult sheep (> 12 months). Fresh fecal specimens were collected from sheep using sterile gloves, and each specimen's information was recorded, including location, date and age. Specimens were transported to the laboratory at low temperatures for further detection.

Sample preparation and DNA extraction

Approximately 300 mg of each fecal specimen was transferred to a 50 ml sterile tube, 20 ml of sterile water was added, and the mixture then stirred with a 1 ml pipette tip to loosen the sample. A 200-300 μl sample was used for DNA extraction with a FastDNA SPIN Kit for Soil (MP Biomedicals, Santa Ana, CA, USA) according to the manufacturer's instructions.

PCR amplification

A 389 bp fragment of the *E. bieneusi* ITS gene was amplified by nested PCR as previously described by Buckholt et al. [29]. Briefly, a 435 bp PCR product was amplified

Table 1 Prevalence of *E. bieneusi* and distribution of ITS genotypes in sheep based on published reports

Year	Country	Province (China)	Prevalence (%)	Genotype (no. of samples)	Reference
2014	Sweden		45.0 (49/109)	BEB6 (32), OEB1 (6), OEB2 (2), BEB6 + OEB1 (4), BEB6 + OEB2 (4), NDb (1)	[28]
2016	Brazil		19.2 (24/125)	BEB6 (11), BEB7 (8), I (2), BEB18 (1), BEB19 (1), LW1(1)	[21]
2014	China	Heilongjiang	4.4 (2/45)	BEB6 (2)	[19]
2015	China	Heilongjiang	13.9 (68/489)	BEB6 (28), CM7 (3), CS-4 (4), BEB6/CM7a (5), BEB6/OEB1a (5), BEB6/NESH4a (3), OEB1(3), BEB6/NESH6a (1), CS-4/EbpCa (1), NESH1(1), NESH2 (1), NESH3 (1), NESH5 (1),	[22]
2015	China	Heilongjiang	22.5 (31/138)	BEB6 (12), Peru6 (5), D (4), O (3), COS-I to COS-VII (one each),	[23]
2015	China	Inner Mongolia	69.3 (260/375)	BEB6 (237), CM7 (23)	[24]
2016	China	Henan	51.9 (161/310)	BEB6 (53), COS-I (12), CM4 (1), CHG3 (5), CHS3 (2), CHS4 (1), CHS5 (1), CHS6 (1), CHS10 (1), CHS12 (1)	[25]
		Liaoning	9.4 (6/64)	BEB6 (3)	
		Heilongjiang	25.0 (10/40)	BEB6 (4), COS-I (2), CHS7 (1), CHS8 (1), CHS9 (1), CHS11 (1)	
2018	China	Qinghai	23.4 (73/312)	BEB6 (31), COS-I (25), NESH5 (11), CHS17 (2), CHS13 (1), CHS14 (1), CHS15 (1), CHS16 (1)	[26]

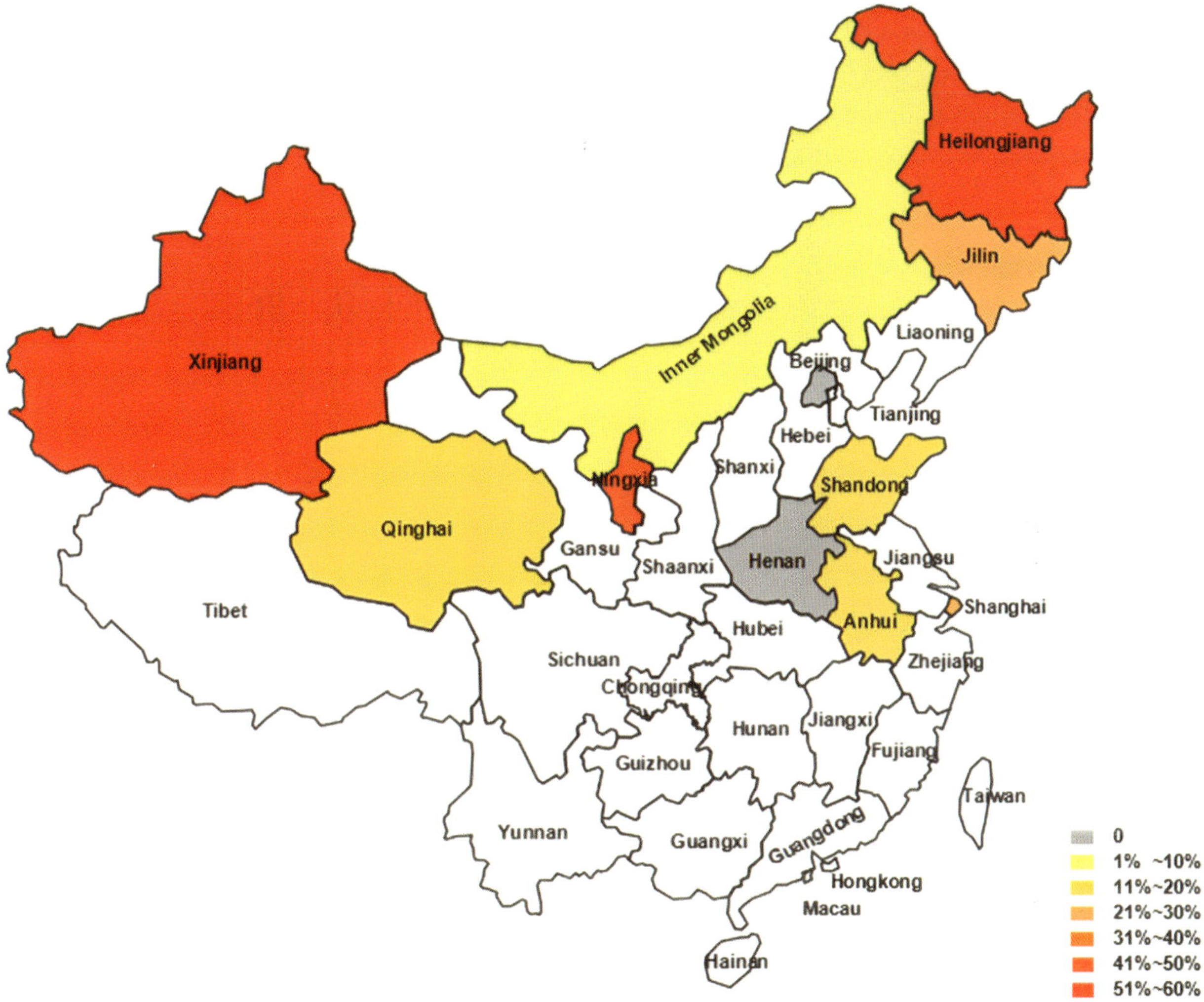

Fig. 1 Geographical map of sampling provinces included in this study. The map was generated using Microsoft Office PowerPoint 2016 software

using the primers EBITS3 (5'-GGT CAT AGG GAT GAA GAG-3') and EBITS4 (5'-TTC GAG TTC TTT CGC GCT C-3') for the primary PCR, and a 389 bp PCR product was amplified using the primers EBITS1 (5'-GCT CTG AAT ATC TAT GGC T-3') and EBITS2.4 (5'-ATC GCC GAC GGA TCC AAG TG-3') for the secondary PCR. Positive and negative controls were included in each PCR reaction. *Ex Taq* DNA Polymerase (TaKaRa Bio Inc., Beijing, China) was used for PCR amplifications. The secondary PCR products were examined by gel electrophoresis on a 1.2% agarose gel containing 4S Green Plus Nucleic Acid Stain (Sangon Biotech, Shanghai, China).

Sequence analysis and phylogenetic construction

Positive samples from the second round of PCR gel electrophoresis were sequenced and analyzed using the BLAST program (http://blast.ncbi.nlm.nih.gov/Blast.cgi). Phylogenetic analysis of *E. bieneusi* was performed using MEGA 7.0 software [30]. All positive samples were sequenced twice, and novel genotypes were designated as previously described by Santín & Fayer [8]. Briefly, all sequences obtained in the present study were analyzed using the BLAST program to determine the *E. bieneusi* genotype based on 243 bp of the ITS gene region. Sequences that differed from published genotypes were considered new genotypes.

Statistical analysis

Differences in infection rates between different regions, provinces and ages were assessed using a Chi-square test with SPSS Version 21.0 software (IBM Corp., Armonk, NY, USA). Differences were considered statistically significant when $P < 0.05$. Prevalence rates and 95% confidence intervals (CI) were also determined. Unique ITS sequences of *E. bieneusi* were submitted to the GenBank database under the accession numbers MH432644-MH432647.

Results

Overall prevalence and genotypic features of *E. bieneusi* in sheep

The overall prevalence of *E. bieneusi* infection in sheep in this study was 20.4% (194/953; 95% CI: 17.8–23.1%). All positive samples were sequenced for *E. bieneusi* genotype determination based on BLAST analyses. Eleven *E. bieneusi* genotypes were identified, including seven previously described genotypes (BEB6, CHG1, CHG3, CHS7, CHS8, COS-I and NESH5) and four novel genotypes (CHHLJS1, CHHLJS2, CHNXS1 and CHXJS1) (Table 2).

Overall, BEB6 (n = 129) was the dominant genotype, followed by CHS8 (n = 32) and CHG1 (n = 14). All other genotypes were present in less than five specimens (Table 2).

Prevalence of *E. bieneusi* in sheep in different regions of China

Of the five regions tested for *E. bieneusi* infections in sheep, northeast China had the highest infection rate (38.5%, 50/130; 95% CI: 30.1–47.4%), followed by northwest China (28.0%, 83/296; 95% CI: 23.0–33.5%), eastern China (17.8%, 58/326; 95% CI: 13.8–22.4%) and northern China (1.8%, 3/166; 95% CI: 0.4–5.2%). *Enterocytozoon bieneusi* infection was not detected in central China (Table 2). A significant difference was observed between different regions (χ^2 = 82.562, df = 4, P < 0.0001). The most common genotype, BEB6, was detected in all *E. bieneusi*-positive regions. In northwest China, we found high prevalence rates of both BEB6 (57.8%, 48/83) and CHS8 (38.6%, 32/83) (Table 2).

Prevalence of *E. bieneusi* in sheep in different provinces in China

Of the 11 provinces tested for *E. bieneusi* in sheep, the highest infection rate was detected in Heilongjiang (51.7%, 31/60; 95% CI: 38.4–64.8%), followed by Ningxia (47.1%, 57/121; 95% CI: 38.0–56.4%), Jilin (27.1%, 19/70; 95% CI: 17.2–39.1%), Shanghai (23.7%, 36/152; 95% CI: 17.2–31.3%), Xinjiang (19.2%, 19/99; 95% CI: 12.0–28.3%), Shandong (13.1%, 16/122; 95% CI: 7.7–20.4%), Anhui (11.5%, 6/52; 95% CI: 4.4–23.4%), Qinghai (9.2%, 7/76; 95% CI: 3.8–18.1%) and Inner Mongolia (2.9%, 3/102; 95% CI: 0.6–8.4%). *Enterocytozoon bieneusi* infection was not detected in Beijing (0/64; 95% CI: 0–5.6%) or Henan (0/35; 95% CI: 0–10.0%) (Table 3). Statistical analysis showed significant differences in infection rates of *E. bieneusi* among the different provinces (χ^2 = 149.446, df = 10, P < 0.0001).

The distribution of *E. bieneusi* genotypes differed among the different provinces. The most common genotype, BEB6, was detected in Heilongjiang (21/31), Inner Mongolia (3/3), Jilin (19/19), Qinghai (6/7), Shanghai (35/36) and Xinjiang (18/19). In contrast, CHG1 (11/16) and CHS8 (32/57) were the dominant genotypes in Shandong and Ningxia, respectively. Four novel genotypes were identified in Heilongjiang (n = 2), Ningxia (n = 1) and Xinjiang (n = 1). More than two genotypes were detected in most provinces, with the exception of Jilin and Inner Mongolia, where only one genotype (BEB6) was found (Table 3).

Prevalence of *E. bieneusi* in different age groups of sheep

Enterocytozoon bieneusi infections were detected in all three age groups. The highest prevalence rate was detected in pre-weaned lambs (25.0%, 73/292; 95% CI: 20.1–30.4%), followed by post-weaned lambs (22.2%, 72/325; 95% CI: 17.8–27.1%) and adult sheep (14.6%, 49/336; 95% CI: 11.0–18.8%), with statistically significant differences among the age groups (χ^2 = 11.438, df = 2, P = 0.003). More than six genotypes were identified in all age groups, and BEB6 was the most common genotype detected in each group (Table 4).

At the province level, infection rates of *E. bieneusi* differed by age group. The most susceptible age group was pre-weaned lambs, and *E. bieneusi* was detected in sheep in this age group in most provinces, including Inner Mongolia (8.1%, 3/31; 95% CI: 1.7–21.9%), Jilin (41.7%, 10/24; 95% CI: 22.1–63.4%), Ningxia (57.5%, 23/40; 95% CI: 40.9–73.0%), Qinghai (12.5%, 3/24; 95% CI: 2.7–32.4%), Shanghai (30.0%, 6/20; 95% CI: 11.9–54.3%) and Xinjiang (38.2%, 13/34; 95% CI: 22.2–56.4%). However, in two

Table 2 Prevalence and genotype distribution of *E. bieneusi* in sheep from different regions of China

Region	No. of specimens	No. positive (%)	95% CI	Genotype (no. of samples)
Central China	35	0[d]	0–10.0	
Eastern China	326	58 (17.8)[c]	13.8–22.4	BEB6 (38), CHG1 (14), CHG3 (5), COS-I (1)
Northern China	166	3 (1.8)[d]	0.4–5.2	BEB6 (3)
Northeast China	130	50 (38.5)[a]	30.1–47.4	BEB6 (40), CHS7 (3), **CHHLJS1** (3), **CHHLJS2** (2), COS-I (2)
Northwest China	296	83 (28.0)[b]	23.0–33.5	BEB6 (48), CHS8 (32), **CHNXS1** (1), **CHXJS1** (1), NESH5 (1)
Total	953	194 (20.4)	17.8–23.1	BEB6 (129), CHS8 (32), CHG1 (14), CHG3 (5), CHS7 (3), COS-I (3), **CHHLJS1** (3), **CHHLJS2** (2), **CHNXS1** (1), **CHXJS1** (1), NESH5 (1)

Note: Different superscript letters within columns represent significant differences between groups (P < 0.05). Novel genotypes identified in this study are indicated in bold

Table 3 Prevalence and genotype distribution of *E. bieneusi* in sheep from different provinces of China

Region	Province	No. of specimens	No. positive (%)	95% CI	Genotype (no. of samples)
Central China	Henan	35	0[e]	0–10.0	
Eastern China	Anhui	52	6 (11.5)[c]	4.4–23.4	CHG1 (3), CHG3 (3)
	Shandong	122	16 (13.1)[c]	7.7–20.4	BEB6 (3), CHG1 (11), CHG3 (2)
	Shanghai	152	36 (23.7)[b]	17.2–31.3	BEB6 (35), COS-I (1)
Northern China	Beijing	64	0[e]	0–5.6	
	Inner Mongolia	102	3 (2.9)[de]	0.6–8.4	BEB6 (3)
Northeast China	Heilongjiang	60	31 (51. 7)[a]	38.4–64.8	BEB6 (21), CHS7 (3), CHHLJS1 (3), COS-I (2), CHHLJS2 (2)
	Jilin	70	19 (27.1)[b]	17.2–39.1	BEB6 (19)
Northwest China	Ningxia	121	57 (47.1)[a]	38.0–56.4	BEB6 (24), CHS8 (32), CHNXS1 (1)
	Qinghai	76	7(9.2)[cd]	3.8–18.1	BEB6 (6), NESH5 (1)
	Xinjiang	99	19 (19.2)[bc]	12.0–28.3	BEB6 (18), CHXJS1 (1)
Total		953	194 (20.4)	17.8–23.1	

Note: Different superscript letters within columns represent significant differences between groups ($P < 0.05$)

provinces, Anhui (13.6%, 3/22; 95% CI: 2.9–34.9%) and Heilongjiang (80.0%, 16/20; 95% CI: 56.3–94.3%), post-weaned lambs had the highest prevalence rate, and in Shandong Province (27.8%, 10/36; 95% CI: 14.2–45.2%) the group with the highest prevalence rate was adult sheep. With the exception of Anhui Province, BEB6 was detected in each group in all provinces (Table 5).

Phylogenetic analysis

Phylogenetic trees were constructed using the novel and known genotypes based on ITS nucleotide sequences as shown in Fig. 2. The results indicated that all genotypes detected in this study belonged to group 2.

Discussion

In the present study, an investigation of *E. bieneusi* was conducted in 11 provinces, which included most areas where sheep are farmed in China. *Enterocytozoon bieneusi* infection was detected in nine provinces, suggesting that *E. bieneusi* is widespread in sheep in China. Compared to studies that used the same testing method, the overall prevalence of *E. bieneusi* in sheep in this study was 20.4%, which is similar to previous reports of *E. bieneusi* in sheep in Brazil (19.2%) [21], but lower than prevalence rates reported in Sweden (68.1%) [28]. The prevalence rate in this study was also higher than a previous report from Iran (10.0%), which was based on the *SSU* rRNA gene [27] (Table 1). Additionally, the prevalence rate of *E. bieneusi* in Heilongjiang in the present study (51.7%) was higher than the previously reported rate of 22.5% found using the same method [23]. However, compared to studies that used different ITS primers, prevalence rates in the present study in Henan (0%), Inner Mongolia (2.9%) and Qinghai (9.2%) were lower than previous reports in Henan (51.9%) [25], Inner Mongolia (69.3%) [24] and Qinghai (23.4%) [26], but higher than previous reports in Heilongjiang (4.4, 13.9 and 25.0%) [19, 22, 25]. The differences between our study and previous studies may be due to differences in detection methods, sampling sites, sampling seasons, sheep age groups or sheep densities. Prevalence rates of *E. bieneusi* in the other provinces, including Ningxia (47.1%), Jilin (27.1%), Shanghai (23.7%), Shandong (13.1%), Xinjiang (19.2%), Anhui (11.5%) and Beijing (0%), have not been previously reported.

In the present study, the prevalence of *E. bieneusi* was assessed in five regions, which include most areas where sheep are bred in China. We did not obtain samples from southeast or southwest China, mainly because goats are the dominant livestock in these areas. The

Table 4 Prevalence and ITS genotype distribution of *E. bieneusi* in different age groups of sheep

Age	No. of specimens	No. positive (%)	95% CI	Genotype (no. of samples)
Pre-weaned lambs	292	73 (25.0)[a]	20.1–30.4	BEB6 (54), CHS8 (12), CHG3 (2), COS-I (1), CHG1 (1), CHHLJS2 (1), CHNXS1 (1), CHXJS1 (1)
Post-weaned lambs	325	72 (22.2)[a]	17.8–27.1	BEB6 (47), CHS8 (11), CHS7 (2), COS-I (2), CHG1 (2), CHG3 (2), CHHLJS1 (2), CHSDS2 (2), NESH5 (1), CHHLJS2 (1)
Adult sheep	336	49 (14.6)[b]	11.0–18.8	BEB6 (28), CHS8 (9), CHG1 (9), CHS7 (1), CHG3 (1), CHHLJS1 (1)
Total	953	194 (20.4)	17.8–23.1	

Note: Different superscript letters within columns represent significant differences between groups ($P < 0.05$)

Table 5 Prevalence and ITS genotype distribution of *E. bieneusi* in different age groups from different provinces

Province	Age	No. of specimens	No. positive (%)	95% CI	Genotype (no. of samples)
Anhui	Pre-weaned lambs	16	2 (12.5)	1.6–38.4	CHG3 (2)
	Post-weaned lambs	22	3 (13.6)	2.9–34.9	CHG1 (2), CHG3 (1)
	Adult sheep	14	1 (7.1)	0.2–33.9	CHG1 (1)
Beijing	Pre-weaned lambs	20	0	0–16.8	
	Post-weaned lambs	22	0	0–15.4	
	Adult sheep	22	0	0–15.4	
Heilongjiang	Pre-weaned lambs	20	12 (60.0)	36.1–80.9	BEB6 (11), CHHLJS2 (1)
	Post-weaned lambs	20	16 (80.0)	56.3–94.3	BEB6 (9), CHS7 (2), COS-I (2), CHHLJS1 (2), CHHLJS2 (1)
	Adult sheep	20	3 (15.0)	3.2–37.9	BEB6 (1), CHS7 (1), CHHLJS1 (1)
Henan	Adult sheep	35	0	0–10.0	
Inner Mongolia	Pre-weaned lambs	37	3 (8.1)	1.7–21.9	BEB6 (3)
	Post-weaned lambs	35	0	0–10.0	
	Adult sheep	30	0	0–11.6	
Jilin	Pre-weaned lambs	24	10 (41.7)	22.1–63.4	BEB6 (10)
	Post-weaned lambs	25	6 (24.0)	9.4–45.1	BEB6 (6)
	Adult sheep	21	3 (14.3)	3.1–36.3	BEB6 (3)
Ningxia	Pre-weaned lambs	40	23 (57.5)	40.9–73.0	CHS8 (12), BEB6 (10), CHNXS1 (1)
	Post-weaned lambs	40	17 (42.5)	27.0–59.1	CHS8 (11), BEB6 (6)
	Adult sheep	41	17 (41.5)	26.3–57.9	CHS8 (9), BEB6 (8)
Qinghai	Pre-weaned lambs	24	3 (12.5)	2.7–32.4	BEB6 (3)
	Post-weaned lambs	32	3 (9.4)	2.0–25.0	BEB6 (2), NESH5 (1)
	Adult sheep	20	1 (5.0)	0.1–24.9	BEB6 (1)
Shandong	Pre-weaned lambs	57	1 (1.8)	0–9.4	CHG1 (1)
	Post-weaned lambs	29	5 (17.2)	5.9–35.8	BEB6 (2), CHG1 (2), CHG3 (1)
	Adult sheep	36	10 (27.8)	14.2–45.2	CHG1 (8), BEB6 (1), CHG3 (1)
Shanghai	Pre-weaned lambs	20	6 (30.0)	11.9–54.3	BEB6 (5), COS-I (1)
	Post-weaned lambs	64	17 (26.6)	16.3–39.1	BEB6 (17)
	Adult sheep	68	13 (19.1)	10.6–30.5	BEB6 (13)
Xinjiang	Pre-weaned lambs	34	13 (38.2)	22.2–56.4	BEB6 (12), CHXJS1 (1)
	Post-weaned lambs	36	5 (13.9)	4.7–29.5	BEB6 (5)
	Adult sheep	29	1 (3.5)	0.1–17.8	BEB6 (1)

prevalence of *E. bieneusi* in northeast China (38.5%) was higher than previously reported (13.9%) [22]. This may be due to differences in sampling sites or sheep age groups. In the present study, we did not detect *E. bieneusi* infection in central China, possibly because only adult sheep were tested in this area (Table 5). Similar results were also reported in China and Sweden [19, 28], where *E. bieneusi* infections were not detected in adult sheep. Therefore, future studies need to increase the number of specimens collected in this area.

In the present study, a higher prevalence of *E. bieneusi* was detected in lambs (23.5%) than in adults (14.6%), which is consistent with many previous studies in Brazil and China [21, 22, 24–26]. The prevalence of *E. bieneusi* in lambs under one year of age was 23.5%, which is similar to the findings of a previous study in Heilongjiang (18.2%) [22], but lower than reported in previous studies in other parts of China [25, 26] and in Sweden [28]. The prevalence in pre-weaned lambs (25.0%) was also similar to a study by Li et al. [19] in Heilongjiang (20.0%) but was significantly lower than previous reports by Ye et al. [24] in Inner Mongolia (77.8%). We also observed differences in adult sheep between this study and previous studies; the reported prevalence in this study (14.6%) was higher than that reported in Brazil (11.1%) by Fiuza et al. [21] and in China (8.7%) by Jiang et al. [22], but was lower than the prevalence reported in Inner Mongolia (62.9%) [24] and in Qinghai (22.7%) [26]. Another report also

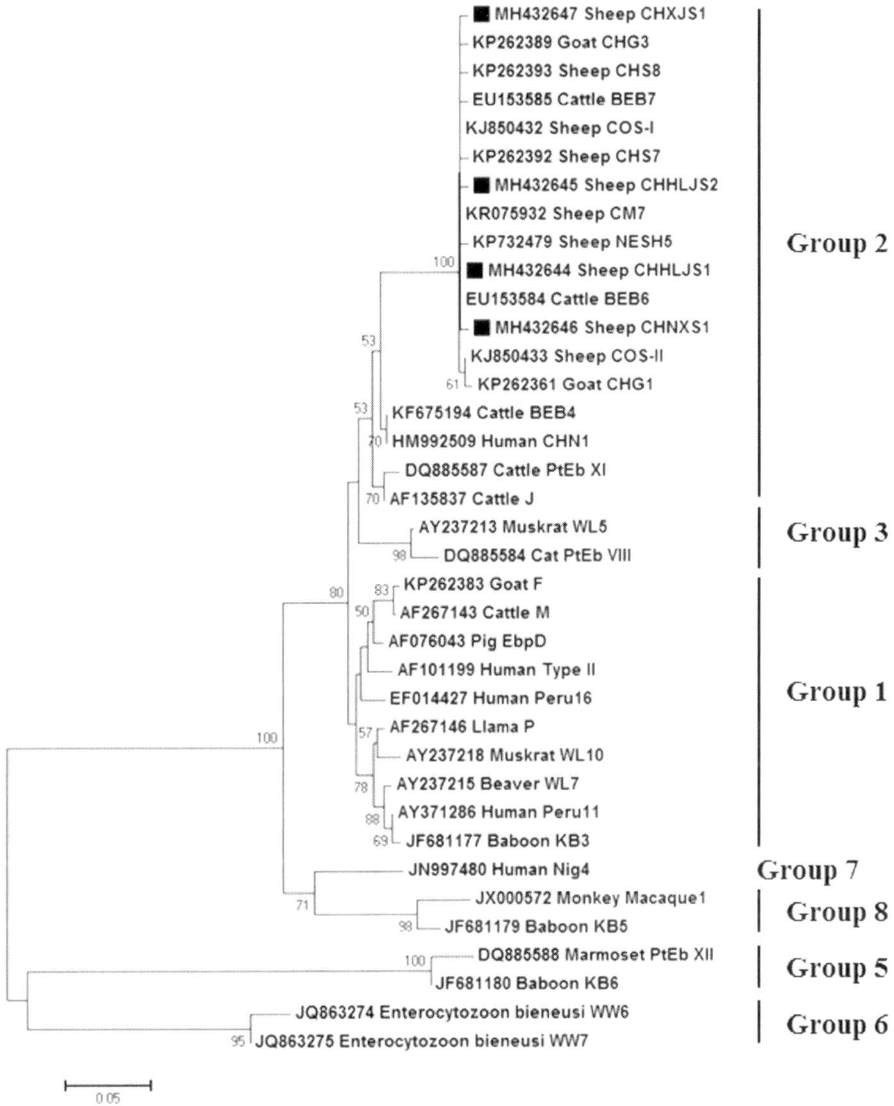

Fig. 2 Phylogenetic analysis of *E. bieneusi* based on ITS gene sequences. The evolutionary history was inferred using the neighbor-joining method and evolutionary analyses were conducted in MEGA 7.0. Bootstrap values > 50% are shown. Filled squares indicate the novel genotypes obtained in the present study

found a higher prevalence of *E. bieneusi* (39.4%) in adult sheep in Liaoning, Henan and Heilongjiang [25]. In contrast, two studies reported no *E. bieneusi* infection in adult sheep in Sweden [28] or Heilongjiang [19]. From these results, it seems that sheep age can affect the *E. bieneusi* infection rate in different regions.

The first reported *E. bieneusi* genotype, BEB6, was described in cattle in the USA [14]. Since then, this genotype has become common in ruminants, including sheep [19, 21–26, 28], goats [31], golden takins [32], deer [20], sika deer [20] and alpacas [33]. In addition, this genotype has also been found in humans [34], cats [15], rhesus macaques [16], yaks [26], horses [35], ducks and geese [36], as well as in urban wastewater [37, 38]. In this study, BEB6 was the most prevalent genotype (66.5%) and was detected in all provinces where *E. bieneusi* infection was found. These results are consistent with previous reports in the same provinces of China, including Heilongjiang [19, 22, 23, 25], Inner Mongolia [24] and Qinghai [26]. Other studies have also reported that BEB6 is the most common genotype in sheep in Sweden [28] and Brazil [21]. In China, BEB6 was also reported to be the most prevalent genotype in other provinces, such as Liaoning and Henan [25]. According to these results, we suggest that BEB6 is a dominant genotype with a widespread geographical distribution in sheep.

In this study, we identified five genotypes (CHG3, CHS7, CHS8, COS-I and NESH5) that were previously reported in sheep in China. CHG3 was previously detected in Henan [25]; CHS7 and CHS8 were previously detected in Heilongjiang [25]; COS-I was previously reported in Heilongjiang [23, 25], Henan [25] and Qinghai [26]; and NESH5 was previously found in Heilongjiang [22] and Qinghai [26]. Similar to these studies, we also found CHS7 and COS-I in Heilongjiang and NESH5 in Qinghai. However, we did not detect genotypes that had been previously reported in some provinces, such as genotype CM7, which was reported in Inner Mongolia and Heilongjiang [22, 24]. Although genotype CHG1 was previously reported in goats in Chongqing, Henan, Shaanxi and Yunnan [25], this study is the first report of this genotype in sheep. Phylogenetic analysis showed that all genotypes belonged to group 2. Although it has been classified as a cattle-specific group [11], some group 2 genotypes have been found in humans, including genotypes BEB6, I and J.

Based on known *E. bieneusi* genotypes [8], four novel genotypes were identified in sheep in this study. Compared to the known genotype BEB6, the novel genotypes CHHLJS1, CHNXS1 and CHXJS1 had two substitutions (A to T at position 155 and A to T at position 178), one substitution (A to G at position 135) and one substitution (A to G at positions 181), respectively. Compared to genotype CHS3, CHHLJS1 had one substitution (G to A at position 86). Phylogenetic analysis showed that all novel genotypes belonged to group 2.

According to the results of our study, there were differences in the geographical distribution of ITS genotypes in sheep. Although BEB6 was the most common genotype in most provinces, we found that CHS8 (56.1%) was the dominant genotype in Ningxia and CHG1 (68.7%) was the dominant genotype in Shandong. In addition, equal occurrences of CHG1 (n = 3) and CHG3 (n = 3) were found in Anhui. In most provinces, more than two genotypes were detected. Similar to previous studies, which reported several genotypes in Heilongjiang [22, 23, 25], we found more than five genotypes in this province (Table 1). Differences in the geographical distribution of *E. bieneusi* genotypes have also been reported in other studies. For example, BEB6 was the only genotype reported in Heilongjiang and Liaoning [19, 25], and only two genotypes (BEB6 and CM7) were previously reported in Inner Mongolia [23]. Moreover, more than five genotypes have been reported in Brazil [21], China [22, 23, 25, 26] and Sweden [28]. However, it seems that the distribution of ITS genotypes was not related to sheep age. In this study, more than six genotypes were detected in all age groups, and the distribution of ITS genotypes was similar between the groups, which is consistent with a previous study in Inner Mongolia [23].

Enterocytozoon bieneusi is an important protozoan parasite that is transmitted *via* water and food. Humans can become infected with microsporidia through human or animal fecal contamination in soil or water [39, 40]. In China, the *E. bieneusi* genotype BEB6 has been detected in wastewater from five cities [37, 41]. In the present study, BEB6 was the most prevalent genotype, indicating that sheep may be a source of *E. bieneusi* contamination in wastewater. However, whether *E. bieneusi* is present in wastewater near farms in these areas is unclear, and more studies are required to further understand the transmission of *E. bieneusi* between sheep and water.

Conclusions

In this study, we assessed the prevalence and genetic diversity of *E. bieneusi* in sheep from 11 provinces across five regions of China. *E. bieneusi* was found in nine provinces, suggesting that *E. bieneusi* is widespread in sheep in China. The overall infection rate was 20.4%, and the highest infection rate was detected in pre-weaned lambs. At the province level, the prevalence in different age groups also differed. Eleven genotypes were detected in sheep in this study, including four novel genotypes. The zoonotic genotype BEB6 was the dominant genotype and may pose a potential threat to humans. We also observed geographical differences in the genotypic features of *E. bieneusi* in sheep, but no differences were found in genotypes among the different age groups. This study covered most areas of China where sheep are bred, and for seven of the provinces this is the first report of *E. bieneusi*. Therefore, this study increases our understanding of the prevalence and genotypic characterization of *E. bieneusi* in sheep in China.

Abbreviations

ITS: Internal transcribed spacer; PCR: Polymerase chain reaction; *SSU* rRNA: Small subunit ribosomal RNA

Acknowledgements

We thank Guodong Mu at Jilin Center for Animal Disease Control and Prevention, Haining Zhou at Ningxia Center for Animal Disease Control and Prevention, Wei Zhu at Tengzhou Animal Husbandry and Veterinary Technology Service Center, and Yibin Hu at Beijing Centre Polytron Technologies Inc. for their help with sample collection. We also thank International Science Editing for editing this manuscript.

Funding

This study was supported in part by The National Key Research and Development Programme of China (grant no. 2018YFD0502305), National Risk Assessment Project for Quality and Safety of Agricultural Products (grant no. GJFP201800703), Shanghai Agriculture Applied Technology Development Program, China (grant no. G20180110), Technical Standard Programme of Shanghai Science and Technology Commission (grant no. 16DZ0501900) and The Key Technology R & D Programme of Ningxia Hui Autonomous Region, China (grant no. 201601).

Authors' contributions

ZC designed the study and revised the manuscript. HY, RM and LC performed the experiments and drafted the manuscript. YH and RA participated in sample collection. YZ, HJ and XZ participated in DNA extraction and PCR amplification. XW and XH participated in data analysis. All authors read and approved the final manuscript.

Competing interests
The authors declare that they have no competing interests.

Author details
[1]Key Laboratory of Animal Parasitology of Ministry of Agriculture, Laboratory of Quality and Safety Risk Assessment for Animal Products on Biohazards (Shanghai) of Ministry of Agriculture, Shanghai Veterinary Research Institute, Chinese Academy of Agricultural Sciences, Shanghai 200241, China. [2]Animal Husbandry and Veterinary Bureau of Changji Hui Autonomous Prefecture, Xinjiang Uyghur Autonomous Region, Changji 831100, Xinjiang, China.

References

1. Didier ES, Weiss LM. Microsporidiosis: current status. Curr Opin Infect Dis. 2006;19:485–92.
2. Didier ES. Microsporidiosis: an emerging and opportunistic infection in humans and animals. Acta Trop. 2005;94:61–76.
3. Keeling P. Five questions about microsporidia. PLoS Pathog. 2009;5: e1000489.
4. Mathis A, Weber R, Deplazes P. Zoonotic potential of the microsporidia. Clin Microbiol Rev. 2005;18:423–45.
5. Matos O, Lobo ML, Xiao L. Epidemiology of *Enterocytozoon bieneusi* infection in humans. J Parasitol Res. 2012;2012:981424.
6. Keeling PJ, Fast NM. Microsporidia: biology and evolution of highly reduced intracellular parasites. Annu Rev Microbiol. 2002;56:93–116.
7. Santín M, Fayer R. Microsporidiosis: *Enterocytozoon bieneusi* in domesticated and wild animals. Res Vet Sci. 2011;90:363–71.
8. Santín M, Fayer R. *Enterocytozoon bieneusi* genotype nomenclature based on the internal transcribed spacer sequence: a consensus. J Eukaryot Microbiol. 2009;56:34–8.
9. Santín M, Fayer R. *Enterocytozoon bieneusi*, *Giardia*, and *Cryptosporidium* infecting white-tailed deer. J Eukaryot Microbiol. 2015;62:34–43.
10. Karim MR, Dong H, Li T, Yu F, Li D, Zhang L, et al. Predomination and new genotypes of *Enterocytozoon bieneusi* in captive nonhuman primates in zoos in China: high genetic diversity and zoonotic significance. PLoS One. 2015;10:e117991.
11. Thellier M, Breton J. *Enterocytozoon bieneusi* in human and animals, focus on laboratory identification and molecular epidemiology. Parasite. 2008; 15:349–58.
12. Guo Y, Alderisio KA, Yang W, Cama V, Feng Y, Xiao L. Host specificity and source of *Enterocytozoon bieneusi* genotypes in a drinking source watershed. Appl Environ Microbiol. 2014;80:218–25.
13. Yue DM, Ma JG, Li FC, Hou JL, Zheng WB, Zhao Q, et al. Occurrence of *Enterocytozoon bieneusi* in donkeys (*Equus asinus*) in China: a public health concern. Front Microbiol. 2017;8:565.
14. Fayer R, Santín M, Trout JM. *Enterocytozoon bieneusi* in mature dairy cattle on farms in the eastern United States. Parasitol Res. 2007;102:15–20.
15. Karim MR, Dong H, Yu F, Jian F, Zhang L, Wang R, et al. Genetic diversity in *Enterocytozoon bieneusi* isolates from dogs and cats in China: host specificity and public health implications. J Clin Microbiol. 2014;52:3297–302.
16. Karim MR, Wang R, Dong H, Zhang L, Li J, Zhang S, et al. Genetic polymorphism and zoonotic potential of *Enterocytozoon bieneusi* from nonhuman primates in China. Appl Environ Microbiol. 2014;80:1893–8.
17. Li J, Luo N, Wang C, Qi M, Cao J, Cui Z, et al. Occurrence, molecular characterization and predominant genotypes of *Enterocytozoon bieneusi* in dairy cattle in Henan and Ningxia, China. Parasit Vectors. 2016;9:142.
18. Li W, Tao W, Jiang Y, Diao R, Yang J, Xiao L. Genotypic distribution and phylogenetic characterization of *Enterocytozoon bieneusi* in diarrheic chickens and pigs in multiple cities, China: potential zoonotic transmission. PLoS One. 2014;9:e108279.
19. Li W, Li Y, Li W, Yang J, Song M, Diao R, et al. Genotypes of *Enterocytozoon bieneusi* in livestock in China: high prevalence and zoonotic potential. PLoS One. 2014;9:e97623.
20. Zhao W, Zhang W, Wang R, Liu W, Liu A, Yang D, et al. *Enterocytozoon bieneusi* in sika deer (*Cervus nippon*) and red deer (*Cervus elaphus*): deer specificity and zoonotic potential of ITS genotypes. Parasitol Res. 2014;113: 4243–50.
21. Fiuza VRDS, Lopes CWG, Cosendey RIJ, de Oliveira FCR, Fayer R, Santín M. Zoonotic *Enterocytozoon bieneusi* genotypes found in Brazilian sheep. Res Vet Sci. 2016;107:196–201.
22. Jiang Y, Tao W, Wan Q, Li Q, Yang Y, Lin Y, et al. Zoonotic and potentially host-adapted *Enterocytozoon bieneusi* genotypes in sheep and cattle in northeast China and an increasing concern about the zoonotic importance of previously considered ruminant-adapted genotypes. Appl Environ Microbiol. 2015;81:3326–35.
23. Zhao W, Zhang W, Yang D, Zhang L, Wang R, Liu A. Prevalence of *Enterocytozoon bieneusi* and genetic diversity of ITS genotypes in sheep and goats in China. Infect Genet Evol. 2015;32:265–70.
24. Ye J, Xiao L, Wang Y, Guo Y, Roellig DM, Feng Y. Dominance of *Giardia duodenalis* assemblage A and *Enterocytozoon bieneusi* genotype BEB6 in sheep in Inner Mongolia, China. Vet Parasitol. 2015;210:235–9.
25. Shi K, Li M, Wang X, Li J, Karim MR, Wang R, et al. Molecular survey of *Enterocytozoon bieneusi* in sheep and goats in China. Parasit Vectors. 2016;9:23.
26. Zhang Q, Cai J, Li P, Wang L, Guo Y, Li C, et al. *Enterocytozoon bieneusi* genotypes in Tibetan sheep and yaks. Parasitol Res. 2018;117:721–7.
27. Askari Z, Mirjalali H, Mohebali M, Zarei Z, Shojaei S, Rezaeian T, et al. Molecular detection and identification of zoonotic Microsporidia spore in fecal samples of some animals with close-contact to human. Iran J Parasitol. 2015;10:381–8.
28. Stensvold CR, Beser J, Ljungström B, Troell K, Lebbad M. Low host-specific *Enterocytozoon bieneusi* genotype BEB6 is common in Swedish lambs. Vet Parasitol. 2014;205:371–4.
29. Buckholt MA, Lee JH, Tzipori S. Prevalence of *Enterocytozoon bieneusi* in swine: an 18-month survey at a slaughterhouse in Massachusetts. Appl Environ Microbiol. 2002;68:2595–9.
30. Kumar S, Stecher G, Tamura K. MEGA7: Molecular Evolutionary Genetics Analysis version 7.0 for bigger datasets. Mol Biol Evol. 2016;33:1870–4.
31. Feng Y, Li N, Dearen T, Lobo ML, Matos O, Cama V, et al. Development of a multilocus sequence typing tool for high-resolution genotyping of *Enterocytozoon bieneusi*. Appl Environ Microbiol. 2011;77:4822–8.
32. Zhao GH, Du SZ, Wang HB, Hu XF, Deng MJ, Yu SK, et al. First report of zoonotic *Cryptosporidium* spp., *Giardia intestinalis* and *Enterocytozoon bieneusi* in golden takins (*Budorcas taxicolor bedfordi*). Infect Genet Evol. 2015;34:394–401.
33. Li W, Deng L, Yu X, Zhong Z, Wang Q, Liu X, et al. Multilocus genotypes and broad host-range of *Enterocytozoon bieneusi* in captive wildlife at zoological gardens in China. Parasit Vectors. 2016;9:395.
34. Wang L, Xiao L, Duan L, Ye J, Guo Y, Guo M, et al. Concurrent infections of *Giardia duodenalis*, *Enterocytozoon bieneusi*, and *Clostridium difficile* in children during a cryptosporidiosis outbreak in a pediatric hospital in China. PLoS Negl Trop Dis. 2013;7:e2437.
35. Qi M, Wang R, Wang H, Jian F, Li J, Zhao J, et al. *Enterocytozoon bieneusi* genotypes in grazing horses in China and their zoonotic transmission potential. J Eukaryot Microbiol. 2016;63:591–7.
36. Zhao W, Yu S, Yang Z, Zhang Y, Zhang L, Wang R, et al. Genotyping of *Enterocytozoon bieneusi* (Microsporidia) isolated from various birds in China. Infect Genet Evol. 2016;40:151–4.
37. Li N, Xiao L, Wang L, Zhao S, Zhao X, Duan L, et al. Molecular surveillance of *Cryptosporidium* spp., *Giardia duodenalis*, and *Enterocytozoon bieneusi* by genotyping and subtyping parasites in wastewater. PLoS Negl Trop Dis. 2012;6:e1809.
38. Ben Ayed L, Yang W, Widmer G, Cama V, Ortega Y, Xiao L. Survey and genetic characterization of wastewater in Tunisia for *Cryptosporidium* spp., *Giardia duodenalis*, *Enterocytozoon bieneusi*, *Cyclospora cayetanensis* and *Eimeria* spp. J Water Health. 2012;10:431–44.
39. Efstratiou A, Ongerth JE, Karanis P. Waterborne transmission of protozoan parasites: review of worldwide outbreaks - an update 2011–2016. Water Res. 2017;114:14–22.
40. Rosado-Garcia FM, Guerrero-Florez M, Karanis G, Hinojosa M, Karanis P. Water-borne protozoa parasites: the Latin American perspective. Int J Hyg Environ Health. 2017;220:783–98.
41. Ye J, Ji Y, Xu J, Ma K, Yang X. Zoonotic *Enterocytozoon bieneusi* in raw wastewater in Zhengzhou, China. Folia Parasitol (Praha). 2017;64:002.

Effectiveness of the Brazilian Visceral Leishmaniasis Surveillance and Control Programme in reducing the prevalence and incidence of *Leishmania infantum* infection

Iara Caixeta Marques da Rocha[1,2], Letícia Helena Marques dos Santos[1], Wendel Coura-Vital[3,4], Gisele Macedo Rodrigues da Cunha[1], Fernanda do Carmo Magalhães[1], Thais Almeida Marques da Silva[1,5], Maria Helena Franco Morais[2], Edward Oliveira[6], Ilka Afonso Reis[7] and Mariângela Carneiro[1,8*]

Abstract

Background: Control strategies adopted by the Brazilian Visceral Leishmaniasis Surveillance and Control Programme (VLSCP) include identifying and culling seropositive infected dogs, early diagnosis and treatment of human cases, chemical control of the vector and population awareness. This study evaluated the effectiveness of the VLSCP on the prevalence and incidence rates of *Leishmania infantum* in children residing in areas under different VLSCP intervention times.

Methods: A quasi-experimental epidemiological study with a panel (two cross-sectional) and a concurrent cohort was performed in three areas of Belo Horizonte, southeast Brazil. The first cross-sectional study (I) was carried out with 1875 children, 478 of which were enrolled in the cohort study. In the second cross-sectional study (II), 413 additional children were included, totalizing 891 children. Laboratory diagnosis was performed by ELISA-rK39. Analyses included multilevel logistic and Poisson regression models.

Results: The incidence rates of *L. infantum* infection were: 14.4% in the area where VLSCP intervention was initiated in 2006 (AI2006); 21.1% in the area where intervention was initiated in 2008 (AI2008); and 11.6% in the area where intervention was initiated in 2010 (AI2010 - control area). A follow-up period of 24 months showed that the persons-time incidence rates in AI2006, AI2008, and AI2010 were: 6.2/100, 10/100, and 5.6/100 persons/24 months, respectively. The final prevalence rates of infection (cross-sectional II - in 2012), compared to the initial rates (cross-sectional I - in 2010), increased 83.7% in AI2006, 74.1% in AI2008, and decreased 5% in AI2010. Analysis of the effectiveness revealed that children residing in AI2008 are more likely to be infected (OR = 1.84; 95% CI: 1.06-3.23) and present a higher risk of infection (IRR = 1.76; 95% CI: 1.05-2.95) compared to those in AI2010. No statistically significant differences were observed in asymptomatic infection (OR and IRR) in AI2006 compared to AI2010.

(Continued on next page)

* Correspondence: mcarneiro@ufmg.br
[1]Laboratório de Epidemiologia das Doenças Infecciosas e Parasitarias, Departamento de Parasitologia, Instituto de Ciências Biológicas, Universidade Federal de Minas Gerais, Belo Horizonte, Minas Gerais, Brazil
[8]Pós-graduação em Ciências da Saúde: Infectologia e Medicina Tropical, Faculdade de Medicina, Universidade Federal de Minas Gerais, Belo Horizonte, Minas Gerais, Brazil
Full list of author information is available at the end of the article

(Continued from previous page)
Conclusions: The VLSCP was not effective at controlling *L. infantum* infection in areas where interventions had respectively been carried out for six and four years. However, it is unclear what the consequences in terms of human infection and diseases would be in the absence of the VLSCP. Efforts to improve the effectiveness of control measures remain a necessary priority.

Keywords: Control programme, Visceral leishmaniasis, Effectiveness, *Leishmania infantum* infection, Quasi-experimental study

Background

Visceral leishmaniasis (VL) is a neglected tropical disease that accounts for approximately 200,000 to 400,000 new cases annually worldwide [1, 2]. In the Americas, the etiological agent is the protozoan *Leishmania* (*Leishmania*) *infantum*, which is transmitted through the bite of the phlebotomine *Lutzomyia longipalpis*, with dogs being its main urban reservoir [3].

In the Americas, VL is present in 12 countries, with 90% of the cases being reported in Brazil (4200–6300 cases per year) and with a fatality rate around 7% [2, 4]. VL urbanization has been documented in Brazil since the 1980s and this trend represents a challenge for control measures in urban areas [5, 6]. The introduction and dispersion of *L. infantum* in urban areas is associated with a complex inter-dependent network and multiple factors such as environmental changes, migration, disorganized population growth and occupation of peripheral urban areas, high urban population density (both human and canine), and inadequate living conditions [4, 6, 7].

The Brazilian Visceral Leishmaniasis Surveillance and Control Programme (VLSCP) strategies include canine serological analysis followed by euthanasia of seropositive dogs, chemical control of the vector, early diagnosis and treatment of human cases, and population awareness [5]. In spite of the implementation of the VLSCP in endemic areas of Brazil, the control interventions have not been successful in interrupting transmission, especially in urban areas [8, 9]. In a systematic review analyzing intervention studies on the effectiveness of VL control programmes that included strategies to reduce the risk of transmission, such as animal reservoir control, vector control with insecticide spraying, or a combination of these interventions, Romero & Boelart [4] concluded that there is a lack of scientific evidence to sustain the effectiveness of these interventions in interrupting the spread of the disease. A randomized community intervention trial evaluating the impact of insecticide spraying and elimination of infected dogs on the incidence of human *L. infantum* infection showed that only dog culling reduced the human incidence, with estimates of effectiveness varying between 27–52%, depending on the analysis performed [10].

The first case of VL in Belo Horizonte, the capital of the state of Minas Gerais, located in southeastern Brazil, was confirmed in 1994 [11]. Since then, there has been significant investment in control measures implemented by the VLSCP [12, 13]. Between 1994 and 2016, 1762 cases were confirmed in Belo Horizonte with the lowest incidence rate of 1.2 cases per 100,000 inhabitants in 1998 and the highest rate of 7.2 cases per 100,000 inhabitants in 2008 [14].

Epidemiological studies in endemic areas highlight a large number of individuals infected by *L. infantum* with no clinical manifestations of the disease [15–20]. Indeed, infection by *L. infantum* affects a significant proportion of the population regardless of the occurrence of cases of the disease in one area [21]. Estimations of prevalence and incidence rates of asymptomatic infection in children appear to reflect recent parasite circulation given that they can indicate transmission cases in an endemic area [5]. Thus, these rates may be used as indicators for evaluation of the effectiveness of the strategies undertaken by the VLSCP in endemic areas [20, 22].

To understand the impact of the VLSCP in reducing the incidence of human VL, it is important to perform effectiveness evaluation under real conditions, i.e. under the routine of implementation and execution of the programme. The aim of the present study was to evaluate the effectiveness of the VLSCP on the prevalence and incidence rates of *L. infantum* infection in children less than ten years of age living in Belo Horizonte. We compared the areas where interventions had been carried out for six (intervention started in 2006) and four years (intervention started in 2008) with an area where the intervention of the VLSCP was being initiated (control area, intervention started in 2010).

Methods

Study area

Located in southeastern Brazil, Belo Horizonte is the capital city of the Brazilian State of Minas Gerais. It has 2,375,151 inhabitants and a population density of 7.2 inhabitants/km^2. It is the sixth most populous city in Brazil, according to the census of the Brazilian Institute of Geography and Statistics [23]. The city is located at 852 m above sea level, 19°49'01"S, 43°57'21"W. The city has a dry winter and a hot and rainy summer, with an average annual temperature of 21 °C, average relative air humidity of 65%, and average annual rainfall of 1500 mm [23].

The study was conducted in three non-randomly selected geographically adjacent areas of Belo Horizonte. These three areas were selected based on the year that the VLSCP actions were initiated. The start date of implementation of the control strategies in each area was defined according to the guidelines and the strategic planning of the municipal public health authority, based on the epidemiological data of each area. In this assessment, the cumulative incidence of human visceral leishmaniasis (HVL) cases, as well as the social and environmental indicators were considered. A description of each area selected to take part in this study is presented below.

Intervention area 2006 (AI 2006)

This is the area where the VLSCP control strategies have been active the longest, as they started in 2006. The area has 20,672 inhabitants [24]. From 2006 to 2012, 13 cases of HVL were notified to the Brazilian Notifiable Disease Information System (Sistema de Informação de Agravos de Notificação, SINAN), and the cumulative incidence was 62.8/100,000 inhabitants [25]. The canine seroprevalence was 9.9% in the first year of intervention and 3.4% in 2012, the last year considered in this study. Vector chemical control was carried out in priority zones throughout all years of the study (2006–2012) [26].

Intervention area 2008 (AI 2008)

The VLSCP started in this area in 2008, which was considered an intermediate intervention time. The area has 22,591 inhabitants [24]. From 2006 to 2012, 11 HVL cases were notified to the SINAN, and the cumulative incidence in the area was 48.7/100,000 inhabitants [25]. The canine seroprevalence decreased from 12.7% in 2008 to 4.1% in 2012. Vector chemical control was carried out in priority zones in 2009, 2010 and 2012 according to strategic planning and epidemiological assessment [26].

Intervention area 2010 (AI 2010)

This area was selected as the control of the present study because the VLSCP was implemented only in 2010. The area has 16,818 inhabitants [24]. From 2006 to 2012, only one case of HVL was reported to the SINAN (in 2008), and the cumulative incidence was 5.9 cases/100,000 inhabitants [25]. In 2010, when the VLSCP started, the canine seroprevalence was 8.6% and decreased to 3.3% in 2012. No chemical vector control was used by the VLSCP until 2012 in this area [26].

Study design

The investigation reported herein involves a quasi-experimental study encompassing a panel study (two cross-sectional) and a concurrent cohort study. The first cross-sectional study (I) established the baseline for the cohort, and the second (II) was carried out at the end of the investigation. Two indicators were estimated for the assessment of the effectiveness of the VLSCP using rK-39 antigen testing (ELISA-rK39): the incidence rate of infection and the difference between the final and the initial prevalence rates of asymptomatic infection. The study was conducted with children since infection in young individuals is an indicator of recent transmission. The inclusion criteria for the cross-sectional study I (baseline) was children aged 2–84 months. The exclusion criterion was applied only for the cohort study, which excluded the seropositive children from the follow-up.

Panel study: Cross-sectional study I

Conducted in 2010, this study established the baseline for the cohort study. It included 1875 children between 2 months and 7 years of age residing in all three areas (AI2006, AI2008, and AI2010). The study estimated the initial seroprevalence of asymptomatic *L. infantum* infection through ELISA-rK39.

Panel study: Cross-sectional study II

Conducted in 2012, this study involved 891 children between 2 months and 10 years of age residing in the three selected areas. At this stage, the final asymptomatic *L. infantum* infection seroprevalence rate was also estimated by ELISA-rK39.

Cohort study

A total of 478 children diagnosed as seronegative for *L. infantum* infection during the first cross-sectional study (2010) were followed-up in the concurrent cohort study. This allowed us to estimate, using ELISA-rK39, the incidence rate of infection by *L. infantum* in 2012 (Fig. 1).

Sampling

Panel Study: Cross-sectional study I (2010)

The sample size estimated for the study (baseline) was established using the following parameters: (i) an incidence among children between 9 months and 6 years of age of 2.7/100 children-years; (ii) type I error probability (α) equivalent to 0.05; (iii) a power for the statistical tests of $(1-\beta) = 0.80$; and (iv) a minimum 30% difference to be detected between the areas. Under these conditions, the sample size estimated for each area was 670 children of this age interval. In total, 1875 children residing in all three areas were assessed during the study.

Panel study: Cross-sectional study II (2012)

The sample size was calculated considering the following parameters: (i) the average prevalence rate of human

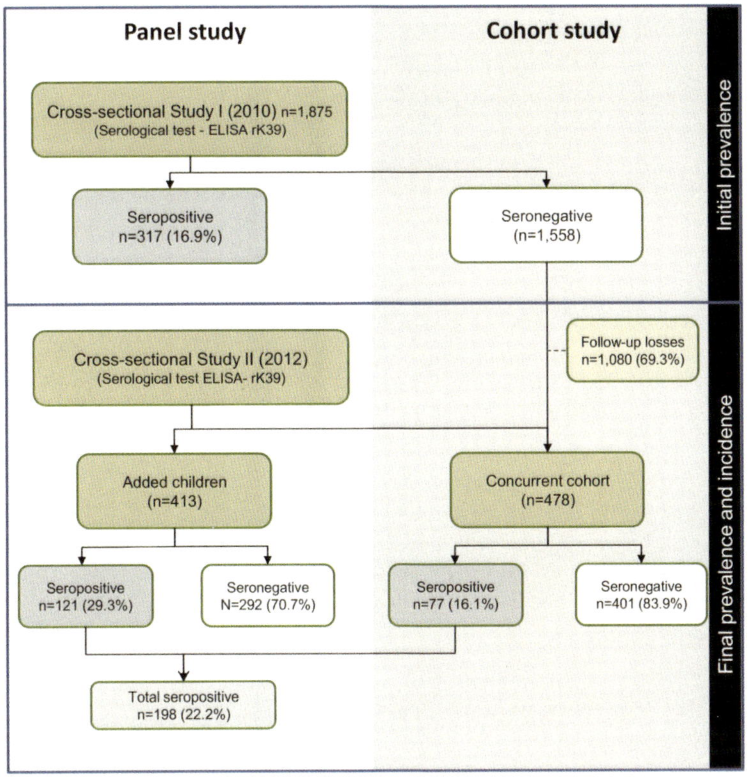

Fig. 1 Study design: panel study (cross-sectional studies I and II) and cohort study. Belo Horizonte, Minas Gerais, Brazil

infection of 15/100 children under 7 years of age, obtained from a previous study conducted in Belo Horizonte (19); (ii) a type I error probability (α) equivalent to 0.05; (iii) estimated precision of 0.05; and (iv) effect of design of 1.5. The sample size was calculated to be composed of approximately 300 children from each area, totalizing 900 children.

Cohort study

The cohort study was designed to follow up all the seronegative children identified in the cross-sectional study I. However, due to the loss of follow-up, it was conducted with all the seronegative children reached during the data collection.

Data and biological sample collection, and serological testing

Throughout the study, the same procedures were used to collect data and blood samples. Initially, the children living in the study area were randomly selected based on the municipal census conducted through the Family Health Programme, a strategy currently adopted by the Brazilian Unified Health System (Sistema Único de Saúde, SUS). These data are periodically updated by community health workers who conduct a census in the areas studied.

Once the children were randomly selected, their parents and/or guardians were contacted by telephone or visited by someone from the team to explain the aims of the study. The data collection was conducted in 2012. The parents or legal guardians that agreed to take part in the study were visited by a team of nurse technicians who collected children's blood samples and performed an interview. Before data collection, a free and informed consent form was signed by each legal guardian. Literate children were also asked to read and sign the informed consent form (adapted for children), thereby agreeing to the terms of the study. The blood was obtained by finger puncture and then transferred to filter paper, according to the protocol described by dos Santos et al. [20].

The ELISA rK-39 tests were carried out using serum obtained from the filter papers, following previously described procedures [21, 27]. The evaluations of rK-39 antigen performance for diagnosis of asymptomatic infection and of the disease showed that the sensitivity ranged between 70–92% and specificity between 77–100% [27–29].

The ELISA-rK39 seropositive children were invited to attend the public health unit for a clinical evaluation. On this occasion, blood samples were collected by venipuncture for complementary laboratory tests. These children were also clinically evaluated for signs and symptoms of VL.

A trained interviewer conducted the interview with the parents or legal guardians using a previously tested, structured questionnaire that sought information regarding the following groups of variables for: children (age, gender, behaviour); household characteristics (number of rooms, number of occupants and intra-domicile characteristics); peri-domicile environment characteristics (presence of backyard, presence and method of garbage disposal, i.e. collected, burned or buried, residual water destination, presence of domestic animals, presence of rubble and manure), knowledge about VL and its vector, and neighbourhood characteristics (presence of animals, trees, backyards and wastelands). Furthermore, we estimated the family income and social class according to the Brazilian socioeconomic classification criteria (Critério de Classificação Socioeconômica do Brasil, CCEB), which takes into account the level of education of the head of the family and the presence of specific domestic goods in the residence [30].

Assessment of the effectiveness of the Visceral Leishmaniasis Surveillance and Control Programme (VLSCP)

The questionnaire data and serological test results were codified and electronically stored in duplicate. The files were then compared and the divergences corrected. The software EpiData version 3.2 (Epidata Association, Odense Denmark, Europe) was used for data entry, and STATA version 12 (Stata Corp., College Station, TX, USA) was used for statistical analyses.

Infection prevalence rates were calculated for each area as a ratio between the number of seropositive children identified by the ELISA-rK39 test and the total number of children analyzed in the area. The percentage prevalence rate change was calculated by comparing the final rate (2012) against the initial rate (2010), according to the following equation:

$$\text{Change (\%)} = \frac{(\text{Final Prevalence} - \text{Initial Prevalence}) \times 100}{\text{Initial Prevalence}}$$

Incidence rates were calculated as the ratio between the numbers of new *L. infantum* seropositive cases, detected by ELISA-rK39, over the total number of children evaluated in the cohort, by area. The person-time incidence rate was estimated as the ratio between the number of new *L. infantum* infection seropositive cases over person-time in the follow-up period (24 months), per area evaluated. The denominator presented the follow-up time of the children evaluated in two time-points (2010 and 2012) plus half of the follow-up time of the children who were lost to the follow-up.

To evaluate the effectiveness of the VLSCP control strategies on the prevalence and incidence of seropositivity by *L. infantum* infection, two statistical models were used: multilevel logistic regression and Poisson regression with estimated robust variance. The multilevel logistic regression model was used in the cross-sectional studies to evaluate the impact of the intervention strategies adopted by the VLSCP on the final sero-prevalence of asymptomatic infection in the studied areas using odds ratio (OR) with a 95% confidence interval (CI). At one level, this model considered the houses and, at a second level, the children's characteristics. The residence was considered at the first level as, in some cases, more than one child from the same household were included in the study and were likely to share similar attributes due to the environment that is common to them. The Poisson regression model with robust variance estimation was used to evaluate the effectiveness of VLSCP intervention strategies on the incidence of new asymptomatic *L. infantum* infection cases in the cohort using the incidence rate ratio (IRR) with 95% CI.

Initially, bivariate analysis was performed in both models. Variables that showed a statistical association ($P < 0.25$) in the bivariate analysis were selected to compose the multivariate models according to the following groups: individual personal variables, socioeconomic, intra- and peri-domicile features, neighborhood, and knowledge of the vector population and the reservoir. Significant variables in all groups ($P < 0.15$) were selected for the multilevel logistic multivariate and Poisson models. Variables with more than two categories were converted into dummy variables. The building of the final models started with the full models, containing all variables, followed by successive discarding (backward selection) of the non-significant variables. The final multilevel logistic model to evaluate effectiveness was adjusted for variables that remained statistically significant ($P < 0.05$), thereby considering the effects of these variables on the prevalence of infection. The multilevel logistic regression was performed using STATA 12's "xtmelogit" function. The final Poisson model with robust variance estimation to evaluate effectiveness was also adjusted for variables that remained significant ($P < 0.05$). This model considered the effects of these variables on the incidence of infection. The Poisson model was carried out using the "vcepoisson (robust) irr" function in STATA version 12.

Results

Study population

To establish the baseline for the study, 1875 children aged 2–84 months (mean: 42.1 months ± 24.7) were evaluated in 2010. Of these, 1558 were seronegative for *L. infantum*. Among those, 478 (31.4%) children were followed in the cohort and assessed again in 2012. The sample analyzed in the cohort study was composed of

160 children from AI2006, 180 children from AI2008 and 138 children from AI2010.

Among the seronegative children, 1080 were lost during the follow-up time. The percentages of losses were similar across all three areas: 71.8% in AI2006, 68.3 % in AI2008, and 67.3 % in AI2010. To characterize this loss, the variables age, gender, occupation and educational level of the household head, household income, presence of dogs, dogs with VL, and property features were compared between those followed and those who were lost during the follow-up. The greatest loss occurred in families with the lower incomes ($P < 0.001$) and lower level of education of the household head ($P = 0.038$).

The sample for the cross-sectional study II was initially composed of the 478 children from the follow-up cases. They were later joined by an additional 413 children, randomly selected, who did not participate in the baseline study, resulting in a sample size of 891 children aged 2–129 months (mean: 62 months ± 27.92). This sample was composed of 287 children from AI2006, 316 children from AI2008 and 288 children from AI2010.

Demographic characteristics of the children evaluated in the cohort and cross-sectional study II according to their area of residence are shown in Table 1. The age distributions of the children followed in the cohort study were statistically different among the areas: AI2010 had the highest proportion of children younger than 72 months (50.7%) and AI2006 and AI2008 had the highest proportion of children > 72 and ≤ 96 months (40.2 and 42.2%, respectively). There was no gender imbalance among the cohort children (Table 1). Considering the cross-sectional study II, the children evaluated presented similar age and gender in the three areas evaluated (Table 1).

Prevalence and incidence rates

In cross-sectional study I, the prevalence rates of asymptomatic *L. infantum* infection detected by ELISA-rK39 were 12.9% (87/675), 14.7% (100/679) and 17.9% (93/521) in AI2006, AI2008 and AI2010, respectively. The prevalence rates in cross-sectional study II were 23.7% (AI2006), 25.6% (AI2008) and 17.0% (AI2010). The relative change percentages showed an increase of 83.7% in AI2006 and 74.1% in AI2008, and a decrease of 5.3% in AI2010 (Table 2).

AI2006 had an incidence ratio (IR) of 14.4% and the person-time incidence rate of 6.2/100 persons/24 months. AI2008 had the highest incidence (IR = 21.1%) and person-time incidence rate of 10/100 persons/24 months. The control area (AI2010) presented the lowest IR (11.6%) and person-time incidence rate (5.6/100 persons/24 months) (Table 2).

Characteristics of the three areas evaluated in the cohort study

In the cohort study, 398 households were visited and information from 478 children was analyzed. Table 3 shows

Table 1 Characteristics of the children living in the three different areas evaluated, Belo Horizonte, Minas Gerais, Brazil

Study	Variable	AI 2006	AI 2008	AI 2010	*P*-value
		n (%)	*n* (%)	*n* (%)	
Cohort	Number of children	160 (33.5)	180 (37.7)	138 (28.9)	
	Age				
	≤ 48 months	13 (8.2)	17 (9.4)	28 (20.3)	0.03
	> 48 and ≤ 72 months	52 (32.7)	61 (33.9)	42 (30.4)	
	> 72 and ≤ 96 months	64 (40.2)	76 (42.2)	46 (33.3)	
	> 96 months	30 (18.9)	26 (14.5)	22 (16.0)	
	Gender				
	Male	78 (48.8)	91 (50.6)	77 (55.8)	0.46
	Female	82 (51.3)	89 (49.4)	61 (44.2)	
Cross-sectional-II	Number of children	287 (32.2)	316 (35.5)	288 (32.3)	
	Age				
	≤ 48 months	84 (29.3)	100 (31.6)	102 (35.4)	0.70
	> 48 and ≤ 72 months	77 (26.8)	91 (28.8)	75 (26.0)	
	> 72 and ≤ 96 months	93 (32.4)	96 (30.4)	81 (28.2)	
	> 96 months	33 (11.5)	29 (9.2)	30 (10.4)	
	Gender				
	Male	137 (47.7)	159 (50.3)	152 (52.8)	0.48
	Female	150 (52.3)	157 (49.7)	136 (47.2)	

Abbreviations: AI2006, area of intervention since 2006; AI2008, area of intervention since 2008; AI2010, area of intervention since 2010; CI, confidence interval

Table 2 Prevalence and incidence of *L. infantum* infection rates in areas with different intervention times by the Brazilian Visceral Leishmaniasis Surveillance and Control Programme, Belo Horizonte, Minas Gerais, Brazil

Areas	Prevalence 2010 (95% CI)	Prevalence 2012 (95% CI)	Change (%)	Incidence 2012 (95% CI)	Person-time incidence[a] (95% CI)
AI2006	12.9 (10.6–15.6)	23.7 (19.1–28.9)	83.7	14.4 (9.8–20.7)	6.2 (4.0–9.1)
AI 2008	14.7 (12.3–17.6)	25.6 (21.1–30.7)	74.1	21.1 (15.8–27.6)	10.0 (7.2–13.6)
AI 2010	17.9 (14.8–21.4)	17.0 (13.1–21.8)	-5.3	11.6 (7.3–18.0)	5.6 (3.3–9.0)

[a]Denominator: Loss/2 + number of children on follow-up for 24 months for each area analyzed. Incidence rate/100 persons-24 months
Abbreviations: AI2006, area of intervention since 2006; AI2008, area of intervention since 2008; AI2010, area of intervention since 2010; CI, confidence interval

the comparison of the families and household characteristics among the three areas evaluated in the cohort study. In all areas analyzed, it was observed that most household heads had completed high school. AI2010 showed the largest number of household heads with higher education, either in the course or completed (23.9%), whereas AI2006 showed the highest percentage of illiterate individuals (12%). According to the CCEB [30], most of the children living in AI2006 (65.5%) and AI2008 (58.7%) belonged to socioeconomic class C or below, with a monthly income below 2.4 of minimum monthly wage (BMMW; in 2012, the Brazilian minimum monthly wage was equivalent to 311 USD). Children from AI2010 belonged mainly (58.4%) to class B2 or lower (monthly income ≤ 4.1 BMMW). Over half of the visited residences in all three areas had dogs, plants in the peri-domicile, and trees in the neighborhood. The presence of chickens was more frequently observed in AI2006 (14.1%) and AI2008 (12.6%), which were the areas with the highest percentage of families from lower socioeconomic classes. Statistically significant differences were found among all three areas concerning "educational level of the head of the family" and "families' socioeconomic class" (Table 3).

Effectiveness of the control strategies adopted by the VLSCP on reducing *L. infantum* incidence rates

The final Poisson model used to evaluate the effectiveness of the control strategies adopted by the VLSCP on reducing *L. infantum* incidence rates showed that children living in AI2008 presented higher IRR (1.82, P = 0.03) than those residing in the control area AI2010 when adjusted according to the child's age, family economic class, and the presence of trees in the neighborhood. In AI2006, the VLSCP interventions showed no statistically significant difference in the IRR of asymptomatic *L. infantum* infection (1.24, P = 0.48) compared with AI2010 when adjusted to the child's age, family economic class, and the presence of trees in the neighborhood (Table 4).

Characteristics of the three areas evaluated in cross-sectional study II

The characteristics of the population evaluated in the second cross-sectional study were very similar to those of the population in the cohort. In cross-sectional study II, 659 households were visited and 891 children participated. Table 5 shows the comparisons of selected characteristics of the families and households among the three areas evaluated in cross-sectional study II. In all areas analyzed, high school was the educational level most frequently completed by the household head. The maximum percentage of household heads with higher education in course or complete was observed in AI2010 (21.8%), whereas AI2006 presented the highest percentage of illiterate individuals (9.2%).

According to the CCEB [30], most of the children living in AI2006 (65.9%) and AI2008 (56.5%) belonged to the socioeconomic class C or lower (≤ 2.4 BMMW). On the other hand, children from AI2010 belonged mainly to the socioeconomic class B or higher (58.4%) (monthly income between 4.1 and 20.8 BMMW). The presence of dogs, plants and trees in the household neighborhood were characteristics commonly found in most households of all three areas (n = 659). The presence of chickens was more frequent in residences of AI2006 (14.8%) and AI2008 (10.8%), which were the ones with the highest rate of families belonging to the lower socioeconomic classes, according to CCEB [30]. Statistically significant differences were found in all three areas for the following variables: level of education of the household head ($P < 0.01$), family's socioeconomic class ($P < 0.01$), the presence of rubble ($P = 0.01$), and the presence of a gully ($P < 0.01$) (Table 5).

Effectiveness of control strategies on reducing the prevalence of asymptomatic *L. infantum* infection

The final multivariate multilevel logistic model used to evaluate the effectiveness of the VLSCP on reducing the prevalence of infection showed that children living in AI2008 were more likely to be infected (OR = 1.94; P = 0.02) than the children from the control area (AI2010) when adjusted for the child's age, socioeconomic class, the presence of trees in the neighborhood and the presence of chickens (Table 6). The chance of children in AI2006 to be infected was not significantly different from those living in AI2010 (OR = 1.71; P = 0.07) when adjusted for the child's age, socioeconomic class, the presence of trees in the neighborhood and the presence of chickens (Table 6).

Table 3 Comparison of the families and household characteristics among the three areas evaluated in the cohort study, Belo Horizonte, Minas Gerais, Brazil

Variable	AI 2006	AI 2008	AI 2010	*P*-value
	n (%)	*n* (%)	*n* (%)	
Number of residences	142 (35.7)	143 (35.9)	113 (28.4)	
Education level of the household head				
Higher education (in course or completed)	15 (10. 6)	7 (4.9)	27 (23.9)	0.001
High-school (completed)	60 (42.3)	77 (53.9)	51 (45.1)	
Foundation (completed)	28 (19.7)	26 (18.2)	16 (14.2)	
Primary school (completed)	22 (15.5)	30 (21.0)	13 (11.5)	
Illiterate	17 (11.9)	3 (2.10)	6 (5.31)	
Socio-economic class (BMMW)				
A1, A2 and B1 (20.8 to 4.2)	16 (11.3)	18 (12.6)	30 (26.6)	0.001
B2 (4.1 to 2.5)	33 (23.2)	41 (28.7)	44 (38.9)	
C1, C2 and D (2.4 to 1.1)	93 (65.5)	84 (58.7)	39 (34.5)	
Chickens				
Present	20 (14.1)	18 (12.6)	10 (8.9)	0.43
Absent	122 (85.9)	125 (87.4)	103 (91.2)	
Dogs				
Present	75 (52.8)	80 (55.9)	60 (53.1)	0.85
Absent	67 (47.2)	63 (44.1)	53 (46.9)	
Peridomiciliar plants				
Present	107 (75.4)	98 (68.5)	87 (77.0)	0.15
Absent	33 (23.24)	45 (31.47)	26 (23.0)	
Neighbourhood trees				
Present	92 (64.8)	89 (62.2)	75 (66.4)	0.78
Absent	50 (35.2)	54 (37.8)	38 (33.6)	
Rubble				
Present	55 (38.7)	39 (27.3)	29 (25.7)	0.06
Absent	85 (59.9)	101 (70.6)	84 (74.3)	
Gully				
Present	46 (32.4)	28 (19.6)	24 (21.2)	0.07
Absent	95 (66.9)	115 (80.4)	88 (77.9)	
Waste				
Present	18 (12.7)	18 (12.6)	21 (18.6)	0.21
Absent	122 (85.9)	125 (87.4)	92 (81.4)	

Abbreviations: AI2006, area of intervention since 2006; AI2008, area of intervention since 2008; AI2010, area of intervention since 2010; BMMW, Brazilian monthly minimum wage; Class A1, A2 and B1 (20.8 to 4.2 BMMW); Class B2, (4.1 to 2.5 BMMW); Class C1, C2 and D (2.4 to 1.1 BMMW)

Table 4 Effectiveness of the control strategies adopted by the Brazilian Visceral Leishmaniasis Surveillance and Control Programme, Belo Horizonte, Minas Gerais, Brazil

Intervention área	IRR[a]	95% CI	*P*-value	IRR[b]	*P*-value	95% CI
AI2010	1					
AI2008	1.82	1.06–3.13	0.03	1.76	0.03	1.05–2.95
AI2006	1.24	0.68–2.25	0.48	1.18	0.59	0.65–2.14

[a]Non-adjusted model
[b]Model adjusted to age of the child, family's socio-economic class and presence of trees in the neighborhood
Abbreviations: AI2006, area of intervention since 2006; AI2008, area of intervention since 2008; AI2010, area of intervention since 2010; CI, confidence interval; IRR, incidence rate ratio

Discussion

The present study showed that the VLSCP was not effective at reducing HVL transmission, as evaluated by the prevalence and incidence of asymptomatic infection by *L. infantum* in children living in areas where the control programme had respectively been carried out for six and four years, compared with the control area where the programme had just been initiated. The prevalence of infection with *L. infantum* showed an increase in AI2006 (83.7%) and AI2008 (74.1%), the two areas where the VLSCP had been previously implemented, and a slight reduction (5%) in the control area AI2010. The incidence and persons-years incidence rates after two years of follow-up were higher in AI2008 (21.1% and 10/100 persons-24 months), followed by AI2006 (14.4% and 6.2/100 persons-24 months) and AI2010 (11.6% and 5.6/100 persons-24 months).

It was expected that the areas AI2006 and AI2008 would present a decrease in the prevalence rates and lower incidence rates of asymptomatic infection compared with the control area (AI2010). Despite the increase of the prevalence rate in AI2006 when compared with the control area (AI2010), after adjustment for confounding factors in the Poisson regression model, the risk of infection (IRR = 1.18) was not statistically significant. AI2008 showed higher final prevalence and incidence rates, and a higher risk of infection (IRR = 1.76) when compared with the control area (AI2010). These results suggest that despite the intervention adopted by the VLSCP in the areas, high transmission occurred among children, especially in AI2008.

A small decrease (5%) was observed in the final prevalence rate in the control area (AI2010) compared with the initial prevalence. Additionally, this area showed the lowest incidence rates of infection compared with the other areas under VLSCP intervention. Despite the short intervention time, the control strategies implemented in this area in 2010 resulted in a small reduction in prevalence. It is likely that the higher socioeconomic level and the healthier environmental conditions and urbanization of this area better supported the control measures in

Table 5 Comparison of the families and household characteristics among the three areas evaluated in the cross-sectional study, Belo Horizonte, Minas Gerais, Brazil

Variables	AI 2006 *n* (%)	AI 2008 *n* (%)	AI 2010 *n* (%)	*P*-value
Number of households	229	223	207	
Education level of the household head				
Higher education in course or completed	21 (9.2)	16 (7.2)	45 (21.8)	0.001
High-school (completed)	103 (45.2)	121 (54.3)	86 (41.7)	
Foundation (completed)	51 (22.4)	40 (17.9)	36 (17.5)	
Primary school (completed)	32 (14.0)	41 (18.4)	27 (13.1)	
Illiterate	21 (9.2)	5 (2.2)	12 (5.8)	
Socio-economic class (BMMW)				
A1, A2 and B1 (20.8 to 4.2)	24 (10.5)	31 (13.9)	49 (23. 7)	0.001
B2 (4.1 to 2.5)	54 (23.6)	66 (29.6)	72 (34.8)	
C1, C2 and D (2.4 to 1.1)	151 (65.9)	126 (56.5)	86 (41.5)	
Chickens				
Present	34 (14.8)	24 (10.8)	18 (8.7)	0.12
Absent	195 (85.1)	199 (89.2)	189 (91.3)	
Dogs				
Present	119 (51.9)	120 (53.8)	104 (50.2)	0.76
Absent	110 (48.0)	103 (46.2)	103 (49.8)	
Peridomicilar plants				
Present	162 (70.7)	145 (65.0)	151 (72.9)	0.02
Absent	65 (28.4)	78 (35.0)	55 (26.6)	
Neighbourhood trees				
Present	148 (64.6)	139 (62.3)	136 (65.7)	0.75
Absent	81 (35.4)	84 (37.7)	71 (34.3)	
Rubble				
Present	93 (40.6)	68 (30.5)	56 (27.1)	0.01
Absent	132 (57.6)	153 (68.6)	151(72.9)	
Gully				
Present	82 (35.8)	49 (22.0)	42 (20.3)	0.001
Absent	144 (62.9)	174 (78.0)	164 (79.2)	
Waste				
Present	35 (15.3)	30 (13.5)	31 (15.0)	0.19
Absent	191(83.4)	193 (86.5)	176 (85.0)	

Abbreviations: AI2006, area of intervention since 2006; AI2008, area of intervention since 2008; AI2010, area of intervention since 2010; BMMW, Brazilian monthly minimum wage; Class A1, A2 and B1 (20.8 to 4.2 BMMW); Class B2, (4.1 to 2.5 BMMW); Class C1, C2 and D (2.4 to 1.1 BMMW)

comparison with the other areas of intervention. Despite the adjustments made to confounding variables in the statistical analysis models, one could infer that epidemiological and intra-urban characteristics in this area

Table 6 Effectiveness of the control strategies adopted by the Brazilian Visceral Leishmaniasis Surveillance and Control Programme in transversal study II, Belo Horizonte, Minas Gerais, Brazil

Intervention área	OR[a]	95% CI	*P*-value	OR[b]	*P*-value	95% CI
AI2010	1					
AI2008	1.94	1.1–3.42	0.02	1.84	0.03	1.06–3.23
AI2006	1.71	1.1–3.42	0.07	1.68	0.07	0.94–2.98

[a]Non-adjusted model
[b]Model adjusted by age of the child, socio-economic class of the family, presence of trees in the neighborhood and presence of chickens.
Abbreviations: AI2006, area of intervention since 2006; AI2008, area of intervention since 2008; AI2010, area of intervention since 2010; OR, odds ratio; CI, confidence interval

may be associated with the reduction in transmission. One ecological study [31] conducted in Belo Horizonte to identify the areas at greater risk for HVL infection and the risk factors involved in transmission corroborate our results. According to the authors, the relative risk of VL was shown to be correlated with lower income and educational level. Since AI2006 and AI2008 presented worse socioeconomic levels and schooling when compared to AI2010, we can expect that these factors may have interfered in the control actions. A point that deserves emphasis is that the baseline prevalence rates of *L. infantum* infection were comparable among the three areas, thus increasing the internal validity of this study, an important condition for programme evaluation studies [32].

A quasi-experimental design, which permits control of external factors or confounding variables without random allocation of the areas under intervention, has been the method of choice to evaluate the effectiveness of health programmes. A panel study (two cross-sectional studies) conducted in the same population in two-time intervals is the best model for demonstrating changes in the prevalence of infection [32], and here, unlike a conventional cross-sectional study, longitudinal measurements of samples of children population were obtained. Even with the limitations associated with losses in the cohort study, caused by the long period between the two evaluations (two years), the analysis of the cohort is of great relevance as it allows for the estimation of incidence, the most appropriate measure in the understanding of disease transmission. In the search for more reliable data, we evaluated incidence after two years of follow-up and a second prevalence with the inclusion of children in the study. This approach allowed us to assess the effectiveness of VLSCP on *L. infantum* infection through different analyses.

Studies that evaluated the strategies adopted by the VLSCP such as the culling of seropositive dogs and insecticide spraying have shown that these measures are not effective in interrupting the human transmission, especially in urban areas. In the study by Souza et al. [22], although the data suggested a small reduction in the incidence of human infection in areas of intervention when compared with the control area, the difference was not statistically significant. The study by Werneck et al. [10] compared different control strategies and showed the low effectiveness of the euthanasia of dogs on the incidence of human infection. On the other hand, a study by Costa et al. [33] pointed towards a protective effect of the euthanasia of infected dogs in the human incidence of *L. infantum* infection associated with intra-domicile spraying. However, spraying the peridomicile, associated or not with canine euthanasia, had no significant protective effect in human transmission. Dietze et al. [34] conducted an intervention study with the aim of determining the impact of the elimination of dogs in controlling the disease. Twelve months after the start of the trial, they observed an increase in HVL seroprevalence in intervention and control areas, whereas canine seroconversion declined in all areas.

The evaluation of the effectiveness of VL control strategies performed herein did not consider VLSCP's indicators of the operational process, such as the number of households visited, the number of examined and euthanized dogs, the time between identification of seropositive dogs and euthanasia, and coverage of insecticide spraying. The assumption was that the programme had been implemented following pre-established strategies based on epidemiological criteria for each area, according to the recommendation of the VLSCP. This assumption can be supported by a study conducted to evaluate the VLSCP activities in Belo Horizonte from 2007 to 2011 [13], which showed a reduction in some indicators of the programme results, such as canine seroprevalence (47.8%) and the incidence of HVL cases (from 7.2 to 3.9/100,000 inhabitants). Additionally, the results showed that more than 85% of the seropositive dogs were euthanized, but only 57.5% of vector control coverage was reached in 2010. Although the authors concluded that the programme objectives were achieved in Belo Horizonte, revision of the proposed actions by the control programme was necessary due to the complexity of the interventions [13].

Problems related to the effectiveness of the VL programme have been pointed out by many authors and include the inaccuracy of the serological test to identify canine infection, the time between the identification of canine infection and euthanasia, substitution of sacrificed dogs by new dogs, absence of an official information system for recording and monitoring canine control activities, insufficient knowledge about the vector behavior, low coverage of insecticide spraying, and the lack of sustainability of the control strategies [9, 33, 35–37]. Although the VLSCP has clear objectives and strategies, it does not propose ways of evaluating its actions. A study conducted to evaluate the control activities demonstrated the importance of evaluating the set of control actions in their routine, through indicators that signal their positive and critical points [13].

The seropositive children identified in the present study were examined by a physician, and new blood samples were collected for other serological (ELISA-rk39 and ELISA with soluble antigen) and molecular (qPCR) tests. No seropositive children at follow-up developed any clinical signs or symptoms of VL and therefore were not treated since the treatment is indicated only for patients with clinical manifestations [5]. These results are in accordance with other studies conducted in Brazil, which clinically monitored asymptomatic individuals with positive results for ELISA-rK39 and revealed that none of the followed individuals developed the disease [18, 19, 38, 39].

A few limitations of the present study need to be mentioned. First, the difficulty in defining *L. infantum* infection cases due to the absence of an accurate diagnostic test for the detection of the asymptomatic infection. The drawback of the diagnostic test is due to the low levels of circulating antibodies in the serum of asymptomatic individuals as the parasitic load is scarce at this stage of the disease [20, 27, 38]. However, given that the same diagnostic procedures were carried out throughout the study, the misclassification bias is probably the same in the different moments and areas evaluated. Secondly, the loss of follow-up was high, and selection bias should be considered. However, the follow-up loss was homogeneous among the three areas, making the data comparable. Conversely, comparison of demographic and socioeconomic characteristics between the participants fully followed-up and those that were lost during the follow-up period revealed socioeconomic differences. The highest proportion of losses was found among participants of the lower socioeconomic classes, as well as among those whose household heads had a lower educational level. It is likely that these families do not own their homes and have greater mobility. In spite of this difference, selection bias may be minimized since the losses were similar among the areas. However, the incidence infection estimates were probably less precise due to the losses during follow-up. The mobility should have little impact on the effectiveness of the programme, as the control measures are implemented in a continuous way with broad actions and focusing on the collective health. Furthermore, in transversal study II, a difference in seroprevalence was observed between the children that were included and those followed in the cohort study. This may be due to age differences, as the children in the follow-up (mean 75 months and median 76 months) were older than the children who were included (mean 47 months and median 47 months). Younger children may be more susceptible to infection. To try to control the age effect, the final model of effectiveness was adjusted by the variable age.

In summary, the present study showed that the prevalence and incidence of *L. infantum* infection increased during the study period in areas under intervention, indicating that the VLSCP was not effective in reducing asymptomatic infection. In contrast, data from the municipal public health services showed that the human disease decreased over the study period in AI2006 and AI2008 (Additional file 1: Table S1). Regarding the areas evaluated, the incidence of VL cases reported to SINAN varied as follows: AI2006, six cases to one case (13 cases during the period); AI2008, two cases to one case (11 cases during the period); AI2010, only one case was reported in the period. Therefore, evaluating the impact of interventions on the incidence of HVL was impracticable due to the small number of clinical cases. It is important to note that indicators involving rare events may cause distortions in the understanding of the results. The importance of the asymptomatic infected individuals in the epidemiology of the disease remains unclear. We would like to point out that the findings must be interpreted with caution since the intervention period analyzed may be too short to draw a conclusive assessment of the effectiveness of the strategies implemented by the VLSCP. The asymptomatic infection in children is probably an indicator of parasite transmission in a given area and does not predict the occurrence of the human disease, as recently demonstrated in a study conducted in Belo Horizonte [21].

The advantages of our study include the evaluation of the effectiveness of the VLSCP without interrupting or interfering with the programme routine. Therefore, assessing the impact of control actions on reducing human infection becomes more real. when it was carried out concomitantly with the actions of the programme.

Conclusions

Evaluation of the strategies adopted by the VLSCP have shown that the control interventions have not been successful in interrupting *L. infantum* transmission, especially in urban areas. The evaluation of effectiveness performed herein showed that the control measures adopted by the VLSCP did not significantly affect asymptomatic infection levels in three urban areas where the programme had been active for different lengths of time. Although the importance of asymptomatic individuals in areas of active transmission needs to be better investigated, it is unclear what the result on infection and illness would be if the VLSCP strategies were absent in the areas analyzed by the present study. There are gaps in the knowledge regarding the urbanization of VL that hamper the effective action of the control programme in Brazil. Therefore, efforts to optimize and improve the effectiveness of control measures remain a necessary priority.

Abbreviations

AI: Area of intervention; CCEB: Critério de Classificação Socioeconômica do Brasil; CI: Confidence interval; HVL: Human visceral leishmaniasis; IR: Incidence rate; BMW: Brazilian minimum wage; OR: Odds ratio; RR: Incidence ratio rate; SINAN: Sistema de Informação de Agravos de Notificação; VL: Visceral leishmaniasis; VLSCP: Visceral Leishmaniasis Surveillance and Control Programme

Acknowledgments

The authors would like to thank the Health Service of Belo Horizonte (Prefeitura de Belo Horizonte) for the help with the municipal census data collection and the logistics necessary to undertake this work. ICMR is grateful to Fundação de Amparo à Pesquisa de Minas Gerais - FAPEMIG for a doctoral research fellowship during 2011–2012. MC is grateful to Conselho Nacional de Desenvolvimento Cientifico e Técnológico - CNPq-Brazil for the research fellowships.

Funding

This study was supported by the following grants: Conselho Nacional de Desenvolvimento Cientifico e Tecnólogico (CNPQ/Universal 78528/2012-4, CNPQ/Universal 448449/2014-5), Brazilian Ministry of Health/National - Leishmaniasis Control Programme/Fundo Nacional de Saúde (no. 25000.204799/2013-65), and Fundação de Amparo à Pesquisa de Minas Gerais - FAPEMIG through the financial support Pesquisador Mineiro (PPM/2016).

Authors' contributions

Conceived the study design: ICMR, LHMS, MHFM and MC. Performed the data collection: ICMR, LHMS, FCM, TAMS and MHFM. Performed the laboratory analysis: GMRC, TAMS and EO. Analyzed the data: ICMR, WCV, IAR and MC. Wrote the original draft: ICMR, WCV, EO, IAR and MC. All authors read and approved the final manuscript.

Competing interests

The authors declare that they have no competing interests.

Author details

[1]Laboratório de Epidemiologia das Doenças Infecciosas e Parasitárias, Departamento de Parasitologia, Instituto de Ciências Biológicas, Universidade Federal de Minas Gerais, Belo Horizonte, Minas Gerais, Brazil. [2]Secretaria Municipal de Saúde de Belo Horizonte, Belo Horizonte, Minas Gerais, Brazil. [3]Departamento de Análises Clínicas, Pós-graduação em Ciências Farmacêuticas, Escola de Farmácia, Universidade Federal de Ouro Preto, Ouro Preto, Minas Gerais, Brazil. [4]Pós-graduação em Ciências Biológicas, Núcleo de Pesquisa em Ciências Biológicas, Universidade Federal de Ouro Preto, Ouro Preto, Minas Gerais, Brazil. [5]Instituto de Ensino e Pesquisa da Santa Casa Belo Horizonte, Belo Horizonte, Minas Gerais, Brazil. [6]Laboratório de Pesquisas Clínicas, Instituto René Rachou, Fundação Oswaldo Cruz, Belo Horizonte, Minas Gerais, Brazil. [7]Departamento de Estatística, Instituto de Ciências Exatas, Universidade Federal de Minas Gerais, Belo Horizonte, Minas Gerais, Brazil. [8]Pós-graduação em Ciências da Saúde: Infectologia e Medicina Tropical, Faculdade de Medicina, Universidade Federal de Minas Gerais, Belo Horizonte, Minas Gerais, Brazil.

References

1. WHO. Leishmaniasis. Geneva: World Health Organization; 2017. http://www.who.int/mediacentre/factsheets/fs375/en/. Accessed 10 Apr 2017.
2. Alvar J, Velez ID, Bern C, Herrero M, Desjeux P, Cano J, et al. Leishmaniasis worldwide and global estimates of its incidence. PLoS One. 2012;7:e35671.
3. Lainson R, Shaw JJ. Epidemiology and ecology of leishmaniasis in Latin-America. Nature. 1978;273:595–600.
4. Romero GA, Boelaert M. Control of visceral leishmaniasis in Latin America a systematic review. PLoS Negl Trop Dis. 2010;4:e584.
5. Ministério da Saúde, Secretaria de Vigilância em Saúde, Brasília. Manual de vigilância e controle da leishmaniose visceral, 1st ed. 2006. http://bvsms.saude.gov.br/bvs/publicacoes/manual_vigilancia_controle_leish_visceral_2006.pdf. Accessed 15 Dec 2016.
6. Harhay MO, Olliaro PL, Costa DL, Costa CH. Urban parasitology: visceral leishmaniasis in Brazil. Trends Parasitol. 2011;27:403–9.
7. Werneck GL. Forum: geographic spread and urbanization of visceral leishmaniasis in Brazil. Introduction. Cad Saúde Pública. 2008;24:2937–40.
8. Costa CH. How effective is dog culling in controlling zoonotic visceral leishmaniasis? A critical evaluation of the science, politics and ethics behind this public health policy. Rev Soc Bras Med Trop. 2011;44:232–42.
9. Dantas-Torres F, Brandao-Filho SP. Visceral leishmaniasis in Brazil: revisiting paradigms of epidemiology and control. Rev Inst Med Trop Sao Paulo. 2006; 48:151–6.
10. Werneck GL, Costa CH, de Carvalho FA, Pires e Cruz Mdo S, Maguire JH, Castro MC. Effectiveness of insecticide spraying and culling of dogs on the incidence of *Leishmania infantum* infection in humans: a cluster randomized trial in Teresina, Brazil. PLoS Negl Trop Dis. 2014;8:e3172.
11. Genaro O, da Costa CA, Williams P, Silva JE, Rocha NM, Lima SL, et al. Occurrence of kala-azar in the urban area of Grande Belo Horizonte, Minas Gerais. Rev Soc Bras Med Trop. 1990;23:121 (In Portuguese).
12. Fiuza VOP, Brandão ST, Pessanha JEM, Menezes FC, Costa IO, Mesquita DM, et al. Perspectivas para a produção de insumos estratégicos para vigilância e controle das leishmanioses. A situação e as necessidades de grandes centros urbanos no Brasil: o exemplo de Belo Horizonte. Rev Soc Bras Med Trop. 2008;3:82–8.
13. Morais MHF, Fiuza VOP, Araújo VOM, Menezes FC, Carneiro M. Evaluation of visceral leishmaniasis control activities in Belo Horizonte, Minas Gerais, Brazil, 2006–2011. Epidemiol Serv Saúde. 2015;24:485–96 (In Portuguese).
14. Prefeitura Municipal de Belo Horizonte. Vigilância epidemiológica da leishmaniose visceral em Belo Horizonte. 2017. http://portalpbh.pbh.gov.br/pbh/ecp/comunidade.do?evento=portlet&pIdPlc=ecpTaxonomiaMenuPortal&app=saude&lang=pt_BR&pg=5571&tax=16045. Accessed 15 July 2017.
15. Caldas AJ, Silva DR, Pereira CC, Nunes PM, Silva BP, Silva AA, et al. *Leishmania* (*Leishmania*) *chagasi* infection in children from an endemic area of visceral leishmaniasis in the São Luis Island-MA, Brazil. Rev Soc Bras Med Trop. 2001;34:445–51 (In Portuguese).
16. Costa CH, Stewart JM, Gomes RB, Garcez LM, Ramos PK, Bozza M, et al. Asymptomatic human carriers of *Leishmania chagasi*. Am J Trop Med Hyg. 2002;66:334–7.
17. Moreno EC, Melo MN, Lambertucci JR, Serufo JC, Andrade AS, Antunes CM, et al. Diagnosing human asymptomatic visceral leishmaniasis in an urban area of the State of Minas Gerais, using serological and molecular biology techniques. Rev Soc Bras Med Trop. 2006;39:421–7.
18. Nascimento Mdo D, Souza EC, da Silva LM, Leal Pda C, Cantanhede Kde L, Bezerra GF, et al. Prevalence of infection by *Leishmania chagasi* using ELISA (rK39 and CRUDE) and the Montenegro skin test in an endemic leishmaniasis area of Maranhão, Brazil. Cad Saude Publica. 2005;21:1801–7 (In Portuguese).
19. Carneiro M, Moreno EC, Goncalves AV, Lambertucci JR, Antunes CMF. Visceral Leishmaniasis: challenges in identifying subclinical *Leishmania* infection. Drug Develop Res. 2011;72:442–50.
20. dos Santos Marques LH, Gomes LI, da Rocha IC, da Silva TA, Oliveira E, Morais MH, et al. Low parasite load estimated by qPCR in a cohort of children living in urban area endemic for visceral leishmaniasis in Brazil. PLoS Negl Trop Dis. 2012;6:e1955.
21. Dos Santos Marques LH, da Rocha ICM, Reis IA, da Cunha GMR, Oliveira E, Pfeilsticker TR, et al. *Leishmania infantum*: illness, transmission profile and risk factors for asymptomatic infection in an endemic metropolis in Brazil. Parasitology. 2017;144:546–56.
22. Souza VMM, Julião FS, Neves RCS, Magalhães PB, Bisinotto TV, Lima AS, et al. Communitary assay for assessment of effectiveness of strategies for prevention and control of human visceral leishmaniasis in the Municipality of Feira de Santana, State of Bahia, Brazil. Epidemiol Serv Saúde. 2008;17:97–106.
23. IBGE. Instituto Brasileiro de Geografia e Estatística. Censo Demográfico 2010. http://www.ibge.gov.br/. Accessed 10 Mar 2017.
24. IBGE. Censo demográfico por setores sensitários. 2010. ftp://ftp.ibge.gov.br/Censos/Censo_Demografico_2010/Sinopse/. Accessed 10 July 2012.
25. SINAN. DATASUS Leishmaniose visceral - casos confirmados notificados no sistema de informação de agravos de notificação. 2016. http://tabnet.datasus.gov.br/cgi/tabcgi.exe?sinannet/cnv/leishvMG.def. Accessed 15 Mar 2017.
26. Morais MHF, Fiuza VOP, de Araújo VEM, Carneiro M. Vigilância e controle da leishmaniose visceral no contexto urbano. Belo Horizonte: FEPMVZ-Editora; 2012.
27. Romero HD, Silva Lde A, Silva-Vergara ML, Rodrigues V, Costa RT, Guimarães SF, et al. Comparative study of serologic tests for the diagnosis of asymptomatic visceral leishmaniasis in an endemic area. Am J Trop Med Hyg. 2009;81:27–33.
28. Maia Z, Lirio M, Mistro S, Mendes CM, Mehta SR, Badaro R. Comparative study of rK39 *Leishmania* antigen for serodiagnosis of visceral leishmaniasis: systematic review with meta-analysis. PLoS Negl Trop Dis. 2012;6:e1484.
29. Pedras MJ, de Gouvea VL, de Oliveira EJ, Rabello A. Comparative evaluation of direct agglutination test, rK39 and soluble antigen ELISA and IFAT for the diagnosis of visceral leishmaniasis. Trans R Soc Trop Med Hyg. 2008;102:172–8.
30. Associação Brasileira de Empresas de Pesquisa. Critério de classificação econômica Brasil. 2012. http://www.abep.org/criterio-brasil. Accessed 12 Aug 2012.
31. de Araujo VE, Pinheiro LC, Almeida MC, de Menezes FC, Morais MH, Reis IA, et al. Relative risk of visceral leishmaniasis in Brazil: a spatial analysis in urban area. PLoS Negl Trop Dis. 2013;7:e2540.
32. Katz MH. Evaluating clinical and public health interventions. A practical guide to study design and statistics. Cambridge: Cambridge University Press; 2010.
33. Costa CH, Tapety CM, Werneck GL. Control of visceral leishmaniasis in urban areas: randomized factorial intervention trial. Rev Soc Bras Med Trop. 2007; 40:415–9 (In Portuguese).
34. Dietze R, Barros GB, Teixeira L, Harris J, Michelson K, Falqueto A, et al. Effect of eliminating seropositive canines on the transmission of visceral leishmaniasis in Brazil. Clin Infect Dis. 1997;25:1240–2.
35. Quinnell RJ, Courtenay O. Transmission, reservoir hosts and control of zoonotic visceral leishmaniasis. Parasitology. 2009;136:1915–34.
36. Nunes CM, Lima VM, Paula HB, Perri SH, Andrade AM, Dias FE, et al. Dog culling and replacement in an area endemic for visceral leishmaniasis in Brazil. Vet Parasitol. 2008;153:19–23.
37. Zuben AP, Donalisio MR. Difficulties in implementing the guidelines of the Brazilian Visceral Leishmaniasis Control Program in large cities. Cad Saúde Publica. 2016;32:e00087415 (In Portuguese).
38. Moreno EC, Goncalves AV, Chaves AV, Melo MN, Lambertucci JR, Andrade AS, et al. Inaccuracy of enzyme-linked immunosorbent assay using soluble and recombinant antigens to detect asymptomatic infection by *Leishmania infantum*. PLoS Negl Trop Dis. 2009;3:e536.
39. de Gouvea VL, de Assis TS, Orsini M, da Silva AR, de Souza GF, Caligiorne R, et al. Combined diagnostic methods identify a remarkable proportion of asymptomatic *Leishmania* (*Leishmania*) *chagasi* carriers who present modulated cytokine profiles. Trans R Soc Trop Med Hyg. 2008;102:548–55.

20

A randomized, blinded, controlled, multi-centered field study assessing the treatment of gastrointestinal nematode infections in cats with fluralaner plus moxidectin spot-on solution

Nadja Rohdich[1*], Eva Zschiesche[1], Oliver Wolf[2], Wolfgang Loehlein[2], Zvezdelina Kirkova[3], Petar Iliev[3], Dhimitër Rapti[4], Rezart Postoli[5], Balázs Capári[6], Róbert Farkas[7] and Rainer K. A. Roepke[1]

Abstract

Background: A spot-on formulation containing fluralaner (280 mg/ml) plus moxidectin (14 mg/ml) (Bravecto® Plus) was developed for the treatment of nematode infections as well as providing 12 weeks of protection against insect and acarine parasites in cats. The effectiveness and safety of this product against feline gastrointestinal nematodes was assessed in naturally-infested, client-owned cats under field conditions in Albania, Bulgaria, Germany and Hungary.

Methods: To be eligible for enrollment in this investigator-blinded study cats had to be at least 10 weeks-old, weigh at least 1.2 kg, be clinically healthy, and have a faecal sample testing positive for nematodes no more than eight days prior to treatment. Cats were stratified into blocks of three in order of presentation at each center and randomly allocated in a 2:1 ratio to be treated topically on Day 0 with fluralaner plus moxidectin (minimum dose rates 40 mg/kg and 2 mg/kg, respectively) or emodepside plus praziquantel (minimum dose rates 3 mg/kg and 12 mg/kg, respectively) (Profender®). Faecal samples were collected from cats prior to treatment and 14 ± 4 days later.

Results: There were 182 cats randomized to the fluralaner plus moxidectin group, and 91 to the emodepside plus praziquantel group. Prior to treatment the most commonly identified nematode egg was *Toxocara cati*, found in 79.1 and 82.4% of cats in the fluralaner plus moxidectin and emodepside plus praziquantel groups, respectively. Eggs of *Toxascaris leonina* were found in 8.2 and 6.6% of cats; of hookworms in 30.8 and 24.2%; and of *Capillaria* spp. in 7.1 and 4.3%, respectively. After treatment, faecal samples from 98.3% of fluralaner plus moxidectin treated and 96.6% of emodepside plus praziquantel-treated cats were free of nematode ova. Geometric mean faecal egg count reductions for *T. cati*, the only eggs found in post-treatment faecal samples, were 99.97% and 99.93%, respectively. Treatment with fluralaner plus moxidectin was non-inferior to emodepside plus praziquantel. Both products were safe and well tolerated by cats treated under field conditions.

Conclusions: This field study confirms that, in addition to 12-week extended duration flea and tick control, fluralaner plus moxidectin provides broad spectrum treatment of nematodes in cats.

Keywords: Bravecto Plus, Cat, Emodepside, Field study, Fluralaner, Hookworms, Lungworms, Moxidectin, Praziquantel, Roundworms

* Correspondence: nadja.rohdich@msd.de
[1]MSD Animal Health Innovation GmbH, Zur Propstei, 55270 Schwabenheim, Germany
Full list of author information is available at the end of the article

Background

Gastrointestinal nematode infections are common in cats in Europe, with an estimated prevalence of up to 40% [1–7]. Cats are universally at risk of infection, although age and access to the outdoors are clear risk factors. In addition to posing a threat to the health of infected cats, the most commonly occurring nematode, *Toxocara cati*, has zoonotic potential. Therefore, there is a need for vigilance and compliance in the implementation of programs to treat feline nematodes. The European Scientific Counsel Companion Animal Parasites (ESCCAP) recommends that adult cats with access to the outdoors be treated for nematodes at least four times per year [8]. Where there is a higher risk of nematode infection (kittens, adult cats with a predominantly outdoor lifestyle), additional treatment may be given [8, 9].

One of the challenges for veterinarians and cat owners is that nematode infections cannot be seen. While parasites (e.g. eggs, larvae) can be detected in faeces, faecal examinations and faecal diagnostic antigen testing are not routine in general practice. However, a recent survey of cats in seven European countries showed co-infection with fleas and gastrointestinal nematodes in 11.9% of tested cats and found access to the outdoors to be a common risk factor for infection with ecto- and endoparasites [5]. While this should not replace routine faecal examination, so that parasiticide treatment is tailored to suit what the cat needs, the presence of ectoparasites can help to serve as a guide that treatment for endoparasites may also be required.

The introduction of the extended duration isoxazoline fluralaner as a topically applied spot-on product has provided cat owners with an option to provide year-round flea and tick control based on application every 12 weeks. The extended duration of activity of fluralaner provides veterinarians with a means to help improve owner compliance with parasite control recommendations, as well as substantially reducing or even removing the risk of parasite-related disease [10]. In a randomized, controlled field study in client-owned cats in the USA, there was an at least 98.6% reduction in flea counts for 12 weeks following a single topical application of fluralaner [11].

Macrocyclic lactones are a diverse family of systemically active, broad spectrum parasiticides that include both avermectins (ivermectin, selamectin and eprinomectin) and milbemycins (milbemycin oxime and moxidectin). The macrocyclic lactones have a spectrum of activity that includes insects, arachnids and nematodes, depending on the agent and species. While macrocyclic lactones have a long half-life and large apparent volume of distribution (greater than the total body water volume), meaning that they are able to penetrate tissues of the body, this varies considerably between agents [12]. Moxidectin, at a dose rate of 1 mg/kg, has been used in cats as a monthly combination product with imidacloprid (for the control of fleas) for the prevention of heartworm disease and treatment of larvae, immature and adult roundworm and hookworm, and the lungworm *Eucoleus aerophilus* (also known as *Capillaria aerophila*) [13, 14]. Now, at a minimum dose rate of 2 mg/kg, moxidectin has been combined with fluralaner into a low-volume, spot-on formulation for cats (Bravecto® Plus, MSD Animal Health). This extended duration, topical product has been approved as being safe and effective for use in cats in Europe and New Zealand, where it is indicated, depending on the geography, for the treatment of flea, tick and ear mite infestations, for the prevention of heartworm disease caused by *Dirofilaria immitis*, and for the treatment of nematode (roundworm, hookworm and lungworm) infections in cats [15, 16]. A field study in Europe demonstrated that a single application of fluralaner plus moxidectin to client-owned cats provided 12 weeks efficacy against fleas and ticks that was superior to the flea control provided by three consecutive monthly applications of fipronil, and non-inferior to fipronil in controlling ticks [17]. To assess the internal parasite control provided by this formulation for cats, a Good Clinical Practice (GCP) compliant field study was initiated in four countries in Europe, Albania, Bulgaria, Germany and Hungary, to evaluate the safety and efficacy against natural infections of gastrointestinal nematodes. In this study, the nematode control provided by a single application of fluralaner plus moxidectin was compared with that provided by a single application of emodepside plus praziquantel (Profender®, Bayer Animal Health).

Methods

Study design

This multi-center study was conducted from June through December, 2015. Cat owners provided informed consent prior to the enrollment of any cat into the study and the initiation of treatment. Individuals involved in treatment assignments and in treatment administration were not masked during the study and were not involved in clinical assessments. The study personnel making clinical observations and parasitologists examining faecal samples were masked to treatment assignments.

Animals

Healthy cats, at least 10 weeks old and weighing at least 1.2 kg, were eligible for inclusion. To qualify, a positive faecal worm egg count was required, collected no more than eight days prior to the day of treatment, for gastrointestinal nematode parasites (roundworms, and/or hookworms, or other). Cats with a chronic medical condition could be included at the discretion of the Investigator. Cats could not have been treated with any anthelmintic or endectocide within 14 days before the start of the study, and treatment with any other drug from these classes was not permitted during the study. Evidence of skin disease, either generalized or at the intended product application site, was a basis for exclusion from the study, as were pregnancy or lactation. Routine health procedures, such as vaccination, and medical care were permitted. Cats were maintained by owners in the home environment or were retained in an animal shelter. If needed, cats were housed individually at the study site or in the animal shelter for collection or correct identification of faecal samples.

Randomization and treatment

Cat enrollment numbers, set in accordance with current anthelmintic evaluation guidelines, planned for a 2:1 ratio randomization of 134 cats to the fluralaner plus moxidectin group and 67 to the emodepside plus praziquantel group [18]. With an estimated drop-out rate of approximately 10%, the number of cats to be included was therefore 150 in the fluralaner plus moxidectin group and 75 in the emodepside plus praziquantel group. In order of presentation at each site, cats eligible for inclusion were stratified by the Investigator into blocks of three and randomly allocated to a treatment group, using computer generated randomization lists. Treatment was administered on a single occasion, on Day 0, taking care to avoid product run-off by parting the hair and applying it directly to the skin, in one or two spots in an area from the base of the skull to between the shoulder blades. The minimum dose rates were 40 mg fluralaner plus 2 mg moxidectin/kg and, according to the manufacturer' instructions, 3 mg emodepside plus 12 mg praziquantel/kg.

Faecal egg counts

Cats were presented for faecal sampling up to 8 days prior to and 14 + 4 days after treatment. Faecal samples from each cat were either sent to a local designated laboratory or were examined on site. Nematode eggs were counted using the modified McMaster method. For flotation, either zinc sulphate solution (Albania, Hungary), sodium chloride solution (Bulgaria), or zinc chloride/sodium chloride solution (Germany) was used. Flotation solutions were adjusted to a specific gravity of 1.3 in Germany and Albania and 1.18 in Bulgaria and Hungary. The sensitivity of counting techniques was 25 (Albania) or 50 eggs per gram of faeces (epg) (Bulgaria, Hungary, Germany). The amount of faeces used for each test was 2 g (Bulgaria), 3 g (Albania, Hungary) or 4 g (Germany). Identification of parasites was based on the distinct morphology of the ova found in the faeces. Hookworms were identified to genus and species in Albania and Germany but not in Bulgaria and Hungary.

Efficacy assessment

The efficacy of each product was calculated for all of the cats that received at least one treatment and were examined according to the protocol (per-protocol (PP) population). The safety of each product was assessed for all cats that were treated (intent-to-treat (ITT) population). The statistical unit was the individual cat. Homogeneity of study groups at inclusion was evaluated descriptively in both the ITT and PP populations as a confirmatory indicator of the quality of randomization and allocation of cats to treatment groups. Pre-treatment means (Day 0) for individual age and weight were calculated for both study groups, as were means, standard errors, minima, and maxima for faecal egg counts (FEC) of each nematode genus and/or species. The comparison of FEC distributions by nematode species was restricted to those animals positive for the respective nematode. Frequency tables were used to compare the distribution of sex, breed and living conditions in both study groups.

The primary efficacy criterion for each group was the percent reduction in FEC for each nematode genus and/or species calculated for geometric and arithmetic means using the formula:

$$\text{Efficacy}\,(\%) = \left(\overline{X}_{g\,(\text{pre-treatment})} - \overline{X}_{g(\text{post-treatment})}\right) / \overline{X}_{g(\text{pre-treatment})} \times 100$$

where X_g is the mean FEC of each group. To address possible zero counts, the geometric means were calculated as follows:

$$X_g = \left(\prod_{i=1}^{n}(X_i + 1)\right)^{\frac{1}{n}} - 1$$

To compensate for the skewed distribution, the FEC was log-transformed and shifted prior to the statistical test: $x_i' = \log(x_i + 1)$. Pre- and post-treatment FECs were compared using a two-sided, two sample t-test for paired samples ($\alpha = 0.05$). Efficacy for a nematode species was claimed if a FEC reduction of at least 90% was demonstrated for each nematode species in 10 cats that were initially positive for that species, and if there was a significant difference between pre- and post-treatment FEC.

Secondary efficacy was based upon the proportion of cats that had FECs of zero post-treatment. Non-inferiority was determined by comparing the percent of nematode-free cats after treatment with fluralaner plus moxidectin with the percent nematode free after treatment with emodepside praziquantel. The Farrington-Manning test of non-inferiority for the risk difference was used with a level of significance of $\alpha = 0.025$ and a tolerated difference of δ

= 0.15 [19]. Both *P*-value and lower 97.5% one-sided confidence limits were calculated. If the lower confidence limit was above -0.15, non-inferiority was concluded. If the lower confidence limit was above 0, superiority of fluralaner plus moxidectin over emodepside plus praziquantel was concluded.

Results

Faecal samples from 838 cats were screened and 273 cats (32.6%) had positive FECs. There were 182 cats included in the fluralaner plus moxidectin group, and 91 cats in the emodepside plus praziquantel group. In the ITT population there were 50 cats from Albania, 60 from Bulgaria, 65 from Germany and 98 from Hungary. More than 90% of enrolled cats in each group were described as either domestic or European, and 61.5% were two years of age or less (11.7% were older than five years), with cats from 11 or 12 weeks of age up to 15 years enrolled in both groups. Ten cats from the ITT population were excluded from the PP population: five cats because the pre-treatment sample was negative (should not have been enrolled), two because of a protocol deviation, one was lost to follow up, and one died in a road traffic accident.

There was homogeneity between the groups for both the ITT and PP populations. In the fluralaner plus moxidectin group, 23% of cats were reported as indoor only, while the equivalent number for the emodepside plus praziquantel group was 14%. For cats reported to be outdoor only, the proportions were 37% and 41%, respectively. The remainder of cats (41% and 45%, respectively) were reported by their owners to spend time both indoors and outdoors. Mean body weights were 4.2 kg and 4.1 kg, respectively, with a minimum of 1.2 kg in each group, and maximum of 6.6 kg in the fluralaner plus moxidectin group and 5.5 kg in the emodepside plus praziquantel group. Males comprised 49% of cats in the fluralaner plus moxidectin group and 53% of cats in the emodepside plus praziquantel group, and neutered cats comprised 28% and 31% of cats in the fluralaner plus moxidectin and emodepside plus praziquantel groups, respectively.

From 273 positive pre-treatment faecal samples the most commonly identified nematode was *T. cati*, eggs of which were identified in 79.1 and 82.4% of the cats in the fluralaner plus moxidectin and emodepside plus praziquantel groups, respectively. The maximum FEC for *T. cati* was 10,100 epg in the fluralaner plus moxidectin group, and 5700 in the emodepside plus praziquantel group (Table 1). Prior to treatment 8.2% of cats in the fluralaner plus moxidectin group and 6.6% of the emodepside plus praziquantel group tested positive for *Toxascaris leonina*. Hookworms were found in 30.8 and 24.2% of cats, respectively. The clinics in Germany and Albania, where hookworms were differentiated to genus and species level, showed that *Ancylostoma tubaeforme* was the most commonly identified genus, found in 21 cats in the fluralaner plus moxidectin group and five cats in the emodepside plus praziquantel group. *Uncinaria stenocephala* was found less commonly; in five and three cats, respectively. *Capillaria* spp. were found in 7.1 and 4.3% of cats, respectively.

Treatment was followed by a reduction in the geometric mean FEC for *T. cati* of 99.97% in the fluralaner plus moxidectin and 99.93% in the emodepside plus praziquantel groups (Table 1). In fact, *T. cati* were the only nematode eggs found in faeces from both groups after treatment. For arithmetic means, the respective reductions in *T. cati* ova were 98.75 and 72.22%, with the substantially lower efficacy in the emodepside plus praziquantel group due to the count in one cat with an FEC of 11,950 epg. Both products were 100% effective in eliminating hookworm ova. In the fluralaner plus moxidectin group, the FECs two weeks after treatment were significantly lower for each parasite ($P < 0.0001$) than baseline counts (Table 2). The primary objectives of (i) at least 90% efficacy per nematode species in 10 cats that were positive for a nematode species before treatment, and (ii) significant differences from baseline for all nematode species were met by fluralaner plus moxidectin treatment. In the fluralaner plus moxidectin group, 98.3% of cats were free of ova of all nematode species that had been present prior to treatment (Table 3). The percent of nematode-free cats in the fluralaner plus moxidectin group was significantly non-inferior to that in the emodepside plus praziquantel group (96.5%). In addition, the lower 97.5% one-sided confidence limit was well above the non-inferiority limit of -0.15, thereby meeting the secondary efficacy objective of the study (Table 3).

The presence of eggs of the lungworm species *Capillaria* spp. in the faeces of study cats allowed assessment of efficacy against this parasite. The results indicate that both fluralaner plus moxidectin and emodepside plus praziquantel were 100% effective in eliminating *Capillaria* spp. ova from the faeces of infected cats.

Both products were well tolerated by cats. Six mild adverse events were reported during the study, four in the fluralaner plus moxidectin group and two in the emodepside plus praziquantel group. Two of the four events (mild alopecia at the application site in one cat and a small area of whitish discoloration of the hair on the neck in one cat) in the fluralaner plus moxidectin group (1% of treated cats in this group) were considered to be probably related to treatment. The other two events involved the withdrawal of the cat that died in a road traffic accident and one cat that developed diarrhea. The two cats from the emodepside plus praziquantel group

Table 1 Geometric (arithmetic) mean faecal egg counts and percent reduction (per protocol population)

Group	Species	Pre-treatment		Post-treatment		Efficacy (%)
		Range	Mean	Range	Mean	
Fluralaner / moxidectin	*Toxocara cati*	25–10,100	407.29 (788.38)	0–1100	0.13 (9.86)	99.97 (98.75)
	Toxascaris leonina	50–2000	126.36 (250.00)	0	0 (0)	100 (100)
	Capillaria spp.	50–800	126.09 (173.21)	0	0 (0)	100 (100)
	Hookworm spp.[a]	50–11,400	252.01 (660.91)	0	0 (0)	100 (100)
Emodepside / praziquantel	*Toxocara cati*	50–5700	280.90 (591.78)	0–11,950	0.20 (164.38)	99.93 (72.22)
	Toxascaris leonina	75– 250	155.47 (170.83)	0	0 (0)	100 (100)
	Capillaria spp.	50–150	95.96 (106.25)	0	0 (0)	100 (100)
	Hookworm spp.[a]	50–1650	201.12 (329.55)	0	0 (0)	100 (100)

[a]Hookworm spp. include *Ancylostoma tubaeforme* and *Uncinaria stenocephala*

had mild diarrhea that was considered to be unrelated to treatment. No serious, treatment-related adverse events occurred in either treatment group.

Discussion

The results of the present study in Europe demonstrate that a single treatment with fluralaner plus moxidectin is highly effective against nematodes that infect cats. The findings are consistent with earlier reports that roundworm and hookworm infections are common in cats (approximately 3 of every 10 cats screened had nematode eggs in faeces), with the roundworm *T. cati* being the most prevalent [1–7]. The study showed that the efficacy of fluralaner and moxidectin was non-inferior to emodepside plus praziquantel. The results of this field study are in line with and further confirm those of a laboratory study in which a topical formulation of imidacloprid in combination with moxidectin (1%) was shown to be effective against experimental infections with *T. cati* and larval stages of *A. tubaeforme* [13].

Infection with respiratory nematodes occurs in cats in Europe. *Aelurostrongylus abstrusus* (3–5% of surveyed cats) and *Capillaria* spp, (1–2%), in particular *Capillaria aerophila* (also known as *Eucoleus aerophilus),* have been reported to be a cause of respiratory disease, as has *Troglostrongylus brevior* [5, 6]. However, prevalence rates vary and can range from around 5 to 20%, with access to the outdoors, but not age, being a risk factor [5]. The methodology in our study focused on nematode ova and not on detecting other faecal parasite stages, and so would not have detected larvae of *A. abstrusus*. Additionally, *Capillaria* eggs found in the faeces may be produced by *C. aerophila*, parasitic in the trachea and bronchi, and/or by *C. putorii* (the cat stomach worm) which inhabits the gastrointestinal tract. Nonetheless, the finding of ova of *Capillaria* spp., not identified to species level, in faecal samples from 6.8% of cats enrolled in our study are in line with earlier reports. In the fluralaner plus moxidectin group, the faeces of 14 cats

Table 2 Number of cats with positive faecal egg counts and, for the fluralaner-moxidectin group, comparison of pre- and post-treatment faecal egg counts, per protocol population

Group	Nematode species	Number positive		Difference post- *vs* pre-treatment[b]		Probability
		Pre-treatment	Post-treatment	Mean	SE	
Fluralaner / moxidectin	*Toxocara cati*	142	3 (97.89%)	5.8920	0.1130	$t_{(141)} = 52.13$; $P < 0.0001$
	Toxascaris leonina	15	0 (100%)	4.8470	0.2520	$t_{(14)} = 19.24$; $P < 0.0001$
	Capillaria spp.	14	0 (100%)	4.8449	0.1996	$t_{(13)} = 24.28$; $P < 0.0001$
	Hookworm spp.[a]	55	0 (100%)	5.5334	0.1534	$t_{(54)} = 36.07$; $P < 0.0001$
Emodepside / praziquantel	*Toxocara cati*	73	2 (97.26%)			
	Toxascaris leonina	6	0 (100%)			
	Capillaria spp.	4	0 (100%)			
	Hookworm spp.[a]	22	0 (100%)			

[a]Hookworm spp. include *Anyclostoma tubaeforme* and *Uncinaria stenocephala*
[b]Differences not calculated for emodepside/praziquantel
Abbreviation: SE, standard error

Table 3 Percent of nematode free cats, with non-inferiority analysis at the post-treatment assessment (per protocol population)

	Presence of faecal eggs		97.5% lower confidence limit	Z-value	P-value
	Yes	No			
Fluralaner / moxidectin	3 (1.70%)	173 (98.30%)	-0.0964	3.2899	0.0005
Emodepside / praziquantel	3 (3.45%)	84 (96.55%)			

Margin = 0.15; Farrington-Manning method

were positive for *Capillaria* spp., with a geometric mean count of 135.34 epg. The complete post-treatment elimination of these ova is consistent with earlier work showing that a topical formulation of moxidectin (combined with imidacloprid) at the dose rate of 1 mg/kg eliminated *Capillaria* spp. ova from infected cats [20, 21]. The results therefore confirm that that moxidectin is highly active against *Capillaria* spp. Similarly, in the emodepside plus praziquantel group, there were no *Capillaria* spp. ova in post-treatment faecal samples, although only four cats were positive pre-treatment when FECs (up to 150 epg) were much lower than in the fluralaner plus moxidectin group (up to 800 epg).

In our study, we did not investigate infections with species of the Dipylidiidae and Taeniidae, which may occur in up to 7% of cats in Europe [5]. The two most commonly recognized of these cestodes, *Dipylidium caninum* and less so *Taenia taeniaformis*, are typically associated with infection in the cat, which is regarded as being epidemiologically insignificant in the transmission of a third tapeworm, *Echinococcus multilocularis* [5, 8]. As neither fluralaner nor moxidectin, nor the families of isoxazolines and macrocyclic lactones to which they belong, have demonstrated evidence of activity against cestode infections, cat owners seeking control of these parasites would need to explore additional treatment options. Elimination of infections with *D. caninum* can be achieved by treatment with praziquantel, while effective flea control presents an ideal means of preventing further infection which occurs through oral ingestion of infected fleas. Praziquantel is also effective in the treatment of infection with *T. taeniaformis*, which is most likely to occur in cats that hunt on a regular basis and so are exposed through consumption of infected intermediate hosts (e.g. rodents) [8]. When treatment of feline cestode infections is required, a praziquantel-containing product administered concomitantly with fluralaner plus moxidectin has been shown to be safe [22, 23].

Regular treatment of gastrointestinal nematodes is recommended not only because of the potential clinical impact of roundworms and hookworms but also as a hygienic measure and to decrease the risk of zoonotic transmission of *T. cati* and *Ancylostoma* spp. [8]. An important benefit of the fluralaner plus moxidectin formulation for cats is that treatment at 12-week intervals not only simplifies the provision of flea and tick control but also, with approximately four treatments per annum, provides broad spectrum treatment of nematodes that is in line with the recommendations of opinion-leading organizations in this field, such as ESCCAP. In higher-risk situations, additional anthelmintic treatments can be built-in to a tailored parasite control program for an individual cat, as required. This simplifies the treatment regimen for the cat owner as well as avoiding potential over-treatment of nematode parasites that may occur when products that require monthly application for tick and/or flea control, such as the combinations of fipronil, (*S*)-methoprene, eprinomectin and praziquantel, imidacloprid and moxidectin, and selamectin with or without sarolaner, are used.

The safety of both fluralaner and moxidectin in cats, as single entity or combination products, has been well established in field and laboratory studies over years of use [11, 13, 14, 17, 20–23]. This study confirmed that fluralaner plus moxidectin (at dose rates from 40–93 mg fluralaner and 2–4.65 mg moxidectin/kg) and emodepside plus praziquantel were safe and well tolerated by cats under field conditions.

Conclusions

This extended duration fluralaner plus moxidectin product, with 12-week efficacy against fleas and ticks, has been confirmed under field conditions to be safe and effective in the treatment of broad range of nematodes in cats.

Abbreviations

epg: eggs per gram of faeces; ESCCAP: European Scientific Counsel Companion Animal Parasites; FEC: faecal egg count; ITT: intent-to-treat; PP: per protocol; $\bar{X}_g$: denotes the mean faecal egg count

Acknowledgments

The authors would like to thank the participating veterinarians and clinics for collecting the data and Dr Bill Ryan of Ryan Mitchell Associates LLC and Dr Linda Horspool for guidance and support with preparation of the manuscript.

Funding

The study was funded by MSD Animal Health.

Authors' contributions

NR, EZ and RKAR authored the study design and protocol. The study was conducted by NR, OW, WL, ZK, IP, DR, RP, BC and RF, and EZ completed the statistical calculations. All authors revised, read and approved the final manuscript.

Competing interests
NR, EZ and RKAR are employees of MSD Animal Health. OW, WL, ZK, PI, DR, RP, BC and RF declare that they have no competing interests.

Author details
[1]MSD Animal Health Innovation GmbH, Zur Propstei, 55270 Schwabenheim, Germany. [2]Loehlein & Wolf Vet Research, Maistrasse 69, 80337 Munich, Germany. [3]Department of Parasitology, Trakia University, Faculty of Veterinary Medicine, Student Campus, 6000 Stara Zagora, Bulgaria. [4]Klinika Veterinare Xhimi, Bulevardi Bajram Curri Nr 2, Tirana, Albania. [5]Faculty of Veterinary Medicine, Agricultural University, Kodër Kamëz, Tirana, Albania. [6]Kapriol Bt, Vak Bottyán St.1, 8330 Suemeg, Hungary. [7]Department of Parasitology and Zoology, Faculty of Veterinary Science, Szent István University, István u. 2, 1078 Budapest VII, Hungary.

References
1. Mircean V, Titilincu A, Vasile C. Prevalence of endoparasites in household cat (*Felis catus*) populations from Transylvania (Romania) and association with risk factors. Vet Parasitol. 2010;171:163–6.
2. Barutzki D, Schaper R. Results of parasitological examinations of faecal samples from cats and dogs in Germany between 2003 and 2010. Parasitol Res. 2011; 109:S45–60.
3. Capári B, Hamel D, Visser M, Winter R, Pfister K, Rehbein S. Parasitic infections of domestic cats, *Felis catus*, in western Hungary. Vet Parasitol. 2013;192:33–42.
4. Knaus M, Rapti D, Shukullari E, Kusi I, Postoli R, Xhaxhiu D, et al. Characterisation of ecto- and endoparasites in domestic cats from Tirana, Albania. Parasitol Res. 2014;113:3361–71.
5. Beugnet F, Bourdeau P, Chalvet-Monfray K, Cozma V, Farkas R, Guillot J, et al. Parasites of domestic owned cats in Europe: co-infestations and risk factors. Parasit Vectors. 2014;25(7):291.
6. Giannelli A, Capelli G, Joachim A, Hinney B, Losson B, Kirkova Z, et al. Lungworms and gastrointestinal parasites of domestic cats: a European perspective. Int J Parasitol. 2017;47:517–28.
7. Symeonidou I, Gelasakis AI, Arsenopoulos K, Angelou A, Beugnet F, Papadopoulos E. Feline gastrointestinal parasitism in Greece: emergent zoonotic species and associated risk factors. Parasit Vectors. 2018;11:4.
8. European Scientific Counsel Companion Animal Parasites. ESCCAP Guideline 1: Worm control in dogs and cats. 3rd edition. 2017. https://www.esccap.org/. Accessed 30 March, 2018.
9. Raue K, Heuer L, Böhm C, Wolken S, Epe C, Strube C. 10-year parasitological examination results (2003 to 2012) of faecal samples from horses, ruminants, pigs, dogs, cats, rabbits and hedgehogs. Parasitol Res. 2017;116:3315–30.
10. Lavan RP, Tunceli K, Zhang D, Normile D, Armstrong R. Assessment of dog owner adherence to veterinarians' flea and tick prevention recommendations in the United States using a cross-sectional survey. Parasit Vectors. 2017;10:284.
11. Meadows C, Guerino F, Sun F. A randomized, blinded, controlled USA field study to assess the use of fluralaner topical solution in controlling feline flea infestations. Parasit Vectors. 2017;10:37.
12. Prichard R, Ménez C, Lespine A. Moxidectin and the avermectins: consanguinity but not identity. Int J Parasitol Drugs Drug Resist. 2012;2:134–53.
13. Arther RG, Charles S, Ciszewski DK, Davis WL, Settje TS. Imidacloprid/moxidectin topical solution for the prevention of heartworm disease and the treatment and control of flea and intestinal nematodes of cats. Vet Parasitol. 2005;133:219–25.
14. Venco L, Mortarino M, Carro C, Genchi M, Pampurini F, Genchi C. Field efficacy and safety of a combination of moxidectin and imidacloprid for the prevention of feline heartworm (*Dirofilaria immitis*) infection. Vet Parasitol. 2008;154:67–70.
15. European Medicines Agency, Committee for Medicinal Products for Veterinary Use. Summary of opinion (initial authorization). 2018. http://www.ema.europa.eu/docs/en_GB/document_library/Summary_of_opinion_-_Initial_authorisation/veterinary/004440/WC500245923.pdf. Accessed 14 June 2018.
16. Ministry for Primary Industries, ACVM register, authorization 13. September 2017. https://eatsafe.nzfsa.govt.nz/web/public/acvm-register. Accessed 14 June 2018.
17. Rohdich N, Zschiesche E, Wolf O, Loehlein W, Pobel T, Gil MJ, et al. Field effectiveness and safety of fluralaner plus moxidectin (Bravecto® Plus) against ticks and fleas: a European randomized, blinded, multicenter field study in naturally-infected client-owned cats. Parasit Vectors. 2018 (In Press).
18. Jacobs DE, Arakawa A, Courtney CH, Gemmell MA, McCall JW, Myers GH, et al. World Association for the Advancement of Veterinary Parasitology (W.A.A.V.P) guidelines for evaluating the efficacy of anthelmintics for dogs and cats. Vet Parasitol. 1994;52:179–202.
19. Farrington CP, Manning G. Test statistics and sample size formulae for comparative binomial trials with null hypothesis of non-zero risk difference or non-unity relative risk. Stat Med. 1990;9:1447–54.
20. Traversa D, Di Cesare A, Di Giulio E, Castagna G, Schaper R, Braun G, et al. Efficacy and safety of imidacloprid 10%/moxidectin 1% spot-on formulation in the treatment of feline infection by *Capillaria aerophila*. Parasitol Res. 2012;111:1793–8.
21. Di Cesare A, Veronesi F, Capelli G, Deuster K, Schaper R, Basano FS, et al. Evaluation of the efficacy and safety of an imidacloprid 10% / moxidectin 1% spot-on formulation (Advocate®, Advantage® Multi) in cats naturally infected with *Capillaria aerophila*. Parasitol Res. 2017;116:55–64.
22. Krüdewagen EM, Remer C, Deuster K, Schunack B, Wolken S, Crafford D, et al. Chemical compatibility and safety of imidacloprid/flumethrin collar (Seresto®) concomitantly used with imidacloprid/moxidectin (Advocate®, Advantage® Multi) and emodepside/praziquantel (Profender®) spot-on formulations. Parasitol Res. 2015;114(Suppl. 1):S55–80.
23. Walther FM, Allan MJ, Roepke RK. Safety of concurrent treatment of cats with fluralaner and emodepside-praziquantel. Parasit Vectors. 2016;9:322.

Seroprevalence and current infections of canine vector-borne diseases in Nicaragua

Andrea Springer[1], Victor M. Montenegro[2], Sabine Schicht[1], Nikola Pantchev[3] and Christina Strube[1*]

Abstract

Background: Vector-borne diseases constitute a major problem for veterinary and public health, especially in tropical regions like Central America. Domestic dogs may be infected with several vector-borne pathogens of zoonotic relevance, which may also severely compromise canine health.

Methods: To assess the prevalence of canine vector-borne diseases in Nicaragua, 329 dogs from seven cities, which were presented to the veterinarian for various reasons, were included in this study. Dogs were examined clinically and diagnostic blood samples were taken for analysis of packed cell volume (PCV) and presence of microfilariae as well as antigen of *Dirofilaria immitis* and antibodies to *Ehrlichia* spp., *Anaplasma* spp. and *Borrelia burgdorferi* (*sensu lato*) by use of a commercially available rapid ELISA. To detect current infections, specific PCRs for the detection of *E. canis*, *A. platys* and *A. phagocytophilum* were carried out on blood samples of the respective seropositive dogs. Microfilaremic blood samples, as well as *D. immitis* antigen positive samples were further subjected to PCR and subsequent sequencing for filarial species identification.

Results: Antibodies against *Ehrlichia* spp. were present in 62.9% of dogs, while *Anaplasma* spp. seroprevalence was 28. 6%. Antibodies against species of both genera were detected in 24.9% of dogs. *Borrelia burgdorferi* (*s.l.*) antibodies were not detected. *Dirofilaria immitis* antigen was present in six animals (1.8%), two of which also showed *D. immitis* microfilariae in buffy coat. In addition to *D. immitis*, *Acanthocheilonema reconditum* was identified by PCR and sequencing in two of four additional microfilaremic blood samples, which were tested negative for *D. immitis* antigen. Current *E. canis* infections as defined by DNA detection were present in 58.5% of *Ehrlichia*-seropositive dogs, while 5.3% of *Anaplasma*-seropositive dogs were PCR-positive for *A. platys*, 2.2% for *A. phagocytophilum* and 16.0% for both *Anaplasma* species. Current *E. canis* infection had a statistically significant negative impact on PCV, whereas no relationship between infection status and clinical signs of disease could be observed.

Conclusions: These results indicate that canine vector-borne diseases are widespread in Nicaragua and that dogs may constitute a reservoir for human infection with *E. canis*, *A. phagocytophilum* and *D. immitis*. Thus, the use of repellents or acaricides to protect dogs from vector-borne diseases is strongly recommended.

Keywords: Vector-borne diseases, Tick-borne diseases, Ticks, Zoonoses, *Rickettsia* spp., *Ehrlichia* spp., *Anaplasma* spp., Central America

Background

Vector-borne pathogens constitute an important problem for veterinary and public health, especially in tropical regions where the climate is ideal for vectors such as ticks and mosquitoes [1]. Domestic dogs may be affected by several vector-borne diseases, including leishmaniosis, babesiosis, ehrlichiosis, anaplasmosis and canine heartworm disease, which may severely compromise canine health. Clinical signs are often unspecific, including fever, lymphadenopathy or weight loss with haematologic abnormalities including anaemia and thrombocytopenia [2]. Co-infections are common in endemic areas and may alter and/or potentiate clinical signs, complicating diagnosis and treatment [3]. However, dogs may also be infected without showing any signs of disease or haematologic abnormalities [4].

* Correspondence: christina.strube@tiho-hannover.de
[1]Institute for Parasitology, Centre for Infection Medicine, University of Veterinary Medicine Hannover, Buenteweg 17, 30559 Hannover, Germany
Full list of author information is available at the end of the article

Many canine vector-borne diseases are of major zoonotic concern, including Lyme borreliosis, granulocytic anaplasmosis, ehrlichiosis and spotted-fever rickettsioses. Dogs may act as reservoirs and sentinels for human infection with these pathogens [4, 5]. In consequence, surveillance of canine vector-borne diseases may reveal infection risks for humans and potential disease emergence foci [2, 6]. For example, *Borrelia burgdorferi* seroprevalence in dogs in the USA was higher in areas with a large number of human Lyme borreliosis cases [7]. Similarly, dogs living in areas associated with human rickettsiosis outbreaks in Costa Rica showed a higher *Rickettsia* seroprevalence than dogs elsewhere [8].

For Central America, prevalence data on canine vector-borne diseases are relatively scarce. In recent years, surveys have been published for Costa Rica [9–11] and Panama [12, 13], demonstrating a high prevalence of *Ehrlichia* spp., followed by *Anaplasma* spp. infections. Furthermore, *Dirofilaria immitis* infections were detected in Costa Rica, with a high regional prevalence in provinces along the Pacific coast [9, 11]. Comparable prevalence rates for *Ehrlichia* spp., *Anaplasma* spp. and *D. immitis* were also detected in Mexico [14]. Regarding Nicaragua, which borders Costa Rica to the north, comparable large-scale studies are lacking. Only a small-scale study (n = 39 dogs) has been conducted so far [15].

Therefore, seroprevalence of antibodies to *Ehrlichia* spp., *Anaplasma* spp. and *B. burgdorferi* (*sensu lato*) as well as antigen of *D. immitis* in dogs from seven different localities in Nicaragua was assessed in this study. Seropositive dogs were further tested by pathogen-specific PCRs for current infections, and relationships with clinical signs were explored.

Methods

Clinical examination and sampling of dogs

From September to October 2013, 329 dogs which were presented at veterinary clinics for various reasons were clinically examined and sampled in seven different cities in western Nicaragua. Four of these cities are located in the Pacific lowlands (Chinandega, León, Managua and Masaya), one at the Pacific coast (Corinto) and two in the central highlands (Jinotega and Juigalpa, Fig. 1). Per city, 31–83 dogs were sampled (Table 1). Most dogs were presented by their owners, whereas only in Managua, 12 dogs from an animal shelter were included in the study. Inclusion criteria for the dogs were the following: more than six months of age; not treated with ivermectin during the last six months nor with doxycycline during the last 12 months; and consent of the owner to use surplus samples for further examinations. Sex, age and breed of each dog were noted and a clinical examination was carried out. Diagnostic blood samples were taken from the cephalic or jugular vein and collected into serum and EDTA tubes. Packed cell volume (PCV) was determined by glass capillary centrifugation of EDTA blood. Remaining EDTA blood and serum was stored at -20 °C for further analyses.

Screening of blood samples for vector-borne pathogens

Canine serum samples were tested for antibodies against *Anaplasma* spp., *Ehrlichia* spp. and *B. burgdorferis* (*s.l.*), as well as antigen of *D. immitis*, by use of a commercially available rapid ELISA (SNAP® 4Dx® Plus, IDEXX Laboratories Inc., Westbrook, ME, USA). According to Stillman et al. [16] the sensitivity and specificity of the test system are 93.2 and 99.2% for *A. phagocytophilum*, 89.2 and 99.2% for *A. platys*, 96.7 and 98.8% for *B. burgdorferi* (*s.l.*), 97.8 and 92.3% for *E. canis*, and 98.9 and 99.3% for *D. immitis*. Furthermore, a cross-reactivity of *E. canis* antigens with anti-*E. chaffeensis* antibodies was shown. Due to documented cross-reactivity between *A. phagocytophilum* and *A. platys* [17], as well as the reactivity to *E. canis*, *E. chaffeensis* and *E. ewingii* [16, 18], we refer to *Anaplasma* spp. and *Ehrlichia* spp. as results in the present study. Additionally, buffy coat of all dogs was investigated microscopically for presence of microfilariae. This technique has a comparable sensitivity to the Knott's test, if at least 25 microfilariae are present per ml of blood sample [19].

To determine which *Anaplasma*- and *Ehrlichia*-seropositive dogs were currently infected (as defined by DNA detection) with *E. canis*, *A. phagocytophilum* and *A. platys*, respectively, species-specific PCRs were carried out. DNA was isolated from blood samples using the Nucleospin® 8 Blood Kit (Macherey-Nagel GmbH & Co. KG, Düren, Germany) according to the manufacturer's instructions.

Samples were tested for *A. phagocytophilum* by employing a nested PCR targeting a 546 bp fragment of the *16S* rRNA gene. Primers used were ge3a and ge10r in a first and ge9f and ge2 in a second PCR round [20]. In each round, the 12.5 µl reaction volume contained 6.25 µl DreamTaq® PCR Mastermix (Thermo Fisher Scientific Inc., Waltham, MA, USA), 0.5 µl of each primer (10 µM each), 4.25 µl deionized water and 1 µl template DNA. In the second round, template DNA was represented by the PCR product of the first round. The thermoprofile was the same for both rounds and consisted of an initial denaturation step at 95 °C for 2 min, followed by 40 cycles at 95 °C for 30 s, 55 °C for 30 s and 72 °C for 1 min, and a final elongation step at 72 °C for 5 min.

To detect *A. platys*, a nested PCR targeting a 678 bp fragment of the *16S* rRNA gene was carried out using primer sets 8F and 1448R for a first and EHR16SR and PLATYS for a second PCR round [21]. Oligonucleotide concentration and reaction set-up were as described above except that 2.5 µl template DNA was used and

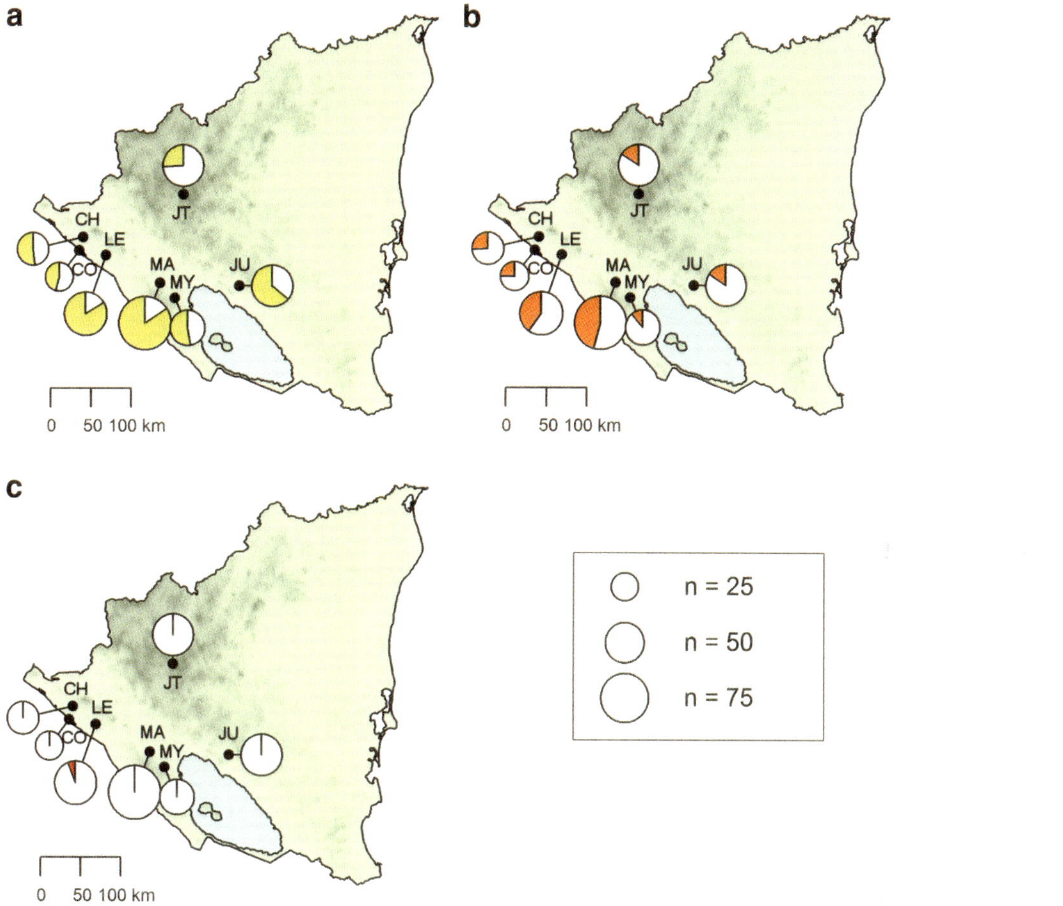

Fig. 1 Seroprevalence of antibodies against *Ehrlichia* spp. (**a**) and *Anaplasma* spp. (**b**) as well as antigen of *Dirofilaria immitis* (**c**) in dogs tested by rapid ELISA in different cities of Nicaragua from September to December 2013. The size of pie charts corresponds to the number of dogs sampled at each site. *Abbreviations*: CH, Chinandega; CO, Corinto; JU, Juigalpa; JT, Jinotega; LE, Léon; MA, Managua; MY, Masaya

the amount of water was adjusted accordingly. The thermoprofile of the first round consisted of an initial denaturation at 95 °C for 2 min, followed by 40 cycles at 95 °C for 1 min, 45 °C for 1 min and 72 °C for 2 min, and final extension at 72 °C for 5 min. The thermoprofile of the second round consisted of an initial denaturation at 95 °C for 1 min, followed by 40 cycles at 95 °C for 30 s, 55 °C for 30 s and 72 °C for 30 s, and a final extension at 72 °C for 5 min.

For detection of *E. canis*, a 389 bp fragment of the *16S* rRNA gene was targeted by nested PCR using primer pairs ECC and ECB in a first and ECAN5 and HE3 in a second PCR round [22, 23]. In the first round, the 25 μl reaction volume contained 12.5 μl DreamTaq® PCR

Table 1 Number of dogs sampled, seroprevalence of *Anaplasma* spp. and *Ehrlichia* spp. and prevalence of *Dirofilaria immitis* antigen as determined by rapid ELISA, at the different sampling locations in Nicaragua

City	Geographical region	No. of dogs sampled	Seroprevalence of *Anaplasma* spp.	Seroprevalence of *Ehrlichia* spp.	Seroprevalence of *Borrelia burgdorferi* (*s.l.*)	Prevalence of *D. immitis*	Prevalence of tick infestation
Corinto	Pacific coast	24	6/24 (25.0%)	11/24 (45.8%)	0	0	5/24 (20.8%)
León	Pacific lowlands	55	22/55 (40.0%)	46/55 (83.6%)	0	6/55 (10.9%)	40/55 (72.7%)
Chinandega	Pacific lowlands	31	8/31 (25.8%)	16/31 (51.6%)	0	0	14/31 (45.2%)
Managua	Pacific lowlands	83	38/83 (45.8%)	70/83 (84.3%)	0	0	36/83 (43.4%)
Masaya	Pacific lowlands	36	4/36 (11.1%)	19/36 (52.8%)	0	0	14/36 (38.9%)
Jinotega	Central highlands	50	8/50 (16.0%)	13/50 (26.0%)	0	0	23/50 (46.0%)
Juigalpa	Central highlands	50	8/50 (16.0%)	32/50 (64.0%)	0	0	27/50 (54.0%)
Total		329	94/329 (28.6%)	207/329 (62.9%)	0/329 (0.0%)	6/329 (1.8%)	159/329 (48.3%)

Mastermix, 0.5 μl of ECC (0.4 μM), 0.5 μl of ECB (10 μM), 9.5 μl deionized water and 2 μl template DNA, while in the second round, 0.5 μl each of primers ECAN5 (0.4 μM) and HE3 (10 μM) as well as 2.5 μl of the PCR-product of the first round were used, and the amount of water was adjusted to 9 μl. The thermoprofile consisted of an initial denaturation at 95 °C for 2 min, followed by 40 cycles at 95 °C for 1 min, 60 °C for 1 min and 72 °C for 1 min, and a final extension at 72 °C for 5 min in the first round. In the second round, a thermoprofile of initial denaturation at 95°C for 1 min, followed by 40 cycles at 95 °C for 30 s, 55 °C for 30 s and 72 °C for 30 s, and a final extension at 72 °C for 5 min was used. In all PCR set-ups, positive and no template controls were included.

Samples which were positive for *D. immitis* antigen in the ELISA or contained microfilariae in buffy coat were subjected to a PCR targeting the internal transcribed spacer (ITS) 1-5.8S rDNA-ITS2 complex by use of primers NC2 and NC5 [24]. The 50 μl reaction volume contained 1 μl *Taq* polymerase (5 PRIME GmbH, Hilden, Germany), 5 μl 10× buffer, 2 μl of each primer (10 μM each), 1 μl deoxynucleotide triphosphates (10 mM each), 37 μl deionized water and 2 μl template DNA. The thermoprofile consisted of an initial denaturation step at 95 °C for 3 min, 30 cycles at 95 °C for 30 s, 55 °C for 30 s, 72 °C for 30 s, followed by final elongation at 72 °C for 10 min. After visualization on 1% agarose gels, bands of the expected size between 1000 and 1500 bp were ligated into a pCR™4-TOPO® TA vector and cloned into One Shot Top10 chemically competent *Escherichia coli* (TOPO® TA Cloning kit, Thermo Fisher Scientific GmbH, Dreieich, Germany). After plasmid extraction and purification (NucleoSpin Plasmid kit, Macherey-Nagel GmbH & Co. KG, Düren, Germany), the insert was sequenced at the Seqlab Sequence Laboratories (Göttingen, Germany).

Statistical analyses

Statistical analyses were conducted in R v. 3.3.1 [25]. To investigate which factors influenced the probability of *Anaplasma* spp. and *Ehrlichia* spp. seropositivity in the rapid ELISA, generalized linear models (GLMs) with binomial error structure and logit-link were constructed (R function 'glm'). Animal age, sex, breed (dichotomized into "with breed"/"mongrel"), city of sampling and tick infestation at the time of examination were included as predictors. Furthermore, *Anaplasma* spp. infection was included as a predictor in the model for *Ehrlichia* spp., and vice-versa, to examine associations between seroprevalence for these pathogens. A third model was constructed to examine which factors influenced the likelihood of a positive result for one or more pathogens in the rapid ELISA in general. Full models were compared to null models containing only an intercept term in a likelihood ratio test (R function 'anova', test = 'chisq'). Model fit was assessed by Hosmer-Lemeshow-tests and inspection of Receiver Operating Characteristic (ROC) curves. Multiple comparisons (Tukey contrasts) between all levels of the factor "city" were performed using the function 'glht' (package *multcomp* [26]), with single-step *P*-value adjustment.

The influence of current infections with *A. platys*, *A. phagocytophilum* and *E. canis* (PCR results) on packed cell volume (PCV) was investigated using a linear mixed model (LMM, package *lme4* [27]). Because animal age and sex may affect PCV in dogs [28], these variables were included as additional fixed factors, while the city of sampling was included as a random factor. Because *A. platys* and *A. phagocytophilum* infections were highly correlated, these factors were investigated in separate models. Full LMMs were compared to null models containing only the random factor in a likelihood ratio test (R function 'anova', test = 'chisq'). To validate LMM assumptions, normality and homogeneity of model residuals were investigated graphically.

The proportion of anorectic dogs was compared between *E. canis*-, *A. platys*- and *A. phagocytophilum*-infected and non-infected dogs using Fisher's exact test.

Since only six dogs were positive for *D. immitis* antigen, these infections were not considered in statistical analyses.

Results

Clinical presentation of dogs

During clinical examinations, tick infestation was noted on 159 of the 329 dogs (48.3%), while flea and lice infestation were noted on 63 (19.1%) and 9 (2.7%) dogs, respectively. Pale mucous membranes were apparent in 129 dogs (39.2%), while anorexia was reported for 19 dogs (5.8%). Two dogs (0.6%) showed apathy, fever, epistaxis and abdominal pain. Lymphadenopathy was noted in one dog (0.3%). Other common clinical anomalies included nail overgrowth (n = 50; 15.2%), alopecia (n = 31; 9.4%), cough (n = 9; 2.7%) and eye discharge (n = 8; 2.4%).

Seroprevalence of Rickettsiales and *D. immitis*

Antibodies against *Ehrlichia* spp. were detected in 62.9% (207/329) of dogs, while *Anaplasma* spp. seroprevalence was 28.6% (94/329). Antibodies against both *Ehrlichia* and *Anaplasma* spp. were detected in 82 animals (24.9%), demonstrating exposure to species of both genera. Antibodies against *B. burgdorferi* (*s.l.*) were not detected. Regional seroprevalences are presented in Table 1 and Fig. 1.

Statistical analyses revealed a significant association of *Ehrlichia* and *Anaplasma* seropositivity; animals that were seropositive for *Ehrlichia* spp. had approximately 5 times higher odds of testing positive for *Anaplasma* antibodies as well, and vice versa (GLM, Table 2, models A and B). Additionally, a significant effect of age on the likelihood of *Ehrlichia* seropositivity was observed, as well as on the likelihood of a positive ELISA result in

Table 2 Results of binomial GLMs testing the influence of different predictor variables on the probability of *Ehrlichia* spp. (Model A) and *Anaplasma* spp. (Model B) seropositivity and for a positive result in the rapid ELISA in general (Model C), amongst 329 dogs from Nicaragua

	Model A: *Ehrlichia* spp. seropositive					Model B: *Anaplasma* spp. seropositive					Model C: SNAP® 4Dx® Plus positive				
	Estimate	SE	*Z*	*P*	OR	Estimate	SE	*Z*	*P*	OR	Estimate	SE	*Z*	*P*	OR
Intercept	-1.85	0.44	-4.26	**<0.001**		-2.25	0.49	-4.55	**<0.001**		-1.13	0.39	-2.91	**0.004**	
Sex (ref. male)	0.09	0.27	0.34	0.735	1.1	0.09	0.27	0.32	0.751	1.09	0.04	0.26	0.15	0.883	1.04
Age	0.11	0.05	2.33	**0.020**	1.11	-0.02	0.05	-0.44	0.663	0.98	0.13	0.05	2.69	**0.007**	1.14
Breed (ref. "with breed")	-0.29	0.29	-0.99	0.321	0.75	-0.13	0.29	-0.43	0.669	0.88	-0.08	0.29	-0.28	0.779	0.92
Anaplasma spp. seropositive	1.61	0.37	4.40	**<0.001**	5	–	–	–	–	–	–	–	–	–	–
Ehrlichia spp. seropositive	–	–	–	–	–	1.62	0.37	4.42	**<0.001**	5.03	–	–	–	–	–
Tick infestation	0.18	0.28	0.65	0.513	1.2	0.05	0.28	0.16	0.871	1.05	0.26	0.27	0.96	0.335	1.3
City[a]															
JU - JT	1.90	0.48	3.93	**0.002**	6.66	-0.59	0.59	-0.99	0.953	0.56	1.28	0.44	2.89	0.058	3.61
MA - JT	2.42	0.47	5.09	**<0.001**	11.21	0.79	0.50	1.56	0.694	2.2	2.36	0.46	5.16	**<0.001**	10.55
MY - JT	1.31	0.52	2.51	0.156	3.7	-0.79	0.71	-1.11	0.922	0.46	0.51	0.49	1.04	0.945	1.66
CO - JT	0.84	0.58	1.46	0.768	2.33	0.35	0.67	0.53	0.998	1.43	0.51	0.54	0.95	0.964	1.67
CH - JT	1.41	0.54	2.64	0.113	4.11	0.21	0.61	0.34	1.000	1.23	1.13	0.50	2.28	0.252	3.09
LE - JT	2.58	0.52	4.98	**<0.001**	13.14	0.46	0.53	0.88	0.975	1.59	2.13	0.48	4.42	**<0.001**	8.43
MA - JU	0.52	0.45	1.17	0.904	1.68	1.37	0.47	2.95	**0.048**	3.95	1.07	0.45	2.38	0.207	2.92
MY - JU	-0.59	0.48	-1.23	0.882	0.55	-0.20	0.68	-0.30	1.000	0.82	-0.78	0.47	-1.65	0.647	0.46
CO - JU	-1.05	0.55	-1.89	0.481	0.35	0.94	0.65	1.44	0.771	2.56	-0.77	0.53	-1.46	0.769	0.46
CH - JU	-0.48	0.50	-0.97	0.959	0.62	0.79	0.59	1.34	0.823	2.21	-0.15	0.48	-0.32	1.000	0.86
LE - JU	0.68	0.49	1.38	0.812	1.97	1.05	0.49	2.14	0.316	2.85	0.85	0.48	1.76	0.575	2.34
MY - MA	-1.11	0.47	-2.36	0.216	0.33	-1.57	0.59	-2.65	0.106	0.21	-1.85	0.48	-3.84	**<0.001**	0.16
CO - MA	-1.57	0.54	-2.91	0.055	0.21	-0.43	0.56	-0.77	0.987	0.65	-1.84	0.54	-3.43	**0.011**	0.16
CH - MA	-1.00	0.50	-2.00	0.413	0.37	-0.58	0.50	-1.16	0.903	0.56	-1.23	0.50	-2.45	0.178	0.29
LE - MA	0.16	0.50	0.32	1.000	1.17	-0.32	0.38	-0.84	0.979	0.73	-0.22	0.51	-0.44	0.999	0.8
CO - MY	-0.46	0.57	-0.82	0.983	0.63	1.14	0.74	1.54	0.712	3.13	0.01	0.55	0.01	1.000	1.0
CH - MY	0.11	0.54	0.20	1.000	1.11	0.99	0.70	1.41	0.785	2.7	0.62	0.52	1.20	0.893	1.86
LE - MY	1.27	0.54	2.36	0.211	3.55	1.25	0.63	1.98	0.418	3.49	1.62	0.53	3.09	**0.033**	5.08
CH - CO	0.57	0.60	0.95	0.964	1.77	-0.15	0.67	-0.22	1.000	0.86	0.62	0.57	1.08	0.933	1.85
LE - CO	1.73	0.60	2.89	0.059	5.65	0.11	0.61	0.18	1.000	1.11	1.62	0.58	2.79	0.077	5.05
LE - CH	1.16	0.55	2.12	0.336	3.2	0.26	0.53	0.49	0.999	1.29	1.00	0.53	1.88	0.489	2.73

Full models were significantly different from null models containing only an intercept: likelihood ratio test, $\chi^2 = 92.3$, $df = 11$, $P < 0.001$ (Model A); $\chi^2 = 53.7$, $df = 11$, $P < 0.001$ (Model B); and $\chi^2 = 60.5$, $df = 11$, $P < 0.001$ (Model C). Significant *P*-values (≤ 0.05) are printed in bold

[a]Multiple comparisons between levels of the factor "City" were performed using Tukey contrasts with single-step *P*-value adjustment.

Abbreviations: JU, Juigalpa; *JT*, Jinotega; *MA*, Managua; *MY*, Masaya; *CO*, Corinto; *CH*, Chinandega; *LE*, Léon; *OR*, odds ratio; *SE*, standard error general (GLM, Table 2, model C), with increasing probability in older dogs. Furthermore, significant differences were observed between the different sampling locations. Particularly, the odds of testing seropositive for *Ehrlichia* spp. were significantly lower in the city of Jinotega compared to Managua, Juigalpa and Léon, whereas for *Anaplasma* spp., a significant difference was only observed between Managua and Juigalpa, with a higher risk in Managua. Considering the results for *Anaplasma* spp., *Ehrlichia* spp. and *D. immitis* together, the odds of testing seropositive for any of these pathogens were significantly higher in Managua and Léon compared to Jinotega, in Managua compared to Corinto and Masaya, and in Masaya compared to Léon (Table 2). In contrast, animal sex and breed (with breed/mongrel) had no influence on seropositivity. Furthermore, tick infestation at the time of presentation was also not associated with seropositivity.

Current infections and their clinical impact

In six dogs (1.8%), which were all sampled at the city of Léon, *D. immitis* antigen was detected. In two of these samples, microfilariae were microscopically observed and confirmed as *D. immitis* by PCR and sequencing. Microfilariae were also observed in four additional samples, which did not test positive for *D. immitis* antigen. In two of these samples, *Acanthocheilonema reconditum* was identified by PCR and sequencing.

Current *E. canis* infection, as determined by amplification of the pathogen's DNA, was detected in 58.5% (121/207) of *Ehrlichia*-seropositive dogs, while *Anaplasma* DNA was detected in 23.4% (22/94) of seropositive samples. Among the 94 animals tested for *Anaplasma* DNA, five dogs (5.3%) were single-infected with *A. platys*, two dogs (2.2%) were single-infected with *A. phagocytophilum* and 15 dogs (16.0%) were co-infected with both species. Among the 85 animals tested by PCR for all three pathogens, four animals (4.7%) were co-infected with *E. canis* and *A. platys*, one animal (1.2%) with *E. canis* and *A. phagocytophilum* and eight animals (9.4%) carried all three pathogens (Table 3).

In the clinical examination, 50.4% (61/121) of dogs with current *E. canis* infection, 75.0% (15/20) of dogs with current *A. platys* infections and 64.7% (11/17) of dogs with current *A. phagocytophilum* showed pale mucous membranes. However, 9 (45.0%) and 6 (35.3%) of these *A. platys*- and *A. phagocytophilum*-infected dogs were co-infected with *E. canis*, respectively. Figure 2 shows the distribution of PCV in non-infected, mono-infected and co-infected dogs in the subset of 85 animals which were tested by PCR for current infections with all three pathogens. In the linear mixed model, only current *E. canis* infection showed a statistically significant negative impact on PCV, while no significant effect of current *A. platys* or *A. phagocytophilum* infection on PCV was found (LMM, Table 4).

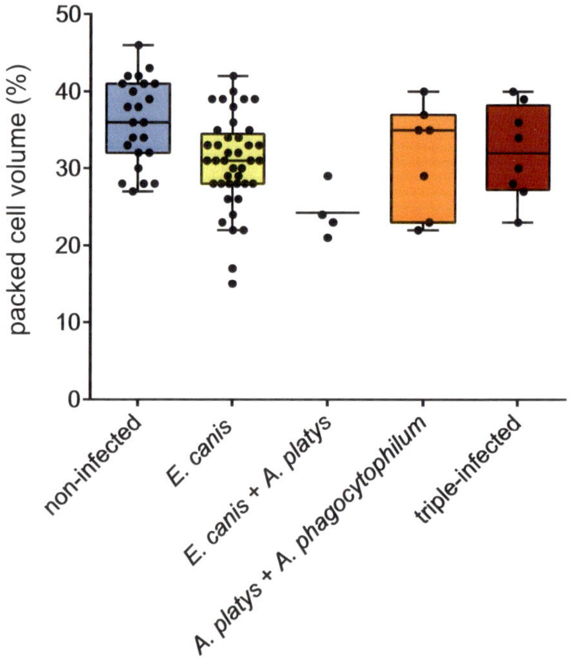

Fig. 2 Packed cell volume of non-infected, mono-infected and co-infected dogs in the subset of animals tested by PCR for current infections (defined as DNA detection) with *Ehrlichia canis* and *Anaplasma* spp. (*n* = 85). Since only one dog each was mono-infected with *A. phagocytophilum* and co-infected with *E. canis* and *A. phagocytophilum*, respectively, these were not plotted. No mono-infections with *A. platys* were found in this data subset. Ends of the boxes define the 25th and 75th percentiles, with a line at the median and whiskers extending to 1.5 the interquartile range or up to the maximum/minimum value

Twelve of 19 dogs for which anorexia was reported were PCR-positive for *E. canis*, with one individual also carrying current *A. platys* and *A. phagocytophilum* infections. However, for neither pathogen there was a significant difference in the occurrence of anorexia among infected and non-infected dogs (Fisher's exact test, $P = 0.1037$, $P = 1$ and $P = 1$, respectively).

Discussion

Dogs may be affected by several vector-borne diseases in the tropics, including important zoonoses. Here, detected

Table 3 Single and multiple infections among the 85 Nicaraguan dogs tested for *Anaplasma* and *Ehrlichia* DNA by PCR

No. of animals	Single infection			Multiple infection			
	Apl	Aph	Ec	Apl + Aph	Apl + Ec	Aph + Ec	Apl + Aph + Ec
85	0 (0.0%)	1 (1.2%)	41 (48.2%)	7 (8.2%)	4 (4.7%)	1 (1.2%)	8 (9.4%)

Abbreviations: Apl, *Anaplasma platys*; Aph, *Anaplasma phagocytophilum*; Ec, *Ehrlichia canis*

Table 4 Results of LMMs testing the influence of animal sex, age and current infections (as defined by DNA detection) with *Ehrlichia canis* and *Anaplasma platys* (Model A) as well as *A. phagocytophilum* (Model B) on packed cell volume (PVC) of 85 dogs from Nicaragua

	Estimate	SE	*df*	*t*	*P*
Model A					
Intercept	37.35	1.89	80	19.79	**<0.001**
Sex (ref. male)	0.15	1.31	80	0.11	0.909
Age	-0.33	0.26	80	-1.24	0.217
E. canis infection	-4.95	1.38	80	-3.58	**<0.001**
A. platys infection	-2.9	1.59	80	-1.83	0.072
Model B					
Intercept	36.75	2.02	80	18.19	**<0.001**
Sex (ref. male)	-0.07	1.33	80	-0.05	0.961
Age	-0.28	0.27	80	-1.03	0.306
E. canis infection	-4.95	1.43	80	-3.47	**<0.001**
A. phagocytophilum infection	-0.7	1.73	80	-0.4	0.688

Full models were significantly different from a null model containing only the random factor "City": likelihood ratio test, $\chi^2 = 15.28$, $df = 4$, $P = 0.004$ (Model A); and $\chi^2 = 11.98$, $df = 4$, $P = 0.017$ (Model B). Significant *P*-values (≤ 0.05) are printed in bold

Abbreviation: SE, standard error

seroprevalence rates among 329 dogs from Nicaragua for *Ehrlichia* spp. and *Anaplasma* spp. were considerably higher than those recently reported for Costa Rica (38.2% and 6.4%, respectively [9]) and Mexico (30.8% and 9.9%, respectively [14]). This could be due to the fact that dogs were only sampled in western parts of Nicaragua, characterized by less rainfall and a higher human population density than the hot and humid Caribbean lowlands in the eastern part of the country. In the abovementioned studies, a higher prevalence of canine vector-borne diseases has also been detected in western compared to central and eastern parts of Costa Rica and Mexico.

Furthermore, *Ehrlichia*- and *Anaplasma*-seropositivity were significantly associated with each other. In experimentally infected dogs it has been shown that concurrent *Ehrlichia*-infection intensifies the humoral immune response to *A. platys* and results in a more persistent *A. platys* infection [29], which may contribute to this phenomenon. Furthermore, both *Ehrlichia* and *A. platys* are predominantly transmitted by the brown dog tick *Rhipicephalus sanguineus* (*s.l.*), which was the most common tick species parasitizing the dogs in this study [30].

Borrelia burgdorferi (*s.l.*) antibodies were not detected, which is in line with the very low seroprevalences reported from Mexico and Costa Rica [9, 14], confirming the fact that Central America is not a Lyme borreliosis endemic region. The expected vector for *B. burgdoferi* (*s.l.*) are ticks of the genus *Ixodes*, which seem to be rather rare as parasites of domestic animals in Nicaragua [30, 31].

Several risk factors for seropositivity for tested vector-borne diseases were explored. A similar study conducted in Costa Rica reported a higher risk of seropositivity for mongrels compared to dogs of a certain breed as well as a significant effect of sex [9], which could not be confirmed in the current study. However, increasing age was identified as a risk factor for *Ehrlichia* spp. seropositivity as well as for a positive ELISA result in general, which most likely reflects cumulative pathogen exposure over the animals' lifetime. Similarly, a significantly lower seropositivity rate of dogs under one year of age compared to older dogs was found in Mexico [14]. Furthermore, significant differences between sampling locations were found. High seroprevalences were found in the capital city, Managua, which differed significantly from the lower rates detected in Jinotega, Masaya and Corinto. However, a general pattern concerning the distribution of seropositivity, e.g. differences between coastal and highland locations, cannot yet be established. Furthermore, data on seroprevalences in the eastern parts of the country are still missing, and should be obtained in future studies.

Dirofilaria immitis antigen was detected in six dogs, which were all sampled in the city of Léon, near the Pacific coast. Similarly, *D. immitis* infections in Costa Rica were almost exclusively detected in districts bordering the Pacific coast [9, 11]. Higher *D. immitis* prevalence in coastal regions has also been observed in Mexico [32]. Additionally, microfilariae in two dogs were identified as *A. reconditum*. In neighbouring Costa Rica, *A. reconditum* infections have been detected in 11.6% of tested dogs, while 15% of dogs showed *D. immitis* infections [11]. In contrast to mosquito-borne dirofilariosis, *A. reconditum* is mainly transmitted by fleas and possibly also by lice as intermediate hosts [33]. Here, approximately 20% of dogs showed flea infestation at the time of examination. Although *A. reconditum* is less pathogenic than *D. immitis*, it is important to acknowledge the presence of this parasite, as it is a differential diagnosis for *D. immitis* if microfilariae are observed in blood samples.

Almost 60% of the *Ehrlichia*-seropositive dogs were currently infected (as defined as DNA detection by PCR in blood samples) with *E. canis*, i.e. at least 36.7% of all 329 dogs. In addition to *E. canis*, *E. ewingii* and *E. chaffeensis* also possess high zoonotic potential and antibodies against these *Ehrlichia* spp. may be detected by the used commercial rapid ELISA. However, we did not test for the presence of *E. ewingii* or *E. chaffeensis* by PCR here, as these pathogens have not been detected in ticks or domestic animals in Central America so far [10, 34, 35]. However, *E. chaffeensis* DNA was isolated from human patients in neighboring Costa Rica [36]. The principal vector of *E. ewingii* and *E. chaffeensis*, *Amblyomma americanum*, has not been reported to occur in Central America [37–39]. Nevertheless, it cannot be entirely excluded that *E. ewingii* and *E. chaffeensis* are present in Nicaragua; this should be considered for future studies as well.

Regarding *Anaplasma* spp., at least 6.6% of all dogs in the present study were currently infected. Both *A. platys* (n = 20), the causative agent of canine cyclic thrombocytopenia, and *A. phagocytophilum* (n = 17), which causes granulocytic anaplasmosis, were detected. In the majority of cases (n = 15), both species were present as co-infections. This result was somewhat surprising. As mentioned above, ixodid ticks, which are known to transmit *A. phagocytophilum*, are rather rare in Central America. Previously, only *A. platys* was reported to infect dogs in Nicaragua [15] and Costa Rica [10]; however, *A. phagocytophilum* has been found at low prevalence in *Rhipicephalus* ticks collected from dogs in Costa Rica [35]. It remains to be proven whether or not ticks other than *Ixodes* spp. may be implicated in the transmission of *A. phagocytophilum*. Nevertheless, the presence of *A. phagocytophilum* in Central America is especially important regarding the zoonotic potential of these pathogens. *Anaplasma phagocytophilum* frequently causes human granulocytic anaplasmosis, while the zoonotic potential of *A. platys* is considered to be low [4].

It cannot be excluded that there were further currently infected dogs amongst the seronegative animals, as antibody titres may not be detectable during the first 16 to 35 days post-infection [29]. However, seronegative animals were not tested by PCR. Therefore, we included only animals tested for current infections with *E. canis* and both *Anaplasma* species when assessing the impact of infections on PCV. In the statistical model, only *E. canis* infection had a significant negative impact on PCV. Likewise, Gaunt et al. [29] detected a significantly lower PCV in *E. canis*-infected dogs, but not in *A. platys*-infected dogs, compared to a control group. However, they reported that co-infection with both pathogens resulted in more severe anaemia than *E. canis* infection alone [29]. Here, only four individuals were co-infected with *E. canis* and *A. platys*, showing on average lower PCV values than those single-infected with *E. canis*. However, this phenomenon was not observed in the group of animals infected with all three pathogens, possibly because animals within this group were in different stages of infection. In general, co-infections may alter and/or exacerbate the clinical presentation of disease [3]; however, infections may also often be asymptomatic [4]. Here, apart from pale mucous membranes, clinical symptoms potentially related to ehrlichiosis or anaplasmosis were only rarely observed, and anorexia, which was frequently reported, was not associated with infection status.

Conclusions

This study provides the first large-scale assessment of canine vector-borne diseases in Nicaragua. Similar to other Central American countries, a high prevalence of *E. canis* was detected, while *D. immitis* infections were rare and *B. burgdorferi* (*s.l.*) infections were not detected. *Anaplasma phagocytophilum* infections were observed almost as frequently as *A. platys* infections. Thus, dogs may constitute a reservoir for *A. phagocytophilum* in Nicaragua, which should not be neglected in the light of the zoonotic potential of this pathogen. Veterinarians and public health officials in Nicaragua should recommend the use of repellents or acaricides to protect dogs from vector-borne diseases, thus reducing the reservoir for human infection as well as the dog owners' exposure to the vectors.

Acknowledgements

The authors wish to thank Ursula Küttler for excellent technical assistance.

Funding

This project was partially funded by IDEXX Laboratories. Study data interpretation is completely independent from the company's opinion and there is no conflict with commercial interests. VMM received funding from the German Academic Exchange Service (DAAD) for a research stay in Germany.

Authors' contributions

VMM collected the blood samples, VMM and SS performed laboratory analyses. CS and VMM designed and coordinated the study. AS performed the statistical analyses and drafted the manuscript. All authors participated in data analysis and interpretation. All authors read and approved the final manuscript.

Competing interests

The authors declare that they have no competing interests.

Author details

[1]Institute for Parasitology, Centre for Infection Medicine, University of Veterinary Medicine Hannover, Buenteweg 17, 30559 Hannover, Germany. [2]Laboratorio de Parasitología, Escuela de Medicina Veterinaria, Universidad Nacional, Campus Benjamín Núñez, Heredia, Costa Rica. [3]IDEXX Laboratories, Moerikestr. 28/3, 71636 Ludwigsburg, Germany.

References

1. Harrus S, Baneth G. Drivers for the emergence and re-emergence of vector-borne protozoal and bacterial diseases. Int J Parasitol. 2005;35:1309–18.
2. Otranto D, Dantas-Torres F, Breitschwerdt EB. Managing canine vector-borne diseases of zoonotic concern: part two. Trends Parasitol. 2009;25:228–35.

3. De Tommasi AS, Otranto D, Dantas-Torres F, Capelli G, Breitschwerdt EB, de Caprariis D. Are vector-borne pathogen co-infections complicating the clinical presentation in dogs? Parasit Vectors. 2013;6:97.
4. Otranto D, Dantas-Torres F, Breitschwerdt EB. Managing canine vector-borne diseases of zoonotic concern: part one. Trends Parasitol. 2009;25:157–63.
5. Day MJ. One health: the importance of companion animal vector-borne diseases. Parasit Vectors. 2011;4:49.
6. Little SE, Heise SR, Blagburn BL, Callister SM, Mead PS. Lyme borreliosis in dogs and humans in the USA. Trends Parasitol. 2010;26:213–8.
7. Duncan AW, Correa MT, Levine JF, Breitschwerdt EB. The dog as a sentinel for human infection: prevalence of *Borrelia burgdorferi* C6 antibodies in dogs from southeastern and mid-Atlantic states. Vector Borne Zoonotic Dis. 2004; 4:221–9.
8. Moreira-Soto A, Carranza MV, Taylor L, Calderón-Arguedas O, Hun L, Troyo A. Exposure of dogs to spotted fever group rickettsiae in urban sites associated with human rickettsioses in Costa Rica. Ticks Tick Borne Dis. 2016; 7:748–53.
9. Montenegro VM, Bonilla MC, Kaminsky D, Romero-Zúñiga JJ, Siebert S, Krämer F. Serological detection of antibodies to *Anaplasma* spp., *Borrelia burgdorferi sensu lato* and *Ehrlichia canis* and of *Dirofilaria immitis* antigen in dogs from Costa Rica. Vet Parasitol. 2017;236:97–107.
10. Rojas A, Rojas D, Montenegro V, Gutiérrez R, Yasur-Landau D, Baneth G. Vector-borne pathogens in dogs from Costa Rica: first molecular description of *Babesia vogeli* and *Hepatozoon canis* infections with a high prevalence of monocytic ehrlichiosis and the manifestations of co-infection. Vet Parasitol. 2014;199:121–8.
11. Rojas A, Rojas D, Montenegro VM, Baneth G. Detection of *Dirofilaria immitis* and other arthropod-borne filarioids by an HRM real-time qPCR, blood-concentrating techniques and a serological assay in dogs from Costa Rica. Parasit Vectors. 2015;8:170.
12. Santamaria A, Calzada JE, Saldaña A, Yabsley MJ, Gottdenker NL. Molecular diagnosis and species identification of *Ehrlichia* and *Anaplasma* infections in dogs from Panama, Central America. Vector Borne Zoonotic Dis. 2014;14: 368–70.
13. Bermúdez CS, Zaldivar AY, Spolidorio MG, Moraes-Filho J, Miranda RJ, Caballero CM, et al. Rickettsial infection in domestic mammals and their ectoparasites in El Valle de Anton, Cocle, Panama. Vet Parasitol. 2011;177:134–8.
14. Movilla R, García C, Siebert S, Roura X. Countrywide serological evaluation of canine prevalence for *Anaplasma* spp., *Borrelia burgdorferi* (*sensu lato*), *Dirofilaria immitis* and *Ehrlichia canis* in Mexico. Parasit Vectors. 2016;9:421.
15. Wei L, Kelly P, Ackerson K, Zhang J, El-Mahallawy HS, Kaltenboeck B, et al. First report of *Babesia gibsoni* in Central America and survey for vector-borne infections in dogs from Nicaragua. Parasit Vectors. 2014;7:126.
16. Stillman BA, Monn M, Liu J, Thatcher B, Foster P, Andrews B, et al. Performance of a commercially available in-clinic ELISA for detection of antibodies against *Anaplasma phagocytophilum*, *Anaplasma platys*, *Borrelia burgdorferi*, *Ehrlichia canis*, and *Ehrlichia ewingii* and *Dirofilaria immitis* antigen in dogs. J Am Vet Med Assoc. 2014;245:80–6.
17. Chandrashekar R, Mainville CA, Beall MJ, O'Connor T, Eberts MD, Alleman AR, et al. Performance of a commercially available in-clinic ELISA for the detection of antibodies against *Anaplasma phagocytophilum*, *Ehrlichia canis*, and *Borrelia burgdorferi* and *Dirofilaria immitis* antigen in dogs. Am J Vet Res. 2010;71:1443–50.
18. O'Connor TP, Hanscom JL, Hegarty BC, Groat RG, Breitschwerdt EB. Comparison of an indirect immunofluorescence assay, western blot analysis, and a commercially available ELISA for detection of *Ehrlichia canis* antibodies in canine sera. Am J Vet Res. 2006;67:206–10.
19. Mylonakis ME, Papadopoulos E, Koutinas AF, Paitaki C, Leontides L. Comparative methodology for the detection and differentiation of circulating microfilariae of *Dirofilaria immitis* in the dog. J Helminthol. 2004;78:137–40.
20. Massung RF, Slater K, Owens JH, Nicholson WL, Mather TN, Solberg VB, et al. Nested PCR assay for detection of granulocytic ehrlichiae. J Clin Microbiol. 1998;36:1090–5.
21. Martin AR, Brown GK, Hugh Dunstan R, Roberts TK. *Anaplasma platys*: an improved PCR for its detection in dogs. Exp Parasitol. 2005;109:176–80.
22. Murphy GL, Ewing SA, Whitworth LC, Fox JC, Kocan AA. A molecular and serologic survey of *Ehrlichia canis*, *E. chaffeensis*, and *E. ewingii* in dogs and ticks from Oklahoma. Vet Parasitol. 1998;79:325–39.
23. Dawson JE, Stallknecht DE, Howerth EW, Warner C, Biggie K, Davidson WR, et al. Susceptibility of white-tailed deer (*Odocoileus virginianus*) to infection with *Ehrlichia chaffeensis*, the etiologic agent of human ehrlichiosis. J Clin Microbiol. 1994;32:2725–8.
24. Newton LA, Chilton NB, Beveridge I, Hoste H, Nansen P, Gasser RB. Genetic markers for strongylid nematodes of livestock defined by PCR-based restriction analysis of spacer rDNA. Acta Trop. 1998;69:1–15.
25. R Core Team. R Foundation for Statistical Computing, Vienna: Austria; 2016. R: A language and environment for statistical computing. http://www.R-project.org/.
26. Hothorn T, Bretz F, Westfall P. Simultaneous inference in general parametric models. Biom J. 2008;50:346–63.
27. Bates D, Mächler M, Bolker B, Walker S. Fitting linear mixed-effects models using lme4. J Stat Softw. 2015;67:1.
28. Latimer KS, editor. Duncan and Prasse's Veterinary Laboratory Medicine: Clinical Pathology. 5th ed. Ames: IA: Wiley-Blackwell; 2011.
29. Gaunt S, Beall M, Stillman B, Lorentzen L, Diniz P, Chandrashekar R, et al. Experimental infection and co-infection of dogs with *Anaplasma platys* and *Ehrlichia canis*: hematologic, serologic and molecular findings. Parasit Vectors. 2010;3:33.
30. Springer A, Montenegro VM, Schicht S, Wölfel S, Schaper SR, Chitimia-Dobler L, Siebert S, Strube C. Detection of *Rickettsia monacensis* and *Rickettsia amblyommatis* in ticks collected from dogs in Costa Rica and Nicaragua. Ticks Tick Borne Dis. 2018;9:1565–72.
31. Bermúdez CSE, Mejía BL, Hernández L, Apanaskevich DA. First records of *Ixodes boliviensis* Neumann, 1904 and *Dermacentor dissimilis* Cooley, 1947 (Ixodida: Ixodidae) as parasites of domestic mammals in Nicaragua. Syst Appl Acarol. 2015;20:462–4.
32. Labarthe N, Guerrero J. Epidemiology of heartworm: what is happening in South America and Mexico? Vet Parasitol. 2005;133:149–56.
33. Pennington NE, Phelps CA. Canine filariasis on Okinawa, Ryukyu Islands. J Med Entomol. 1969;6:59–67.
34. Romero LE, Meneses AI, Salazar L, Jiménez M, Romero JJ, Aguiar DM, et al. First isolation and molecular characterization of *Ehrlichia canis* in Costa Rica, Central America. Res Vet Sci. 2011;91:95–7.
35. Campos-Calderón L, Ábrego-Sánchez L, Solórzano-Morales A, Alberti A, Tore G, Zobba R, et al. Molecular detection and identification of Rickettsiales pathogens in dog ticks from Costa Rica. Ticks Tick Borne Dis. 2016;7:1198–202.
36. Norman R, Daniela C, Priscilla M. Molecular detection of *Ehrlichia chaffeensis* in humans, Costa Rica. Emerg Infect Dis. 2015;21:532.
37. Bermúdez CSE, Castro A, Esser H, Liefting Y, García G, Miranda RJ. Ticks (Ixodida) on humans from central Panama, Panama (2010–2011). Exp Appl Acarol. 2012;58:81–8.
38. Esser HJ, Herre EA, Blüthgen N, Loaiza JR, Bermúdez SE, Jansen PA. Host specificity in a diverse Neotropical tick community: an assessment using quantitative network analysis and host phylogeny. Parasit Vectors. 2016;9:1–14.
39. Troyo A, Calderón-Arguedas Ó, Alvarado G, Vargas-Castro LE, Avendaño A. Ectoparasites of dogs in home environments on the Caribbean slope of Costa Rica. Rev Bras Parasitol Vet. 2012;21:179–83.

Permissions

All chapters in this book were first published in P&V, by BioMed Central; hereby published with permission under the Creative Commons Attribution License or equivalent. Every chapter published in this book has been scrutinized by our experts. Their significance has been extensively debated. The topics covered herein carry significant findings which will fuel the growth of the discipline. They may even be implemented as practical applications or may be referred to as a beginning point for another development.

The contributors of this book come from diverse backgrounds, making this book a truly international effort. This book will bring forth new frontiers with its revolutionizing research information and detailed analysis of the nascent developments around the world.

We would like to thank all the contributing authors for lending their expertise to make the book truly unique. They have played a crucial role in the development of this book. Without their invaluable contributions this book wouldn't have been possible. They have made vital efforts to compile up to date information on the varied aspects of this subject to make this book a valuable addition to the collection of many professionals and students.

This book was conceptualized with the vision of imparting up-to-date information and advanced data in this field. To ensure the same, a matchless editorial board was set up. Every individual on the board went through rigorous rounds of assessment to prove their worth. After which they invested a large part of their time researching and compiling the most relevant data for our readers.

The editorial board has been involved in producing this book since its inception. They have spent rigorous hours researching and exploring the diverse topics which have resulted in the successful publishing of this book. They have passed on their knowledge of decades through this book. To expedite this challenging task, the publisher supported the team at every step. A small team of assistant editors was also appointed to further simplify the editing procedure and attain best results for the readers.

Apart from the editorial board, the designing team has also invested a significant amount of their time in understanding the subject and creating the most relevant covers. They scrutinized every image to scout for the most suitable representation of the subject and create an appropriate cover for the book.

The publishing team has been an ardent support to the editorial, designing and production team. Their endless efforts to recruit the best for this project, has resulted in the accomplishment of this book. They are a veteran in the field of academics and their pool of knowledge is as vast as their experience in printing. Their expertise and guidance has proved useful at every step. Their uncompromising quality standards have made this book an exceptional effort. Their encouragement from time to time has been an inspiration for everyone.

The publisher and the editorial board hope that this book will prove to be a valuable piece of knowledge for researchers, students, practitioners and scholars across the globe.

List of Contributors

Maryna Golovchenko and Nataliia Rudenko
Institute of Parasitology, Biology Centre, Czech Academy of Sciences, Branišovská 31, CZ-37005 České Budějovice, Czech Republic

Pavlina Vechtova, Jarmila Sterbova, Jan Sterba, Marie Vancova, Ryan O. M. Rego, Martin Selinger, Martin Strnad and Libor Grubhoffer
Institute of Parasitology, Biology Centre, Czech Academy of Sciences, Branišovská 31, CZ-37005 České Budějovice, Czech Republic
Faculty of Science, University of South Bohemia, Branišovská 1760, CZ-37005 České Budějovice, Czech Republic

Ai-Ling Tian and Fu-Kai Zhang
State Key Laboratory of Veterinary Etiological Biology, Key Laboratory of Veterinary Parasitology of Gansu Province, Lanzhou Veterinary Research Institute, Chinese Academy of Agricultural Sciences, Lanzhou, Gansu Province 730046, People's Republic of China

Xing-Quan Zhu
State Key Laboratory of Veterinary Etiological Biology, Key Laboratory of Veterinary Parasitology of Gansu Province, Lanzhou Veterinary Research Institute, Chinese Academy of Agricultural Sciences, Lanzhou, Gansu Province 730046, People's Republic of China
College of Veterinary Medicine, Yangzhou University, Yangzhou, Jiangsu Province 225009, People's Republic of China
Jiangsu Co-innovation Center for the Prevention and Control of Important Animal Infectious Diseases and Zoonoses, Yangzhou, Jiangsu Province 225009, People's Republic of China

MingMin Lu, XiaoWei Tian, WenJuan Wang and Xiang Rui Li
College of Veterinary Medicine, Nanjing Agricultural University, Nanjing 210095, People's Republic of China

Guillermo Calderón-Mantilla and Evangelia Petsalaki
European Molecular Biology Laboratory-European Bioinformatics Institute, Wellcome Genome Campus, Hinxton CB10 1SD, UK

Si-Yang Huang
College of Veterinary Medicine, Yangzhou University, Yangzhou, Jiangsu Province 225009, People's Republic of China
Jiangsu Co-innovation Center for the Prevention and Control of Important Animal Infectious Diseases and Zoonoses, Yangzhou, Jiangsu Province 225009, People's Republic of China

Hany M. Elsheikha
Faculty of Medicine and Health Sciences, School of Veterinary Medicine and Science, University of Nottingham, Sutton Bonington Campus, Loughborough LE12 5RD, UK

Shankari Prasad Datta and Srimonti Sarkar
Department of Biochemistry, Bose Institute, P 1/12 CIT Road Scheme VII M, Kolkata, West Bengal 700054, India

Avisek Mondal
Department of Biochemistry, Bose Institute, P 1/12 CIT Road Scheme VII M, Kolkata, West Bengal 700054, India
Present Address: Section on Developmental Genetics, Eunice Kennedy Shriver National Institute of Child Health and Human Development, NIH, Bethesda, Maryland, USA

Kuladip Jana
Division of Molecular Medicine, Bose, Institute, P 1/12 CIT Road Scheme VII M, Kolkata, West Bengal 700054, India

Sandipan Ganguly
Division of Parasitology, National Institute of Cholera and Enteric Diseases, P-33, CIT Road, Scheme XM, Beliaghata, Kolkata, West Bengal 700010, India

Caroll Stoore, Constanza Andrade, Christian Hidalgo, Felipe Corrêa, Mauricio Jiménez and Rodolfo Paredes
Escuela de Medicina Veterinaria, Facultad de Ciencias de la Vida, Universidad Andres Bello, Santiago, Chile

Marcela Hernandez
Laboratorio de Biología Periodontal, Facultad de Odontología, Universidad de Chile, Santiago, Chile

Facultad de Ciencias de la Salud, Universidad Autonoma de Chile, Santiago, Chile

Jan Hattendorf
Swiss Tropical and Public Health Institute, Socinstrasse 57, 4002 Basel, Switzerland
University of Basel, Petersplatz 1, 4001 Basel, Switzerland

Stefanie Knopp
Swiss Tropical and Public Health Institute, Socinstrasse 57, 4002 Basel, Switzerland
University of Basel, Petersplatz 1, 4001 Basel, Switzerland
Wolfson Wellcome Biomedical Laboratories, Department of Life Sciences, Natural History Museum, Cromwell Road, London SW7 5BD, UK

David Rollinson
Wolfson Wellcome Biomedical Laboratories, Department of Life Sciences, Natural History Museum, Cromwell Road, London SW7 5BD, UK

Shaali M Ame, Said M Ali and Faki Bakar
Public Health Laboratory Ivo-de Carneri, Chake-Chake, Pemba, United Republic of Tanzania

Iddi S Khamis, Mwanaidi A Khamis and Fatma Kabole
Neglected Diseases Programme, Ministry of Health, Unguja, United Republic of Tanzania

Bobbie Person
SchistosomiasisConsortium for Operational Research and Evaluation, 145 Coverdell Center, The University of Georgia, 500 D.W. Brooks Drive, Athens, Georgia 30602, USA

Sharon Tirosh-Levy, Yuval Gottlieb and Amir Steinman
Koret School of Veterinary Medicine, The Robert H. Smith Faculty of Agriculture, Food and Environment, The Hebrew University of Jerusalem, Rehovot, Israel

Dmitry A. Apanaskevich
United States National Tick Collection, James H. Oliver, Jr Institute of Coastal Plain Sciences, Georgia Southern University, Statesboro, Georgia, USA

Kosta Y. Mumcuoglu
Parasitology Unit, Department of Microbiology and Molecular Genetic, The Kuvin Centre for the Study of Infectious and Tropical Diseases, Hebrew University-Hadassah Medical School, Jerusalem, Israel

Mojca Kristan and Jo Lines
Department of Disease Control, London School of Hygiene and TropicalMedicine, London, UK

Tarekegn A. Abeku
Malaria Consortium, London, UK

Muhammad Majeed, Hatem Soliman, Gokhlesh Kumar, Mansour El-Matbouli and Mona Saleh
Clinical Division of Fish Medicine, University of Veterinary Medicine, Vienna, Austria

Veronique Dermauw
Department of Biomedical Sciences, Institute of Tropical Medicine, Nationalestraat 155, 2000 Antwerp, Belgium

Pierre Dorny
Department of Biomedical Sciences, Institute of Tropical Medicine, Nationalestraat 155, 2000 Antwerp, Belgium
Laboratory of Parasitology, Faculty of Veterinary Medicine, Ghent University, Salisburylaan 133, B-9820 Merelbeke, Belgium

Chiara Trevisan
Department of Biomedical Sciences, Institute of Tropical Medicine, Nationalestraat 155, 2000 Antwerp, Belgium
Department of Veterinary and Animal Sciences, Faculty of Health and Medical Sciences, University of Copenhagen, Dyrlægevej, 100 Frederiksberg, Denmark

Brian Lassen
Department of Veterinary and Animal Sciences, Faculty of Health and Medical Sciences, University of Copenhagen, Dyrlægevej, 100 Frederiksberg, Denmark
Institute of Veterinary Medicine and Animal Sciences, Estonian University of Life Sciences, Kreutzwaldi 1, 51006 Tartu, Estonia

Smaragda Sotiraki
Veterinary Research Institute, HAO-DEMETER, Campus Thermi, 57001 Thessaloniki, Greece

Minerva Laranjo-González
IRTA, Centre de Recerca en Sanitat Animal (CReSA, IRTA-UAB), Campus de la Universitat Autònoma de Barcelona, 08193 Bellaterra, Spain

Ziqi Wang
University of Florida College of Medicine, Gainesville, Florida, USA

Age Kärssin
Veterinary and Food laboratory, Kreutzwaldi 30, 51006 Tartu, Estonia
Institute of Veterinary Medicine and Animal Sciences, Estonian University of Life Sciences, Kreutzwaldi 1, 51006 Tartu, Estonia

Pikka Jokelainen
Institute of Veterinary Medicine and Animal Sciences, Estonian University of Life Sciences, Kreutzwaldi 1, 51006 Tartu, Estonia
Laboratory of Parasitology, Department of Bacteria, Parasites and Fungi, Infectious Disease Preparedness, Statens Serum Institute, Copenhagen, Denmark
Faculty of Veterinary Medicine, University of Helsinki, Helsinki, Finland

Aleksandar Cvetkovikj and Jovana Stefanovska
Department of Parasitology and Parasitic Diseases, Faculty of Veterinary Medicine, Ss. Cyril and Methodius University in Skopje, Lazar Pop Trajkov 5-7, 1000 Skopje, Former Yugoslav Republic of Macedonia

Andrea S. Winkler, Annette Abraham and Veronika Schmidt
Centre for Global Health, Department of Neurology, Technical University Munich, Ismaninger Strasse 22, 81675 Munich, Germany
10Centre for Global Health, Department of Community Medicine and Global Health, Institute of Health and Society, University of Oslo, Kirkeveien 166, 0450 Oslo, Norway

Branko Bobić and Olgica Djurković-Djaković
Centre of Excellence for Food- and Vector-borne Zoonoses, Institute for Medical Research, University of Belgrade, Belgrade, Serbia

Carmen Michaela Cretu
Department of Parasitology, Carol Davila University of Medicine and Pharmacy, Colentina Clinical Hospital, Bucharest, Romania

Cozma Vasile
Department of Parasitology, University of Agricultural Sciences and Veterinary Medicine Cluj-Napoca, Cluj-Napoca, Romania

Dimitris Arvanitis
Department of Microbiology, 424 Military General Hospital, Thessaloniki, Greece

Gunita Deksne
Institute of Food Safety, Health and Environment, Riga, Latvia
Faculty of Biology, University of Latvia, Riga, Latvia

Ilievski Boro
Institute for Pathology, Medical Faculty, University "Ss. Cyril and Methodius", Skopje, Former Yugoslav Republic of Macedonia

István Kucsera
Department of Parasitology, National Institute for Public Health, Budapest, Hungary

Jacek Karamon
Department of Parasitology and Invasive Diseases, National Veterinary Research Institute in Pulawy, Pulawy, Poland

Břetislav Koudela
Department of Pathology and Parasitology, Faculty of Veterinary Medicine, University of Veterinary and Pharmaceutical Sciences Brno, Palackého tř. 1946/1, 61242 Brno, Czech Republic
Central European Institute of Technology, University of Veterinary and Pharmaceutical Sciences Brno, Palackého tř. 1946/1, 61242 Brno, Czech Republic

Maja Jurhar Pavlova
Institute for Microbiology and Parasitology, Medical faculty, University "Ss. Cyril and Methodius", Skopje, Former Yugoslav Republic of Macedonia

Marian Varady
Institute of Parasitology, Slovak Academy of Sciences, Košice, Slovakia

Marina Pavlak
Department of Veterinary Economics and Epidemiology, Faculty of Veterinary Medicine, University of Zagreb, Zagreb, Croatia

Mindaugas Šarkūnas
Lithuanian University of Health Sciences, Kaunas, Lithuania

Miriam Kaminski
Department of Neurology, Klinikum rechts der Isar, Technical University Munich, Ismaninger Straße 22, 81675 Munich, Germany

Dagny Stojčević Jan
Department of Parasitology and Parasitic Diseases with Clinic, Faculty of Veterinary Medicine, University of Zagreb, Zagreb, Croatia

Zorica Dakić
Parasitological Laboratory, Department of Microbiology, Clinical Center of Serbia, Belgrade, Serbia

Sarah Gabriël
Department of Veterinary Public Health and Food Safety, Faculty of Veterinary Medicine, Ghent University, Salisburylaan 133, 9820 Merelbeke, Belgium

Brecht Devleesschauwer
Department of Veterinary Public Health and Food Safety, Faculty of Veterinary Medicine, Ghent University, Salisburylaan 133, 9820 Merelbeke, Belgium
Department of Epidemiology and Public Health, Sciensano, Brussels, Belgium

Rousseau Djouaka
International Institute of Tropical Agriculture, Cotonou 08 BP 0932, Benin

Genevieve Tchigossou and Romaric Akoton
International Institute of Tropical Agriculture, Cotonou 08 BP 0932, Benin
University of Abomey Calavi, BP 526 Cotonou, Benin

Kabirou Moutairou and Akadiri Yessoufou
University of Abomey Calavi, BP 526 Cotonou, Benin.

Helen Irving
Liverpool School of Tropical Medicine, Pembroke Place, Liverpool L3 5QA, UK

Jacob M Riveron and Charles S Wondji
Liverpool School of Tropical Medicine, Pembroke Place, Liverpool L3 5QA, UK
LSTM Research Unit at the Centre for Research in Infectious Diseases (CRID), Yaoundé, Cameroon

Seun Atoyebi
Cell Biology and Genetics Unit, Department of Zoology, University of Ibadan, Ibadan, Oyo State, Nigeria

Mark A. Freeman
Ross University School of Veterinary Medicine, Basseterre, Saint Kitts and Nevis

Árni Kristmundsson
Institute for Experimental Pathology, University of Iceland, Reykjavík, Iceland

Clarer Jones and Donath Tarimo
Department of Parasitology and Medical Entomology, Muhimbili University of Health and Allied Sciences, Dar es Salaam, Tanzania

Billy Ngasala
Department of Parasitology and Medical Entomology, Muhimbili University of Health and Allied Sciences, Dar es Salaam, Tanzania
Department of Women's and Children's Health International Maternal and Child Health (IMCH), Uppsala Universitet, Uppsala, Sweden

Yahya A. Derua
National Institute for Medical Research, Dar es Salaam, Tanzania

Lisa Reimer
Liverpool School of Tropical Medicine, Liverpool, UK

Moses Bockarie
European and Development Countries Clinical Trials Partnership, Cape Town, South Africa

Mwelecele N. Malecela
WHO Regional Office for Africa, Brazzaville, Republic of the Congo

Frédéric Jourdain and Marie Picard
Research Unit MiVEGEC, French National Research Institute for Sustainable Development, IRD-CNRS-Montpellier University, Montpellier, France

Tatiana Sulesco
Institute of Zoology, Ministry of Education, Culture and Research, Chisinau, Moldova

Nabil Haddad
Laboratory of Immunology and Vector Borne Diseases, Lebanese University, Fanar, Lebanon

Zoubir Harrat
Laboratoire Éco-épidémiologie Parasitaire et Génétique des Populations, Institut Pasteur d'Algérie, Algiers, Algeria

Samer Saleh Sawalha
Ministry of Health, Public Health General Directorate, Environmental Health Department, Vector Control Unit, Ramallah, Palestine

Filiz Günay
Faculty of Science, Biology Department, Ecology Section, Vector Ecology Research Group Laboratories, Hacettepe University, Ankara, Turkey

Khalil Kanani
Parasitic and Zoonotic Diseases Department, Vector-Borne Diseases Programmes Manager, MOH, Amman, Jordan

Taher Shaibi
Reference Laboratory of Parasites and Vector Borne Diseases, NCDC Libya, and Zoology Department, Faculty of Science, University of Tripoli, Tripoli, Libya

Denys Akhramenko
State Body I.I. Mechnikov Ukrainian Anti-Plague Research Institute of Ministry of Health, Odessa, Ukraine

M'hammed Sarih
Laboratoire des Maladies Vectorielles, Institut Pasteur du Maroc, Casablanca, Morocco

Enkelejda Velo
Control of Infectious Diseases Department, Institute of Public Health, Tirana, Albania

Lusine Paronyan
Vector-borne and Parasitic Diseases Epidemiology Department, NCDC, Ministry of Health, Yerevan, Armenia

Igor Pajovic
Biotechnical Faculty, University of Montenegro, Podgorica, Montenegro

Chafika Faraj
Laboratoire d'Entomologie Médicale, Institut National d'Hygiéne, Rabat, Morocco

Irakli Sikharulidzec and David Putkaradze
Zooentomology Laboratory, National Center for Disease Control and Public Heath, Tbilisi, Georgia

Jelena Maric
P.I.Veterinary Institute of the Republic of Srpska "Dr. Vaso Butozan", Banja Luka, Bosnia and Herzegovina

Golubinka Bosevska and Elizabeta Janceska
Laboratory for virology and molecular diagnostics, Institute of Public Health of R. Macedonia, Skopje, Former Yugoslav Republic of Macedonia

Ali Bouattour
Université de Tunis El Manar, Institut Pasteur de Tunis, LR11IPT03 Service d'Entomologie Médicale, Tunis, Tunisia

Afrim Hamidi and Kurtesh Sherifi
Faculty of Agriculture and Veterinary Sciences, University of Prishtina, Pristina, Republic of Kosovo

Bülent Alten
Faculty of Science, Biology Department, Ecology Section, Vector Ecology Research Group Laboratories, Hacettepe University, Ankara, Turkey

Dušan Petrić
Faculty of Agriculture, Laboratory for Medical and Veterinary Entomology, University of Novi Sad, Novi Sad, Serbia

Vincent Robert
French National Research Institute for Sustainable Development, Research Unit MiVEGEC, IRD-CNRS-Montpellier University, Montpellier, France

Mercedes María Noel Reynoso, Alejandro Lucia, Eduardo Nicolás Zerba and Raúl Adolfo Alzogaray
UNIDEF-CITEDEF-CONICET- CIPEIN, Juan B. de La Salle 4397, (1603) Villa Martelli, Buenos Aires, Argentina

Magalla Bastian Chalitha Lakmal Somarathne, Yasanthi Illika Nilmini Silva Gunawardene, Naduvilath Vishvanath Chandrasekharan, Arjuna Nisantha Bandara Ellepola and Ranil Samantha Dassanayake Magalla Bastian Chalitha Lakmal Somarathne, Naduvilath Vishvanath Chandrasekharan and Ranil Samantha Dassanayake
Department of Chemistry, Faculty of Science, University of Colombo, Colombo 03 00300, Sri Lanka

Yasanthi Illika Nilmini Silva Gunawardene
Molecular Medicine Unit, Faculty of Medicine, University of Kelaniya, Ragama 11010, Sri Lanka

Arjuna Nisantha Bandara Ellepola
Department of Bioclinical Sciences, Faculty of Dentistry, Health Sciences Center, University of Kuwait, Kuwait City, Kuwait

Kei Owada
School of Medicine, The University of Queensland, QLD, South Brisbane, Australia
Children's Health and Environment Program, Child Health Research Centre, The University of Queensland, QLD, South Brisbane, Australia

Colleen L Lau
Children's Health and Environment Program, Child Health Research Centre, The University of Queensland, QLD, South Brisbane, Australia
Research School of Population Health, Australian National University, ACT, Canberra, Australia

Ricardo J Soares Magalhães
Children's Health and Environment Program, Child Health Research Centre, The University of Queensland, QLD, South Brisbane, Australia
Spatial Epidemiology Laboratory, School of VeterinaryScience, The University of Queensland, QLD, Gatton, Australia

Archie C A Clements
Research School of Population Health, Australian National University, ACT, Canberra, Australia

Lydia Leonardo
Department of Parasitology, College of Public Health, University of the Philippines Manila, Manila, Philippines

Laith Yakob
Department of Disease Control, London School of Hygiene and Tropical Medicine, London, UK

Mark Nielsen
School of Psychology, The University of Queensland, QLD, St Lucia, Australia
Faculty of Humanities, University of Johannesburg, Auckland Park, South Africa

Hélène Carabin
Department of Biostatistics and Epidemiology, College of Public Health, University of Oklahoma Health Sciences Center, Oklahoma, USA

Vikas Taank and Wenshuo Zhou
Department of Biological Sciences, Old Dominion University, Norfolk, VA, USA

Hameeda Sultana and Girish Neelakanta
Department of Biological Sciences, Old Dominion University, Norfolk, VA, USA
Center for Molecular Medicine, College of Sciences, Old Dominion University, Norfolk, VA, USA

Xuran Zhuang and Utpal Pal
Department of Veterinary Medicine, Virginia-Maryland Regional College of Veterinary Medicine, University of Maryland, College Park, MD, USA

John F. Anderson
Department of Entomology, Connecticut Agricultural Experiment Station, New Haven, CT, USA

Heng Yang, Rongsheng Mi, Long Cheng, Yan Huang, Yehua Zhang, Haiyan Jia, Xiaoli Zhang, Xu Wang, Xiangan Han and Zhaoguo Chen
Key Laboratory of Animal Parasitology of Ministry of Agriculture, Laboratory of Quality and Safety Risk Assessment for Animal Products on Biohazards (Shanghai) of Ministry of Agriculture, Shanghai Veterinary Research Institute, Chinese Academy of Agricultural Sciences, Shanghai 200241, China

Rui An
Animal Husbandry and Veterinary Bureau of Changji Hui Autonomous Prefecture, Xinjiang Uyghur Autonomous Region, Changji 831100, Xinjiang, China

Letícia Helena Marques dos Santos, Gisele Macedo Rodrigues da Cunha and Fernanda do Carmo Magalhães
Laboratório de Epidemiologia das Doenças Infecciosas e Parasitárias, Departamento de Parasitologia, Instituto de Ciências Biológicas, Universidade Federal de Minas Gerais, Belo Horizonte, Minas Gerais, Brazil

Iara Caixeta Marques da Rocha
Laboratório de Epidemiologia das Doenças Infecciosas e Parasitárias, Departamento de Parasitologia, Instituto de Ciências Biológicas, Universidade Federal de Minas Gerais, Belo Horizonte, Minas Gerais, Brazil
Secretaria Municipal de Saúde de Belo Horizonte, Belo Horizonte, Minas Gerais, Brazil

Thais Almeida Marques da Silva
Laboratório de Epidemiologia das Doenças Infecciosas e Parasitárias, Departamento de Parasitologia, Instituto de Ciências Biológicas, Universidade Federal de Minas Gerais, Belo Horizonte, Minas Gerais, Brazil
5Instituto de Ensino e Pesquisa da Santa Casa Belo Horizonte, Belo Horizonte, Minas Gerais, Brazil

Mariângela Carneiro
Laboratório de Epidemiologia das Doenças Infecciosas e Parasitárias, Departamento de Parasitologia, Instituto de Ciências Biológicas, Universidade Federal de Minas Gerais, Belo Horizonte, Minas Gerais, Brazil

Pós-graduação em Ciências da Saúde: Infectologia e Medicina Tropical, Faculdade de Medicina, Universidade Federal de Minas Gerais, Belo Horizonte, Minas Gerais, Brazil

Maria Helena Franco Morais
Secretaria Municipal de Saúde de Belo Horizonte, Belo Horizonte, Minas Gerais, Brazil

Wendel Coura-Vital
Departamento de Análises Clínicas, Pós-graduação em Ciências Farmacêuticas, Escola de Farmácia, Universidade Federal de Ouro Preto, Ouro Preto, Minas Gerais, Brazil
Pós-graduação em Ciências Biológicas, Núcleo de Pesquisa em Ciências Biológicas, Universidade Federal de Ouro Preto, Ouro Preto, Minas Gerais, Brazil

Edward Oliveira
Laboratório de Pesquisas Clínicas, Instituto René Rachou, Fundação Oswaldo Cruz, Belo Horizonte, Minas Gerais, Brazil

Ilka Afonso Reis
Departamento de Estatística, Instituto de Ciências Exatas, Universidade Federal de Minas Gerais, Belo Horizonte, Minas Gerais, Brazil
Pós-graduação em Ciências da Saúde: Infectologia e Medicina Tropical, Faculdade de Medicina, Universidade Federal de Minas Gerais, Belo Horizonte, Minas Gerais, Brazil

Nadja Rohdich, Eva Zschiesche and Rainer K. A. Roepke
MSD Animal Health Innovation GmbH, Zur Propstei, 55270 Schwabenheim, Germany

Oliver Wolf and Wolfgang Loehlein
Loehlein and Wolf Vet Research, Maistrasse 69, 80337 Munich, Germany

Zvezdelina Kirkova and Petar Iliev
Department of Parasitology, Trakia University, Faculty of Veterinary Medicine, Student Campus, 6000 Stara Zagora, Bulgaria

Dhimitër Rapti
Klinika VeterinareXhimi, Bulevardi Bajram Curri Nr 2, Tirana, Albania

Rezart Postoli
Faculty of Veterinary Medicine, Agricultural University, Kodër Kamëz, Tirana, Albania

Balázs Capári
Kapriol Bt, Vak Bottyán St.1, 8330 Suemeg, Hungary

Róbert Farkas
Department of Parasitology and Zoology, Faculty of Veterinary Science, Szent István University, István u. 2, 1078 Budapest VII, Hungary

Andrea Springer, Sabine Schicht and Christina Strube
Institute for Parasitology, Centre for Infection Medicine, University of Veterinary Medicine Hannover, Buenteweg 17, 30559 Hannover, Germany

Victor M. Montenegro
Laboratorio de Parasitología, Escuela de Medicina Veterinaria, Universidad Nacional, Campus Benjamín Núñez, Heredia, Costa Rica

Nikola Pantchev
IDEXX Laboratories, Moerikestr. 28/3, 71636 Ludwigsburg, Germany

Index